Osseointegrated Oral implants

Osseointegrated Oral implants

Mechanisms of Implant Anchorage, Threats and Long-Term Survival Rates

Editor

Tomas Albrektsson

MDPI • Basel • Beijing • Wuhan • Barcelona • Belgrade • Manchester • Tokyo • Cluj • Tianjin

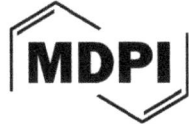

Editor
Tomas Albrektsson
Göteborg University
Sweden.

Editorial Office
MDPI
St. Alban-Anlage 66
4052 Basel, Switzerland

This is a reprint of articles from the Special Issue published online in the open access journal *Journal of Clinical Medicine* (ISSN 2077-0383) (available at: https://www.mdpi.com/journal/jcm/special_issues/Osseointegrated_Oral_implants).

For citation purposes, cite each article independently as indicated on the article page online and as indicated below:

LastName, A.A.; LastName, B.B.; LastName, C.C. Article Title. *Journal Name* **Year**, *Article Number*, Page Range.

ISBN 978-3-03936-640-8 (Hbk)
ISBN 978-3-03936-641-5 (PDF)

Cover image courtesy of Tomas Albrektsson.

© 2020 by the authors. Articles in this book are Open Access and distributed under the Creative Commons Attribution (CC BY) license, which allows users to download, copy and build upon published articles, as long as the author and publisher are properly credited, which ensures maximum dissemination and a wider impact of our publications.

The book as a whole is distributed by MDPI under the terms and conditions of the Creative Commons license CC BY-NC-ND.

Contents

About the Editor ix

Preface to "Osseointegrated Oral implants" xi

Chih-Hao Chen, Benjamin R. Coyac, Masaki Arioka, Brian Leahy, U. Serdar Tulu,
Maziar Aghvami, Stefan Holst, Waldemar Hoffmann, Antony Quarry, Oded Bahat,
Benjamin Salmon, John B. Brunski and Jill A. Helms
A Novel Osteotomy Preparation Technique to Preserve Implant Site Viability and
Enhance Osteogenesis
Reprinted from: *J. Clin. Med.* **2019**, *8*, 170, doi:10.3390/jcm8020170 1

Xingting Han, Dong Yang, Chuncheng Yang, Sebastian Spintzyk, Lutz Scheideler, Ping Li,
Dichen Li, Jürgen Geis-Gerstorfer and Frank Rupp
Carbon Fiber Reinforced PEEK Composites Based on 3D-Printing Technology for Orthopedic
and Dental Applications
Reprinted from: *J. Clin. Med.* **2019**, *8*, 240, doi:10.3390/jcm8020240 15

Jung-Yoo Choi, Tomas Albrektsson, Young-Jun Jeon and In-Sung Luke Yeo
Osteogenic Cell Behavior on Titanium Surfaces in Hard Tissue
Reprinted from: *J. Clin. Med.* **2019**, *8*, 604, doi:10.3390/jcm8050604 33

Xing Yin, Jingtao Li, Waldemar Hoffmann, Angelines Gasser, John B. Brunski
and Jill A. Helms
Mechanical and Biological Advantages of a Tri-Oval Implant Design
Reprinted from: *J. Clin. Med.* **2019**, *8*, 427, doi:10.3390/jcm8040427 43

Holger Zipprich, Paul Weigl, Eugenie König, Alexandra Toderas, Ümniye Balaban and
Christoph Ratka
Heat Generation at the Implant–Bone Interface by Insertion of Ceramic and Titanium Implants
Reprinted from: *J. Clin. Med.* **2019**, *8*, 1541, doi:10.3390/jcm8101541 57

Michele Stocchero, Yohei Jinno, Marco Toia, Marianne Ahmad, Evaggelia Papia,
Satoshi Yamaguchi and Jonas P. Becktor
Intraosseous Temperature Change during Installation of Dental Implants with Two Different
Surfaces and Different Drilling Protocols: An In Vivo Study in Sheep
Reprinted from: *J. Clin. Med.* **2019**, *8*, 1198, doi:10.3390/jcm8081198 75

Dirk U. Duddeck, Tomas Albrektsson, Ann Wennerberg, Christel Larsson and Florian Beuer
On the Cleanliness of Different Oral Implant Systems: A Pilot Study
Reprinted from: *J. Clin. Med.* **2019**, *8*, 1280, doi:10.3390/jcm8091280 89

Christoph Ratka, Paul Weigl, Dirk Henrich, Felix Koch, Markus Schlee and Holger Zipprich
The Effect of In Vitro Electrolytic Cleaning on Biofilm-Contaminated Implant Surfaces
Reprinted from: *J. Clin. Med.* **2019**, *8*, 1397, doi:10.3390/jcm8091397 107

Markus Schlee, Loubna Naili, Florian Rathe, Urs Brodbeck and Holger Zipprich
Is Complete Re-Osseointegration of an Infected Dental Implant Possible? Histologic Results of
a Dog Study: A Short Communication
Reprinted from: *J. Clin. Med.* **2020**, *9*, 235, doi:10.3390/jcm9010235 121

Teresa Lombardi, Federico Berton, Stefano Salgarello, Erika Barbalonga, Antonio Rapani, Francesca Piovesana, Caterina Gregorio, Giulia Barbati, Roberto Di Lenarda and Claudio Stacchi
Factors Influencing Early Marginal Bone Loss around Dental Implants Positioned Subcrestally: A Multicenter Prospective Clinical Study
Reprinted from: *J. Clin. Med.* **2019**, , 1168, doi:10.3390/jcm8081168 129

Simone Marconcini, Enrica Giammarinaro, Ugo Covani, Eitan Mijiritsky, Xavier Vela and Xavier Rodríguez
The Effect of Tapered Abutments on Marginal Bone Level: A Retrospective Cohort Study
Reprinted from: *J. Clin. Med.* **2019**, *8*, 1305, doi:10.3390/jcm8091305 143

Ron Doornewaard, Maarten Glibert, Carine Matthys, Stijn Vervaeke, Ewald Bronkhorst and Hugo de Bruyn
Improvement of Quality of Life with Implant-Supported Mandibular Overdentures and the Effect of Implant Type and Surgical Procedure on Bone and Soft Tissue Stability: A Three-Year Prospective Split-Mouth Trial
Reprinted from: *J. Clin. Med.* **2019**, *8*, 773, doi:10.3390/jcm8060773 153

.Markus Schlee, Florian Rathe, Urs Brodbeck, Christoph Ratka, Paul Weigl and Holger Zipprich
Treatment of Peri-Implantitis—Electrolytic Cleaning Versus Mechanical and Electrolytic Cleaning—A Randomized Controlled Clinical Trial—Six-Month Results
Reprinted from: *J. Clin. Med.* **2019**, *8*, 1909, doi:10.3390/jcm8111909 171

Alberto Monje, Angel Insua and Hom-Lay Wang
Understanding Peri-Implantitis as a Plaque-Associated and Site-Specific Entity: On the Local Predisposing Factors
Reprinted from: *J. Clin. Med.* **2019**, *8*, 279, doi:10.3390/jcm8020279 185

Tomas Albrektsson
Are Oral Implants the Same As Teeth?
Reprinted from: *J. Clin. Med.* **2019**, *8*, 1501, doi:10.3390/jcm8091501 205

Maria Menini, Paolo Pesce, Domenico Baldi, Gabriela Coronel Vargas, Paolo Pera and Alberto Izzotti
Prediction of Titanium Implant Success by Analysis of microRNA Expression in Peri-Implant Tissue. A 5-Year Follow-Up Study
Reprinted from: *J. Clin. Med.* **2019**, *8*, 888, doi:10.3390/jcm8060888 209

Pierluigi Coli and Lars Sennerby
Is Peri-Implant Probing Causing Over-Diagnosis and Over-Treatment of Dental Implants?
Reprinted from: *J. Clin. Med.* **2019**, *8*, 1123, doi:10.3390/jcm8081123 221

David Reinedahl, Bruno Chrcanovic, Tomas Albrektsson, Pentti Tengvall and Ann Wennerberg
Ligature-Induced Experimental Peri-Implantitis—A Systematic Review
Reprinted from: *J. Clin. Med.* **2018**, *7*, 492, doi:10.3390/jcm7120492 235

David Reinedahl, Silvia Galli, Tomas Albrektsson, Pentti Tengvall, Carina B. Johansson, Petra Hammarström Johansson and Ann Wennerberg
Aseptic Ligatures Induce Marginal Peri-Implant Bone Loss—An 8-Week Trial in Rabbits
Reprinted from: *J. Clin. Med.* **2019**, *8*, 1248, doi:10.3390/jcm8081248 245

Ricardo Trindade, Tomas Albrektsson, Silvia Galli, Zdenka Prgomet, Pentti Tengvall and Ann Wennerberg
Bone Immune Response to Materials, Part I: Titanium, PEEK and Copper in Comparison to Sham at 10 Days in Rabbit Tibia
Reprinted from: *J. Clin. Med.* **2018**, *7*, 526, doi:10.3390/jcm7120526 265

Ricardo Trindade, Tomas Albrektsson, Silvia Galli, Zdenka Prgomet, Pentti Tengvall and Ann Wennerberg
Bone Immune Response to Materials, Part II: Copper and Polyetheretherketone (PEEK) Compared to Titanium at 10 and 28 Days in Rabbit Tibia
Reprinted from: *J. Clin. Med.* **2019**, *8*, 814, doi:10.3390/jcm8060814 281

Rune J. Christiansen, Henrik J. Münch, Charlotte M. Bonefeld, Jacob P. Thyssen, Jens J. Sloth, Carsten Geisler, Kjeld Søballe, Morten S. Jellesen and Stig S. Jakobsen
Cytokine Profile in Patients with Aseptic Loosening of Total Hip Replacements and Its Relation to Metal Release and Metal Allergy
Reprinted from: *J. Clin. Med.* **2019**, *8*, 1259, doi:10.3390/jcm8081259 299

Adrien Naveau, Kouhei Shinmyouzu, Colman Moore, Limor Avivi-Arber, Jesse Jokerst and Sreenivas Koka
Etiology and Measurement of Peri-Implant Crestal Bone Loss (CBL)
Reprinted from: *J. Clin. Med.* **2019**, *8*, 166, doi:10.3390/jcm8020166 315

Luis Amengual-Peñafiel, Manuel Brañes-Aroca, Francisco Marchesani-Carrasco, María Costanza Jara-Sepúlveda, Leopoldo Parada-Pozas and Ricardo Cartes-Velásquez
Coupling between Osseointegration and Mechanotransduction to Maintain Foreign Body Equilibrium in the Long-Term: A Comprehensive Overview
Reprinted from: *J. Clin. Med.* **2019**, *8*, 139, doi:10.3390/jcm8020139 335

About the Editor

Tomas Albrektsson started working together with p-I Brånemark in the development of osseointegrated implants in 1967. Since then, Albrektsson has published some 400 scientific papers in peer reviewed journals and presented more than 1300 lectures to professional audiences. He has a current h-index (Scopus) of 86. Albrektsson has received numerous awards and honorary memberships, as well as two honorary doctorates. Currently, Albrektsson works as an emeritus professor at the Biomaterials Department of the University of Gothenburg, and as a visiting professor at the Prosthodontic Department, University of Malmö, Sweden.

Preface to "Osseointegrated Oral implants"

Osseointegrated Oral Implants: Mechanisms of Implant Anchorage, Threats and Long Term Survival Rate

Osseointegrated oral implants were first used clinically in 1965 at the Gothenburg University of Sweden, and then only in small numbers. There, the original osseointegration team, of which I was a participant, worked clinically and experimentally under the leadership of P-I Branemark to test osseointegration principles not only in the oral cavity but also as craniofacial and orthopedic implants [1–7]. Other pioneers of the early days were Willi Schulte of Tübingen University, Germany, and André Schroeder of Bern University, Switzerland, who published their first papers on bone-anchored oral implants in 1976, in all probability without knowing about Brånemark´s earlier work [8,9]. These three University-employed innovators became the fathers of the most used oral implant systems of our day—the Nobel, the Dentsply and the Straumann implants.

The present volume represents the state-of-the-art in oral implants today. Some interpretations may be too old and others too untested to survive the scrutiny of time. However, this is how scientific ideas usually develop. The pioneering team behind osseointegration was convinced that titanium was inert and that its incorporation in bone simulated a simple wound healing phenomenon [2,10], hypotheses that today are recognized as being incorrect. Nevertheless, the very good clinical results achieved with moderately rough osseointegrated oral implants with a 10 year survival rate in the range of 96–99% [11] meant that other hypotheses could be verified, despite some errors in interpretations. We learned countless lessons from the early work behind modern oral implants. In a similar manner, I personally consider those who believe marginal bone loss around oral implants to be solely dependent on bacteria to be on the wrong track, which does not preclude the future value of some of the findings of this research.

New valuable findings on osseointegration include a most interesting paper by Chen et al. [12], who present evidence that a novel type of osteotomy may preserve implant site viability by using a very low drill speed with the potential advantage of minimal tissue violence. Han et al. [13] present an in vitro study using 3D printed carbon fiber reinforced PEEK material that, in the future, may provide possibilities for applications in oral implantology, on the condition that the in vitro findings of the biocompatibility of this material can be supported by in vivo analyses. An animal study by Choi et al. [14] evaluates osteogenic cell behavior in a new manner by using ultrastructural techniques and immune flourescence analyses during the first 10 days after implant placement. The notion that oral implants must be rounded bodies belonged to our old convictions. In this volume, we learn about the potential advantages of changing the implant design to a tri-oval one. Implants with this design displayed significantly enhanced implant stability in the bone when tested in animal studies [15].

Zipprich et al. [16] point out that the insertion of ceramic implants may cause more interfacial heat than the placement of titanium implants, indicative of the need to use a very slow drill speed with the ceramic devices. Stocchero et al. [17] analyze intraosseous temperatures when performing undersized drilling and report a negative impact on the bone some distance away from the implant. Duddeck et al. [18] demonstrate that our commercially available oral implants may be contaminated, perhaps having an effect on clinical outcomes.

The effects of a novel type of electrolytical cleaning technique for implant surfaces decontaminated by biofilms is presented in two papers [19,20]. It proved possible not only to clean away the biofilm in vitro but also to re-establish osseointegration of a previously infected implant in a dog model. To the knowledge of the editor this is the first time we have seen evidence of re-osseointegration under such circumstances.

Three papers test potential improvements of osseointegrated implants in clinical settings. Lombardi et al. [21] evaluate factors that influence marginal bone loss during the first year after implantation, a time when most clinical scientists do not talk about peri-implantitis but, instead, of bone remodeling. Greater initial marginal bone loss was seen with deep insertion protocols, thin peri-implant mucosa and short abutments. Marconcini et al. [22] describe the tapered abutments that were found to result in minimal marginal bone loss in a one year retrospective study. Doornewaard et al. [23] present a three year prospective study of implant-supported mandibular overdentures in a split mouth model. The equicrestal implant placement was reported to yield significantly higher implant surface exposure.

Threats to osseointegration include marginal bone loss that, if continuous, may result in clinical failure. Currently, the most quoted reason for such unwanted marginal bone loss is what some investigators call peri-implantitis, allegedly behind all marginal bone loss after the first year of implantation. Schlee et al. [24] analyze their previously described electrolytical cleaning method and suggest that 100 million oral implants around the world may be infected and threatened by failure. I judge this great number of implants suffering from risk of failure to be unrealistic and rather based on unsuitable criteria for disease. However, the potential for re-osseointegration in case of marginal bone loss may, nevertheless, be of substantial aesthetical importance. The electrolytical cleaning technique was not improved by simultaneous mechanical cleaning based on a 6 month randomized study [24]. Monje and co-workers [25] describe the peri-implantitis site-specific entity and present a traditional overview of predisposing factors for ailment. As previously indicated, I do not personally believe that implants and teeth are the same [26], nor do I agree with all bacterial interpretations of these papers. An overly strong immune reaction may likewise lead to marginal bone resorption. Having said so, bacterial attacks may follow secondary to strong immune reactions. Certainly, time will tell more about the right and wrong than our present reasoning.

The last part of this book is centered on immunological findings of osseointegrated implants, discussed in 8 different papers. Menini et al. [27] present a follow up of a previously published paper [28] that claimed plaque causes inflammation but not marginal bone loss. In the new paper, they demonstrate that some specific mRNA signatures appear to protect from bone resorption despite plaque accumulation. Coli and Sennerby [29] question the use of tests like probing depth and bleeding on probing that have been taken over from periodontology, but never independently assessed with respect to oral implants. Reinedahl et al. [30,31] demonstrate significant immune reactions to ligatures around titanium implants. Marginal bone resorption was demonstrated despite lack of implant plaque and all implants having been placed in a bacteria free environment in the tibia of research animals. These strong and adverse immune reactions to the implant/ligature compound caused marginal bone loss due to the immune system control of the osteoblast/osteoclast balance, thereby contradicting hundreds of previously published papers suggesting a direct bacterial attack due to the ligatures. Bacterial attacks in such cases may largely represent a secondary phenomenon only.

Trindade et al. [32], in a previous experimental publication, demonstrated that titanium gives rise to immune reactions. In two separate papers, Trindade et al. [33,34] confirm these observations, but the authors notice an even stronger immune reaction to materials such as copper and PEEK at 28 days of follow up in an in vivo study. It seems that the body accepts mild immune reactions, like those emanating from titanium implants, and reacts either by preventing osseointegration, like in the case of copper and PEEK, or resulting in marginal bone loss around already integrated implants if provoked by very strong/imbalanced immune reactions [35]. Christiansen et al. [36] examine marginal bone loss in total hip replacement cases and report a significantly different cytokine profile compared to the situation without bone loss, suggesting an association with innate and adaptive immunity. Naveau et al. [37] point out that osseointegration is a foreign body reaction, indicative of an immune response to oral implants in the normal clinical situation. Amengual-Peñafiel et al. [38] agree with these observations and refer to the functioning oral implant as being in a state of foreign body equilibrium. This is a new way to look at an oral implant that is in opposition both with the notion that titanium is inert and, further, with those who see titanium implants as similar to teeth

All in all, this book contains a collection of research that clearly increases our knowledge of osseointegration. The papers in this book will be repeatedly quoted and serve as inspiration for further research efforts in our discipline of oral implantology.

Gothenburg, Sweden June 10th, 2020

Tomas Albrektsson Professor emeritus of Dept of Biomaterials, University of Gothenburg, Sweden

Visiting professor of Dept of Prosthodontics, University of Malmö, Sweden

Tomas Albrektsson
Guest Editors

References.

1. Brånemark, P.I.; Breine, U.; Adell, R.; Hansson, B.O.; Lindström, J.; Ohlsson, Å. Intraosseous anchorage of dental prostheses I Experimental findings. *Scand. J. Plast. Reconstr. Surg.* **1969**, *3*, 81–100.
2. Brånemark, P.I.; Hansson, B.O.; Adell, R.; Breine, U.; Lindström, J.; Hallén, O. Osseointegrated implants in the treatment of the edentulous jaw. *Scand. J. Plast. Reconstr. Surg.* **1977**, *16*, 1–99.
3. Tjellström, A.; Lindström, J.; Nylén, O.; Albrektsson, T.; Brånemark, P.-I.; Birgersson, B.; Nero, H.; Sylvan, C.The bone anchored auricular episthesis. *Laryngoscope* **1981**, *91*, 811–815.
4. Tjellström, A.; Rosenhall, U.; Lindström, J.; Hallén, O., Albrektsson, T.; Brånemark, P. I. Five-year experience with skin penetrating bone-anchored implants in the temporal bone. *Acta Otolaryngol.* **1983**, *95*, 568–575.
5. Carlsson, L.; Albrektsson, B.J.; Albrektsson, T.; Jacobsson, M.; Macdonald, W.; Regnér, L.; Weidenhielm, L.R. Stepwise introduction of a bone- conserving osseointegrated hip arthroplasty using RSA and a randomized study: I Preliminary observations - 52 patients followed for 3 years. *Acta Orthop. Scand.* **2006**, *77*, 549–558.
6. Carlsson, L.; Albrektsson, T.; Albrektsson, B.J.; Jacobsson, M.; Macdonald, W.; Regnér, L.; Weidenhielm, L.R. Stepwise introduction of a bone-conserving osseointegrated hip arthroplasty using RSA and a randomized study II. Clinical proof of concept - 40 patients followed for 2 years. *Acta Orthop. Scand.* **2006**, *77*, 559–566.
7. Brånemark, R.; Hagberg, K.; Kulbacka-Ortiz, K.; Berlin, Ö.; Rydevik, B. Osseointegrated percutaneous prosthetic system for the treatment of patients with transfemoral amputation: A prospective five-year follow-up of patient reported outcomes and complications. *J. Am. Orthop. Surg.* **2019**, *15*, 743–751.

8. Schulte, W.; Heimke, G. The Tübinger immediate implant. *Quintessence* **1976**, *27*, 17–23.
9. Schroeder, A.; Pohler, O.; Sutter, F. Tissue reaction to an implant of a titanium hollow cylinder with a titanium surface spray layer. *Schweiz. Monatschr. Zahnheilkunde* **1976**, *86*, 713–717.
10. Albrektsson, T.; Brånemark, P.I.; Hansson, H.A.; Kasemo, B.; Larsson, K.; Lundström, I.; McQueen, D.H.; Skalak, R. The interface zone of inorganic implants in bone. *Ann. Biomed. Eng.* **1983**, *11*, 1–41.
11. Wennerberg, A.; Albrektsson, T.; Chrcanovic, B. Long-term clinical outcome of implants with different surface modifications. *Eur. J. Oral Implatol.* 2018, *11* (Suppl. 1), S123–S136.
12. Chen, C.; Coyar, B.; Arioka, M.; Leahy, B.; Tulu, U.; Aghvami, M.; Holst, S.; Hoffman, W.; Quarry, A.; Bahat Om Salmon, B.; et al. A novel osteotomy preparation technique to preserve implant site viability and enhance osteogenesis. *J. Clin. Med.* 2019;8: 170, doi:10.3390/jcm8020170.
13. Han, X.; Yang, D.; Yang, C.; Spintzyk, S.; Scheideler, L.; Li, P.; Li, D.; Geis-Gerstoffer, J.; Rupp, F. Carbon fiber reinforced PEEK composite based on 3D-printing technology for orthopedic and dental application. *J. Clin. Med.* 2019;8: 240, doi:10.3390/jcm8020240.
14. Choi, J.; Albrektsson, T.; Jeon, Y.; Luke Yeo, I. Osteogenic cell behavior on titanium surfaces in hard tissue. *J. Clin. Med.* **2019**, *8*, 604, doi:10.3390/jcm8050604.
15. Yin, X.; Li, J.; Hoffman, W.; Gasser, A.; Brunski, J.; Helms, J. Mechanical and biological advantages of a tri-oval implant design. *J. Clin. Med.* **2019**, *8*, 427:doi:10.3390/jcm8040427.
16. Zipprich, H.; Weigl, P.; Künig, E.; Toderas, A.; Balaban, Ü.; Ratka, C. Heat generation at the implant-bone interface by insertion of ceramic and titanium implants. *J. Clin. Med.* **2019**, *8*, 1581:doi:10.3390/jcm8101541.
17. Stocchero, M.; Jinno, Y.; Toia, M.; Ahmad, M.; Papia, E.; Yamaguchi, S.; Becktor, J. Intraosseous temperature change during installation of dental implants with two different surfaces and different drilling protocols: An in vivo study in sheep. *J. Clin. Med.* **2019**, *8*, 1198:https://doi.org/10.3390/jcm8081198.
18. Duddeck, D.; Albrektsson, T.; WEnnerberg, A.; Larsson, C.; Beuer, F. On the cleanliness of different oral implant systems: A pilot study. *J. Clin. Med.* **2019**, *8*, 1280, doi:10.3390/jcm8091280.
19. Ratka, C.; Weigl, P.; Henrich, D.; Koch, F.; Schlee, M.; Zipprich, H. The effect of in-vitro electrolytic cleaning on biofilm contaminated implant surfaces. *J. Clin. Med..*) 1397, doi:10.3390/jcm8091397 -.
20. Schlee, M.; Naili l Rathe, F.; Brodbeck, U.; Zipprich, H. Is complete re-osseointegration of an infected dental implant possible? Histologic results of a dog study: A short communication. *J. Clin. Med.* **2020**, *9*, 235:doi:10.3990/jcm9010235.
21. Lombardi, T.; Berton, F.; Salgarello, S.; Barbalonga, E.; Rapani, A.; Piovesana, F.; Gregorio, F.; Barbati, G.; DiLenarda, R.; Stacchi, C. Factors influencing early marginal bone loss around dental implants positioned under bone level; A multicenter prospective clinical study. *J. Clin. Med.* 2019, 8, 1168, doi:10.3390/jcm8081168.
22. Marconcini, S.; Giammarinaro, E.; Covani, U.; Mijiritsky, E.; Vela, X.; Rodriguez, X. The effect of tapered abutments on marginal bone level: A retrospective cohort study. *J. Clin. Med.* **2019**, *8*, 1305, doi:10.3390/jcm8091305.
23. Doorneward, R.; Glibert, M.; Matthys, C.; Vervaeke, S.; Bronkhorst, E.; De Bruyn, H. Improvement of quality of life with implant-supported mandibular overdentures and the effect of implant type and surgical procedure on bone and soft tissue stability: A three-year prospective split-mouth trial. *J. Clin. Med.* **2019**, *8*, 773:https://doi.org/10.3390/jcm8060773.
24. Schlee, M.; Rathe, F.; Brodbeck, U.; Ratka, C.; Weigl, P.; Zipprich, H. Treatment of peri-implantitis—Electrolytical cleaning versus mechanical and electrolytical cleaning—A randomized controlled clinical trial—Six month results. *J. Clin. Med.* 1909, doi:10.3390/jcm8111909.
25. Monje, A.; Insua, A.; Wang, H.L. Understanding peri-implantitis as a site specific entity: On the local predisposing factors. *J. Clin. Med.* **2019**, *8*, 279, doi:10.3390/jcm8020279.
26. Albrektsson, T. Are oral implants the same as teeth? *J. Clin. Med.* **2019**, *8*, 1501, doi:10.3390/jcm8091501.
27. Menini, M.; Pesce, P.; Baldi, D.; Vargas, G.C.; Pera, P.; Izotti, A. Prediction of titanium implant success by analysis of micro-RNA expression in peri-implant tissue. A 5-year follow up study. *J. Clin. Med.* **2019**, *8*, 888, doi:10.3390/jcm8060888.

28. Menini, M.; Setti, P.; Pera, F.; Pesce, P. Peri-implant tissue health and bone resorption in patients with immediately loaded implant-supported full-arch prostheses. *Int. J. Prosth.* **2018**, *31*, 327–333.
29. Coli, P.; Sennerby, L. Is peri-implant probing causing over –diagnosis and over-treatment of dental implants? *J. Clin. Med.* **2019**, *8*, 1123, doi:10.3390/jcm8081123.
30. Reinedahl, D.; Chrcanovic, B.; Albrektsson, T.; Tengvall, P.; WEnnerberg, A. Ligature induced experimental peri-implantitis- a systematic review. *J. Clin. Med.* **2018**, *7*, 492–501, doi:10.3390/jcm7120492.
31. Reinedahl, D.; Galli, S.; ALbrektsson, T. Aseptic ligatures induce marginal bone loss: An 8 week trial in rabbits. *J. Clin. Med.* **2019**, *8*, 1248, doi:10.3390/jcm8081248.
32. Trindade, R.; Albrektsson, T.; Galli, S.; Prgomet, Z.; Tengvall, P.; Wennerberg, A. Osseointegration and foreign body reaction: Titanium implants activate the immune system and suppress bone resorption during the first 4 weeks after implantation. *Clin. Implant. Dent. Rel. Res.* **2018**, *20*, 526, doi:10.3390/jcm7120526.
33. Trindade, R.; Albrektsson, T.; Galli Sm Prgomet, E.; Tengvall, P.; Wennerberg, A. Bone immune response to materials: Part I: Titanium, Peek and copper in comparison to sham at 10 days in rabbit tibia. *J. Clin. Med.* 2018. 7, 526.
34. Trindade, R.; Albrektsson, T.; Galli, S.; Prgomet, Z.; Tengvall, P.; Wennerberg, A. Bone immune response to materials Part II. Copper and polyetheretherketone(PEEK) compared to titanium at 10 and 28 days in rabbit tibia. *J. Clin. Med.* **2019**, *8*, 814, doi:10.3390/jcm8060814.
35. Albrektsson, T.; Dahlin, C.; Reinedahl, D.; Tengvall, P.; Trindade, R.; Wennerberg, A. An imbalance of the immune system instead of a disease behind marginal bone loss aorund oral implants: Position paper. *Int. J. Oral Maxillofac. Implants* 2020, 35, doi:10.11607//jomi.8218, in press.
36. Christiansen, R.; Münch, H.; Bonefeld, C.; Thyssen, J.; Sloth, J.; Geisler, C.; Söballe, K.; Jellesen, M.; Jakobsen, S. Cytokine profile in patients with aseptic loosening of total hip replacements and its relation to metal release and metal allergy. *J. Clin. Med.* **2019**, *8*, 1259, doi:10.3390/jcm8081259.
37. Naveau, A.; Shinmyouzu, K.; Moore, C.; Avivi-Arber, L.; Jokerst, J.; Koka, S. Etiology and measurement of peri-implant crestal bone loss (CBL). *J. Clin. Med.* **2019**, *8*, 166, doi:10.3390/jcm8020166.
38. Amengual-Peñafiel, L.; Brañes-Aroca, M.; Marchesani-Carrasco, F.; Jara-Sepulveda, M.; Parada-Pozas, L.; Cartes-Velásquez, R. Coupling between osseointegration and mechaotransduction to maintain foreign body equilibrium long term: A comprehensive overview. *J. Clin. Med.* **2019**, *8*, 139, doi:10.3390/jcm8020139.

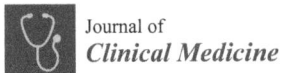

Article

A Novel Osteotomy Preparation Technique to Preserve Implant Site Viability and Enhance Osteogenesis

Chih-Hao Chen [1,2,†], Benjamin R. Coyac [1,†], Masaki Arioka [1,3,†], Brian Leahy [1], U. Serdar Tulu [1], Maziar Aghvami [1], Stefan Holst [4,5], Waldemar Hoffmann [4], Antony Quarry [4], Oded Bahat [6], Benjamin Salmon [7,8], John B. Brunski [1] and Jill A. Helms [1,*]

1. Division of Plastic and Reconstructive Surgery, Department of Surgery, Stanford University School of Medicine, Stanford, CA 94305, USA; chchen5027@gmail.com (C.-H.C.); benjamin_coyac@hotmail.fr (B.R.C.); amasaki@stanford.edu (M.A.); bleahy94@gmail.com (B.L.); serdartulu@stanford.edu (U.S.T.); maziara@stanford.edu (M.A.); brunsj6@stanford.edu (J.B.B.)
2. Craniofacial Research Center, Department of Plastic and Reconstructive Surgery, Chang Gung Memorial Hospital, Chang Gung University School of Medicine, Taoyuan 33305, Taiwan
3. Department of Clinical Pharmacology, Faculty of Medical Sciences, Kyushu University, Fukuoka 812-8582, Japan
4. Nobel Biocare Services AG P.O. Box, CH-8058 Zürich-Flughafen, Switzerland; stefan.holst@nobelbiocare.com (S.H.); waldemar.hoffmann@nobelbiocare.com (W.H.); antony.quarry@nobelbiocare.com (A.Q.)
5. Department of Prosthodontics, School of Dentistry, Johann-Wolfgang Goethe University, 60438 Frankfurt, Germany
6. Private Practice, Beverly Hills, CA 90210, USA; odedbahat@gmail.com
7. Paris Descartes-Sorbonne Paris Cité University, EA2496 Montrouge, France; benjamin.salmon@parisdescartes.fr
8. Dental Medicine Department, Bretonneau Hospital, HUPNVS, AP-HP, 75018 Paris, France
* Correspondence: jhelms@stanford.edu; Tel.: +1-650-736-3640
† These authors contributed equally to this work.

Received: 6 January 2019; Accepted: 27 January 2019; Published: 1 February 2019

Abstract: The preservation of bone viability at an osteotomy site is a critical variable for subsequent implant osseointegration. Recent biomechanical studies evaluating the consequences of site preparation led us to rethink the design of bone-cutting drills, especially those intended for implant site preparation. We present here a novel drill design that is designed to efficiently cut bone at a very low rotational velocity, obviating the need for irrigation as a coolant. The low-speed cutting produces little heat and, consequently, osteocyte viability is maintained. The lack of irrigation, coupled with the unique design of the cutting flutes, channels into the osteotomy autologous bone chips and osseous coagulum that have inherent osteogenic potential. Collectively, these features result in robust, new bone formation at rates significantly faster than those observed with conventional drilling protocols. These preclinical data have practical implications for the clinical preparation of osteotomies and alveolar bone reconstructive surgeries.

Keywords: osteogenesis; osteotomy; bone healing; bone chips; drilling tool design

1. Introduction

The medical and dental professions, with few exceptions, adapted commercially available tools for use that were developed for drilling other materials [1]. For example, bone-cutting tools, which are largely predicated on the design of metal-cutting instruments. Metal drills are end-cutting tools, e.g., only the tip of the drill is engaged in producing a hole, and the same is true for the vast majority of bone-cutting drills [2]. Metal drills and most bone drills are also designed to cut at a high rotational velocity, which means that the drill can be advanced with minimal axial thrust force [3]. Metal and bone drills generally have a relatively small rake angle, which means that particles generated by cutting are typically scattered from the site to avoid obstructing the drill. Metal drilling typically requires a lubricant that serves as a coolant [4]; in bone cutting, these functions are replaced by saline irrigation [5].

We studied the biological responses to osteotomy site preparation in multiple animal species [6–9] including humans [10], and these analyses, coupled with computational and finite element modeling [5], prompted us to reconsider the design of a bone-cutting tool, optimized for osteotomy site preparation. The resulting tool, called the OsseoShaper, is designed to limit osteocyte death caused by mechanical and thermal damage, and simultaneously retain osseous coagulum/bone chips generated by bone cutting. For this study, cutting tools were downscaled to accommodate the smaller size of the rat maxillae; however, the ratio of cutting-tool diameter and bone surface area was representative of what is used clinically. The purpose of this study was then to compare osteotomies produced by a downscaled OsseoShaper versus a conventional drill in terms of heat generation, osteocyte viability, bone remodeling, and onset of new bone formation.

2. Materials and Methods

2.1. Animals and Experimental Plan

Stanford APLAC approved all procedures (#13146), which conform to ARRIVE guidelines. In total, 18 female Wistar rats (Charles River Laboratories) were used in this study. All animals underwent ovariectomy (OVX) and bilateral maxillary first molar (M1) extraction when they were seven weeks old. Animals were then maintained for eight weeks, during which time the osteoporotic phenotype developed [11,12] and the extraction socket completed its healing [9]. All animals were then subjected to bilateral osteotomy site preparation in the healed M1 location. Animals were sacrificed at intervals of 0.5 days, three days, and seven days. Before surgery, general anesthesia was reached via intraperitoneal injection of ketamine (100 mg/kg) (Vedco, Inc., St. Joseph, MO, USA) and xylazine (10 mg/kg) (Akorn, Inc., Lake Forest, IL, USA), while analgesia was reached via subcutaneous injection of Buprenorphine SR (0.5 mg/kg). After surgery, rats recovered in a controlled, 37 °C environment, fed a soft food diet for the duration of the experiment and housed in groups of two. Weight changes were <10%. No adverse events (e.g., uncontrolled pain, infection, prolonged inflammation) were encountered.

2.2. Ovariectomy and Tooth Extraction

To align our experimental model with the average patient receiving a dental implant, e.g., >50 years old [13], seven-week-old female rats underwent OVX [14]. This produced in our animal model an osteopenic/osteoporotic phenotype, which is representative of patients over 50 years of age [15]. In brief, a dorsal midline incision was made between the mid-back and tail base. The peritoneal cavity was accessed through bilateral muscle layer incisions, the ovary was identified, and the connection between the fallopian tube and the uterine horn was suture-ligated. After bilateral removal of the ovaries, the wounds were closed layer by layer.

In parallel with the OVX, bilateral maxillary first molars (M1) were extracted. This further aligned our experimental model with patients, in which the majority of dental implants are placed in healed extraction sites [16]. In brief, micro-forceps were used to loosen and remove the tooth in toto. Bleeding was controlled by local compression. Healing of the extraction site was confirmed using histology and micro-computed tomographic (μCT) imaging. By post-extraction day 21 (PED21), the extraction site was fully healed, as shown by the fact that the bone volume/total volume (BV/TV) of the extraction site was equivalent to adjacent, pristine bone [10].

2.3. Osteotomy Site Preparation

To directly compare two surgical drilling tools for their ability to maintain osteotomy site viability, rats were anesthetized before a full thickness periosteal flap was elevated at the M1 tooth extraction site. A handpiece (KaVo Dental, Uxbridge, UK) with saline irrigation was used to produce a pilot 1.0-mm drill hole, followed by step-wise enlargement using progressively larger drill diameters (Table 1). In the OsseoShaper protocol, the same type of pilot drill was used to produce a pilot osteotomy; thereafter, a downscaled prototype of the OsseoShaper was used to enlarge the osteotomy to the same final maximum diameter as was achieved with the conventional surgical drill protocol. The mini OsseoShaper was used without irrigation. Drill speeds were adjusted to result in the same radial velocity for all drills and to compensate for slightly different diameters. Each osteotomy was made with a new drill. After osteotomy, tension-free primary closure of the periosteal flap was achieved using tissue glue (VetClose, Henry Schein, Dublin, OH, USA).

Table 1. Surgical drill parameters.

Company	External Diameter	Product Identifier
OsteoMed	1.0 mm	220-0065
OsteoMed	1.3 mm	220-0064
OsteoMed	1.6 mm	220-0116
Downscaled prototype of the OsseoShaper	1.0 mm (apex) 1.6 mm (crest)	Non-commercial prototype

2.4. Tissue Collection and Processing

Tissues were collected at post-osteotomy day (POD) 0.5 to evaluate micro-damage and programmed cell death caused by surgical drilling, as well as at POD3 and POD7, when new bone formation is initiated [7]. In brief, animals were euthanized; then, the entire maxillae were dissected free from other tissues and transferred to 4% paraformaldehyde (PFA) and stored at 4 °C overnight. After fixation, samples were decalcified in ethylenediaminetetraacetic acid (EDTA), embedded in paraffin, and sectioned at an 8-μm thickness for analyses. Tissue sections were deparaffinized in Citrisolv (Decon Labs, Inc., King of Prussia, PA, USA) and hydrated via a series of decreasing concentrations of ethanol before staining or other histological/cellular activity analyses.

2.5. Histology

For aniline blue staining, sections were treated with a saturated solution of picric acid followed by a 5% phosphotungstic acid solution and staining in 1% aniline blue. Slides were then dehydrated and mounted using Permount (Fisher Scientific, Hampton, NH, USA). For pentachrome staining, sections were pre-treated with 6% nitric acid and stained with toluidine blue solution for 5 min (0.5 g toluidine blue in 100 mL of distilled water at pH 1 to 1.5, adjusted with 0.5% HCl). Picrosirius red staining [17] was used to detect collagenous osteoid matrix. Tissues were stained with picrosirius red then viewed under polarized light. Tightly aligned fibrillary collagen molecules appear red compared to less organized collagen fibrils that show a color of shorter (green–yellow) wavelengths.

2.6. Quantification of Programmed Cell Death

Terminal deoxynucleotidyl transferase deoxyuridine triphosphate (dUTP) nick end labeling (TUNEL) staining (Roche Diagnostics GmbH, Mannheim, Germany) was performed according to the manufacturers' guidelines. Following deparaffinization and rehydration, paraffin sections were stained by incubating slides in permeabilization solution for 8 min, adding TUNEL reaction mixture, then incubating at 37 °C in the dark. Between these steps, paraffin sections were washed with phosphate-buffered saline (PBS). To quantify the extent of apoptotic osteocytes, TUNEL-stained tissue sections from 4–6 different samples were analyzed. Each section was photographed using a Leica digital image system at 20× magnification. The number of TUNEL-labeled osteocytes corresponding to apoptotic cells was determined, and the cells grouped according to their distance from the cut edge. The corresponding area for each group was then calculated. The number of apoptotic cells per unit area was calculated by dividing the number of apoptotic cells to the corresponding area (cell/mm^2).

2.7. Tartrate-Resistant Acid Phosphatase (TRAP) Activity

Identification of osteoclasts was done using TRAP staining. TRAP activity was observed using a leukocyte acid phosphatase staining kit (catalog #386A-1KT, Sigma-Aldrich, St. Louis, MO, USA). Tissue sections were processed according to the manufacturer's instructions. To quantify the TRAP activity, TRAP-stained tissue sections were photographed using a Leica digital image system at 10× magnification. The TRAP^{+ve} area corresponding to osteoclasts was determined within the radial zone extending 300 µm from the cutting edge. The TRAP^{+ve} ratio was calculated by dividing the TRAP^{+ve} pixels by the total pixels of the region of interest.

2.8. Immunostaining

To localize, within the osteotomies, cells that had initiated differentiation down an osteogenic lineage, immunostaining was performed using standard procedures [18]. In brief, following deparaffinization, endogenous peroxidase activity was quenched by 3% hydrogen peroxide for 5 min, and then washed in PBS. Slides were blocked with 5% goat serum (Vector S-1000) for 1 h at room temperature. The appropriate primary antibody was added and incubated overnight at 4 °C, then washed in PBS. The primary antibodies used in this study were Osterix (1:1200; ab22552, Abcam, Cambridge, MA, USA) and Cathepsin K (1:200; ab19027, Abcam, Cambridge, MA, USA). Samples were incubated with appropriate biotinylated secondary antibodies (Vector BA-x) for 30 min, then washed in PBS. An avidin/biotinylated enzyme complex (Kit ABC Peroxidase Standard Vectastain PK-4000, Vectorlabs, Burlingame, CA, USA) was added and incubated for 30 min, and a 3,3′-diaminobenzidine (DAB) substrate kit (Kit Vector Peroxidase substrate DAB SK-4100, Vectorlabs, Burlingame, CA, USA) was used to develop the color reaction. Phalloidin immunostaining was performed using Palloidin Control, DyLight 488 conjugate (1:300; PI21833, Invitrogen, Grand Island, NY, USA).

2.9. Histomorphometric Analyses

Histomorphometric measurements were performed using ImageJ software v.1.51 (NIH, Bethesda, MD, USA). To quantify the amount of new bone formation in the osteotomy site as a function of time, a minimum of four osteotomy sites were analyzed. For each osteotomy site, a minimum of six aniline blue-stained histologic sections that spanned the distance from the furcation to the apex were used to quantify new bone formation. Each section was photographed using a Leica digital image system at 20× magnification. To calculate the percentage of new bone formation, the number of aniline blue^{+ve} pixels within an osteotomy was measured and divided by the number of the total pixels in the same osteotomy area.

2.10. Micro-Computed Tomography (µCT)

Scanning and analyses followed published guidelines [19]. Three-dimensional µCT imaging was performed at various times after surgery. In brief, samples were fixed in 4% PFA at 4 °C overnight. Then, they were transferred to 70% ethanol solution for µCT scanning before the decalcification process. A µCT tomography data-acquisition system (VivaCT 40, Scanco, Brüttisellen, Switzerland) at 10.5-µm voxel size (70 kV, 115 µA, 300 ms of integration time) was used for scanning and reconstruction. Bone morphometry was performed using the acquisition system's analysis software (Scanco). Multiplanar reconstruction and volume rendering were carried out using Avizo (FEI, Hillsboro, OR, USA) and ImageJ v1.51 (NIH, Bethesda, MD, USA) software, before being imported into Adobe Photoshop and Illustrator (CC2017, Adobe, San Jose, CA, USA).

2.11. Calculation of Osteotomy Surface Roughness

To calculate the irregularity of the osteotomy walls, the Shape Filter plugin for ImageJ was employed [20]. Ten transverse sections were used to outline the contours of osteotomies using ImageJ. The contours were then converted to black-and-white images, and the plugin was used to obtain the convexity and solidity values. Convexity measured the surface roughness of a two-dimensional (2D) shape and was defined as H/P, where H was the perimeter of convex hull of the shape, and P was the perimeter of the contour. Solidity was defined as C/A, where C was the area occupied by the contour, and A was the area occupied by the convex hull of the contour. The perimeter of the contour was defined as the total length of the shape's perimeter. Shapes such as a square have equal lengths of convex hulls and perimeter of the contours, which results in a convexity = 1. A star, however, has a pentagon convex hull (consider the shape when surrounded by a rubber band) while the perimeter of the contour is the star shape itself. Since the perimeter of the star contour (P) is larger than the convex hull (H), its convexity (H/P) is <1 and, therefore, its surface is rougher compared to a same-sized pentagon.

2.12. Heat Transfer During Drilling

The temperature produced when cutting with a conventional protocol involving multiple drills was compared to site preparation with the mini OsseoShaper. Sawbones 35 (Pacific Research Laboratory, Vashon Island, DC, USA) was used. Drills and drilling protocols used are as listed in Table 1. Thermal radiation was measured immediately after drilling via an infrared camera (SEEK CompactPRO, Seek Thermal Application, Santa Barbara, CA, USA). The drilling protocol was repeated six times in new Sawbones. Means and standard deviations were reported.

The temperature distribution during drilling was also calculated in MATLAB using a finite difference method. Details of the heat transfer model are described in Reference [5]. The differences between the conventional drill and mini OsseoShaper models can be summarized as follows: in the conventional high-speed drilling, the heat flux was applied to the drill hole's boundary where the tip of the drill was located, and the tip was moved vertically. Below the drill tip, the value of the heat flux was set to zero, and irrigation was applied above the drill tip. In the OsseoShaper low-speed drilling, the heat flux was applied to the drill hole's boundary at and above the tip due to the tapered shape of the drill, such that the points of engagement between the drill and the bone increased over time as the drill was moved vertically.

2.13. Statistical Analyses

Results were presented in the form of means ± standard deviations, with N equal to the number of samples analyzed. Student's t-tests were performed. Significance was set at $p < 0.05$, and all statistical analyses were performed with SPSS software (IBM, Armonk, NY, USA).

3. Results

3.1. A New Surgical Drilling Tool That Cuts Efficiently at Very Low Speeds

Most osteotomies are produced through the stepwise enlargement of an initial pilot drill hole with sequentially larger diameter drills [21], all coupled with the use of copious irrigation [22]. We recapitulated that clinical scenario in a rat model, by producing osteotomies using surgical drills with progressively larger diameters. The final drill was 1.6 mm in diameter and was run at 1000 rpm with irrigation (Figure 1A). In osteotomies produced with the downscaled prototype of OsseoShaper, the same pilot drill hole was produced and then followed by a single drill, the OsseoShaper (Figure 1A). The OsseoShaper was run at 50 rpm without irrigation.

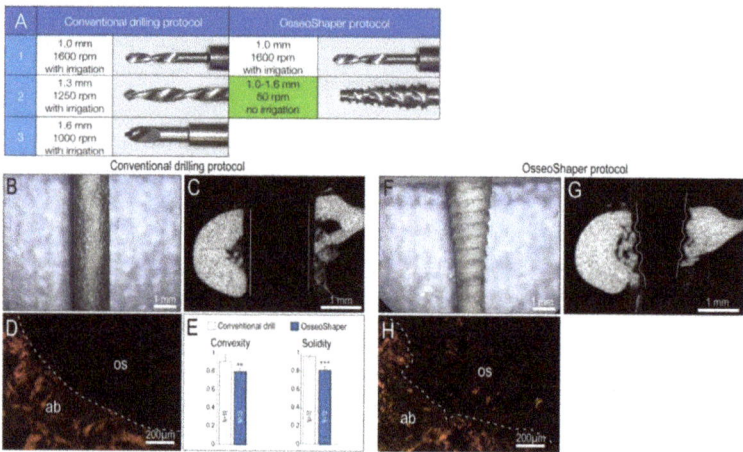

Figure 1. Osteotomy site preparation with OsseoShaper requires fewer steps and, unlike conventional drills, produces a rough surface. (**A**) All osteotomy site preparations began with the use of a 1.0-mm pilot drill run at 1600 rpm plus irrigation; afterward, the conventional osteotomy procedure used a 1.3-mm drill (1250 rpm plus irrigation) followed by a 1.6-mm drill (1000 rpm plus irrigation). The OsseoShaper protocol used the same 1.0-mm pilot drill at 1600 rpm plus irrigation, and was then followed by the OsseoShaper run at 50 rpm without irrigation. Using a conventional drill (**B**) in plexiglass demonstrates the shape and texture of a cut surfaces, and (**C**) in bone, μCT sections illustrate the parallel walls of the osteotomy. (**D**) Picrosirius red staining of a representative transverse tissue section demonstrates the resulting smooth cut surface. (**E**) Quantification of surface texture, as expressed by convexity and solidity, resulting from a conventional drilling protocol. Using an OsseoShaper (**F**) in plexiglass demonstrates a tapered shape with a threaded surface, (**G**) which is validated by μCT imaging. (**H**) Picrosirius red staining of a representative transverse tissue section demonstrates the textured cut surface and the retention of collagen containing osseous coagulum. Solid and dotted lines show the edge of the osteotomy. Two asterisks indicate $p < 0.01$. Three asterisks indicate $p < 0.001$. Scale bars (**B,C,F,G**) = 1 mm, and (**D,H**) = 200 μm. Abbreviations: ab, alveolar bone; os, osteotomy.

A conventional surgical drill is designed to cut only at its tip, which produces a smooth-walled osteotomy, visible both in plexiglass (Figure 1B) and μCT section of bone (Figure 1C). Analyses using picrosirius red staining revealed, under polarized light, the collagen organization at the cut edge when a conventional drill was employed (Figure 1D). Quantification of surface texture, as expressed by convexity and solidity, resulting from a conventional drilling protocol demonstrated the smoother cut edge (Figure 1E). By contrast, the OsseoShaper was designed with a cutting flute running its length; this resulted in a heteromorphic, textured osteotomy surface, visible both in plexiglass (Figure 1F) and in μCT (Figure 1G). Picrosirius red staining demonstrates the textured cut surface and the retention of collagen containing osseous coagulum (Figure 1H).

3.2. The OsseoShaper Allows the Retention of Viable, Autologous Bone Chips in the Osteotomy

Conventional drills have a rake angle that ranges from 0 to approximately 5°, the consequence of which is the production of small (<30 μm) bone particles. In addition, conventional drills are typically run at rotational velocities of 800 rpm or higher [23]. Finally, conventional drills are designed to rotate in the same direction, regardless of whether they are being advanced or withdrawn from the osteotomy. Collectively, these attributes result in minimal retention of particulate matter, as can be visualized when cutting Sawbone in vitro (Figure 2A). Coupled with irrigation, the majority of bone debris is typically removed from the osteotomy (Figure 2B).

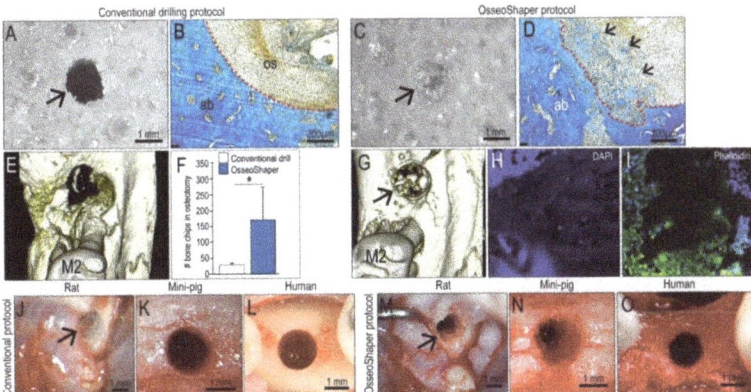

Figure 2. OsseoShaper-produced osteotomies retain more viable bone chips and osseous coagulum. Gross view of a hole produced in 0.32 g/cc Sawbone prepared with (**A**) a conventional drilling protocol versus (**C**) OsseoShaper. Representative transverse sections stained with aniline blue in the osteotomy sites using (**B**) a conventional drilling protocol and (**D**) OsseoShaper protocol. Micro-CT imaging of an osteotomy prepared with (**E**) a conventional drilling protocol versus (**G**) an OsseoShaper. (**F**) Quantification of bone chips in the osteotomy by μCT imaging ($N = 5$). Representative tissue sections of bone chips produced by the OsseoShaper using (**H**) 4′,6-diamidino-2-phenylindole (DAPI) and (**I**) phalloidin staining. Intra-operative view of an osteotomy prepared with conventional drills versus the OsseoShaper in rats (**J,M**), in mini-pigs (**K,N**), and in patients (**L,O**). Arrows indicate the osteotomy. Small arrows in (**D**) indicate the osteoid matrix. Dotted lines show the edge of the osteotomy. Asterisk indicates $p < 0.05$. Scale bars = 1 mm (**A,C,J–O**) and 200 μm (**B,E**). Abbreviations: as indicated previously.

By comparison, the rake angle on a mini OsseoShaper produces osseous coagulum and relatively large (~100 μm) bone chips; additionally, the OsseoShaper is designed to be reversed upon removal. These features result in the collection of bone chips in the cutting flutes, which are then transferred into the osteotomy while the tool is being withdrawn. These events can be visualized when cutting Sawbone (Figure 2C), and upon histologic examination of the osteotomy using aniline blue staining to detect osteoid matrix (Figure 2D).

Micro-CT imaging was used to quantify the volume of osseous coagulum and bone chips retained in the osteotomy. These analyses verified that OsseoShaper osteotomies retained significantly more osseous material than did conventionally prepared osteotomies (Figure 2E,F,G). A closer examination of the bone chips produced by the OsseoShaper using 4′,6-diamidino-2-phenylindole (DAPI; to detect viable cells) and phalloidin staining (to detect actin filaments) revealed that a subset of chips retained viable osteocytes within the osseous matrix (Figure 2H) and that the majority of chips were surrounded by viable cells (Figure 2I). Clinically, bone chips were only visible in the OsseoShaper-prepared osteotomy sites; this aspect was consistent among species, including rats, mini-pigs, and humans (Figure 2J–O).

3.3. The Mini OsseoShaper Preserves Peri-Implant Bone by Limiting Heat Transfer and Minimizing Thermal Apoptosis

A zone of osteocyte death is produced by conventional drilling [6,7,10]. For example, cutting at 1000 rpm with irrigation produced a ~250-μm-wide, circumferential distribution of TUNEL[+ve], apoptotic osteocytes (Figure 3A, quantified in C). By comparison, minimal osteocyte apoptosis was detected after OsseoShaper site preparation (Figure 3B, quantified in C).

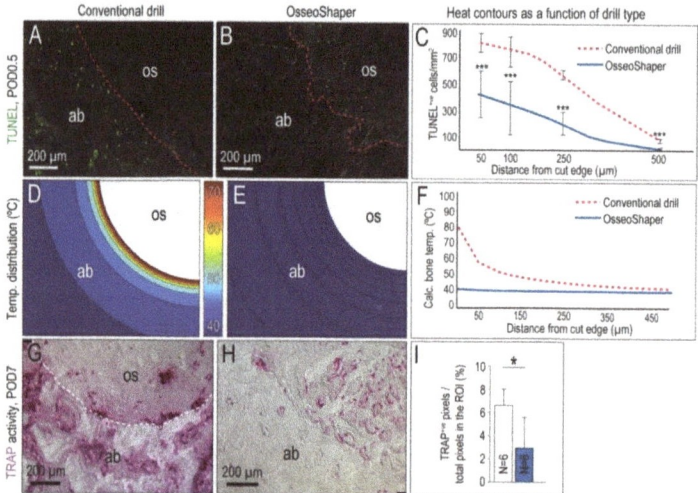

Figure 3. The OsseoShaper generates less heat, which results in a smaller zone of cell death and less tartrate-resistant acid phosphatase (TRAP)-mediated bone remodeling than conventional drills. (**A**) Representative tissue section from an osteotomy prepared using standard drills, where terminal deoxynucleotidyl transferase deoxyuridine triphosphate (dUTP) nick end labeling (TUNEL)$^{+ve}$ cells are apoptotic osteocytes. (**B**) Equivalent tissue section from an osteotomy prepared using the OsseoShaper, where the majority of apoptotic cells are detected in the osseous coagulum. (**C**) Distribution of TUNEL^{+ve} cells as a function of distance from cut edge of osteotomy. Computational models were used to map the distribution of heat in bone as a function of distance from the cut edge, in osteotomies produced using (**D**) conventional drills and (**E**) using the OsseoShaper. (**F**) Calculated temperatures in bone, expressed as a function of radial distance from conventional drills (dotted red line) and from the OsseoShaper (blue line) ($N = 6$). (**G**) Representative transverse tissue section from an osteotomy produced with conventional drills, analyzed on for TRAP activity on post-osteotomy day 7 (POD7). (**H**) TRAP activity on a representative transverse tissue section from an OsseoShaper-produced osteotomy. (**I**) Quantification of TRAP^{+ve} pixels/total pixels in the region of interest (ROI). A dotted line is used to indicate the cut edge of the osteotomy. Asterisk indicates $p < 0.05$. Scale bars = 200 µm. Abbreviations: as indicated previously.

A computational model was used to calculate peak temperatures produced by both types of cutting tools, taking into account the speed at which the drills were run, the density of the bone being cut, and, in the case of conventional drill protocols, the use of irrigation [5]. In the case of conventional protocols, a peak temperature of ~80 °C was generated at the cut edge, despite the use of copious irrigation (Figure 3D; quantified in F). Temperatures decreased as a function of distance from the cut edge but nevertheless, temperatures were >40 °C within a ~150-µm circumferential zone (Figure 3A and [6]).

By comparison, the mini OsseoShaper generated significantly lower (~40 °C) peak temperatures (Figure 3E; quantified in F). Even without the use of irrigation, calculated temperatures immediately adjacent to the cut edge remained in the physiologic range (Figure 3F), well below temperatures known to cause osteocytes necrosis, i.e., 45 °C [24].

An in vitro method supported our conclusion that drilling with the mini OsseoShaper produced less heat. Using Sawbones, site preparation was carried out following the same protocol as used for the site preparation in the rat maxilla (Figure 1A) and, immediately thereafter, the temperature of each drill was measured using an infrared camera (Figure S1, Supplementary Materials). The same method was used to measure heat radiating from the mini OsseoShaper. In the conventional protocol, the heat radiating from conventional drills was significantly higher for each step compared to the heat radiating from the mini OsseoShaper (Figure S1).

Osteocyte death is typically accompanied by peri-implant bone resorption [6,7]. In the case of osteotomies produced with conventional drills, the osteoclast marker TRAP was detected throughout the bone adjacent to the osteotomy edge, as well as in the osteotomy itself (Figure 3G). By contrast, mini OsseoShaper osteotomies exhibited minimal TRAP-mediated bone resorption (Figure 3H). The TRAP activity that was detected reflected new bone remodeling in the osteotomy (Figure 3H; quantified in I).

3.4. In Mini OsseoShaper Osteotomies, New Bone Formation Is Accelerated

The OsseoShaper was designed to retain osseous coagulum, e.g., mineralized particles including cortical and trabecular bone chips, blood, and stroma that have inherent osteogenic potential [25,26]. On POD3, evidence of this retained osseous coagulum was abundant; compared to conventionally prepared osteotomies, those prepared with the mini OsseoShaper were filled with aniline blue^{+ve} osteoid matrix (compare Figure 4A,B). This matrix served as a nidus for new bone formation and remodeling, as demonstrated by significantly higher Cathepsin K (Figure 4C,D; quantified in E) and Osterix (Figure 4F,G) expression in the mini OsseoShaper osteotomies. By POD7, mini OsseoShaper osteotomies were filled with new bone at a time point when conventionally prepared osteotomies had not yet started to repair (Figure 4H,I; quantified in J).

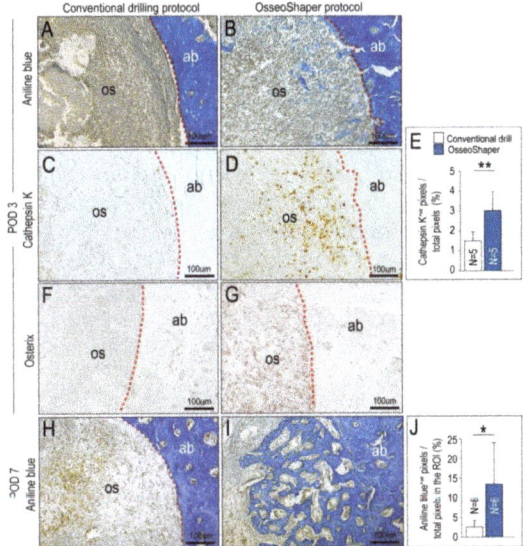

Figure 4. OsseoShaper drilling protocol promotes alveolar bone healing. Representative transverse tissue sections stained with aniline blue on post-osteotomy day 3 (POD3) following osteotomy site preparation with (**A**) conventional drills versus (**B**) the Nobel OsseoShaper. Note the presence of osseous coagulum in the osteotomy site prepared with the OsseoShaper. Adjacent tissue sections immunostained with Cathepsin K in the osteotomy sites of (**C**) conventional drills versus (**D**) the Nobel OsseoShaper. (**E**) Quantification of Cathepsin K^{+ve} pixels/total pixels in the osteotomy site. Adjacent tissue sections immunostained with Osterix in the osteotomy sites of (**F**) conventional drills versus (**G**) the OsseoShaper. (**H**) Tissue sections stained with aniline blue show minimal new bone formation in conventional drill group, while (**I**) osteotomies in the OsseoShaper group show more new bone formation on POD7. (**J**) Quantification of aniline blue^{+ve} pixels/total pixels in the osteotomy site. Dotted lines show the edge of the osteotomy. One asterisk indicates $p < 0.05$. Two asterisks indicate $p < 0.01$. Scale bars = 100 μm. Abbreviations: as indicated previously.

4. Discussion

Most reconstructive surgeries involve the cutting and removal of bone tissue [27] and, ideally, the goal is to resect a well-defined volume of bone and leave behind a cut edge that is favorable to early cell attachment and matrix deposition [28,29]. Clinicians universally agree that the preservation of cell viability is of utmost importance [30–32], and that high-speed rotating instruments can compromise this viability because they create thermal and mechanical trauma [33–37]. Irrigation can reduce some of the heat generated by high-speed rotatory surgical drills [22,38], but irrigation also removes bone chips, connective tissue stroma, blood, and stem-cell populations, collectively referred to as osseous coagulum, which have osteogenic potential [39–42].

The importance of preserving bone viability led to the development of a wide variety of new cutting tools for bone [43]. For example, gas and solid-state lasers use linear thermal absorption to ablate osteoid tissues and, while they are effective at removing the bone, they also generate heat and consequently show many of the same detrimental effects as drilling [44,45]. Plasma ablation lasers avoid some of these problems by creating energy pulses in very small (i.e., μm) zones that result in very high (several thousand Kelvin) temperatures over a very short (picosecond) duration. The result is limited thermal damage to the bone [46]; technical constraints, however, limit the use of these lasers in most clinical practices [47].

The OsseoShaper was designed to efficiently cut bone at a low (<50 rpm) velocity. This low-speed drilling results in less bone being cut per unit time and, therefore, less heat evolution per unit time (Figure 3). Less heat generation by the OsseoShaper translates into less of a temperature rise in the bone, which obviates the need for a coolant (Figure 3). The biological sequelae of lower heat generation by the mini OsseoShaper was shown by analyses for osteocyte apoptosis and osteoclast activity; because of the minimal temperature rise, few osteocytes underwent programmed cell death, which translated into less peri-implant bone resorption (Figure 3). Clinicians are fully aware that a viable osteotomy site is critical for new bone formation, and this point is perhaps best illustrated by the extent to which surgeons will go to reduce heat produced by rotary cutting tools. Here, we show that improved osteotomy site viability is indeed directly related to enhanced osteogenesis, which we believe will logically translate into a faster osseointegration of an implant placed into such osteotomies.

4.1. A Unique Design That Enables Retention of Bone Chips and Osseous Coagulum in an Osteotomy Site

Most drills produce bone chips and osseous coagulum, which has inherent osteogenic material that can stimulate new bone formation [25,26]. Most of this osteogenic material is flushed out of the site by irrigation [25], which is required to cool conventional drills. The rake angle of the OsseoShaper produces larger bone chips than conventional drilling protocols.

Most conventional drills rotate clockwise, whether advancing or withdrawing the tool and, coupled with the high rotational velocity, effectively disperse the bone chips and osseous coagulum. The OsseoShaper slowly rotates clockwise when advanced and is then reversed upon withdrawal; this design feature effectively retains bone chips and osseous coagulum in the osteotomy site (Figure 2). This feature was also visible in osteotomy site preparation performed in mini-pig and human individuals (Figure 2). Historic studies demonstrated that such bone chips that remain in situ are highly osteogenic [48].

Cutting flute placement affects the roughness of the osteotomy. Compared to the smooth-walled osteotomies produced by conventional drills, osteotomies produced by the OsseoShaper are textured (Figure 1). Some investigators speculated that a textured surface represents an optimal site for new bone deposition because it mimics the bone surface left behind after osteoclast-mediated remodeling [49].

Clinicians recognize that a bone graft from a patient has osteogenic potential and, therefore, a variety of methods were developed in an attempt to collect this autologous material [50]. Most, if not all, of these collection methods necessitate removal of the autologous bone chips from the body and storage ex vivo. In doing so, the bone graft material is potentially subjected to desiccation, temperature changes, e.g., deviations from 37 °C, and bacterial contamination. Use of the OsseoShaper negates these concerns; bone chips remain in situ and, in doing so, their viability is likely to be enhanced and/or preserved.

4.2. A Streamlined Protocol for Osteotomy Site Preparation

In conventional drilling protocols, a pilot hole is first produced; then, the osteotomy is gradually enlarged through the use of progressively larger diameter drills. A pilot hole is also created before use of the OsseoShaper, after which the final sized osteotomy is produced in a single step (Figure 1). In conventional drilling protocols, the use of multiple drills increases the chance of deviating from the intended axis of the osteotomy, which in turn impacts the axis of the implant placed into the osteotomy [51]. By reducing the number of surgical drills required to produce the final osteotomy, the alignment error is also effectively reduced [52], and subsequent implant placement will follow the axis of the last drill.

5. Conclusions

In our study, we present a new drill design that is meant to efficiently cut bone at a very low rotational speed, obviating the need for irrigation as a coolant and a lubricant. Osteocyte viability is maintained by the low-speed cutting that produces little heat. Autologous bone chips are generated and maintained on site thanks to the lack of irrigation, coupled with the unique design of the cutting flutes. This osseous coagulum has inherent osteogenic capacities. Collectively, a robust formation of new bone is observed with the new drill design, at rates significantly faster than those observed with conventional drilling protocols. These data have practical applications for clinical implant site preparation and alveolar bone reconstruction.

Supplementary Materials: The following are available online at http://www.mdpi.com/2077-0383/8/2/170/s1, Figure S1: Thermal radiation measurements of conventional and Osseoshaper protocols in Sawbones.

Author Contributions: Conceptualization, S.H. and A.Q.; methodology, J.A.H. and J.B.B.; data generation, C.-H.C., B.R.C., M.A. (Masaki Arioka), B.L., U.S.T., M.A. (Maziar Aghvami), B.S., W.H., A.Q., and O.B.; writing—original draft preparation, C.-H.C., B.R.C., M.A. (Masaki Arioka), J.B.B., and J.A.H.; writing—review and editing, C.-H.C., B.R.C., M.A. (Masaki Arioka), J.B.B., W.H., and J.A.H. All authors read and approved the manuscript.

Funding: This work was supported by NIH R01 DE024000-12 to J.A.H. and J.B.B. and a grant from Nobel Biocare Services AG, Kloten, Switzerland (grant number 2015-1400).

Acknowledgments: Special thanks to Audrey Schmitt, DDS, MSc (periodontist, private practice, Rouen, France) for providing surgical photographs from a conventional osteotomy site preparation. J.A.H. and J.B.B. are paid consultants for Nobel Biocare.

Conflicts of Interest: The authors declare no conflicts of interest.

References

1. Jackson, C.J.; Ghosh, S.K.; Johnson, W. On the evolution of drill-bit shapes. *J. Mech. Work Technol.* **1989**, *18*, 231–267. [CrossRef]
2. Pandey, R.K.; Panda, S.S. Drilling of bone: A comprehensive review. *J. Clin. Orthop. Trauma* **2013**, *4*, 15–30. [CrossRef] [PubMed]
3. Abouzgia, M.B.; James, D.F. Measurements of shaft speed while drilling through bone. *J. Oral. Maxillofac. Surg.* **1995**, *53*, 1308–1315, Discussion in **1995**, *53*, 1315–1316. [CrossRef]
4. Yan, P.; Rong, Y.M.; Wang, G. The effect of cutting fluids applied in metal cutting process. *Proc. Inst. Mech. Eng. B* **2016**, *230*, 19–37. [CrossRef]
5. Aghvami, M.; Brunski, J.B.; Serdar Tulu, U.; Chen, C.H.; Helms, J.A. A Thermal and Biological Analysis of Bone Drilling. *J. Biomech. Eng.* **2018**, *140*. [CrossRef]
6. Cha, J.Y.; Pereira, M.D.; Smith, A.A.; Houschyar, K.S.; Yin, X.; Mouraret, S.; Brunski, J.B.; Helms, J.A. Multiscale analyses of the bone-implant interface. *J. Dent. Res.* **2015**, *94*, 482–490. [CrossRef] [PubMed]
7. Wang, L.; Aghvami, M.; Brunski, J.; Helms, J. Biophysical regulation of osteotomy healing: An animal study. *Clin. Implant Dent. Relat. Res.* **2017**, *19*, 590–599. [CrossRef] [PubMed]

8. Pei, X.; Wang, L.; Chen, C.; Yuan, X.; Wan, Q.; Helms, J.A. Contribution of the PDL to osteotomy repair and implant osseointegration. *J. Dent. Res.* **2017**, *96*, 909–916. [CrossRef]
9. Li, J.; Yin, X.; Huang, L.; Mouraret, S.; Brunski, J.B.; Cordova, L.; Salmon, B.; Helms, J.A. Relationships among bone quality, implant osseointegration, and Wnt signaling. *J. Dent. Res.* **2017**, *96*, 822–831. [CrossRef]
10. Chen, C.H.; Pei, X.; Tulu, U.S.; Aghvami, M.; Chen, C.T.; Gaudilliere, D.; Arioka, M.; Maghazeh Moghim, M.; Bahat, O.; Kolinski, M.; et al. A comparative assessment of implant site viability in humans and rats. *J. Dent. Res.* **2018**, *97*, 451–459. [CrossRef]
11. Chen, C.H.; Wang, L.; Serdar Tulu, U.; Arioka, M.; Moghim, M.M.; Salmon, B.; Chen, C.T.; Hoffmann, W.; Gilgenbach, J.; Brunski, J.B.; et al. An osteopenic/osteoporotic phenotype delays alveolar bone repair. *Bone* **2018**, *112*, 212–219. [CrossRef] [PubMed]
12. Arioka, M.; Zhang, X.; Li, Z.; Tulu, U.S.; Liu, Y.; Wang, L.; Yuan, X.; Helms, J.A. Osteoporotic changes in the periodontium impair alveolar bone healing. *J. Dent. Res.* **2019**. [CrossRef]
13. Mangano, F.; Mortellaro, C.; Mangano, N.; Mangano, C. Is low serum vitamin d associated with early dental implant failure? A retrospective evaluation on 1625 implants placed in 822 patients. *Mediators Inflamm.* **2016**. [CrossRef] [PubMed]
14. Kalu, D.N. The ovariectomized rat model of postmenopausal bone loss. *Bone Miner.* **1991**, *15*, 175–191. [CrossRef]
15. Cummings, S.R.; Melton, L.J. Epidemiology and outcomes of osteoporotic fractures. *Lancet* **2002**, *359*, 1761–1767. [CrossRef]
16. Chen, S.T.; Beagle, J.; Jensen, S.S.; Chiapasco, M.; Darby, I. Consensus statements and recommended clinical procedures regarding surgical techniques. *Int. J. Oral Maxillofac. Implants* **2009**, *24*, 272–278.
17. Yin, X.; Li, J.; Chen, T.; Mouraret, S.; Dhamdhere, G.; Brunski, J.B.; Zou, S.; Helms, J.A. Rescuing failed oral implants via Wnt activation. *J. Clin. Periodontol.* **2015**. [CrossRef] [PubMed]
18. Minear, S.; Leucht, P.; Jiang, J.; Liu, B.; Zeng, A.; Fuerer, C.; Nusse, R.; Helms, J.A. Wnt proteins promote bone regeneration. *Sci. Transl. Med.* **2010**, *2*. [CrossRef]
19. Bouxsein, M.L.; Boyd, S.K.; Christiansen, B.A.; Guldberg, R.E.; Jepsen, K.J.; Muller, R. Guidelines for assessment of bone microstructure in rodents using micro-computed tomography. *J. Bone Miner. Res.* **2010**, *25*, 1468–1486. [CrossRef]
20. Wagner, T.; Lipinski, H.G. IJBlob: An ImageJ library for connected component analysis and shape analysis. *J. Open Res. Softw.* **2013**, *1*, 6–8.8
21. Wang, L.; Wu, Y.; Perez, K.C.; Hyman, S.; Brunski, J.B.; Tulu, U.; Bao, C.; Salmon, B.; Helms, J.A. Effects of Condensation on Peri-implant Bone Density and Remodeling. *J. Dent. Res.* **2017**, *96*, 413–420. [CrossRef] [PubMed]
22. Isler, S.C.; Cansiz, E.; Tanyel, C.; Soluk, M.; Selvi, F.; Cebi, Z. The effect of irrigation temperature on bone healing. *Int. J. Med. Sci.* **2011**, *8*, 704–708. [CrossRef] [PubMed]
23. Almeida, K.P.; Delgado-Ruiz, R.; Carneiro, L.G.; Leiva, A.B.; Calvo-Guirado, J.L.; Gomez-Moreno, G.; Malmstrom, H.; Romanos, G.E. Influence of Drilling Speed on Stability of Tapered Dental Implants: An Ex Vivo Experimental Study. *Int. J. Oral Maxillofac. Implants* **2016**, *31*, 795–798. [CrossRef] [PubMed]
24. Dolan, E.B.; Haugh, M.G.; Tallon, D.; Casey, C.; McNamara, L.M. Heat-shock-induced cellular responses to temperature elevations occurring during orthopaedic cutting. *J. R. Soc. Interface* **2012**, *9*, 3503–3513. [CrossRef] [PubMed]
25. Robinson, R.E. The osseous coagulum for bone induction technique. A review. *J. Calif. Dent. Assoc.* **1970**, *46*, 18–27. [PubMed]
26. Robinson, E. Osseous coagulum for bone induction. *J. Periodontol.* **1969**, *40*, 503–510. [CrossRef]
27. Preston, C.F.; Fulkerson, E.W.; Meislin, R.; Di Cesare, P.E. Osteotomy about the knee: Applications, techniques, and results. *J. Knee Surg.* **2005**, *18*, 258–272. [CrossRef]
28. Yeniyol, S.; Jimbo, R.; Marin, C.; Tovar, N.; Janal, M.N.; Coelho, P.G. The effect of drilling speed on early bone healing to oral implants. *Oral Surg. Oral Med. Oral Pathol. Oral Radiol.* **2013**, *116*, 550–555. [CrossRef]
29. Giro, G.; Marin, C.; Granato, R.; Bonfante, E.A.; Suzuki, M.; Janal, M.N.; Coelho, P.G. Effect of drilling technique on the early integration of plateau root form endosteal implants: an experimental study in dogs. *J. Oral Maxillofac. Surg.* **2011**, *69*, 2158–2163. [CrossRef]
30. Miron, R.J.; Gruber, R.; Hedbom, E.; Saulacic, N.; Zhang, Y.; Sculean, A.; Bosshardt, D.D.; Buser, D. Impact of bone harvesting techniques on cell viability and the release of growth factors of autografts. *Clin. Implant Dent. Relat. Res.* **2013**, *15*, 481–489. [CrossRef]

31. Maus, U.; Andereya, S.; Gravius, S.; Siebert, C.H.; Schippmann, T.; Ohnsorge, J.A.; Niedhart, C. How to store autologous bone graft perioperatively: an in vitro study. *Arch. Orthop. Trauma Surg.* **2008**, *128*, 1007–1011. [CrossRef] [PubMed]
32. Laursen, M.; Christensen, F.B.; Bunger, C.; Lind, M. Optimal handling of fresh cancellous bone graft: different peroperative storing techniques evaluated by in vitro osteoblast-like cell metabolism. *Acta Orthop. Scand.* **2003**, *74*, 490–496. [CrossRef] [PubMed]
33. Davidson, S.R.; James, D.F. Drilling in bone: Modeling heat generation and temperature distribution. *J. Biomech. Eng.* **2003**, *125*, 305–314. [CrossRef] [PubMed]
34. Eriksson, A.R.; Albrektsson, T. Temperature threshold levels for heat-induced bone tissue injury: A vital-microscopic study in the rabbit. *J. Prosthet. Dent.* **1983**, *50*, 101–107. [CrossRef]
35. Lundskog, J. Heat and bone tissue. An experimental investigation of the thermal properties of bone and threshold levels for thermal injury. *Scand. J. Plast. Reconstr. Surg.* **1972**, *9*, 1–80. [PubMed]
36. Eriksson, A.; Albrektsson, T.; Grane, B.; McQueen, D. Thermal injury to bone. A vital-microscopic description of heat effects. *Int. J. Oral Surg.* **1982**, *11*, 115–121. [CrossRef]
37. Matthews, L.S.; Hirsch, C. Temperatures measured in human cortical bone when drilling. *J. Bone Joint. Surg. Am.* **1972**, *54*, 297–308. [CrossRef] [PubMed]
38. Tawy, G.F.; Rowe, P.J.; Riches, P.E. Thermal damage done to bone by burring and sawing with and without irrigation in knee arthroplasty. *J. Arthroplasty* **2016**, *31*, 1102–1108. [CrossRef]
39. Gazdag, A.R.; Lane, J.M.; Glaser, D.; Forster, R.A. Alternatives to autogenous bone graft: Efficacy and indications. *J. Am. Acad Orthop. Surg.* **1995**, *3*, 1–8. [CrossRef]
40. Khan, S.N.; Cammisa, F.P., Jr.; Sandhu, H.S.; Diwan, A.D.; Girardi, F.P.; Lane, J.M. The biology of bone grafting. *J. Am. Acad Orthop. Surg.* **2005**, *13*, 77–86. [CrossRef]
41. Burchardt, H. Biology of bone transplantation. *Orthop. Clin. North Am.* **1987**, *18*, 187–196. [PubMed]
42. Chen, T.; Li, J.; Cordova, L.A.; Liu, B.; Mouraret, S.; Sun, Q.; Salmon, B.; Helms, J. A WNT protein therapeutic improves the bone-forming capacity of autografts from aged animals. *Sci. Rep.* **2018**, *8*, 119. [CrossRef] [PubMed]
43. Bertollo, N.; Walsh, W.R. Drilling of bone: Practicality, limitations and complications associated with surgical drill-bits. *Biomech. Appl.* **2011**. [CrossRef]
44. Lustmann, J.; Ulmansky, M.; Fuxbrunner, A.; Lewis, A. Photoacoustic injury and bone healing following 193nm excimer laser ablation. *Lasers Surg. Med.* **1992**, *12*, 390–396. [CrossRef] [PubMed]
45. Vogel, A.; Venugopalan, V. Mechanisms of pulsed laser ablation of biological tissues. *Chem. Rev.* **2003**, *103*, 577–644. [CrossRef] [PubMed]
46. Leucht, P.; Lam, K.; Kim, J.B.; Mackanos, M.A.; Simanovskii, D.M.; Longaker, M.T.; Contag, C.H.; Schwettman, H.A.; Helms, J.A. Accelerated bone repair after plasma laser corticotomies. *Ann. Surg.* **2007**, *246*, 140–150. [CrossRef] [PubMed]
47. Romanos, G.E.; Gupta, B.; Yunker, M.; Romanos, E.B.; Malmstrom, H. Lasers use in dental implantology. *Implant Dent.* **2013**, *22*, 282–288. [CrossRef] [PubMed]
48. Rivault, A.F.; Toto, P.D.; Levy, S.; Gargiulo, A.W. Autogenous bone grafts: osseous coagulum and osseous retrograde procedures in primates. *J. Periodontol.* **1971**, *42*, 787–796. [CrossRef]
49. Bell, S.; Ajami, E.; Davies, J.E. An improved mechanical testing method to assess bone-implant anchorage. *J. Vis. Exp.* **2014**. [CrossRef]
50. Young, M.P.; Worthington, H.V.; Lloyd, R.E.; Drucker, D.B.; Sloan, P.; Carter, D.H. Bone collected during dental implant surgery: A clinical and histological study. *Clin. Oral Implants Res.* **2002**, *13*, 298–303. [CrossRef]
51. Schneider, D.; Marquardt, P.; Zwahlen, M.; Jung, R.E. A systematic review on the accuracy and the clinical outcome of computer-guided template-based implant dentistry. *Clin. Oral Implants Res.* **2009**, *20* (Suppl. 4), 73–86. [CrossRef] [PubMed]
52. Horwitz, J.; Zuabi, O.; Machtei, E.E. Accuracy of a computerized tomography-guided template-assisted implant placement system: an in vitro study. *Clin. Oral Implants Res.* **2009**, *20*, 1156–1162. [CrossRef] [PubMed]

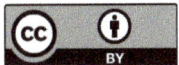

© 2019 by the authors. Licensee MDPI, Basel, Switzerland. This article is an open access article distributed under the terms and conditions of the Creative Commons Attribution (CC BY) license (http://creativecommons.org/licenses/by/4.0/).

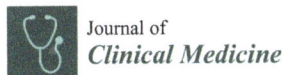

Article

Carbon Fiber Reinforced PEEK Composites Based on 3D-Printing Technology for Orthopedic and Dental Applications

Xingting Han [1], Dong Yang [2], Chuncheng Yang [2], Sebastian Spintzyk [1], Lutz Scheideler [1], Ping Li [1], Dichen Li [2,*], Jürgen Geis-Gerstorfer [1] and Frank Rupp [1]

1. Section Medical Materials Science and Technology, University Hospital Tübingen, Osianderstr. 2–8, D-72076 Tübingen, Germany; xingting.han@student.uni-tuebingen.de (X.H.); Sebastian.Spintzyk@med.uni-tuebingen.de (S.S.); lutz.scheideler@med.uni-tuebingen.de (L.S.); ping.li@uni-tuebingen.de (P.L.); juergen.geis-gerstorfer@med.uni-tuebingen.de (J.G.-G.); Frank.Rupp@med.uni-tuebingen.de (F.R.)
2. State Key Laboratory for Manufacturing System Engineering, School of Mechanical Engineering, Xi'an Jiaotong University, Xi'an 710054, China; yangdong2015@stu.xjtu.edu.cn (D.Y.); yang.chun.cheng@stu.xjtu.edu.cn (C.Y.)
* Correspondence: dcli@mail.xjtu.edu.cn; Tel.: +86-029-8339-9510

Received: 11 January 2019; Accepted: 5 February 2019; Published: 12 February 2019

Abstract: Fused deposition modeling (FDM) is a rapidly growing three-dimensional (3D) printing technology and has great potential in medicine. Polyether-ether-ketone (PEEK) is a biocompatible high-performance polymer, which is suitable to be used as an orthopedic/dental implant material. However, the mechanical properties and biocompatibility of FDM-printed PEEK and its composites are still not clear. In this study, FDM-printed pure PEEK and carbon fiber reinforced PEEK (CFR-PEEK) composite were successfully fabricated by FDM and characterized by mechanical tests. Moreover, the sample surfaces were modified with polishing and sandblasting methods to analyze the influence of surface roughness and topography on general biocompatibility (cytotoxicity) and cell adhesion. The results indicated that the printed CFR-PEEK samples had significantly higher general mechanical strengths than the printed pure PEEK (even though there was no statistical difference in compressive strength). Both PEEK and CFR-PEEK materials showed good biocompatibility with and without surface modification. Cell densities on the "as-printed" PEEK and the CFR-PEEK sample surfaces were significantly higher than on the corresponding polished and sandblasted samples. Therefore, the FDM-printed CFR-PEEK composite with proper mechanical strengths has potential as a biomaterial for bone grafting and tissue engineering applications.

Keywords: fused deposition modeling; polyether ether ketone; biocomposite; orthopedic implant; oral implant; mechanical properties; wettability; topography; biocompatibility; cell adhesion

1. Introduction

Cranio-maxillofacial defects related to tumors, traumas, infections, or congenital deformities are highly challenging tasks for oral and maxillofacial surgeons to reconstruct [1,2]. When bone losses are too severe for human body routine mechanisms to regenerate, autologous grafts are the first considerations due to the simultaneous osteogenic, osteoinductive, and osteoconductive properties [3]. However, the shape of the donor sites, bone graft resorption, and infection restrict the application of autografts [4]. Currently, the most popular orthopedic/dental artificial materials are metals like titanium (Ti) and its alloys. These materials have many advantages, such as excellent biocompatibility, corrosion resistance, and mechanical strength [5]. However, there are some critical drawbacks of Ti, one of which is stress-shielding, which may occur at the interface between Ti and bone during load transfer and result in surrounding bone loss [6]. In addition, the radiopacity of Ti alloys in the CT and MR scan images and the release of harmful metal ions hinder the application of metals [7]. Due to the limitations observed in metallic biomaterials, polymers have been explored in recent years as potential alternative materials for bone replacement.

In the last few years, polyether ether ketone (PEEK) has been investigated widely in oral and cranio-maxillofacial surgery. Possible applications are dental implants, skull implants, osteosynthesis plates, and bone replacement material for nasal, maxillary, or mandibular reconstructions (Figure 1) [8–11]. PEEK is considered an alternative material for Ti due to its excellent biocompatibility, radiolucency, chemical resistance, low density (1.32 g/cm^3), and mechanical properties resembling human bone. PEEK is a polyaromatic semi-crystalline thermoplastic polymer with an elastic modulus of 3–4 GPa (Table 1), which is much lower than that of Ti (102–110 GPa) and very close to the human trabecular bone (1 GPa) [8,12]. Moreover, the mechanical strengths of PEEK can be enhanced by the incorporation of other materials (e.g., carbon fibers) [8]. Normally, carbon fiber reinforced polyether ether ketone (CFR-PEEK) has an elastic modulus close to the human cortical bone (14 GPa), depending on the amount of reinforced carbon fiber and manufacturing methods. CFR-PEEK is considered as a promising candidate to replace metallic materials because of the inherited advantages of PEEK and improved mechanical properties [13,14].

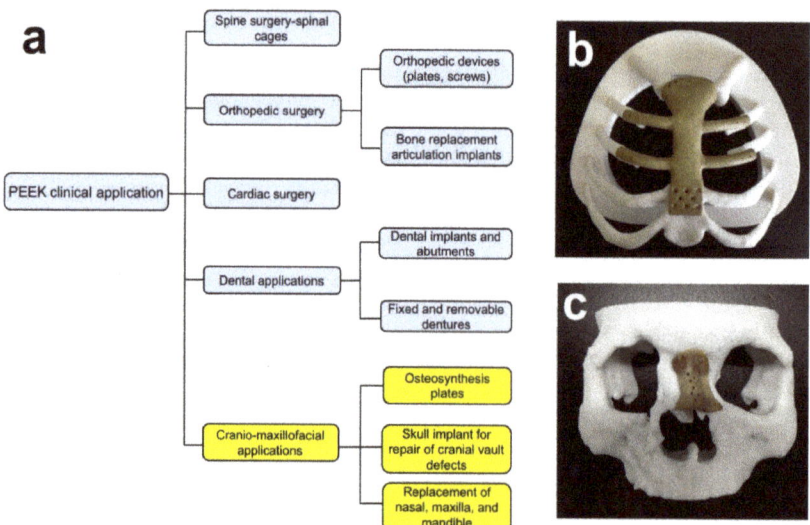

Figure 1. (a) Clinical applications of PEEK; Fused deposition modeling (FDM)-printed PEEK (b) breastbone and (c) nasal reconstructions.

Table 1. The elastic modulus of different materials and human tissues.

Materials	Elastic Modulus (GPa)	References
PEEK	3–4	[8]
Ti	102–110	[8]
Zirconia	210	[15]
Cortical bone	14	[8]
Trabecular bone	1	[15]

Additive manufacturing (AM) is a layer-by-layer manufacturing method, fabricating specimens by fusing or depositing materials, such as metals, ceramics, plastics, or even living cells [16]. This technique is becoming popular in orthopedic surgery for fabricating patient-specific implants due to the low cost, the feasibility of complex architectures, and the short production time [17]. Selective laser sintering (SLS) has been the most popular AM technology for fabricating PEEK in the past decades [18,19]. Compared with SLS, fused deposition modeling (FDM) is one of the fastest growing three-dimensional (3D) printing methods due to the lower costs, easier use (filament vs. powder), and reduced risk of material contamination or degradation. Furthermore, it has increasingly been applied to the manufacturing of PEEK and its composites in recent years [20]. However, due to the semicrystalline structure and high melting temperature of PEEK (compared with other FDM filament materials like polylactic acid (PLA) and acrylonitrile butadiene styrene (ABS)), it is difficult to process PEEK objects by FDM printing and the process is liable to cause excessive thermal stress and thermal cracks [8,18]. Yang et al. and Wu et al. have already measured the mechanical properties of FDM-printed pure PEEK and found that compared with some traditional manufacturing methods (i.e., injection molding), FDM-printed PEEK had lower mechanical strengths, which were influenced by layer thickness, printing speed, ambient temperature, nozzle temperature, and heat treatment [21,22]. FDM-printed PEEK composites, to the best of our knowledge, have not yet been studied.

Compared with Ti, the unmodified PEEK is bioinert and has limited osteoconductive properties, which may influence the osseointegration after implantation [23,24]. Surface topographical modification is one of the mechanical surface modification methods to increase the biological performance of cranio-maxillofacial implants [25]. Surface roughness may influence cell adhesion, and a roughened surface usually has a more extensive surface area which offers more binding sites for cell attachment [26]. Some studies have already analyzed the influence of surface roughness on the bioactivity of PEEK and its composites [26–28]. However, in these reports, PEEK and its composites were all manufactured by traditional techniques like milling, injection modeling, and compression molding. For the FDM-manufactured PEEK, most studies only analyzed the manufacturing process and mechanical properties of pure PEEK, without PEEK composites [17,18,22]. According to our knowledge, tests of the mechanical properties of FDM-printed CFR-PEEK are still lacking. Therefore, the aim of this study was to evaluate the mechanical properties and microstructures of PEEK and CFR-PEEK samples manufactured by FDM. Specific attention was paid to the question of whether the FDM printing process has introduced or produced toxic substances and to the influence of surface treatments on the cell adhesion on sample surfaces.

2. Materials and Methods

2.1. Sample Preparation and Surface Modification

2.1.1. Sample Preparation

A 3D printing system for PEEK material and its composite from Jugao-AM Tech. Corp. (Xi'an, China) was used to prepare all test specimens. In the printing process, the PEEK material was heated and transformed into a semi liquid state inside the nozzle. Then, the feedstock filament was forced to pass through the nozzle where it was melted and deposited in the form of a thin layer onto the platform. After one layer was finished, the platform went down along the z-axis equal to the pre-setting layer thickness. The desired geometry of the final complex objects was built layer-by-layer under the control of a computer. The extrusion temperature was set at 420 °C, and the printing speed was 40 mm/s. The bead width of each printing line was 0.4 mm, and the layer thickness was 0.2 mm (Table 2). Moreover, the PEEK filaments, as the material for 3D printing in this paper, were reprocessed from pellets (450G, VICTREX Corp., Thornton Cleveleys, UK), and 5% milled carbon fibers with a length of 80–150 μm and a diameter of 7 μm (Nanjing WeiDa Composite Material Co. Ltd., Nanjing, China) were chosen as the reinforcements. Before printing, a special fixative paper (Mingtai 3D Technology Co., Ltd., Shenzhen, China) was applied to the print bed for the objects' adhesion and warping improvement. After printing the samples and cooling them down to room temperature, the samples were placed into a furnace (101-0 s, Shaoxing SuPo Instrument Corp., Shaoxing, China) for the heat treatment (tempering) process. After heating for 2 h at 300 °C, the samples were cooled down to room temperature to decrease shrinkage distortion and residual stress to obtain good mechanical performance of the parts.

Table 2. Technical specifications of the FDM printer.

Parameters	Technical Specifications
Nozzle diameter	0.4 mm
Bead width	0.4 mm
Layer thickness	0.2 mm
Printing speed	40 mm/s
Raster angle	Consistent with the longest edge
Ambient temperature	20 °C
Nozzle temperature	420 °C

The dimension of the PEEK and CFR-PEEK samples for testing the mechanical properties (tensile, bending, and compressive tests) was according to ISO standards. The dog-bone shape tensile testing specimens (90 mm × 5 mm × 4 mm) were printed according to ISO 527-1 standard [29], and the cuboid bending specimens (80 mm × 10 mm × 4 mm) were printed according to ISO 178 standard (Figure 2) [30]. According to ISO 604 standard, two sample groups were manufactured for testing compressive strength and compressive modulus, respectively [31]. The round-shaped PEEK and CFR-PEEK disc samples for the wettability, roughness, microstructure, and biological tests were produced with a diameter of 14 mm and a thickness of 1 mm.

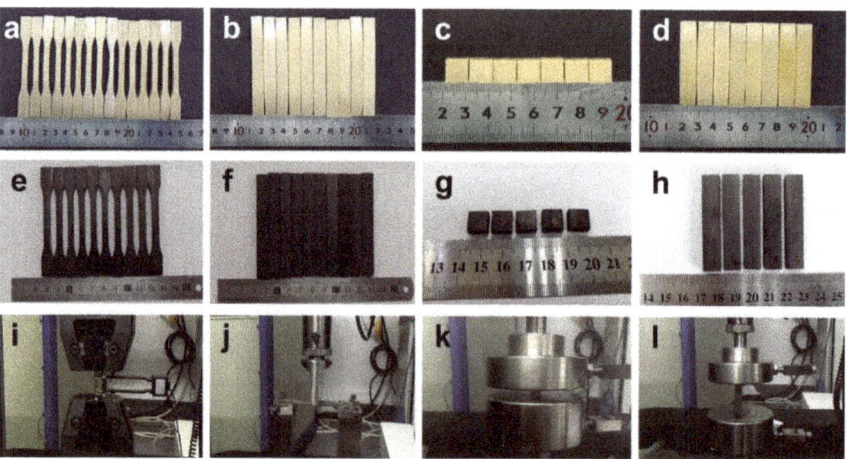

Figure 2. Pure PEEK and CFR-PEEK samples for testing mechanical properties: (**a,e**) tensile samples of PEEK and CFR-PEEK; (**b,f**) bending samples of PEEK and CFR-PEEK; (**c,g**) compressive samples (compressive strength) of PEEK and CFR-PEEK; (**d,h**) compressive samples (compressive modulus) of PEEK and CFR-PEEK; (**i**) tensile test; (**j**) bending test; (**k,l**) compressive tests of strength and modulus.

Ti disc samples (Grade: 4, Straumann AG, Basel, Switzerland) with 15 mm diameter and 1 mm thickness were prepared from Ti sheet metal (Straumann AG, Basel, Switzerland) with a punching tool. The Ti samples were used as an additional control group for the wettability, roughness, and biological tests. All titanium discs underwent a surface treatment, which was consistent with the polished PEEK and CFR-PEEK.

2.1.2. Sample Surface Modification

After printing, the PEEK and CFR-PEEK disc samples for wettability, roughness, microstructure, and biological tests were divided into three groups: as-printed (untreated) group, polished group, and sandblasted group (n = 12 per group). The untreated group included the directly printed samples, without any surface treatment. For the polished and sandblasted groups, all the discs were manually polished with a series of SiC abrasive papers up to P4000 (Buehler, Lake Bluff, IL, USA) by a polisher (Buehler, Coventry, UK). Then, the samples of the sandblasted group were further modified using a sandblasting machine (P-G 400, Harnisch + Rieth, Winterbach, Germany) with 120 μm alumina (Al_2O_3) particles (Cobra, Renfert, Hilzingen, Germany) under the pressure of 0.1 MPa at a distance of 50 mm for 15 s.

All Ti disc surfaces were modified using the same processes as for PEEK and CFR-PEEK samples by a series of SiC abrasive papers (1200, 2500, 4000 grit, Buehler, Lake Bluff, IL, USA) by a polisher (Buehler, Coventry, UK). After polishing, all the samples were cleaned with deionized (DI) water by an ultrasonic cleaner (Sonorex Super RK102H, Bandelin, Berlin, Germany) to remove residual Al_2O_3 particles on the sample surfaces.

2.2. Mechanical Properties Test

Mechanical tests were carried out using an electro-hydraulic servo mechanical testing machine (CMT4304, MTS Corp., Eden Prairie, MN, USA) according to ISO standards. ISO 527-1: 2012 (Plastics—Determination of tensile properties), ISO 178: 2010 (Plastics—Determination of flexural properties), and ISO 604: 2002 (Plastics—Determination of compressive properties) were applied for the tensile, bending, and compressive tests, respectively [29–31]. Six samples were tested for each batch with a 1 mm/min testing speed, and the test was performed at an ambient temperature of 20 °C.

2.3. Surface Characterization

To determine the surface morphology, samples of PEEK and CFR-PEEK from the untreated, polished, and sandblasted groups (n = 2 per group) were sputtered with a 20 nm thick Au–Pd coating (SCD 050, Baltec, Lübeck, Germany) and characterized by a scanning electron microscope (SEM) (LEO 1430, Zeiss, Oberkochen, Germany) at 200× and 2000× magnification.

The surface topography of the discs (n = 6 per group) was analyzed by a profilometer (Perthometer Concept S6P, Mahr, Göttingen, Germany). For each sample, 121 profiles were measured over a 3 mm × 3 mm area. The arithmetic mean height (Sa) and root mean square height (Sq) were calculated based on these topographies by software (MountainsMap Universal 7.3, Digital Surf, Besançon, France).

The water contact angle (WCA) was measured at room temperature on six samples per group using a drop shape analyzer (DSA 10-MK 2, Kruess, Hamburg, Germany). Drops of 2 μL of distilled water were deposited on the respective disc surfaces using an automatic pipette. After 20 s wetting time, the contact angle at the air–water–substrate interface was quantified from the drop geometry using DSA software (version 1.90.0.11, Kruess, Hamburg, Germany).

2.4. Biological Tests

Biological tests consisted of an extract test and a direct contact test to analyze the cytotoxicity and of the investigation of cell attachment to the different samples (n = 9 per group). Two materials (PEEK and CFR-PEEK) with three different surfaces each (untreated, polished, and sandblasted) were tested. In each test, n = 3 samples were used for each surface modification. All tests were performed three times in independent experiments. Directly before the biological tests, samples were ultrasonically cleaned with DI water for 15 min and sterilized with 70% ethanol and 100% ethanol (15 min each). Subsequently, the samples were dried on filter paper in a sterile workbench (Lamin Air HB2472, Burgdorf, Switzerland).

2.4.1. Cell Culture

L929 fibroblasts (DSMZ GmbH, Braunschweig, Germany) were cultured in DMEM medium (21063-029, Gibco, Paisley, UK) containing 10% fetal bovine serum (FBS, Life Technologies, Carlsbad, CA, USA), 1% penicillin/streptomycin (15140-122, Life Technologies Co., Carlsbad, CA, USA), and 1% GlutaMAX (Life Technologies Co., Paisley, UK) in 75 cm^2 sterile cell culture flasks (Costar, Corning, Tewksbury, MA, USA). The cells were maintained in an incubator under a humidified atmosphere with 5% CO_2 at 37 °C. The DMEM culture medium was renewed twice a week. When cells reached confluence, Trypsin (GIBCO, Paisley, UK) was used to detach cells from the bottom of flasks, and 1/10 of the total cells were transferred into a new flask.

2.4.2. Test for In Vitro Cytotoxicity

The in vitro cytotoxicity test of PEEK and CFR-PEEK was performed by an extract method based on ISO 10993-5 [32]. Extracts were derived from soaking the samples with DMEM cell culture medium for 24 h at 37 °C. The ratio between the sample surface area and extraction vehicle volume was 3 cm^2/mL. In the meantime, the cells were precultured for 24 h. The seeding concentration of L929 cells was 30,000 cells/cm^2 in 200 µL DMEM medium per well in a 96-well plate (Cellstar 655180, Greiner Bio-One, Frickenhausen, Germany). After 24 h, the culture medium was removed from the cells and replaced by 150 µL extracts obtained from the respective sample groups. Three concentrations of each extract were tested: (a) undiluted (150 µL extracts), (b) 1:3 diluted with medium (50 µL extracts + 100 µL medium), and (c) 1:10 diluted (15 µL extracts + 135 µL medium). Ti samples were used as the negative control, and copper (Cu) samples were used as the positive control. After culturing for an additional 24 h, the extracts in all groups were replaced by 100 µL fresh DMEM medium to avoid artifacts in the following assay caused by blue color in the Cu extracts. The cytotoxicity was quantitatively analyzed by CCK-8 assay (Dojindo Molecular Technologies, Inc., Rockville, MD, USA). The volume of CCK-8 solution added to each test well was 10 µL. After incubating for 2 h, the optical density (OD) value was measured by a microplate ELISA reader (Tecan F50, Tecan Austria, Groedig, Austria) at 450 nm wavelength. The metabolic activity of L929 cells in the different test groups in comparison to the negative control was calculated according to the following formula:

$$\text{Cell metabolic activity (\%)} = (OD_t - OD_b)/(OD_{nc} - OD_b)\,100\%, \tag{1}$$

where the OD value is the absorbance value of the respective test group (OD_t), blank control group (OD_b), and negative control group (OD_{nc}).

2.4.3. Cell Adhesion and Spreading

L929 cells were seeded on PEEK, CFR-PEEK, and Ti samples in 12-well plates (REF 3512, Costar, Kennebunk, ME, USA) with a density of 30,000 cells/cm^2 and incubated in 2.4 mL DMEM medium at 37 °C and 5% CO_2. After incubation for 24 h, cell adhesion was terminated by rinsing with Hank's balanced salt solution (HBSS, Biochrom AG, Berlin, Germany). Adhering cells were vital stained for 10 min in a solution of 25 µg/mL fluorescein diacetate (FDA) and 1.25 µg/mL ethidium bromide (EB) (Sigma-Aldrich Chemie GmbH, Taufkirchen, Germany) in HBSS. For each sample, a minimum of six typical surface areas of every magnification (25×, 100×, 200×, and 400×) was documented by an Optishot-2 fluorescence microscope (Nikon, Tokyo, Japan) equipped with a digital camera (550D, Canon, Tokyo, Japan). Cell adhesion and spreading were assessed by measuring the density of the vital-stained cells (cells/cm^2) and the mean area of sample surface covered by cells (% of Ti) using a photo editing software (ImageJ, v1.8.0, National Institutes of Health, Bethesda, MD, USA).

2.5. *Statistical Analysis*

SPSS Version 21 (SPSS INC, Chicago, IL, USA) was used for analyzing the data. Shapiro–Wilk and Levene tests were applied to assess the assumptions of data normal distribution and homogeneity of variances. The results of the mechanical properties of each parameter were tested using the Student's *t*-test of unpaired data with equal variance. One-way analysis of variance (ANOVA) was used for the cell density, and cell adhesion and spreading followed by Tukey post-hoc test ($\alpha = 0.05$). The contact angle and roughness data were analyzed by Kruskal–Wallis analysis ($\alpha = 0.05$) for the disobedience of the data normality or homogeneity of variances.

3. Results

3.1. Mechanical Properties

Table 3 shows the results of mechanical tests for the FDM-printed PEEK and CFR-PEEK samples. From Table 3, it is observed that the PEEK samples with reinforced carbon fiber had significantly better strengths than the bare PEEK in the tensile and bending tests ($p < 0.05$). As for the compressive test, there was no statistical difference between the two materials in compressive strength.

Table 3. Mechanical properties (means ± standard deviation) of PEEK and CFR-PEEK.

Groups	Tensile Strength (MPa)	Tensile Modulus (GPa)	Bending Strength (MPa)	Bending Modulus (GPa)	Compressive Strength (MPa)	Compressive Modulus (GPa)
PEEK	95.21 ± 1.86 [a]	3.79 ± 0.27 [a]	140.83 ± 1.97 [a]	3.56 ± 0.13 [a]	138.63 ± 2.69 [a]	2.79 ± 0.11 [a]
CFR-PEEK	101.41 ± 4.23 [b]	7.37 ± 1.22 [b]	159.25 ± 13.54 [b]	5.41 ± 0.51 [b]	137.11 ± 3.43 [a]	3.51 ± 2.12 [b]

Different lowercase letters in the same column indicate significantly different groups ($p < 0.05$).

3.2. Surface Characterization

To understand how topological factors affect cell adhesion and spreading, the surface morphology of PEEK and CFR-PEEK composite was determined using SEM. Figure 3 presents the SEM images of untreated, polished, and sandblasted PEEK and CFR-PEEK samples. Printing borders, as shown in Figure 3a,d were formed on the surface due to the deposition between two printing lines. The clear peaks and valleys, which completely disappeared after polishing and sandblasting, could be identified on both untreated PEEK and CFR-PEEK sample surfaces. The polished surfaces displayed the smoothest morphology, although a few defects remained on the polished CFR-PEEK surfaces (Figure 3b,e). The surfaces of specimens, however, after sandblasting treatment possessed surface topography features in the micrometer scale with a homogeneous distribution of protuberances and cavities (Figure 3c,f).

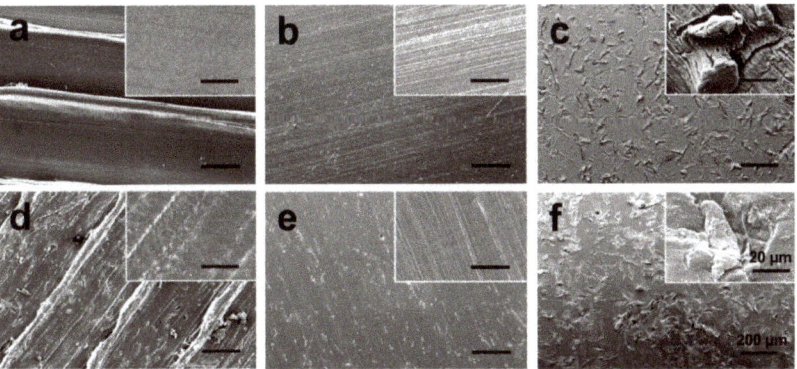

Figure 3. SEM images of PEEK and CFR-PEEK composite: (**a**) untreated PEEK; (**b**) polished PEEK; (**c**) sandblasted PEEK; (**d**) untreated CFR-PEEK; (**e**) polished CFR-PEEK; (**f**) sandblasted CFR-PEEK. Bars represent 200 μm and 20 μm (inserts), respectively.

Figure 4 illustrates the roughness of specimens of different groups. It is obvious that the untreated specimens displayed the roughest surfaces, both for PEEK and CFR-PEEK materials with the Sa value of 17.67 ± 5.7 µm and 32.36 ± 17.02 µm, which were significantly higher than the values of the polished and sandblasted groups ($p < 0.05$). The Sa values of sandblasted PEEK (0.85 ± 0.14 µm) and CFR-PEEK (0.97 ± 0.26 µm) samples were slightly higher than those of the polished surfaces (0.42 ± 0.26 µm and 0.67 ± 0.42 µm). In contrast, the polished Ti samples showed a very smooth surface (0.2 ± 0.04 µm), which was more homogenous compared with that of the polished PEEK and CFR-PEEK samples. The same trend could also be seen in the Sq data.

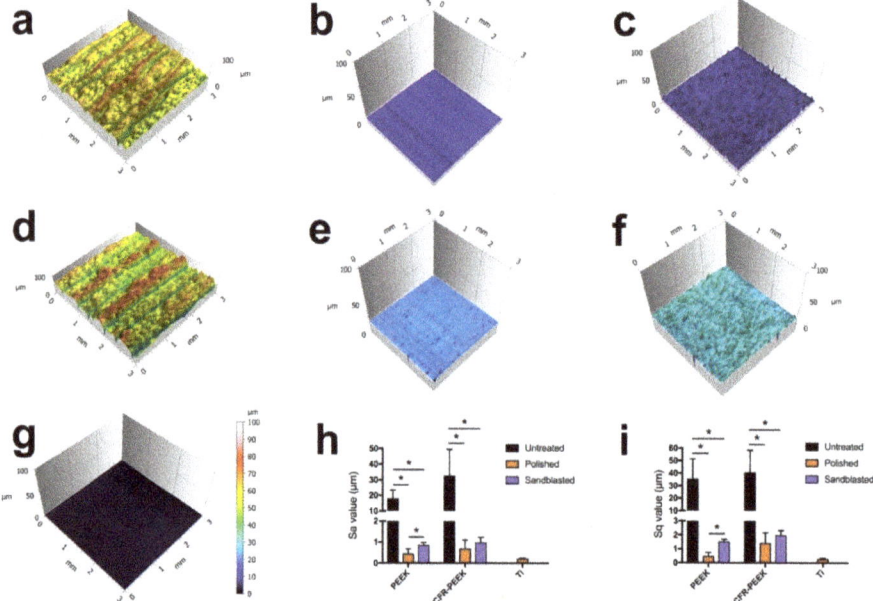

Figure 4. Reconstructed three-dimensional (3D) surface topographies of analyzed samples, and Sa and Sq values: (**a**) untreated PEEK; (**b**) polished PEEK; (**c**) sandblasted PEEK; (**d**) untreated CFR-PEEK; (**e**) polished CFR-PEEK; (**f**) sandblasted CFR-PEEK; (**g**) polished Ti; (**h**,**i**) Sa and Sq values of as-printed, polished, and sandblasted PEEK and CFR-PEEK samples, the polished Ti was used as an additional reference. The data are presented as means ± standard deviation, * $p < 0.05$.

The result of contact angle analysis is shown in Figure 5. Data revealed that the untreated surfaces of pure PEEK reflected an obvious hydrophobic response to water with a mean contact angle of 105 ± 26°. The polished PEEK specimens exhibited a hydrophilic behavior (78 ± 3°). After sandblasting, the contact angle rose slightly (88 ± 7°), but the difference was not significant ($p > 0.05$). As for the CFR-PEEK samples, the untreated group also indicated the most hydrophobic sample surface (92 ± 12°) compared with polished (82 ± 5°) and sandblasted (75 ± 3°) specimens. Both PEEK and CFR-PEEK samples, whether with or without surface modifications, revealed a more hydrophobic response to water compared to Ti (51 ± 5°).

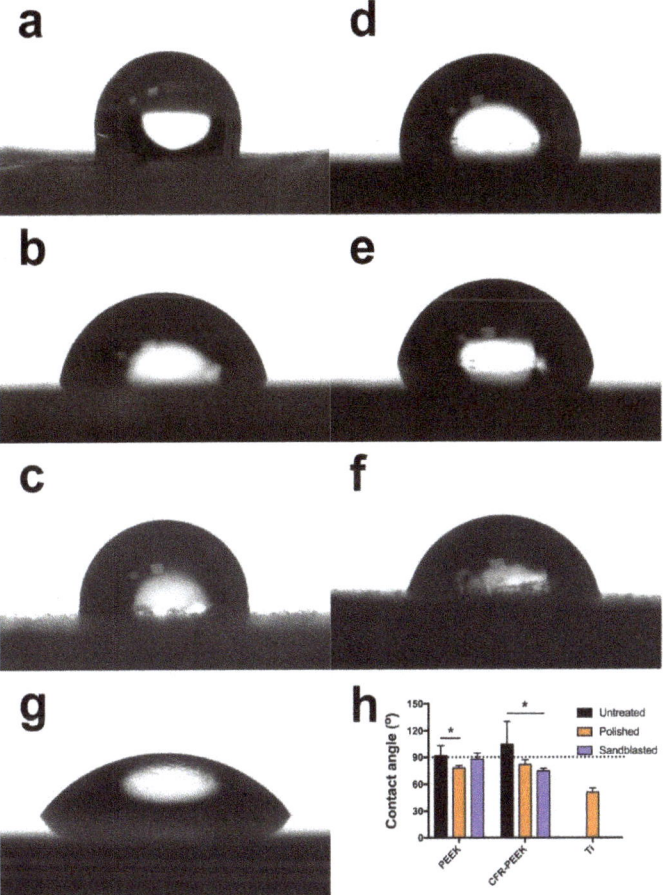

Figure 5. Water contact angle measured on untreated, polished, and sandblasted PEEK and CFR-PEEK samples: (**a**) untreated PEEK; (**b**) polished PEEK; (**c**) sandblasted PEEK; (**d**) untreated CFR-PEEK; (**e**) polished CFR-PEEK; (**f**) sandblasted CFR-PEEK. (**g**) Ti (additional reference); (**h**) quantitative contact angle values (means ± standard deviation). The dotted line indicates the contact angle of 90°, which is the division of hydrophilicity and hydrophobicity, * $p < 0.05$.

3.3. Cytotoxicity

Cell metabolic activity is expressed as a percentage of the mean OD value of cells cultured with extracts of the negative control (Ti), as displayed in Figure 6i,j. The data showed high cell viability in the cultures treated with 1:1, 1:3, and 1:10 extract concentrations of both tested materials, PEEK and CFR-PEEK, independent of the respective surface treatment (PEEK: untreated: 98 ± 23%, 106 ± 17%, 97 ± 22%; polished: 105 ± 25%, 106 ± 16%, 102 ± 15%; sandblasted: 106 ± 33%, 114 ± 27%, 98 ± 37%; CFR-PEEK: untreated: 98 ± 20%, 100 ± 28%, 97 ± 23%; polished: 102 ± 27%, 97 ± 31%, 105 ± 25%; sandblasted: 99 ± 38%, 100 ± 33%, 96 ± 23%). All extracts of PEEK and CFR-PEEK samples showed no toxicity after 24 h incubation. Cell viability in all cultures was significantly above the 70% level regarded as toxicity threshold according to ISO 10993-5 [32]. The results were confirmed by morphology analysis as seen in Figure 6a–h. Cells in the 100% extracts of the PEEK and CFR-PEEK groups exhibited a similar appearance as the negative control (Ti) group with distinct fibroblastic profiles. On the contrary, a large number of dead cells appeared in the positive group with a cell survival rate of 1 ± 2%.

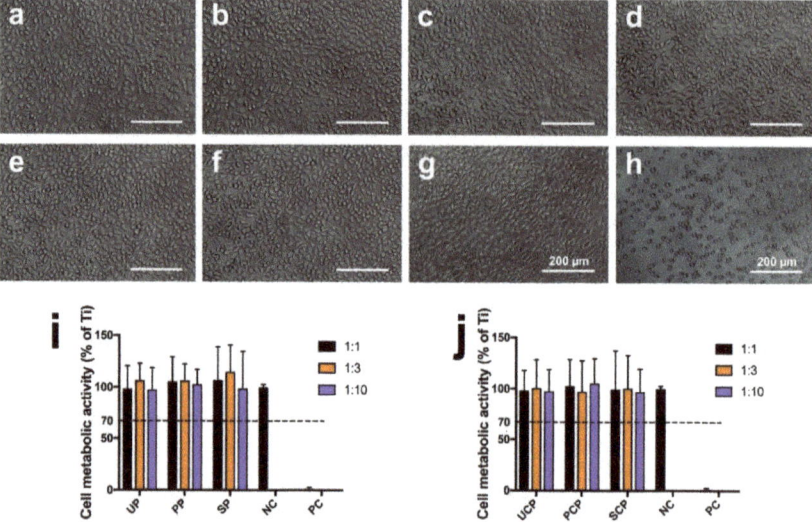

Figure 6. Cytotoxicity tests of L929 cells of PEEK and CFR-PEEK 100% extracts: (a) untreated PEEK; (b) polished PEEK; (c) sandblasted PEEK; (d) untreated CFR-PEEK; (e) polished CFR-PEEK; (f) sandblasted CFR-PEEK; (g) negative control (Ti); (h) positive control (Cu). (i,j) shows the quantitative result of the CCK-8 test in the culture media with different extract concentrations of PEEK and CFR-PEEK. The data are presented as means ± standard deviation. UP: untreated PEEK; PP: polished PEEK; SP: sandblasted PEEK; NC: negative control; PC: positive control; UCP: untreated CFR-PEEK; PCP: polished CFR-PEEK; SCP: sandblasted CFR-PEEK. The dotted line indicates the toxicity threshold of 70% cell viability according to ISO 10993-5.

3.4. Cell Adhesion and Spreading

Cell viability, attachment, and spreading were examined through a LIVE/DEAD staining assay, as shown in Figure 7. Compared with polished and sandblasted samples, untreated samples indicated more attached cells on the surfaces, both for PEEK and CFR-PEEK materials (Figure 7a–f). In addition, many cells attached in lines in the valleys resulting from the FDM manufacturing process (Figure 7a,d). Figure 7h,i reveals the quantitative cell density and quantification of the mean surface area covered by cells. Cell density on the sample surfaces of untreated PEEK and CFR-PEEK was significantly higher than on the corresponding polished and sandblasted groups ($p < 0.05$), where density was close to the Ti group. Moreover, the untreated groups showed higher cell coverage compared to the modified surfaces. The polished groups showed the lowest cell attachment for PEEK as well as CFR-PEEK samples.

Figure 8 shows the attached L929 cells around PEEK (Figure 8a–c), CFR-PEEK (Figure 8d–f), and Ti (Figure 8g) samples of the direct contact test after culturing for 24 h. The cells on PEEK and CFR-PEEK samples showed fibroblastic features and distinct profiles unaffected by the different materials and surface modifications. Moreover, the cell number was also similar to the negative control (Ti), which confirmed that the PEEK and CFR-PEEK materials were not toxic.

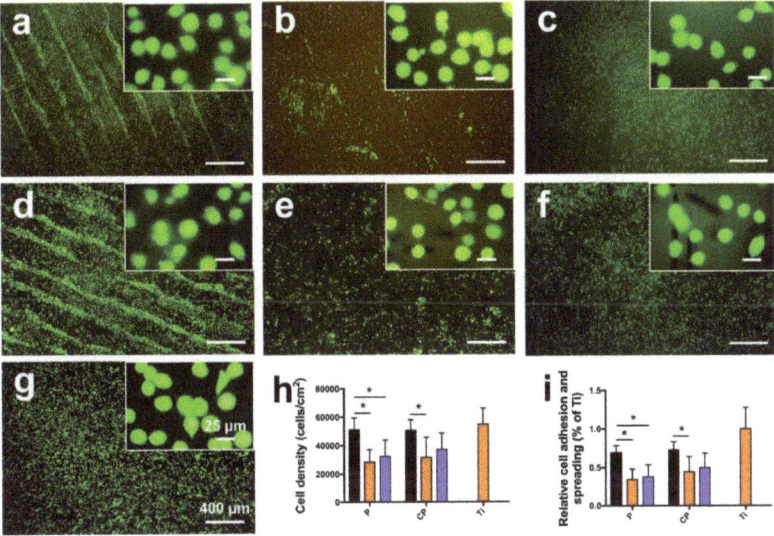

Figure 7. LIVE/DEAD staining of L929 cells on PEEK and CFR-PEEK samples after culturing for 24 h, with Ti as an additional control. (**a**) untreated PEEK; (**b**) polished PEEK; (**c**) sandblasted PEEK; (**d**) untreated CFR-PEEK; (**e**) polished CFR-PEEK; (**f**) sandblasted CFR-PEEK; (**g**) Ti. (**h**,**i**) shows the quantitative cell density and quantification of the mean surface area covered by cells. The data are presented as means ± standard deviation, * $p < 0.05$. P: PEEK; CP: CFR-PEEK; black bar: untreated group; orange bar: polished group; blue bar: sandblasted group. Cytotoxic effects, indicated by dead (red stained) cells, are not detectable.

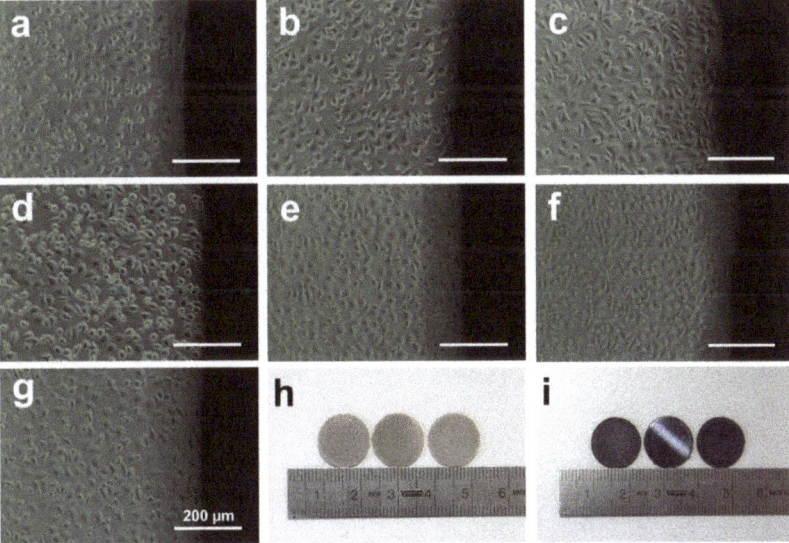

Figure 8. Microscopic images of L929 cells observed around samples of direct contact test after culturing for 24 h. (**a**) untreated PEEK; (**b**) polished PEEK; (**c**) sandblasted PEEK; (**d**) untreated CFR-PEEK; (**e**) polished CFR-PEEK; (**f**) sandblasted CFR-PEEK; (**g**) Ti; (**h**) PEEK samples (untreated, polished, and sandblasted); (**i**) CFR-PEEK samples (untreated, polished, and sandblasted).

4. Discussion

This study aimed to investigate the mechanical properties of FDM-printed PEEK composite, the influence of manufacturing on the materials' cytotoxicity, and the impact of surface topography and wettability on cell adhesion. To the best of our knowledge, there is currently no literature on these topics, whereas the manufacturing parameters and mechanical properties of FDM-processed bare PEEK and the SLS-printed PEEK composite have already been published elsewhere [18,21,33–35]. According to the manufacturing principles of FDM, only thermoplastic filaments can be used, like PLA, ABS, and PEEK [33]. However, it is a great challenge to fabricate ideal-performance PEEK objects through FDM equipment due to its high melting temperature (above 300 °C), high melting expansion, and especially the semicrystalline property, in particular for PEEK composites [22,34]. In this study, FDM-printed CFR-PEEK composite was successfully fabricated, and the mechanical properties were first measured. Moreover, the influence of the surface topography and roughness on biocompatibility and cell adhesion of FDM-printed PEEK and CFR-PEEK was also estimated for the first time.

The mechanical results indicated that the pure PEEK showed low strength in tensile, bending, and compressive tests. However, the addition of 5% carbon fiber into the PEEK matrix improved the mechanical strengths (Table 3), showing values similar to those of human cortical bone (elastic modulus: 14 GPa) [8] Normally, the mechanical properties of additively manufactured PEEK were obviously lower than the traditionally produced parts (i.e., injection molding) [21]. Although some studies have been done on PEEK composites by adding reinforcement fillers using SLS technology, the mechanical properties of FDM-printed PEEK composites were still insufficient, compared with their cast counterparts as a bone replacement material for severe cranio-maxillofacial defects [34,35]. The manufacturing conditions of the FDM process, such as layer thickness, printing speed, ambient temperature, nozzle temperature, and heat treatment, can produce a significant impact on the mechanical properties of PEEK samples [21,22]. In this study, the tensile strength of bare PEEK was 95.21 ± 1.86 MPa with an elastic modulus of 3.79 ± 0.27 GPa, which was comparable to the injection-molded pure PEEK (100 MPa and 4 GPa) [21]. While the tensile strength and elastic modulus of CFR-PEEK composites reached 101.41 ± 4.23 MPa and 7.37 ± 1.22 GPa, which were much higher than the injection-molded pure PEEK, the similar trend could also be seen in the bending and compressive tests. This result indicates that the printing conditions used in this study were suitable for PEEK and CFR-PEEK manufacturing. Deng et al. and Wu et al. have measured the mechanical properties of FDM-printed pure PEEK and found that the mechanical strength of printed PEEK samples was significantly lower than the traditionally produced objects, whereas in this study the values were quite similar [18,21]. One proper explanation for the excellent mechanical properties in this research is the application of post heat treatment (tempering). Theoretically, heat treatment methods can increase the degree of crystallinity and relieve the residual stress and shrinkage distortion, which will increase the mechanical performance of PEEK parts [22]. Therefore, the mechanical strengths of PEEK composite could be tailored by carbon fibers to mimic human cortical bone, thus avoiding stress shielding [8].

Polishing and sandblasting are common surface processing methods in dentistry to get a smooth or rough surface. However, the FDM-printed sample surfaces were much rougher compared with sandblasted ones, as shown in Figures 3 and 4. This finding can be related to the working principle of FDM. Thermoplastic materials are extruded by the printing nozzle, which can move across the building platform in x- and y-axes, to generate a 2D layer line by line. Then, a 3D object is built up by melting the successive 2D layers together. The crosswise oriented, threadlike inner structure of the specimen results in some unfilled areas between lines and layers, and also in the original printing structures on sample surfaces [36]. In this study, the sandblasted samples showed slightly rougher surfaces than the polished ones. Compared with some previous studies, the sandblasting parameters (i.e., distance and pressure) in this research had to be set lower in order not to perforate the layer-by-layer manufacturing pattern [26,27,37]. In other studies, using traditional methods to fabricate PEEK and its composite samples like injection molding or milling, the interior of the blocks was homogenous without layers or unfilled areas. The samples in this study were produced using FDM technology, laying down objects in layers with a thickness of 0.2 mm. If a higher sandblasting pressure or closer distance were applied to modify the sample, the upper surface layer would be exfoliated (Figure 9). Therefore, based on the parameters used for sandblasting in this study, the sandblasted sample surfaces were slightly rougher than the polished ones, but not obviously different.

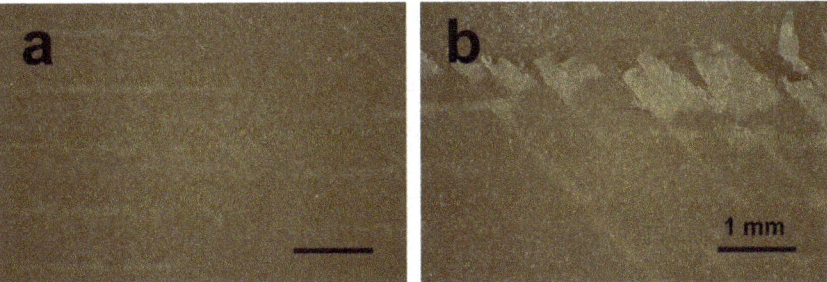

Figure 9. Optical micrographs of sandblasted PEEK samples (**a**) under 0.1 MPa pressure; (**b**) under 0.5 MPa pressure.

It is recognized that the surface wettability of biomaterials is important for their bioactivities, such as cell adhesion and spreading [38]. Therefore, the hydrophilicity of the samples was evaluated by the static sessile drop method, and the results are shown in Figure 5. Both PEEK and CFR-PEEK materials, before surface modification, represented a hydrophobic response to water (contact angle between 90–110°), which is typical for PEEK materials [8,39]. After polishing and sandblasting, both samples exhibited slightly hydrophilic behavior with contact angles below 90°. Commonly, wettability is closely related to the surface topography and chemical composition of a material [39]. The higher water contact angle in the untreated group in this study could be explained by the printing structures produced by FDM (Figures 3 and 4). On highly roughened surfaces, the peaks and valleys prevent the water droplet from spreading on the surface, which can result in increased contact angles since the peaks and valleys on the sample surfaces constitute "geometrical barriers" for the droplet spreading [37,40]. According to the study undertaken by Ourahmoune et al., the surface morphology strongly influences the hydrophilic behavior of PEEK and its composites [37]. For the polished and sandblasted samples, since the differences of roughness values between these two groups were not obvious, the water contact angles were similar.

Due to its chemical inertness, PEEK provides inherent good biocompatibility, and this is also one of its advantages that favors its clinical use [8]. However, for the FDM-printed PEEK using a relatively new technology to fabricate PEEK using AM, studies focusing on the possible introduction of toxic substances during the printing process are still lacking, especially for its composites. According to ISO 10993-5, a reduction of cell viability by more than 30% indicates a cytotoxic effect [32]. In this study (Figure 6), the cell metabolic test of PEEK and CFR-PEEK samples showed that more than 96% of cells survived in all sample groups tested, independent of the respective surface modification. This result was comparable to the negative control group (Ti). The cytotoxicity results indicated that there were no toxic effects generated by the printing process. Moreover, after surface treatment, some carbon fibers were exposed on the surface of CFR-PEEK samples. However, this exposure has not led to increased cytotoxicity. Zhao et al. investigated FDM-printed pure PEEK and obtained a similar result that no toxic substances were introduced during the printing process [17].

Cell adhesion and spreading are closely related to surface properties, that is, composition, roughness, morphology, and wettability [41]. In addition to chemical composition, surface roughness and morphology play a critical role in the biological responses of biomaterial surfaces. In this study, the untreated PEEK and CFR-PEEK sample surfaces exhibited significantly more cell attachment than the polished and sandblasted samples, where the attachment level was close to the Ti surfaces. The as-printed PEEK and CFR-PEEK showed a higher cell density which might be due to the special 3D-printed structures. As shown in Figure 3a,d and Figure 4a,d, the clear ridges and valleys on the surfaces could be identified on both PEEK and CFR-PEEK sample surfaces. These special printing structures could enlarge the surface area significantly compared with polished and sandblasted surfaces. Significantly more spaces are available for cells to attach and spread on this geometrical morphology. For many engineering applications, a post-printing process is always needed to eliminate the manufactured structures [39]. However, to improve the cell attachment and spreading, a rough surface as generated by FDM seems beneficial, which could not be achieved by sandblasting. It was obvious that the cells accumulated in the surface grooves resulting from the manufacturing process (Figure 7a,d). Figure 4a,d showed the reconstructed 3D surface topographies of the as-printed PEEK and CFR-PEEK samples. The cells could slide into the valleys on the sample surfaces and attach there. As for both the polished and sandblasted surfaces, the originally printed surface structures were removed and the surfaces showed a lower cell density, but the cells appeared more homogeneously attached. After polishing and sandblasting, the exposure of carbon fibers on the surface of CFR-PEEK samples did not improve the cell attachment significantly. This finding confirmed that reinforced carbon fibers could improve the mechanical properties of FDM-printed PEEK, but would not influence the cytotoxicity and cell adhesion. In this study, the biological response of FDM-printed PEEK was investigated at a basic level, including cytotoxicity and cell adhesion. In future studies, more biological tests (e.g., in vitro cell metabolic activity, proliferation, and in vivo osseointegration) should be applied to evaluate bioactivities.

To sum up, the results indicate that the FDM-printed CFR-PEEK has excellent mechanical properties compared with the printed bare PEEK. In addition, no toxic substances were introduced during the FDM printing process. FDM technology can yield a highly roughened surface suitable for cells to attach.

5. Conclusions

In this study, the mechanical properties of FDM-printed, carbon fiber reinforced PEEK composite were systematically studied for the first time, including tensile, bending, and compressive tests. The experimental results confirmed that samples printed from pure PEEK material showed mechanical properties comparable to traditionally manufactured PEEK objects, obtained by extrusion techniques for example. On the contrary, the printed CFR-PEEK specimen represented significantly improved mechanical properties compared to printed pure PEEK. FDM technology could be used to provide more satisfactory mechanical strength of PEEK and its composites. Therefore, it is an appropriate method for matching the mechanical properties of PEEK composites with carbon fibers to mimic human cortical bone and avoid stress shielding in clinical applications, like dental implants, skull implants, osteosynthesis plates, and bone replacement material for nasal, maxillary, or mandibular reconstructions.

Additionally, the impact of the surface topography and roughness of FDM-printed PEEK and its composites on biocompatibility and cell adhesion was also estimated for the first time. Laboratory experiments here clearly showed that no toxic substances were introduced during the FDM manufacturing process of pure PEEK and CFR-PEEK. Surface treatments leading to partial exposure of the fiber compound in the bulk material did not lead to increased cytotoxicity. FDM-manufactured surfaces had highly rough topographies, which could not be achieved by typical dental sandblasting processes. This structure was more suitable for cells to attach and spread compared with polished and sandblasted surfaces, resulting in a cell density comparable to that on Ti sample surfaces. Although tests carried out in this study are limited, it is expected that the CFR-PEEK composite with its enhanced mechanical properties has great potential to be used as an orthopedic or dental implant material in bone repair, regeneration, and tissue engineering applications.

Author Contributions: Conceptualization, S.S., L.S., and F.R.; Formal analysis, X.H.; Methodology, X.H., D.Y., C.Y., and P.L.; Project administration, D.L. and J.G.-G.; Writing—original draft, X.H.; Writing—review and editing, X.H., S.S., L.S., J.G.-G., and F.R.

Funding: This research was supported by the National Natural Science Foundation of China (No. 51835010). The China Scholarship Council (CSC) is gratefully acknowledged for the financial support of Xingting Han (Grant 201606280045) and Ping Li (Grant 201608440274).

Acknowledgments: The authors would like to thank Ernst Schweizer for his assistance in the SEM analysis.

Conflicts of Interest: The authors declare no conflict of interest.

References

1. Ren, Z.H.; Wu, H.J.; Tan, H.Y.; Wang, K.; Zhang, S. Transfer of anterolateral thigh flaps in elderly oral cancer patients: Complications in oral and maxillofacial reconstruction. *J. Oral Maxillofac. Surg.* **2015**, *73*, 534–540. [CrossRef] [PubMed]
2. Rohner, D.; Guijarro-Martínez, R.; Bucher, P.; Hammer, B. Importance of patient-specific intraoperative guides in complex maxillofacial reconstruction. *J. Cranio-Maxillofac. Surg.* **2013**, *41*, 382–390. [CrossRef] [PubMed]
3. Bauer, T.W.; Muschler, G.F. Bone Graft Materials: An Overview of the Basic Science. *Clin. Orthop. Relat. Res.* **2000**, *371*, 10–27. [CrossRef]
4. Hallman, M.; Thor, A. Bone substitutes and growth factors as an alternative/complement to autogenous bone for grafting in implant dentistry. *Periodontol. 2000* **2008**, *47*, 172–192. [CrossRef] [PubMed]
5. Zhao, Y.; Wong, S.M.; Wong, H.M.; Wu, S.; Hu, T.; Yeung, K.W.K.; Chu, P.K. Effects of Carbon and Nitrogen Plasma Immersion Ion Implantation on In vitro and In vivo Biocompatibility of Titanium Alloy. *ACS Appl. Mater. Interfaces* **2013**, *5*, 1510–1516. [CrossRef] [PubMed]
6. Bougherara, H.; Bureau, M.N.; Yahia, L. Bone remodeling in a new biomimetic polymer-composite hip stem. *J. Biomed. Mater. Res. Part A* **2010**, *92*, 164–174. [CrossRef]
7. Wang, H.; Lu, T.; Meng, F.; Zhu, H.; Liu, X. Enhanced osteoblast responses to poly ether ether ketone surface modified by water plasma immersion ion implantation. *Colloids Surf. B Biointerfaces* **2014**, *117*, 89–97. [CrossRef]
8. Najeeb, S.; Zafar, M.S.; Khurshid, Z.; Siddiqui, F. Applications of polyetheretherketone (PEEK) in oral implantology and prosthodontics. *J. Prosthodont. Res.* **2016**, *60*, 12–19. [CrossRef]
9. Panayotov, I.V.; Orti, V.; Cuisinier, F.; Yachouh, J. Polyetheretherketone (PEEK) for medical applications. *J. Mater. Sci. Mater. Med.* **2016**, *27*, 118. [CrossRef]
10. Schwitalla, A.; Müller, W.-D. PEEK Dental Implants: A Review of the Literature. *J. Oral Implantol.* **2013**, *39*, 743–749. [CrossRef]
11. Trindade, R.; Albrektsson, T.; Galli, S.; Prgomet, Z.; Tengvall, P.; Wennerberg, A. Bone Immune Response to Materials, Part I: Titanium, PEEK and Copper in Comparison to Sham at 10 Days in Rabbit Tibia. *J. Clin. Med.* **2018**, *7*, 526. [CrossRef] [PubMed]
12. Sandler, J.; Werner, P.; Shaffer, M.S.P.; Demchuk, V.; Altstädt, V.; Windle, A.H. Carbon-nanofibre-reinforced poly (ether ether ketone) composites. *Compos. Part A Appl. Sci. Manuf.* **2002**, *33*, 1033–1039. [CrossRef]
13. Devine, D.M.; Hahn, J.; Richards, R.G.; Gruner, H.; Wieling, R.; Pearce, S.G. Coating of carbon fiber-reinforced polyetheretherketone implants with titanium to improve bone apposition. *J. Biomed. Mater. Res. Part B Appl. Biomater.* **2013**, *101*, 591–598. [CrossRef] [PubMed]
14. Lu, T.; Liu, X.; Qian, S.; Cao, H.; Qiao, Y.; Mei, Y.; Chu, P.K.; Ding, C. Multilevel surface engineering of nanostructured TiO_2 on carbon-fiber-reinforced polyetheretherketone. *Biomaterials* **2014**, *35*, 5731–5740. [CrossRef] [PubMed]
15. Lee, W.; Koak, J.; Lim, Y.; Kim, S.; Kwon, H.; Kim, M. Stress shielding and fatigue limits of poly-ether-ether-ketone dental implants. *J. Biomed. Mater. Res. Part B Appl. Biomater.* **2012**, *100*, 1044–1052. [CrossRef] [PubMed]
16. Ventola, C.L. Medical Applications for 3D Printing: Current and Projected Uses. *Pharm. Ther.* **2014**, *39*, 704–711.
17. Zhao, F.; Li, D.; Jin, Z. Preliminary investigation of poly-ether-ether-ketone based on fused deposition modeling for medical applications. *Materials* **2018**, *11*, 288. [CrossRef]

18. Deng, X.; Zeng, Z.; Peng, B.; Yan, S.; Ke, W. Mechanical properties optimization of poly-ether-ether-ketone via fused deposition modeling. *Materials* **2018**, *11*, 216. [CrossRef]
19. Zhao, X.; Xiong, D.; Liu, Y. Improving surface wettability and lubrication of polyetheretherketone (PEEK) by combining with polyvinyl alcohol (PVA) hydrogel. *J. Mech. Behav. Biomed. Mater.* **2018**, *82*, 27–34. [CrossRef]
20. Punchak, M.; Chung, L.K.; Lagman, C.; Bui, T.T.; Lazareff, J.; Rezzadeh, K.; Jarrahy, R.; Yang, I. Outcomes following polyetheretherketone (PEEK) cranioplasty: Systematic review and meta-analysis. *J. Clin. Neurosci.* **2017**, *41*, 30–35. [CrossRef]
21. Wu, W.; Geng, P.; Li, G.; Zhao, D.; Zhang, H.; Zhao, J. Influence of layer thickness and raster angle on the mechanical properties of 3D-printed PEEK and a comparative mechanical study between PEEK and ABS. *Materials* **2015**, *8*, 5834–5846. [CrossRef] [PubMed]
22. Yang, C.; Tian, X.; Li, D.; Cao, Y.; Zhao, F.; Shi, C. Influence of thermal processing conditions in 3D printing on the crystallinity and mechanical properties of PEEK material. *J. Mater. Process. Technol.* **2017**, *248*, 1–7. [CrossRef]
23. Rabiei, A.; Sandukas, S. Processing and evaluation of bioactive coatings on polymeric implants. *J. Biomed. Mater. Res. Part A* **2013**, *101*, 2621–2629. [CrossRef] [PubMed]
24. Ma, R.; Tang, T. Current strategies to improve the bioactivity of PEEK. *Int. J. Mol. Sci.* **2014**, *15*, 5426–5445. [CrossRef] [PubMed]
25. Gittens, R.A.; Olivares-Navarrete, R.; McLachlan, T.; Cai, Y.; Hyzy, S.L.; Schneider, J.M.; Schwartz, Z.; Sandhage, K.H.; Boyan, B.D. Differential responses of osteoblast lineage cells to nanotopographically-modified, microroughened titanium–aluminum–vanadium alloy surfaces. *Biomaterials* **2012**, *33*, 8986–8994. [CrossRef] [PubMed]
26. Deng, Y.; Liu, X.; Xu, A.; Wang, L.; Luo, Z.; Zheng, Y.; Deng, F.; Wei, J.; Tang, Z.; Wei, S. Effect of surface roughness on osteogenesis in vitro and osseointegration in vivo of carbon fiber-reinforced polyetheretherketone– Nanohydroxyapatite composite. *Int. J. Nanomed.* **2015**, *10*, 1425–1447. [PubMed]
27. Elawadly, T.; Radi, I.A.W.; El Khadem, A.; Osman, R.B. Can PEEK Be an Implant Material? Evaluation of Surface Topography and Wettability of Filled Versus Unfilled PEEK With Different Surface Roughness. *J. Oral Implantol.* **2017**, *43*, 456–461. [CrossRef] [PubMed]
28. Wu, X.; Liu, X.; Wei, J.; Ma, J.; Deng, F.; Wei, S. Nano-TiO_2/PEEK bioactive composite as a bone substitute material: In vitro and in vivo studies. *Int. J. Nanomed.* **2012**, *7*, 1215.
29. *ISO 527-1: 2012 Plastics—Determination of Tensile Properties—Part 1: General Principles*; International Organization for Standardization: Geneva, Switzerland, 2012.
30. *ISO 178: 2010 Plastics—Determination of Flexural Properties*; International Organization for Standardization: Geneva, Switzerland, 2010.
31. *ISO 604: 2002 Plastics—Determination of Compressive Properties Plastiques*; International Organization for Standardization: Geneva, Switzerland, 2002.
32. *ISO 10993-5: 2009 Biological Evaluation of Medical Devices—Part 5: Tests for In Vitro Cytotoxicity*; International Organization for Standardization: Geneva, Switzerland, 2009.
33. Rinaldi, M.; Ghidini, T.; Cecchini, F.; Brandao, A.; Nanni, F. Additive layer manufacturing of poly (ether ether ketone) via FDM. *Compos. Part B Eng.* **2018**, *145*, 162–172. [CrossRef]
34. Yan, M.; Tian, X.; Peng, G.; Li, D.; Zhang, X. High temperature rheological behavior and sintering kinetics of CF/PEEK composites during selective laser sintering. *Compos. Sci. Technol.* **2018**, *165*, 140–147. [CrossRef]
35. Stepashkin, A.A.; Chukov, D.I.; Senatov, F.S.; Salimon, A.I.; Korsunsky, A.M.; Kaloshkin, S.D. 3D-printed PEEK-carbon fiber (CF) composites: Structure and thermal properties. *Compos. Sci. Technol.* **2018**, *164*, 319–326. [CrossRef]
36. Xu, Y.; Unkovskiy, A.; Klaue, F.; Rupp, F.; Geis-Gerstorfer, J.; Spintzyk, S.; Xu, Y.; Unkovskiy, A.; Klaue, F.; Rupp, F.; et al. Compatibility of a Silicone Impression/Adhesive System to FDM-Printed Tray Materials—A Laboratory Peel-off Study. *Materials* **2018**, *11*, 1905. [CrossRef] [PubMed]
37. Ourahmoune, R.; Salvia, M.; Mathia, T.G.; Mesrati, N. Surface morphology and wettability of sandblasted PEEK and its composites. *Scanning* **2014**, *36*, 64–75. [CrossRef] [PubMed]
38. Gittens, R.A.; Scheideler, L.; Rupp, F.; Hyzy, S.L.; Geis-Gerstorfer, J.; Schwartz, Z.; Boyan, B.D. A review on the wettability of dental implant surfaces II: Biological and clinical aspects. *Acta Biomater.* **2014**, *10*, 2907–2918. [CrossRef] [PubMed]

39. Al Qahtani, M.S.A.; Wu, Y.; Spintzyk, S.; Krieg, P.; Killinger, A.; Schweizer, E.; Stephan, I.; Scheideler, L.; Geis-Gerstorfer, J.; Rupp, F. UV-A and UV-C light induced hydrophilization of dental implants. *Dent. Mater.* **2015**, *31*, e157–e167. [CrossRef] [PubMed]
40. Rupp, F.; Gittens, R.A.; Scheideler, L.; Marmur, A.; Boyan, B.D.; Schwartz, Z.; Geis-Gerstorfer, J. A review on the wettability of dental implant surfaces I: Theoretical and experimental aspects. *Acta Biomater.* **2014**, *10*, 2894–2906. [CrossRef] [PubMed]
41. Zhu, X.; Chen, J.; Scheideler, L.; Reichl, R.; Geis-Gerstorfer, J. Effects of topography and composition of titanium surface oxides on osteoblast responses. *Biomaterials* **2004**, *25*, 4087–4103. [CrossRef]

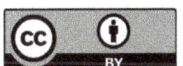

© 2019 by the authors. Licensee MDPI, Basel, Switzerland. This article is an open access article distributed under the terms and conditions of the Creative Commons Attribution (CC BY) license (http://creativecommons.org/licenses/by/4.0/).

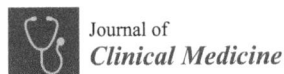

Article

Osteogenic Cell Behavior on Titanium Surfaces in Hard Tissue

Jung-Yoo Choi [1], Tomas Albrektsson [2,3], Young-Jun Jeon [1] and In-Sung Luke Yeo [4,*]

1. Dental Research Institute, Seoul National University, Seoul 03080, Korea; jychoi55@snu.ac.kr (J.-Y.C.); yoowjs@snu.ac.kr (Y.-J.J.)
2. Department of Biomaterials, Sahlgrenska Academy, University of Gothenburg, 40530 Gothenburg, Sweden; tomas.albrektsson@biomaterials.gu.se
3. Department of Prosthodontics, Faculty of Odontology, Malmö University, 21118 Malmö, Sweden
4. Department of Prosthodontics, School of Dentistry and Dental Research Institute, Seoul National University, 101 Daehak-ro, Jongro-gu, Seoul 03080, Korea
* Correspondence: pros53@snu.ac.kr; Tel.: +82-2-2072-2661; Fax: +82-2-2072-3860

Received: 12 April 2019; Accepted: 28 April 2019; Published: 2 May 2019

Abstract: It is challenging to remove dental implants once they have been inserted into the bone because it is hard to visualize the actual process of bone formation after implant installation, not to mention the cellular events that occur therein. During bone formation, contact osteogenesis occurs on roughened implant surfaces, while distance osteogenesis occurs on smooth implant surfaces. In the literature, there have been many in vitro model studies of bone formation on simulated dental implants using flattened titanium (Ti) discs; however, the purpose of this study was to identify the in vivo cell responses to the implant surfaces on actual, three-dimensional (3D) dental Ti implants and the surrounding bone in contact with such implants at the electron microscopic level using two different types of implant surfaces. In particular, the different parts of the implant structures were scrutinized. In this study, dental implants were installed in rabbit tibiae. The implants and bone were removed on day 10 and, subsequently, assessed using scanning electron microscopy (SEM), immunofluorescence microscopy (IF), transmission electron microscopy (TEM), focused ion-beam (FIB) system with Cs-corrected TEM (Cs-STEM), and confocal laser scanning microscopy (CLSM)—which were used to determine the implant surface characteristics and to identify the cells according to the different structural parts of the turned and roughened implants. The cell attachment pattern was revealed according to the different structural components of each implant surface and bone. Different cell responses to the implant surfaces and the surrounding bone were attained at an electron microscopic level in an in vivo model. These results shed light on cell behavioral patterns that occur during bone regeneration and could be a guide in the use of electron microscopy for 3D dental implants in an in vivo model.

Keywords: osteogenesis; cell plasticity; dental implants; electron microscopy; scanning transmission electron microscopy; bone-implant interface

1. Introduction

Dental implants are cylindrical prosthetics with screw threads, usually made of titanium (Ti), which are used to replace missing teeth and to support the mastication function of artificial teeth. However, the biological contact with the surface of dental implants is different from that with natural teeth. Osseointegration, the direct contact between bone and implant, is viewed as a hard tissue encapsulation, a foreign body immune reaction that isolates the implant; this bone response is generally accepted as a bio-affinitive reaction to a biocompatible material [1]. To enhance the activity of osteogenic cells in bone integration, the physical and chemical characteristics of the implant surface—including the surface energy, wettability, and topography—are modified, because direct enhancement of the bone surface is much more difficult [2–11]. Such surface treatments can be, in reality, an enhancement to encase the foreign body in hard connective tissue [1,12,13]. Therefore, it is necessary to investigate the in vivo biological response to implant surfaces at the cellular level.

To control the variables, and thereby produce a sound scientific result, in vitro studies using purified cell lines and flat Ti discs with modified surfaces can be performed. However, promising in vitro results in cell responses to such Ti discs do not guarantee obtainment of the desired reactions for Ti implants with the same modified surfaces in in vivo environments. The Ti implants used today to treat patients are screw-shaped, rather than flat disc-shaped. Screw threads have macro- and microstructures—such as roots, flanks, and crests—which the homogeneous Ti disc surfaces for the in vitro experiments are unable to simulate [14]. The cell lines for in vitro tests are usually osteoblast-like cells, rather than human osteogenic cells, and the in vivo environment is very different from an in vitro cell culture medium [5,8,15]. Nonetheless, osteoblastic cell lines in in vitro tests form a simplified system which does not take into account aspects such as immune responses [16]. Therefore, translational evidence is required to create a bridge between the in vitro cell results and the in vivo tissue results—that is, the cellular response to a Ti implant surface in the in vivo environment.

This study aimed to observe Ti implants and the surrounding bone in contact with such implants at the electron microscopic level to identify the in vivo cell responses to the implant surfaces

2. Materials and Methods

2.1. In Vivo Study

This study was approved by the Ethics Committee of the Animal Experimentation of the Institutional Animal Care and Use Committee (CRONEX-IACUC 201702003; Cronex, Hwasung, Korea). All experiments were conducted in accordance with the ARRIVE guidelines for reporting in vivo animal experiments [17]. A total of 8 male New Zealand white rabbits (age: 1–2 years; body weight: 2.6–3.0 kg) with no signs of disease were used. The rabbits were anaesthetized via intramuscular injection of tiletamine/zolazepam (15 mg/kg; Zoletil 50, Virbac Korea Co., Ltd., Seoul, Korea) and xylazine (5 mg/kg; Rompun, Bayer Korea Ltd., Seoul, Korea). Before surgery, the skin over the area of the proximal tibia was shaved and washed with betadine, and an antibiotic (Cefazolin, Yuhan Co., Seoul, Korea) was intramuscularly administered. Lidocaine was locally injected into each surgical site. The skin was incised, and the tibiae were exposed after muscle dissection and periosteal elevation. Drills and profuse sterile saline irrigation were used to prepare the implant sites on the flat tibial surface. The drilling was performed with a final diameter of 4.0 mm at the upper cortical bone, in which the implants were installed in cortical bone and medullary space. Only the V-shaped parts of the threads were engaged (Figure 1A). A total of 5 rabbits received acid-etched (SLA) implants only. Each rabbit received 4 SLA implants, 2 on each side of the rabbit tibia. Three rabbits received turned implants only, each receiving 4 turned implants, 2 on each side of the tibia. The cover screw was covered. The muscle and fascia were sutured with absorbable 4–0 Vicryl sutures, and the outer dermis was closed with a nylon suture. The rabbits were separately housed after surgery. All rabbits were sacrificed via an intravenous overdose of potassium chloride after 10 days of bone healing. After 10 days [1,18,19], the tibiae were exposed, all of the inserted implants were removed through unscrewing, and the surrounding bone was surgically removed en bloc with an adjacent bone collar and immediately placed in Karnovsky's solution for cell fixation in falcon tubes, while the specimens for fluorescence immunocytochemistry were preserved in Roswell Park Memorial Institute (RPMI) media and fetal bovine serum (Gibco, Thermo Fisher Scientific, Waltham, MA, USA) in cell culture dish.

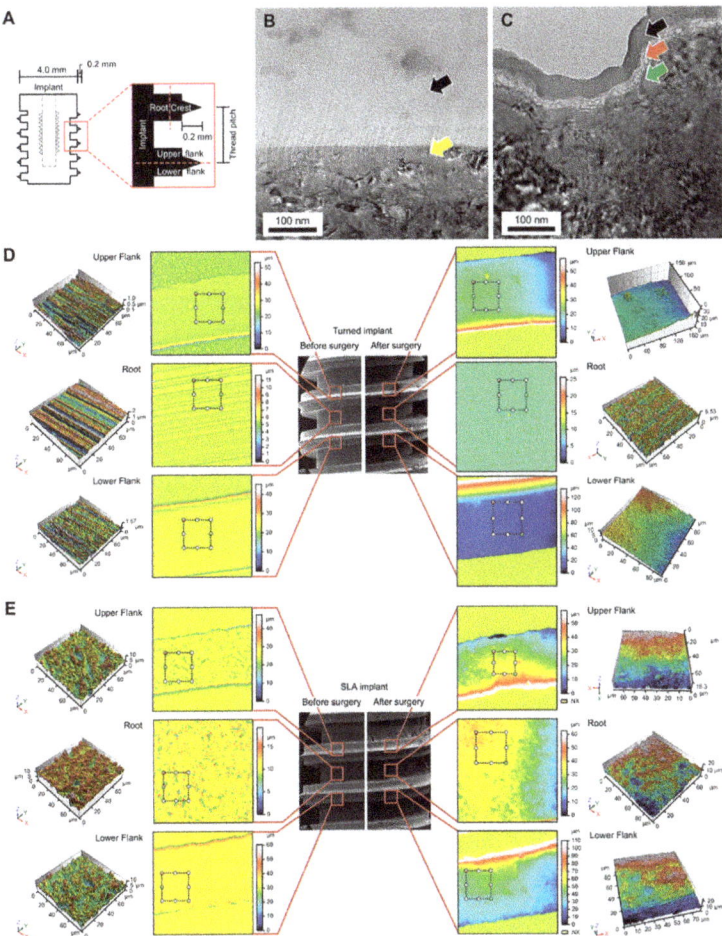

Figure 1. (**A**) Simplified diagram of, and terminology regarding, the screw-shaped implants used in this study. The inner half, close to the minor diameter of the implant, was defined as the root area. The outer half, close to the major diameter of the implant, was called the crest area. The upper half of the thread was defined as the upper flank (UF), and the lower half was the lower flank (LF). (**B**) Cs-corrected transmission electron microscopy (Cs-STEM) analysis retrieved from focused ion beam specimens of the turned and (**C**) acid-etched (SLA) implants on day 10. There were no cells detected on the turned surface (yellow arrow) beneath the Pt-coated layer (black arrow), whereas, cells were detected on SLA surface (red arrow). (**D**) Confocal laser scanning microscopy (CLSM) of the turned and (**E**) SLA surfaces measured in root, UF, and LF. The turned implant revealed a smooth texture, and no cells were seen after in vivo experiment. The SLA implants displayed cell attachment in the root area, depicted as irregular structure of grey color on top of roughened topography in the 3D mapping of the CLSM.

2.2. Sample Preparation and Implant Surface Modification

Herein, 26 Ti sandblasted, large-grit, and SLA implants and 18 turned implants were used (Deep Implant System, Inc., Seongnam, Korea). The implants were made of grade 4 commercially pure Ti by computer numerical control (CNC) machining. The implant surface was called 'turned' when the surface had no further modification after CNC machining. The SLA surface was made by sandblasting the implant surface with 250–500 μm alumina particles and by etching the surface with HCl/H_2SO_4

acid mixture. All of the implants were 4.0 mm in diameter and 5.0 mm in length. A total of 20 SLA implants were used in an in vivo study, and 6 were used in the surface analysis, while 12 turned implants were used in the in vivo analysis, and 6 were used in the surface analysis.

2.3. Surface Characteristics

Among the 6 SLA implants and 6 turned implants used in the surface analysis, 2 of each type of implant were used for scanning electron microscopy (SEM; Hitachi S-4700, Hitachi, Tokyo, Japan), 2 were used for confocal laser scanning microscopy (CLSM; LSM 800, Carl Zeiss AG, Oberkochen, Germany), and the remaining 2 implants were used for focused ion beam (FIB; Helios 650, FEI, Hillsboro, OR, USA) and Cs-corrected transmission electron microscopy (Cs-STEM; JEM-ARM200F, Cold FEG, FEOL Ltd., Tokyo, Japan), which are capable of producing transmission electron microscopy (TEM) images directly from an undecalcified specimen. SEM was used to observe the topographical features, while CLSM was used to analyze the surface roughness levels. The measured area roughness parameters included the average height deviation value (S_a) and the developed surface area ratio (S_{dr}). FIB and Cs-STEM were used to observe the undecalcified implant surface directly without any resin embedding.

2.4. Scanning Electron Microscopy (SEM) Analysis

The retrieved implant specimens and surrounding bony specimens were fixed with Karnovsky's solution and washed in 0.1 M phosphate buffer saline (PBS) 3 times every 15 min. The specimens were dehydrated through a graded 70–100% ethanol series and then treated with hexamethyldisilazane for 15 min. The surrounding bone specimens were cut in half around the round hole in which the implant had been inserted, after degradation with 80% ethanol using rotary discs within an appropriate amount of time. Prior to the SEM analysis, the implant and bone specimens were sputter coated with a thin film of platinum to protect the implant and bony surfaces. All specimens were handled with Ti forceps and surgical gloves in a clean laboratory environment. Each implant and bone sample was attached using adhesive carbon tape, as well as aluminum tape, on the SEM sample stub. The samples were inserted into a Hitachi S-4700 (Hitachi, Tokyo, Japan), which was operated at 20 kV.

2.5. Immunofluorescence Microscopy (IF) Analysis

Prior to the sacrifice of the rabbit tibiae, the implants were removed from each tibia and, along with the surrounding bone, the specimens were preserved for 3 h in the refrigerator in the RPMI media, which contained penicillin (50 U/mL) and streptomycin (50 µg/mL). The cells underwent immunostaining and were incubated for 15 min with a protein block (DAKO, Agilent, Santa Clara, CA, USA, X0909) to remove non-specific binding protein. The cells were then incubated for 30 min with a diluted osteocalcin primary antibody (1:100 dilution in 3% bovine serum albumin (BSA), #MA120788, Thermo Fisher Scientific, USA). After being rinsed in PBS, these cells were incubated for 1 h with a diluted secondary antibody (1:200 diluted goat anti-mouse IgG-FITC in 3% BSA, #A10530, Thermo Fisher Scientific, Waltham, MA, USA) in a dark room and washed with PBS. Subsequently, nuclear counterstaining was performed using Hoechst 33342 (Thermo Fisher Scientific, Waltham, MA, USA) (1:10,000 dilution) for 5 min. After the counterstaining, the images were obtained by fluorescence microscopy using Axio Observer.A1 (Carl Zeiss, Jena, Germany).

2.6. Transmission Electron Microscopy (TEM) Analysis

Prior to sacrifice, the implants were removed, and the cells were isolated with a cell scraper and fixed in Karnovsky's solution. After sacrifice, the cells from the bony structures around the area where implants had been placed were collected and fixed in Karnovsky's solution. They were washed in 0.1 M PBS 3 times every 15 min. The specimens were dehydrated through a graded 70–100% ethanol series, exchanged with propylene oxide, and embedded in a mixture of Epon 812 and Araldite. Ultrathin sections (70 nm) were cut using a Leica EM UC6 Ultramicrotome (Leica, Vienna, Austria). A ribbon of serial ultrathin sections from each bony specimen and implant were collected on copper grids and stained with uranyl acetate and lead citrate. The serial fields were photographed at ×500 magnification using a JEOL 1400-Flash electron microscope (JEOL, Tokyo, Japan) operated at 120 kV.

2.7. TEM Sample Preparation by Focused Ion Beam (FIB)

The implant specimens were fixed with Karnovsky's solution and washed in 0.1 M PBS 3 times every 15 min. The specimens were dehydrated through a graded 70–100% ethanol series and finally treated with hexamethyldisilazane for 15 min. A Helios 650 (FEI, Hillsboro, OR, USA) dual-beam FIB system was used for the TEM sample preparation. The specimens were deposited with a platinum layer to protect the implant and bony surfaces prior to milling. A Ga^+ ion beam accelerated voltage of 30 kV was used for milling. The TEM sample (under 100 nm) was attached to a Cu TEM grid. The TEM analysis at Cs-STEM was observed using a JEM-AFM200F (Cold FEG, JEOL, Tokyo, Japan).

3. Results

3.1. Parts of the Implant

The distribution of the main locations of cells was classified into three major structures within the implant: The root, the lower flank (LF), and the upper flank (UF). The implants used in this study were specially designed: The sharp V-shape parts for the firm engagement of bone, and the square area between the threads for the biologic response with no physical intervention such as stress (Figure 1A).

3.2. TEM Sample Preparation by Focused Ion Beam (FIB)

Surface characteristics along with cell attachment were probed using Cs-TEM from the FIB system. The cells were detected directly from an undecalcified specimen without the need to undergo cell isolation. The cells on the turned surface were unseen (Figure 1B), while on the SLA surface, organic matter was detected under the Pt-coated layer (Figure 1C).

3.3. Confocal Laser Scanning Microscopy (CLSM) Analysis of the Implant

The different topographical features [10,20,21] of the implants may affect cell attachment. Therefore, CLSM was used to measure the height parameters (S_a), as well as the hybrid parameters (S_{dr}), for the root, UF, and LF areas. The S_a values for the turned surface were 0.163 µm, 0.086 µm, and 0.098 µm, and the S_{dr} values were 10.3%, 8.2%, and 12.1% in the root, UF, and LF, respectively (Figure 1D). On the SLA surfaces, the S_a values were 1.14 µm, 1.17 µm, and 1.09 µm, and the S_{dr} values were 237%, 235%, and 239% for the root, UF, and LF, respectively. The S_a and S_{dr} values differed in terms of surface characteristics, with the SLA being higher; however, based on the different structural components, no differences were found in either the S_a or S_{dr}. After the cells were fixed, the 3D topographical mapping of the cells also showed higher cell quantities in the root area of the SLA implants (Figure 1E). To see the correlation of the surrounding bone and the retrieved implant, the topographical parameters of the bone were also tested, but unfortunately, due to the sputtering of the Pt, the parameters could not be calculated in the bone area.

3.4. Scanning Electron Microscopy (SEM) Analysis of the Implant

In our research, the cell attachment and spreading varied depending on the structural differences in the implant thread. Cells were not attached in turned surfaces in all parts of the implants (Figure 2A). In the root area of SLA implants, an active cellular event took place. The cells were aggregated and spread out effectively, with their cellular processes extended. The fibrin of the cell could be detected. In the crest area, osteocytes and their processes were observed on both the UF and LF. However, they were not as active as the cells in the root area, in which the cells maintained a round shape, insufficiently spreading, and were in a static form (Figure 2B).

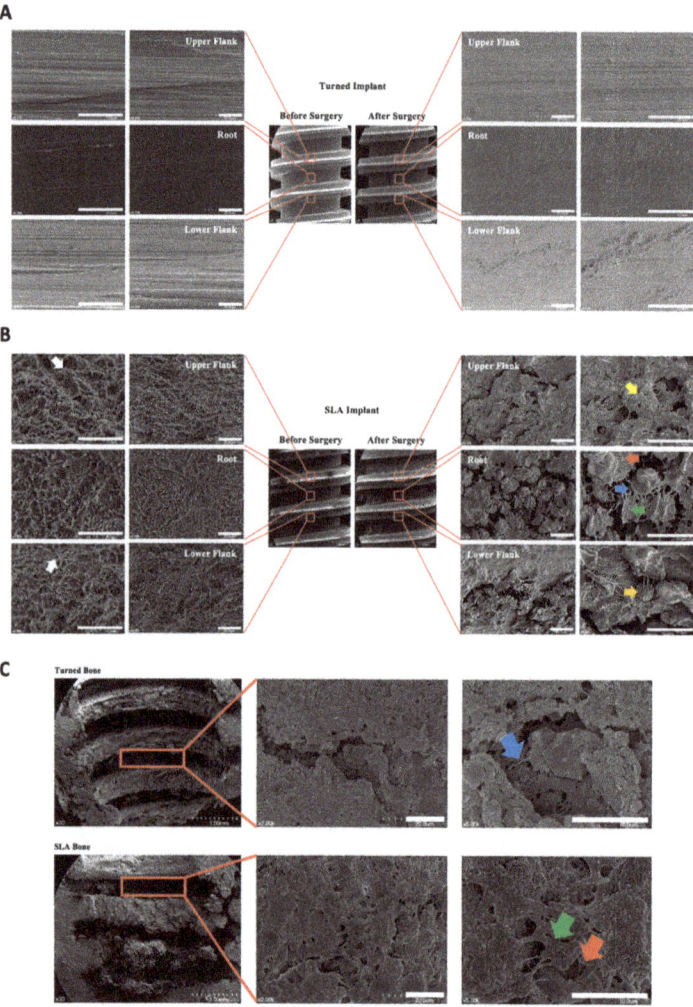

Figure 2. (**A**) Scanning Electron Microscopy (SEM) analysis of the turned implants. The smooth surface is displayed with many turned grooves. No cells were attached after 10 days. (**B**) SEM analysis of sandblasted, large-grit, and SLA implants. The surface characteristics of the SLA implants, which are typically porous, with honeycomb shapes (white arrow); the rather sharp peaks (left top white arrow) are definite, and the texture of the surface is rough. On the right-hand-side, the cells (green arrow) are shown to be mainly attached and actively spread out in the root area, with their filopodia extended (blue arrow). The fibrin can be seen on the cells (red arrow). In the UF, osteocytes and their processes are seen (yellow arrow). In the LF, the cell process is being extended, getting ready to migrate. The round cells are in static status (orange arrow). (**C**) SEM analysis of the surrounding bone of the removed turned and SLA implants at day 10. In the upper row, the overall image reveals traces of the smooth implant surface; thus, the bone texture is rather regular. The formation of the fibrin network is shown beneath some active cells (blue arrow). The lower row demonstrates the surrounding bone of the removed SLA implant. The texture of the bone is rather rough compared with that of the turned implant. The red blood cells can be seen underneath the cells. The mineralization grains (green arrow) are shown, and collagen (red arrow) is depicted well with striped bands. Scale bars = 10 μm.

3.5. Scanning Electron Microscopy (SEM) Analysis of the Surrounding Bone of the Retrieved Implant

The SEM analysis of the surrounding bone of the retrieved turned implants revealed a fibrin network among the cells, whereas a striped pattern of supposed collagen bands was elucidated in the SLA implants. In the area where the bone was in contact with the UF and LF, a bone matrix was formed, while the crest area of the thread showed a fibrin network and an active cellular response. In the surrounding bone of the SLA-retrieved implants, the texture of the bone surface was rougher compared to that of the turned implants. Red blood cells were embedded, and a mineralization process had occurred in the crest area where the collagen bands were visible; cell folding could be observed with granules (Figure 2C).

3.6. Immunofluorescence Microscopy (IF) Analysis

Among the cells attached on the SLA surfaces, osteogenic cells needed to be identified because they are the key cells in bone formation. Accordingly, the attachment of osteogenic cells to the implant surface was confirmed through the use of osteocalcin—antibody targeted for rabbits in vivo. Immunofluorescence microscopy enabled the development of images of osteogenic cells on the SLA implants and the surrounding bone after 10 days, and consequently, confirmed the existence of osteogenic cells on the implant surface. While osteogenic cells were detected on the implant surface, the surrounding bone showed few osteogenic cells (Figure 3A).

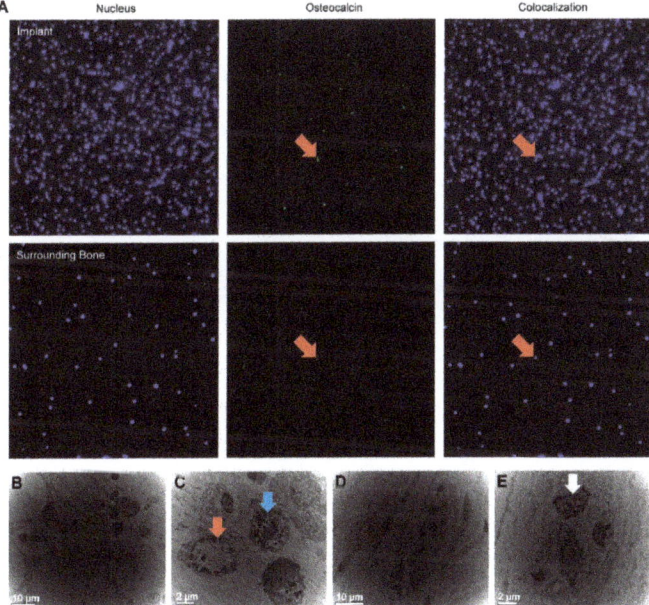

Figure 3. (**A**) Immunofluorescence microscopy (IF) of the SLA implants and surrounding bone on day 10, including nucleus, marker, and colocalization. Osteogenic cells (red arrow) are attached to the SLA implant surface rather than to the surrounding bone, which showed few osteogenic cells. The magnification of the photographs is ×200. (**B**) Transmission electron microscopy (TEM) analysis of retrieved SLA implant at day 10. (**C**) Macrophages (blue arrow) and osteogenic cell (red arrow) can be seen in the SLA implants. (**D**) TEM analysis of surrounding bone on day 10. (**E**) In the surrounding bone, osteocytes (white arrow) were detected.

3.7. Transmission Electron Microscopy (TEM) Analysis

The samples were also scrutinized by TEM. The TEM images of the SLA implants revealed macrophages and osteogenic cells (Figure 3B,C), while in the surrounding bone, osteocytes were detected (Figure 3D,E).

4. Discussion

In the present study, we aimed to determine the cell activity that occurs during the bone-forming process. We targeted the challenges concerning the lack of actual visualization of bone formation, and put much effort into presenting data on the active process in a bony environment with an actual 3D implant structure rather than the flat Ti discs used in in vitro studies. Our experimental data showed that a positive cell reaction occurred on the SLA surfaces, whereas the turned surfaces lacked cell adhesion. Meanwhile, the surrounding bone of the turned surface implants exhibited active cellular events. This may be confirmation of contact osteogenesis on the SLA surfaces. Whilst distance osteogenesis appears to occur around the smooth turned surfaces, it is well known that rougher turned surfaces (that were not investigated in this paper) also display contact osteogenesis [19,22–24].

According to the IF results seen, confirmation of osteogenic cells on the roughened implant surfaces might be further evidence of contact osteogenesis. However, further investigation is required to determine why only few osteogenic cells were detected on the bone surface—which is considered to be the place for distance osteogenesis. In addition, although limitations exist, in that cell classification is difficult in FIB specimens, the results reveal further evidence of contact osteogenesis on the SLA surface. Investigations are needed to better understand the link between such a phenomenon and the higher clinical long-term survival rate of implants with the SLA surfaces (over 95%), compared to that of turned implants (81–91%) [25,26].

The cells on the Ti implant surfaces seemed to be able to read the configuration of the structural parts of the implant. Considering the fact that implant geometry is a major factor in the initial stability of an implant inserted into bone and that osseointegration contributes to the subsequent stability, such SEM results imply that the initial, or primary, stability is associated with the shape of the crest area and that the secondary, or biological, stability is mainly connected to the cellular behavior at the root area [27,28].

Under the circumstances of immobility, exogenous foreign material such as Ti implants, exhibit bone demarcation instead of implant rejection; hence, the stability-enhancing structures of an implant may be of particular importance [29]. Cylindrical implants without threads have uniform but weak attachment to the bone, which is especially weak to shear stress. This weakness may have been one reason why the cylindrical implants displayed a lot of bone resorption in situ [30]. With regards to the electron microscopic images captured in the in vivo environment of this study, all the implant components shown, including the thread structure and microtopography, are important in the cellular response during the osseointegration process. Altering the surface roughness of a material may affect the biological processes regulating the behavioral mechanisms (e.g., cell activity, adhesion) of osteoblastic/immune cells, such extracellular protein deposition at the moment of implantation has an influence on the cellular behavior which later leads to differences in in vivo outcomes [31,32]. This study was qualitative. Quantitative investigations are necessary for various modified surfaces. Recently, implants made of other materials—including ceramic and polyetheretherketone (PEEK)—have been developed, the surfaces of which need to be further investigated with respect to this in vivo cellular response [33,34].

This study successfully presented direct evidence of the behavior of osteogenic cells on the implant surface in an in vivo environment at the electron microscopic level. According to the interpreted data herein, in the bone surrounding dental implants, cell behavior is determined by the treated surface of the implant, whereas cells attached to the SLA implants seem to be able to read the configuration of different implant structures and develop an attachment pattern that conforms to those structures.

Author Contributions: Conceptualization, J.-Y.C. and Y.-J.J.; Methodology, J.-Y.C., Y.-J.J., and T.A.; Software, J.-Y.C.; Validation, J.-Y.C., T.A., and I.-S.L.Y.; Formal Analysis, J.-Y.C. and Y.-J.J.; Investigation, J.-Y.C.; Resources, J.-Y.C., T.A., Y.-J.J., and I.-S.L.Y.; Data Curation, J.-Y.C., T.A., Y.-J.J., and I.-S.L.Y.; Writing—Original Draft Preparation, J.-Y.C.; Writing—Review & Editing, J.-Y.C., T.A., and I.-S.L.Y.; Visualization, J.-Y.C., T.A., Y.-J.J., and I.-S.L.Y.; Supervision, I.-S.L.Y.; Project Administration, J.-Y.C. and I.-S.L.Y.; Funding Acquisition, I.-S.L.Y.

Funding: This work was supported by a National Research Foundation of Korea (NRF) grant funded by the Ministry of Science, ICT and Future Planning, the Korean Government [No. NRF-2016R1A2B4014330].

Conflicts of Interest: The authors declare that there are no conflicts of interest regarding the publication of this paper.

References

1. Trindade, R.; Albrektsson, T.; Galli, S.; Prgomet, Z.; Tengvall, P.; Wennerberg, A. Osseointegration and foreign body reaction: Titanium implants activate the immune system and suppress bone resorption during the first 4 weeks after implantation. *Clin. Implant Dent. Relat. Res.* **2018**, *20*, 82–91. [CrossRef] [PubMed]
2. Kohles, S.S.; Clark, M.B.; Brown, C.A.; Kenealy, J.N. Direct assessment of profilometric roughness variability from typical implant surface types. *Int. J. Oral Maxillofac. Implants* **2004**, *19*, 510–516.
3. Yeo, I.S.; Han, J.S.; Yang, J.H. Biomechanical and histomorphometric study of dental implants with different surface characteristics. *J. Biomed. Mater. Res. B Appl. Biomater.* **2008**, *87*, 303–311. [CrossRef] [PubMed]
4. Choi, J.Y.; Lee, H.J.; Jang, J.U.; Yeo, I.S. Comparison between bioactive fluoride modified and bioinert anodically oxidized implant surfaces in early bone response using rabbit tibia model. *Implant Dent.* **2012**, *21*, 124–128. [CrossRef]
5. Kang, H.K.; Kim, O.B.; Min, S.K.; Jung, S.Y.; Jang, D.H.; Kwon, T.K.; Min, B.M.; Yeo, I.S. The effect of the dltiddsywyri motif of the human laminin alpha2 chain on implant osseointegration. *Biomaterials* **2013**, *34*, 4027–4037. [CrossRef]
6. Koh, J.W.; Kim, Y.S.; Yang, J.H.; Yeo, I.S. Effects of a calcium phosphate-coated and anodized titanium surface on early bone response. *Int. J. Oral Maxillofac. Implants* **2013**, *28*, 790–797. [CrossRef] [PubMed]
7. Kwon, T.K.; Lee, H.J.; Min, S.K.; Yeo, I.S. Evaluation of early bone response to fluoride-modified and anodically oxidized titanium implants through continuous removal torque analysis. *Implant Dent.* **2012**, *21*, 427–432. [CrossRef]
8. Yeo, I.S.; Min, S.K.; Kang, H.K.; Kwon, T.K.; Jung, S.Y.; Min, B.M. Identification of a bioactive core sequence from human laminin and its applicability to tissue engineering. *Biomaterials* **2015**, *73*, 96–109. [CrossRef] [PubMed]
9. Wennerberg, A.; Albrektsson, T.; Chrcanovic, B. Long-term clinical outcome of implants with different surface modifications. *Eur. J. Oral Implantol.* **2018**, *11* (Suppl. 1), S123–S136. [PubMed]
10. Wennerberg, A.; Albrektsson, T. On implant surfaces: A review of current knowledge and opinions. *Int. J. Oral Maxillofac. Implants* **2010**, *25*, 63–74. [PubMed]
11. Choi, J.Y.; Jung, U.W.; Kim, C.S.; Jung, S.M.; Lee, I.S.; Choi, S.H. Influence of nanocoated calcium phosphate on two different types of implant surfaces in different bone environment: An animal study. *Clin. Oral Implants Res.* **2013**, *24*, 1018–1022. [CrossRef] [PubMed]
12. Albrektsson, T.; Chrcanovic, B.; Molne, J.; Wennerberg, A. Foreign body reactions, marginal bone loss and allergies in relation to titanium implants. *Eur. J. Oral Implantol.* **2018**, *11* (Suppl. 1), S37–S46.
13. Albrektsson, T. On implant prosthodontics: One narrative, twelve voices-1. *Int. J. Prosthodont.* **2018**, *31*, s11–s14.
14. Choi, J.Y.; Kang, S.H.; Kim, H.Y.; Yeo, I.L. Control variable implants improve interpretation of surface modification and implant design effects on early bone responses: An in vivo study. *Int. J. Oral Maxillofac. Implants* **2018**, *33*, 1033–1040. [CrossRef] [PubMed]
15. Min, S.K.; Kang, H.K.; Jang, D.H.; Jung, S.Y.; Kim, O.B.; Min, B.M.; Yeo, I.S. Titanium surface coating with a laminin-derived functional peptide promotes bone cell adhesion. *Biomed. Res. Int.* **2013**, *2013*, 638348. [CrossRef]
16. Araújo-Gomes, N.; Romero-Gavilán, F.; Sánchez-Pérez, A.M.; Gurruchaga, M.; Azkargorta, M.; Elortza, F.; Martinez-Ibañez, M.; Iloro, I.; Suay, J.; Goñi, I. Characterization of serum proteins attached to distinct sol-gel hybrid surfaces. *J. Biomed. Mater. Res. B Appl. Biomater.* **2018**, *106*, 1477–1485. [CrossRef]

17. Kilkenny, C.; Browne, W.J.; Cuthi, I.; Emerson, M.; Altman, D.G. Improving bioscience research reporting: The arrive guidelines for reporting animal research. *Vet. Clin. Pathol.* **2012**, *41*, 27–31. [CrossRef]
18. Trindade, R.; Albrektsson, T.; Galli, S.; Prgomet, Z.; Tengvall, P.; Wennerberg, A. Bone immune response to materials, part i: Titanium, peek and copper in comparison to sham at 10 days in rabbit tibia. *J. Clin. Med.* **2018**, *7*, 526. [CrossRef]
19. Choi, J.Y.; Sim, J.H.; Yeo, I.L. Characteristics of contact and distance osteogenesis around modified implant surfaces in rabbit tibiae. *J. Periodontal Implant Sci.* **2017**, *47*, 182–192. [CrossRef] [PubMed]
20. Wennerberg, A.; Albrektsson, T. Effects of titanium surface topography on bone integration: A systematic review. *Clin. Oral Implants Res.* **2009**, *20* (Suppl. 4), 172–184. [CrossRef]
21. Yeo, I.S. Reality of dental implant surface modification: A short literature review. *Open Biomed. Eng. J.* **2014**, *8*, 114–119. [CrossRef] [PubMed]
22. Albrektsson, T.; Brånemark, P.I.; Hansson, H.A.; Lindström, J. Osseointegrated titanium implants. Requirements for ensuring a long-lasting, direct bone-to-implant anchorage in man. *Acta Orthop. Scand.* **1981**, *52*, 155–170. [CrossRef]
23. Davies, J.; Turner, S.; Sandy, J.R. Distraction osteogenesis—A review. *Br. Dent. J.* **1998**, *185*, 462–467. [CrossRef] [PubMed]
24. Davies, J.E. Mechanisms of endosseous integration. *Int. J. Prosthodont.* **1998**, *11*, 391–401.
25. Buser, D.; Janner, S.F.; Wittneben, J.G.; Brägger, U.; Ramseier, C.A.; Salvi, G.E. 10-year survival and success rates of 511 titanium implants with a sandblasted and acid-etched surface: A retrospective study in 303 partially edentulous patients. *Clin. Implant Dent. Relat. Res.* **2012**, *14*, 839–851. [CrossRef]
26. Adell, R.; Lekholm, U.; Rockler, B.; Brånemark, P.I. A 15-year study of osseointegrated implants in the treatment of the edentulous jaw. *Int. J. Oral Surg.* **1981**, *10*, 387–416. [CrossRef]
27. Kwon, T.K.; Kim, H.Y.; Yang, J.H.; Wikesjö, U.M.; Lee, J.; Koo, K.T.; Yeo, I.S. First-order mathematical correlation between damping and resonance frequency evaluating the bone-implant interface. *Int. J. Oral Maxillofac. Implants* **2016**, *31*, 1008–1015. [CrossRef]
28. Meredith, N. Assessment of implant stability as a prognostic determinant. *Int. J. Prosthodont.* **1998**, *11*, 491–501.
29. Donath, K.; Laass, M.; Günzl, H.J. The histopathology of different foreign-body reactions in oral soft tissue and bone tissue. *Virchows Arch. A Pathol. Anat. Histopathol.* **1992**, *420*, 131–137. [CrossRef]
30. Chrcanovic, B.R.; Albrektsson, T.; Wennerberg, A. Reasons for failures of oral implants. *J. Oral Rehabil.* **2014**, *41*, 443–476. [CrossRef]
31. Romero-Gavilán, F.; Gomes, N.C.; Ródenas, J.; Sánchez, A.; Azkargorta, M.; Iloro, I.; Elortza, F.; García Arnáez, I.; Gurruchaga, M.; Goñi, I.; et al. Proteome analysis of human serum proteins adsorbed onto different titanium surfaces used in dental implants. *Biofouling* **2017**, *33*, 98–111. [CrossRef] [PubMed]
32. Dodo, C.G.; Senna, P.M.; Custodio, W.; Paes Leme, A.F.; Del Bel Cury, A.A. Proteome analysis of the plasma protein layer adsorbed to a rough titanium surface. *Biofouling* **2013**, *29*, 549–557. [CrossRef]
33. Bormann, K.H.; Gellrich, N.C.; Kniha, H.; Schild, S.; Weingart, D.; Gahlert, M. A prospective clinical study to evaluate the performance of zirconium dioxide dental implants in single-tooth edentulous area: 3-year follow-up. *BMC Oral Health* **2018**, *18*, 181. [CrossRef] [PubMed]
34. Najeeb, S.; Zafar, M.S.; Khurshid, Z.; Siddiqui, F. Applications of polyetheretherketone (peek) in oral implantology and prosthodontics. *J. Prosthodont. Res.* **2016**, *60*, 12–19. [CrossRef] [PubMed]

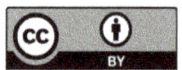

© 2019 by the authors. Licensee MDPI, Basel, Switzerland. This article is an open access article distributed under the terms and conditions of the Creative Commons Attribution (CC BY) license (http://creativecommons.org/licenses/by/4.0/).

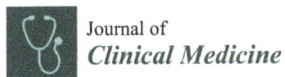

Article

Mechanical and Biological Advantages of a Tri-Oval Implant Design

Xing Yin [1,2], Jingtao Li [1,2], Waldemar Hoffmann [3], Angelines Gasser [3], John B. Brunski [2] and Jill A. Helms [2,*]

[1] State Key Laboratory of Oral Diseases & National Clinical Research Center for Oral Diseases, West China Hospital of Stomatology, Sichuan University, Chengdu 610041, China; yinxing@scu.edu.cn (X.Y.); lijingtao86@163.com (J.L.)
[2] Division of Plastic and Reconstructive Surgery, Department of Surgery, Stanford School of Medicine, Stanford, CA 94305, USA; brunsj6@stanford.edu
[3] Nobel Biocare Services AG, P.O. Box, Zurich-Airport, 8058 Zurich, Switzerland; waldemar.hoffmann@nobelbiocare.com (W.H.); angelines.gasser@nobelbiocare.com (A.G.)
* Correspondence: jhelms@stanford.edu

Received: 2 February 2019; Accepted: 25 March 2019; Published: 28 March 2019

Abstract: Of all geometric shapes, a tri-oval one may be the strongest because of its capacity to bear large loads with neither rotation nor deformation. Here, we modified the external shape of a dental implant from circular to tri-oval, aiming to create a combination of high strain and low strain peri-implant environment that would ensure both primary implant stability and rapid osseointegration, respectively. Using in vivo mouse models, we tested the effects of this geometric alteration on implant survival and osseointegration over time. The maxima regions of tri-oval implants provided superior primary stability without increasing insertion torque. The minima regions of tri-oval implants presented low compressive strain and significantly less osteocyte apoptosis, which led to minimal bone resorption compared to the round implants. The rate of new bone accrual was also faster around the tri-oval implants. We further subjected both round and tri-oval implants to occlusal loading immediately after placement. In contrast to the round implants that exhibited a significant dip in stability that eventually led to their failure, the tri-oval implants maintained their stability throughout the osseointegration period. Collectively, these multiscale biomechanical analyses demonstrated the superior in vivo performance of the tri-oval implant design.

Keywords: dental implant; osseointegration; alveolar bone remodeling/regeneration; bone biology; finite element analysis (FEA); biomechanics

1. Introduction

Implants have undergone a nearly continual transformation since their inception. Variations in fabrication materials, surface texture, coating, and taper have yielded implants that osseointegrated and are clinically successful [1–5]. Most dental implants, however, still have a circular cross-section, which reflects their origins as titanium screws [6,7].

A non-circular cross-section may have advantages. When placed into a cylindrical osteotomy, conventional implants typically have a uniform bone-implant contact (BIC), and the resulting peri-implant strains are uniformly distributed around its circumference [8]. Although the relationship is not straightforward [9], it is generally presumed that the greater the amount of bone-implant contact (BIC) the better is implant stability [10].

A non-circular, e.g., tri-oval shaped implant, on the other hand, would be predicted to engage bone on its vertices, or tri-oval maxima, which would provide mechanical stability and result in peri-implant strains concentrated at these regions.

Depending on the extent of tri-ovality, there would also be sites of minimal BIC. An extensive literature has shown that new woven bone first forms in areas where BIC is absent [8,11–14].

In previous studies, we demonstrated that when an implant is placed with high insertion torque (IT), then peri-implant bone is compressed and osteocytes within this bone begin to die [8,15,16].

Some proposed embodiments of dental implants have had non-circular cross-sectional shapes to reduce "friction between the bone and implant during insertion" [17,18]. Once the implant is in place, however, it is not friction but rather peri-implant stresses and strains that appear to be most important: Inserting an implant creates strains in peri-implant tissues [11,19,20], and the magnitude of these strains has a direct, quantifiable impact on the behavior of cells and tissues in the peri-implant environment [20,21].

In areas where an implant contacts bone, the stiff interface stabilizes the implant [15]. There is a biological downside to this relationship, though: if the implant is placed with high IT, then the stiff interfacial bone is compressed to a greater extent, and the result is higher strain. Cells within the bone matrix, i.e., osteocytes, respond to this high strain by dying [8,15,16].

The converse is also true: in areas of low strain, fewer peri-implant osteocytes die and bone resorption is minimal [22]. If the peri-implant bone is "soft", e.g., has a trabecular microstructure, then cells in the low strain environment tend to proliferate. Ultimately, these cells can differentiate into osteoblasts and osseointegration ensues [22].

Once osteocytes have died, necrotic bone is resorbed via an osteoclast-mediated process [8,15]. Thereafter, new bone formation ensues [8,23]. The resorption of dead peri-implant bone, however, jeopardizes implant stability. We speculated that there could be a way to avoid this by purposefully creating a combination of high strain and low strain peri-implant environments that would ensure both mechanical engagement in the surrounding bone, i.e., primary stability, and rapid osseointegration, respectively. In a tri-oval implant design, the maxima regions would theoretically correspond to areas of higher strain and provide initial mechanical stability. The minima regions of the tri-oval design would theoretically correspond to areas of low strain and constitute pro-osteogenic zones where new bone formation would contribute to secondary implant stability. Here, we tested the veracity of this theory by comparing outcomes of tri-oval and round implants placed into healed maxillary sites according to a well-established in vivo mouse model of oral implant osseointegration.

2. Materials and methods

2.1. Implant Design

Implants were manufactured from CP Titanium Grade 4 with a TiUnite surface (Nobel Biocare AB, Goteborg, Sweden). Geometries for round (control) and tri-oval implants are described in Supplemental Table S1.

2.2. Animals and Tooth Extraction Surgeries

Procedures were approved by Stanford Committee on Animal Research (protocol #13146) and conformed to the ARRIVE guidelines. Wild-type C57BL/6 mice (Jackson Laboratory, Bar Harbor, ME, USA, #003291) were housed in a temperature-controlled environment with 12h light/dark cycles. In total, 96 eight-week-old male mice were used.

2.3. Implant Placement, Osteotomy Site Preparation, and Experimental Groups

Extraction of bilateral maxillary 1st molars (mxM1) was performed using forceps. Bleeding was controlled by local pressure. Extraction sockets were allowed to fully heal for four weeks [22]. Pain control was ensured by daily delivery of analgesics. Immediately following surgery mice received sub-cutaneous injections of buprenorphine (0.05–0.1 mg/kg) for analgesia once a day for a total of three days. Animals were fed with regular hard chow diet. Daily monitoring revealed no evidence of prolonged inflammation during healing at the surgical sites. No antibiotics were given to the operated animals.

Following anesthesia, osteotomy sites were produced using a dental engine (NSK, Tokyo, Japan) and a 0.45mm diameter drill bit at 800 rpm (Drill Bit City, Prospect Heights, IL, USA). Aseptic saline was used for irrigation during the drilling process.

A split-mouth design was employed for this study, wherein each mouse received one round implant and one tri-oval implant. See Supplemental Table S2 for the distribution of groups and analyses performed in each group. Implants were placed either below the occlusal plane or at the level of occlusion.

2.4. Implant Insertion Torque Measurement

To compare the insertion torque (IT) of the round and tri-oval implants, two independent experimental setting were performed. In one experimental design, holes (0.45mm diameter) were produced in a uniform block of poplar wood and then round and tri-oval implants were inserted all the way into the wood block. The IT was then recorded by attaching the implants to a miniature torque cell (MRT Miniature Flange Style Reaction Torque Transducer, Interface Inc., Scottsdale, AZ, USA). Poplar wood had an elastic modulus of 10.9 GPa [24], which is on the same order of magnitude as dense bone (e.g., 10–20 GPa) [25].

In another experimental design, the IT was measured directly on mice [26]. Osteotomies (0.45 mm in diameter) were prepared in the healed maxillary tooth extraction sites and the implants were inserted. The animals were sacrificed immediately after implant placement. The mandible was removed to fully expose the inserted implant, and the IT was then measured by connecting the implant to a pre-calibrated hand-held gauge (Tonichi, Tokyo, Japan).

The rationale for comparing insertion torques (IT) of round and trioval implants in wood was not to imply that wood is an excellent substitute test material for bone; rather it was because (a) wood offered a uniform material allowing side-by-side IT tests of round and trioval implants under identical conditions, and (b) the IT tests in wood could be conducted using a sensitive miniature torque transducer that could not be used in vivo.

2.5. Lateral Stability Testing, Finite Element Modeling, and Calculation of Elastic Modulus

A lateral stiffness test (LST) of implants in alveolar bone was carried out using maxillae samples retrieved on PID 0, 3, 7, 14, and 20. The LST was based on an assumed linear relationship between a lateral force exerted on the top of an implant and the resulting lateral displacement of the implant in bone. Our experience with this method, including modeling with finite element analysis indicates that this assumption is valid for displacements in the range of about 0 to 50 μm [15,27].

To carry out LST, the animals were sacrificed and the skulls, with the maxillae removed and sectioned in half sagittally, were submerged in 100% ethanol. The half-maxilla containing the implants was then rigidly clamped to a solid support so that the implant was positioned between a linear actuator (Ultra Motion Digit D-A.083-AB-HT17075-2-K-B/3, Mattituck, NY, USA) equipped with an in-line 10 N force transducer (Honeywell Model 31), and a displacement transducer (MG-DVRT-3, Lord MicroStrain, Williston, VT, USA). A tare load of 0.05 N was applied to one side of the implant while the stylus of the displacement transducer was positioned against the diametrically-opposite side of the implant. Under software command, the actuator was triggered to deliver three cycles of a displacement vs. time waveform with a peak displacement of about 30 μm (Figure 1M). The force was applied, and the resulting lateral displacement of the implant was measured at a consistent height of ~0.5 mm above the crest of the maxillary bone. Previous tests and calculations show that under the force conditions in this test, there is negligible deformation of the titanium implant, meaning that virtually all lateral displacement arises from displacements in the peri-implant tissue. Lateral force and lateral displacement of the implant were recorded and stored to disc for later data analysis and calculation of the ratio between force and displacement, i.e., lateral stiffness (in Newtons/micron).

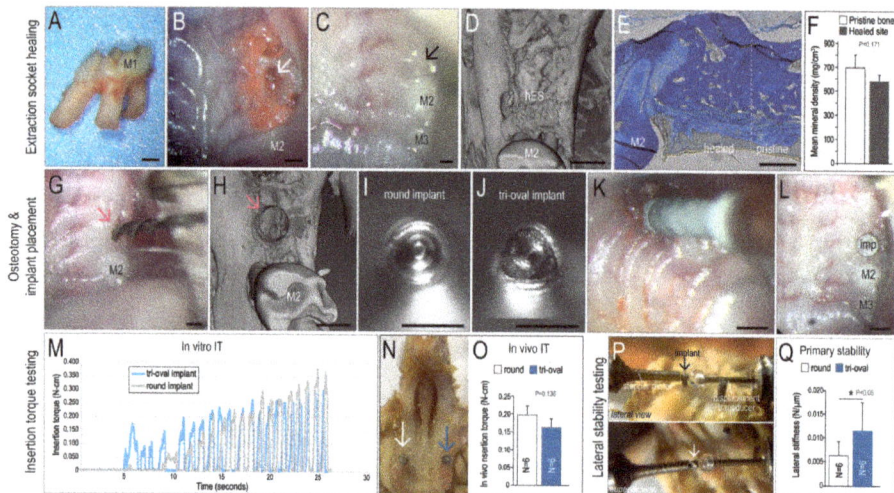

Figure 1. Tri-oval implants placed in type III bone with the same insertion torque exhibit higher primary stability as compared to conventional round implants. (**A**) Maxillary first molars (M1) were extracted from skeletally mature (8-week-old) male mice. (**B**) Intraoral photos of extraction socket (white arrow) and (**C**) Healed extraction site (black arrow). (**D**) Representative micro-CT imaging and (**E**) Representative aniline blue staining of the healed extraction socket on PED28. (**F**) Quantification of mean bone mineral density (BMD) on PED28, where the BMD of the healed extraction site was equivalent to surrounding pristine alveolar bone. (**G**) Osteotomies (0.45 mm dia.; pink arrow) were produced in the healed extraction sites using dental drill. (**H**) Representative micro-CT image of the prepared osteotomy site. (**I**) Geometries of the round and (**J**) tri-oval implants in cross-section. (**K**) Implant placement surgery. (**L**) Implants were positioned at the height of the gingiva. (**M**) In vitro IT testing and (**N**) In vivo IT testing where the white arrow indicates a round implant; blue arrow indicates a tri-oval implant. (**O**) Quantification of in vivo IT for round (white) and tri-oval (blue) implants. (**P**) Lateral stability testing of round and tri-oval implants (arrows) in the mouse maxillae; a stepper motor laterally displaces the implant a known amount while the force to do so is measured by a transducer. (**Q**) Tri-oval implants are significantly more stable than round implants at the time of insertion. Abbreviations: M1, maxillary first molar; M2, maxillary second molar; M3, maxillary third molar; hES, healed extraction site; PED, post-extraction day; imp, implant; IT, insertion torque. Scale bars = 500 µm.

Finite element (FE) modeling provided insight into the relationship between the experimentally-measured lateral stiffness and the elastic properties of the surrounding peri-implant bone [28]. Based on stiffness values from lateral stability testing at post-implant day 3 (PID3), a FE model was used to estimate the elastic modulus of peri-implant tissue. A computer-aided design (CAD) file of each implant was obtained from the manufacturer (Nobel Biocare AB, Göteborg, Sweden) and imported into COMSOL Multiphysics 5.3 when formulating models of the lateral stiffness testing (LST). Each implant was installed to full depth (i.e., eight threads) into a 0.45 mm drill hole made completely through a cylinder (2 mm diameter, 1.45 mm height) of uniform bone having a Young's elastic modulus and Poisson's ratio selected so that the lateral stiffness computed from the FE model matched the experimentally-measured lateral stiffness. A no-slip boundary condition was applied between implant and bone, and the side and bottom surfaces of the bone cylinder were fixed in space. In the FE model simulating LST, a 0.2N lateral load was applied on the side of the implant's top portion, at a height of 0.58 mm above the surface of the bone. The direction of the applied force was perpendicular to the long axis of the implant. The resulting displacement of the implant in the same direction of the lateral force was measured from the displacement output. The ratio of the applied lateral force to the measured lateral displacement at 0.58 mm above the surface of the bone was defined as the lateral stiffness. A typical FE model formulated as described above involved about 238,000 degrees of freedom. To match the results from a given experimental stiffness test of a round or tri-oval implant, the Young's elastic modulus of the bone in the model was parametrically changed until there was a match in lateral stiffness between the FE model and the actual experiment. These FE models demonstrated that the lateral stiffness strongly depended on the Young's elastic modulus of the peri-implant bone.

2.6. Calculating Elastic Modulus of Peri-Implant Bone as a Function of Lateral Stability

Implant insertion caused dynamic tissue remodeling, which could potentially change the tissue elastic modulus in the peri-implant region. Although the changes in peri-implant elastic modulus could not be measured directly on mice, we used FE modeling to generate estimates basing on stiffness values from lateral stability testing at PID3. In the round implant cases, the mean lateral stiffness was 0.00198 N/μm, which corresponded to a modulus of ~2.6 MPa for the peri-implant bone. In the tri-oval implant cases, the mean lateral stiffness was 0.00689 N/μm, which corresponded to a modulus of ~9.2 MPa, a 3.5 times stiffer peri-implant bone than in the case of the round implants.

2.7. Sample Preparation, Tissue Processing, and Histology

Mice were euthanized on PID 3, 7, 10, 14, and 20. For those animals whose implants were to be subjected to mechanical testing, maxillae were harvested with skin and superficial muscles removed, fixed in 100% ethanol, and then subjected to lateral stiffness testing. In cases where implants were evaluated by histology/histomorphometry, tissues were fixed in 4% paraformaldehyde overnight at 4 °C then decalcified in 19% EDTA.

After complete demineralization, specimens were dehydrated through an ascending ethanol series and underwent clearing in xylene prior to paraffin embedding. Before immersion in xylene, implants were gently removed from the samples. Eight-micron-thick longitudinal sections were cut and collected on Superfrost-plus slides [27]. Tissue sections prepared for histology, immunohistochemistry, and immunofluorescence were prepared by one individual then quantified by a blinded individual.

Aniline blue staining was performed to detect osteoid matrix. Tissues sections were also stained with the acidic dye, picrosirius red, to discriminate tightly packed and aligned collagen molecules. Viewed under polarized light, well-aligned fibrillary collagen molecules present polarization colors of longer wavelengths (red) as compared to less organized collagen fibrils that show colors of shorter (green-yellow) wavelengths [27].

2.8. Histomorphometry

Maxillae were embedded in paraffin and sectioned in the transverse planes. The space occupied by the 0.5mm implant was represented across ~60 tissue sections, each of which were 8 μm thick. Of those 60 sections, a minimum of four Aniline blue-stained tissue sections were used for the quantification of new peri-implant bone formation. Each section was photographed using a Leica digital imaging system at 5× and 10× magnification. The digital images were analyzed using ImageJ software 1.4 (National Institute of Mental Health, Bethesda, MD, USA). The percentage of aniline blue-positive new bone (%NB) was calculated using the area occupied by aniline-blue-positive pixels divided by the total number of pixels in the defined region of interest (ROI). Pixel counts from these individual tissue sections were performed in triplicate then averaged for each sample.

2.9. TUNEL Staining, Alkaline Phosphatase Activity, and Tartrate Resistant Acid Phosphatase Activity

TUNEL staining was performed as described by the manufacturer. Briefly, sections were incubated in proteinase K buffer (20 μg/mL in 10 mM Tris pH 7.5), applied to a TUNEL reaction mixture (In Situ Cell Death Detection Kit, Roche, Mannheim, Germany), and mounted with DAPI mounting medium (Vector Laboratories, Burlingame, CA, USA). Slides were viewed under an epifluorescence microscope.

Alkaline phosphatase (ALP) activity was detected by incubation in nitro blue tetrazolium chloride (NBT; Roche, Mannheim, Germany), 5-bromo-4-chloro-3-indolyl phosphate (BCIP; Roche, Mannheim, Germany), and NTM buffer (100 mM NaCl, 100 mM Tris pH 9.5, 5 mM MgCl). After its development, the slides were dehydrated in a series of ethanol and xylene and subsequently cover-slipped with Permount mounting media (Thermo Fisher Scientific, Waltham, MA, USA).

Tartrate-resistant acid phosphatase (TRAP) activity was observed using a leukocyte acid phosphatase staining kit (Sigma, St. Louis, MO, USA). After its development, the slides were dehydrated in a series of ethanol and xylene and subsequently cover-slipped with Permount mounting media (Thermo Fisher Scientific, Waltham, MA, USA).

2.10. Micro-CT Imaging

Scanning and analyses followed published guidelines [29]. Ex vivo high-resolution acquisitions (VivaCT 40, Scanco, Brüttisellen, Switzerland) at 10.5 µm voxel size (55 kV, 145 µA, 347 ms integration time), were performed on post-extraction days 28 and immediately after drill preparation. Multiplanar reconstruction and volume rendering were carried out using OsiriX software (version 5.8, Pixmeo, Bernex, Switzerland).

2.11. Statistical Analyses

For lateral stiffness tests, results are presented as the mean ± 95% confidence interval. In testing for differences among five means in the stiffness tests for the round or the tri-oval implants at PID 0 through 20, we used one-way ANOVA with PID time as the factor. In comparing the stiffness of round vs. tri-oval implants at any given time point (PID), Student's t-test was used to quantify differences. $p \leq 0.05$ was significant.

3. Results

3.1. Tri-oval Implants Exhibit Higher Primary Stability Compared to Round Implants

Most dental implants are placed into healed sites [30]; to recapitulate this clinical condition, maxillary first molars (mxM1) were extracted from skeletally mature mice (Figure 1A,B). Within seven days, soft tissue healing was complete (Figure 1C). After four weeks, sites were evaluated clinically, by µCT imaging (Figure 1D), and by histology (Figure 1E), which together confirmed complete healing (Figure 1F).

A split-mouth design was then used: osteotomies were produced in healed sites (Figure 1G,H) and two implants were placed, one round (Figure 1I) and the other tri-oval (Figure 1J). All implants were placed ~0.5 mm above the alveolar bone crest and below the plane of occlusion (Figure 1K,L). Insertion torque (IT) was measured using in vitro and in vivo methods. Both analyses indicated that IT values were equivalent between the round and tri-oval implants (Figure 1M,N,O). Primary stability was measured (Figure 1P) and these lateral stability tests demonstrated that tri-oval implants had significantly higher primary stability than round implants (Figure 1Q). How was this greater primary stability achieved?

3.2. The Maxima of a Tri-Oval Implant Provide Higher Stability

Computational models were generated to determine whether a difference in contributed to the higher primary stability of tri-oval implants. These analyses showed that the threads of a round implant penetrated ~25 µm into bone whereas for a tri-oval implant, the maxima penetrated ~45 µm into bone (Figure 2A). Despite the fact that minima regions were not in contact with bone, a tri-oval implant still had a larger calculated BIC (Figure 2B).

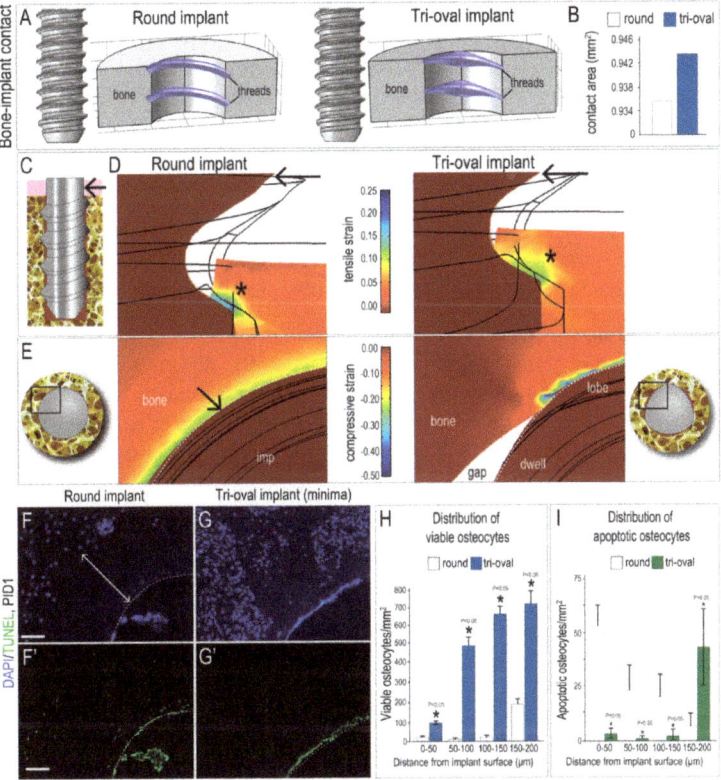

Figure 2. Compared to a round implant, the minima of a tri-oval implant are associated with significantly lower strains and a significantly smaller zone of osteocyte death. (**A**) FE modeling of round (left) and tri-oval (right) implants in bone, using CAD files of the actual implants used in vivo. In a transverse plane, the threads of each type of implant (blue) penetrate the bone, which is modeled as a solid material. (**B**) The calculated bone-implant contact area due to thread penetration. (**C**) Formulation of a FE model of laterally-loaded implant in bone. (**D**) Peri-implant strains surrounding laterally-loaded round and tri-oval implants in the sagittal plane. (**E**) Peri-implant strains arising from initial misfit of the round and tri-oval implants as seen in the transverse plane; only the maxima of the tri-oval implant penetrate the bone. (**F**) DAPI staining of interfacial bone surrounding a representative round implant and (**G**) a representative tri-oval implant; white arrow denotes a circumferential osteocyte-free zone and dotted white line demarcates the osteotomy edge. (**F′**, **G′**) TUNEL staining on adjacent tissue sections. Quantification of the distribution of (**H**) viable and (**I**) apoptotic osteocytes as a function of distance from implant. Abbreviations: imp, implant; PID, post-implant day. Scale bars = 50 μm.

We used FE modeling to understand how the difference in BIC affected peri-implant strains and, in turn, lateral stiffness of the implants. Lateral loading was simulated in the FE model (arrow, Figure 2C) and in both cases the resulting strains concentrated at sites of BIC (Asterix, Figure 2D). The magnitude of these strains, however, was higher in the round implant case (Figure 2D). This meant that when exposed to the same lateral force, the stability of the tri-oval implant was greater than that for the round implant.

The distribution of the peri-implant strains was different, depending on the implant geometry. For example, the round implants had a circumferential zone of high strain whereas the tri-oval implants had strains concentrated only at the maxima; the minima (gaps) had no strain (Figure 2E).

We correlated these strain distributions with biological sequelae. Surrounding round implants was a ~150 μm circumferential zone in which no viable DAPI^{+ve} osteocytes were detectable (white arrow, Figure 2F). Most dying TUNEL^{+ve} osteocytes were found within this same zone (Figure 2F'). Around tri-oval implants, the tri-oval maxima had a similar distribution of dead and dying cells, but in the minima, viable osteocytes were abundant (Figure 2G; quantified in 2H). Dying osteocytes were significantly lower (Figure 2G'; quantified in I). The distribution of DAPI^{+ve} versus dead and TUNEL^{+ve} osteocytes was calculated (Figure 2H, I and Supplemental Figure S1); these data demonstrated that bone viability in the tri-oval minima—which comprised approximately 50% of the circumference of the implant—was significantly higher around the round implants.

3.3. Tri-oval Implants Exhibit Less Bone Resorption, which Allows them to Maintain their Stability Over Time

Peri-implant TRAP activity was more abundant around the round implants (Figure 3A) compared to the tri-oval implants (Figure 3B; quantified in Figure 3C). Resorption removes mineralized matrix, which reduces the elastic modulus of bone and leads to implant instability (white bars, Figure 3D). The tri-oval implants showed no significant loss in stability (blue bars, Figure 3D). Therefore, minimal TRAP activity observed around the tri-oval implants correlated with their greater stability after 3 days.

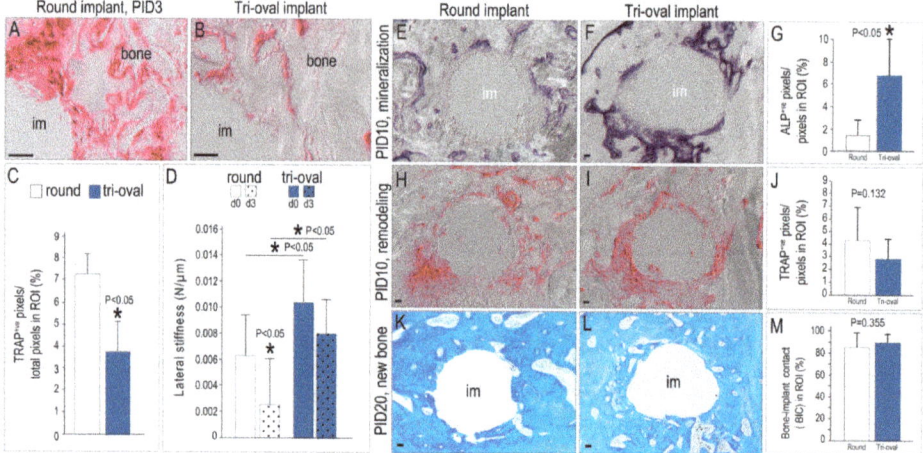

Figure 3. Tri-oval implants exhibits less bone resorption but more robust mineralization. (**A**) TRAP staining of interfacial tissues surrounding a representative round implant on PID3. (**B**) TRAP staining of the minima region around a tri-oval implant on PID3. (**C**) TRAP staining was quantified around the entire circumference of round and tri-oval implants. (**D**) Lateral stiffness test of round and tri-oval implants on PID0 and 3. (**E**) ALP staining of interfacial tissues surrounding a representative round and (**F**) a tri-oval implant on PID10, quantified in (**G**). (**H**) TRAP staining of interfacial tissues surrounding a representative round and (**I**) a tri-oval implant on PID10, quantified in (**J**). (**K**) Aniline blue staining of interfacial tissues surrounding a representative round and (**L**) a tri-oval implant on PID20; quantified in (**M**). Abbreviations as previously stated. Scale bars = 50 μm.

Eventually, both round and tri-oval implants showed evidence of new peri-implant bone mineralization (Figure 3E,F), although the amount of ALP activity was significantly greater around the tri-oval implants (quantified in Figure 3G). This new bone underwent normal remodeling (Figure 3H,I; quantified in Figure 3J). By PID20, both the round and tri-oval implants were fully surrounded by bone (Figure 3K,L; quantified in Figure 3M).

3.4. Tri-Oval Implants Exhibit Superior Osseointegration Compared to Conventional Round Implants

In the experiments conducted thus far, tri-oval implants exhibited better primary stability than round implants, yet both eventually were surrounded by bone. This result was not unexpected because in both cases, implants were placed sub-occlusally, and in previous studies we have shown that sub-occlusal round implants osseointegrate efficiently and effectively [31,32]. Moreover, no differences in quantity of bone or in lateral stability were detected at PID14 (Figure 4B).

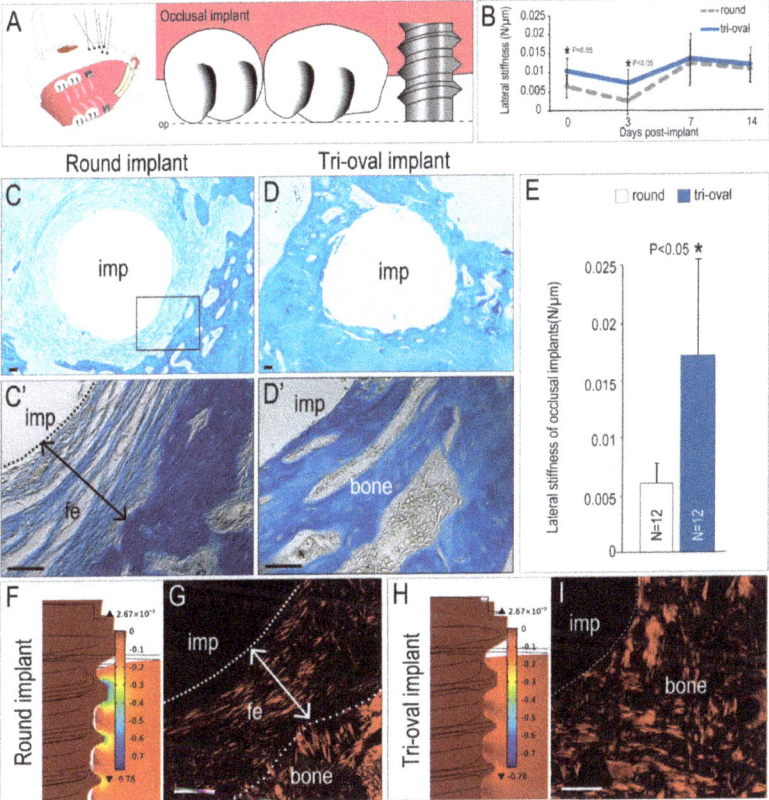

Figure 4. Stability over time as the function of implant geometry. (**A**) Schematic of an occlusal, or functional implant. (**B**) Quantification of lateral stability of sub-occlusal round and tri-oval implants at different timepoints. Aniline blue-stained tissue sections from PID20 through an (**C,C′**) occlusal round implant and (**D,D′**) an occlusal tri-oval implant. (**E**) Quantification of lateral stability of occlusal round and tri-oval implants on PID20. (**F**) In round occlusal implants, FE modeling of peri-implant strain on PID3 and (**G**) picrosirius-red stained tissues from PID20. (**H**) In tri-oval occlusal implants, FE modeling of peri-implant strain on PID3 and (**I**) picrosirius red-stained tissues from PID20. Abbreviations: op, occlusal plane; imp, implant; fe, fibrous encapsulation. Scale bars = 50 μm.

We wondered if the fact that significantly better primary stability exhibited by the tri-oval implant would have a long-term benefit if the implants were immediately loaded. Both the round and tri-oval implants were subjected to functional loading, immediately after placement, which was achieved by positioning the very top of the implant at the same height as the adjacent molar (Figure 4A). The difference in outcome was dramatic: whereas the round implants underwent fibrous encapsulation (Figure 4C,C′), these tri-oval implants osseointegrated (Figure 4D,D′).

Lateral stability results were consistent with histologic/histomorphometric analyses: the soft interfacial tissues surrounding the round implant cases offered little support and consequently, the round implants exhibited poor secondary stability (i.e., small values of lateral stiffness). In comparison, the stiffer interfacial tissues around the tri-oval implants translated into larger lateral stiffness and thus higher secondary stability (Figure 4E).

3.5. The Magnitude of Interfacial Strain is a Key Influence on Whether an Implant will Undergo Fibrous Encapsulation or Osseointegration

Why did these round occlusal implants fail? The key to answering this question lies in the observation that the same round implants can osseointegrate, provided they are placed sub-occlusally to reduce loading (Figure 3). Thus, the round implants failed because they lacked sufficient primary stability (Figure 1Q). We sought to link this observation about stiffness at PID0 with the fates of the implants on PID20, and to do so, we turned again to FE modeling.

Implant stability is a function of the elastic modulus of peri-implant tissue; in other words, the stiffer the tissue, the less the implant will move under loading. FE modeling was used to back-calculate the peri-implant bone modulus that corresponded to the experimentally-measured lateral stability (see Materials and methods). At PID0 and PID3, the peri-implant tissues surrounding trioval implants were 3.5 times stiffer than those surrounding round implants. Using these modulus values, FE models demonstrated that peri-implant strains at PID0 and PID3 were significantly higher around the round occlusal implant (Figure 4F). For example, at the crestal thread tips of an occlusally-loaded round implant, principal compressive strain magnitudes reached >50% (Figure 4F). On the other hand, identically-loaded tri-oval implants were surrounded by stiffer peri-implant tissue and the resulting strains at PID0 and PID3 were less than 10% (Figure 4H). Collectively, these data provide critical insights as to why a round implant with significantly less primary stability underwent fibrous encapsulation when subjected to immediate loading (Figure 4G), whereas a tri-oval implant, with statistically higher primary stability, underwent osseointegration when subjected to the same immediate loading conditions (Figure 4I).

4. Discussion

We coupled mechanical testing with computational studies and histologic/immunohistologic analyses to assess how altering an implant's geometry affected its ability to osseointegrate. We tested implants that were placed below the level of the occlusal plane, and those placed in function. In both scenarios, the tri-oval implants out-performed the round implants. Evidence supporting this conclusion came from mechanical, computational, and biological analyses.

4.1. The Maxima of a Tri-Oval Implant aid in Mechanical Stability

Compared to round implants, the tri-oval implants exhibited better primary stability, which was achieved without using a higher IT (Figure 1). The larger stability was achieved because the maxima of the tri-oval implant penetrated a greater distance into bone than did the threads of the round implant (Figure 2). Based on our data, one might legitimately ask if the novel tri-oval implant design would be negated simply by undersizing the osteotomy for the round implant. In this thought experiment, the threads of the round implant would penetrate deeper into bone and as a result the implant would presumably demonstrate better initial stability. But just as reliably, this scenario would also increase IT [8], peri-implant strain [11], and its associated micro-damage [8,15,33]. In turn, this micro-damage would increase the spatial extent of peri-implant bone resorption (Figure 3) during the early post-operative stages of bone remodeling, which would lower the net modulus of the peri-implant bone and result in a transient decrease of initial stability–as seen for example at PID 3 (Figure 4B).

Clinical observations are consistent with this line of reasoning: in multiple studies, sub-occlusal implants showed a decline in mean ISQ values between weeks 1-4 [34–36]. Friberg also reported a decrease in stability for a majority of sub-occlusal implants [37,38]. Our preclinical study appears to be the first to provide direct molecular, cellular, histologic, and mechanical data to explain how this transient "dip" in implant stability actually occurs.

4.2. The Minima of a Tri-Oval Implant Create a Pro-Osteogenic Environment

Fifty percent of the peri-tri-oval implant environment had very low/no strain (Figure 2E), where damage to the mineralized matrix is minimized, osteocyte death is minimal, and bone resorption is reduced [8,15,33]. Together these events culminated in significantly more new bone around the tri-oval implants (Figures 2 and 3). A similar finding has been reported using a canine implant model, where investigators demonstrated that new woven bone forms first in regions where there is a gap in the bone-implant contact [12]. We find that areas of low/no strain strongly support osteoblast differentiation and new mineralized matrix deposition, provided the osteogenic potential of the bone is good [22].

4.3. Clinical Implications of this Study

Round-shaped implants can osseointegrate, even when subjected to loading immediately after placement. Why, then, did we observe that round implants failed to undergo osseointegration? The answer is straightforward: in those cases where round implants became encapsulated in fibrous tissue it was because loading was allowed on an implant that lacked sufficient primary stability (Figure 1). If the same implant—with the same degree of instability—was buried, then by PID20 it was surrounded by new bone (Figure 3). These data indicate the importance of an "unloaded" healing period proposed by Branemark [39]. What if the healing period is eliminated? Our data predict that healing periods between implant placement and loading could be shortened- or eliminated—without jeopardizing long-term implant success if osteocyte death was minimized during site preparation, and the implant had a geometry that provided both mechanical stability and a pro-osteogenic environment.

5. Conclusions

These multiscale biomechanical analyses demonstrated that the novel tri-oval implant design provided mechanically and biologically favorable environment for peri-implant bone formation and promoted osseointegration.

Supplementary Materials: The following are available online at http://www.mdpi.com/2077-0383/8/4/427/s1, Figure S1. Method to determine the distribution of apoptotic osteocytes. (**A**) Using differential interference contrast (DIC), the peri-implant environment of round implants was visualized. (**B**) DAPI staining identified viable osteocytes in four zones circumscribing the implant. (**C**) Co-staining with TUNEL identified apoptotic osteocytes in four zones circumscribing the implant. (**D–F**) The same procedure was used to analyze the minima regions of tri-oval implants. Abbreviations: imp, implant. Scale bars = 50 µm.; Table S1. Osteotomy and implant parameters; Table S2. Osteotomy and implant parameters.

Author Contributions: Conceptualization: X.Y. and J.A.H.; methodology: X.Y. and J.A.H.; validation: X.Y., J.L., and J.A.H.; data curation: X.Y., J.L., and J.A.H.; formal analysis: X.Y., J.L., W.H., A.G., and J.B.B.; investigation: X.Y. and J.L.; writing—original draft preparation: X.Y. and J.A.H; writing—review and editing: X.Y., J.L., W.H., A.G., J.B.B., and J.A.H.; funding acquisition: X.Y., J.B.B., and J.A.H. All authors gave final approval and agree to be accountable for all aspects of the work.

Funding: This research project was supported by grants from National Natural Science Foundation of China (81801019), China Postdoctoral Science Foundation (2018M640929) and Sichuan Science and Technology Program (2019JDRC0099) to X.Y. and National Institutes of Health (DE 024000) to J.B.B. and J.A.H. In addition, funds from Nobel Biocare Services AG (Kloten, Switzerland) were used to support this research (2015-1400).

Conflicts of Interest: The authors declare no conflict of interest. J.B.B. and J.A.H. are paid consultants for Nobel Biocare. All other authors declare no potential conflicts of interest with respect to the authorship and/or publication of this article.

References

1. Wennerberg, A.; Albrektsson, T.; Chrcanovic, B. Long-term clinical outcome of implants with different surface modifications. *Eur. J. Oral Implantol.* **2018**, *11* (Suppl. 1), S123–S136.
2. Gurzawska, K.; Dirscherl, K.; Jorgensen, B.; Berglundh, T.; Jorgensen, N.R.; Gotfredsen, K. Pectin nanocoating of titanium implant surfaces—An experimental study in rabbits. *Clin. Oral Implants Res.* **2017**, *28*, 298–307. [CrossRef] [PubMed]
3. Cardoso, M.V.; de Rycker, J.; Chaudhari, A.; Coutinho, E.; Yoshida, Y.; Van Meerbeek, B.; Mesquita, M.F.; da Silva, W.J.; Yoshihara, K.; Vandamme, K.; et al. Titanium implant functionalization with phosphate-containing polymers may favour in vivo osseointegration. *J. Clin. Periodontol.* **2017**, *44*, 950–960. [CrossRef] [PubMed]
4. Cardoso, M.V.; Chaudhari, A.; Yoshihara, K.; Mesquita, M.F.; Yoshida, Y.; Van Meerbeek, B.; Vandamme, K.; Duyck, J. Phosphorylated Pullulan Coating Enhances Titanium Implant Osseointegration in a Pig Model. *Int. J. Oral Maxillofac. Implants* **2017**, *32*, 282–290. [CrossRef]
5. Becker, W.; Hujoel, P.; Becker, B.E.; Wohrle, P. Survival rates and bone level changes around porous oxide-coated implants (TiUnite). *Clin. Implants Dent. Relat. Res.* **2013**, *15*, 654–660. [CrossRef] [PubMed]
6. Branemark, P.I.; Adell, R.; Breine, U.; Hansson, B.O.; Lindstrom, J.; Ohlsson, A. Intra-osseous anchorage of dental prostheses. I. Experimental studies. *Scand. J. Plast. Reconstr. Surg.* **1969**, *3*, 81–100. [CrossRef]
7. Buser, D.; Sennerby, L.; De Bruyn, H. Modern implant dentistry based on osseointegration: 50 years of progress, current trends and open questions. *Periodontology 2000* **2017**, *73*, 7–21. [CrossRef] [PubMed]
8. Cha, J.Y.; Pereira, M.D.; Smith, A.A.; Houschyar, K.S.; Yin, X.; Mouraret, S.; Brunski, J.B.; Helms, J.A. Multiscale analyses of the bone-implant interface. *J. Dent. Res.* **2015**, *94*, 482–490. [CrossRef] [PubMed]
9. Degidi, M.; Perrotti, V.; Strocchi, R.; Piattelli, A.; Iezzi, G. Is insertion torque correlated to bone-implant contact percentage in the early healing period? A histological and histomorphometrical evaluation of 17 human-retrieved dental implants. *Clin. Oral Implants Res.* **2009**, *20*, 778–781. [CrossRef] [PubMed]
10. Meredith, N.; Book, K.; Friberg, B.; Jemt, T.; Sennerby, L. Resonance frequency measurements of implant stability in vivo. A cross-sectional and longitudinal study of resonance frequency measurements on implants in the edentulous and partially dentate maxilla. *Clin. Oral Implants Res.* **1997**, *8*, 226–233. [CrossRef]
11. Wazen, R.M.; Currey, J.A.; Guo, H.; Brunski, J.B.; Helms, J.A.; Nanci, A. Micromotion-induced strain fields influence early stages of repair at bone-implant interfaces. *Acta Biomater.* **2013**, *9*, 6663–6674. [CrossRef] [PubMed]
12. Berglundh, T.; Abrahamsson, I.; Lang, N.P.; Lindhe, J. De novo alveolar bone formation adjacent to endosseous implants. *Clin. Oral Implants Res.* **2003**, *14*, 251–262. [CrossRef] [PubMed]
13. Futami, T.; Fujii, N.; Ohnishi, H.; Taguchi, N.; Kusakari, H.; Ohshima, H.; Maeda, T. Tissue response to titanium implants in the rat maxilla: Ultrastructural and histochemical observations of the bone-titanium interface. *J. Periodontol.* **2000**, *71*, 287–298. [CrossRef] [PubMed]
14. Sandborn, P.M.; Cook, S.D.; Spires, W.P.; Kester, M.A. Tissue response to porous-coated implants lacking initial bone apposition. *J. Arthroplast.* **1988**, *3*, 337–346. [CrossRef]
15. Wang, L.; Wu, Y.; Perez, K.C.; Hyman, S.; Brunski, J.B.; Tulu, U.; Bao, C.; Salmon, B.; Helms, J.A. Effects of Condensation on Peri-implant Bone Density and Remodeling. *J. Dent. Res.* **2017**, *96*, 413–420. [CrossRef] [PubMed]
16. Suarez, D.R.; Valstar, E.R.; Rozing, P.M.; van Keulen, F. Fracture risk and initial fixation of a cementless glenoid implant: The effect of numbers and types of screws. *Proc. Inst. Mech. Eng. H J. Eng. Med.* **2013**, *227*, 1058–1066. [CrossRef]
17. Carlsson, L.; Engman, F.; Fromell, R.; Jörneus, L. Threaded Implant for Obtaining Reliable Anchoring in Bone. EP 1 030 622 B2, 14 May 2014.
18. Reams, J.W.; Goodman, R.E.; Rogers, D.P. Reduced Friction Screw-Type Dental Implant. US5902109, 11 May 1999.
19. Torcasio, A.; Zhang, X.; Van Oosterwyck, H.; Duyck, J.; van Lenthe, G.H. Use of micro-CT-based finite element analysis to accurately quantify peri-implant bone strains: A validation in rat tibiae. *Biomech. Model. Mechanobiol.* **2012**, *11*, 743–750. [CrossRef]
20. Leucht, P.; Kim, J.B.; Wazen, R.; Currey, J.A.; Nanci, A.; Brunski, J.B.; Helms, J.A. Effect of mechanical stimuli on skeletal regeneration around implants. *Bone* **2007**, *40*, 919–930. [CrossRef]

21. Leucht, P.; Monica, S.D.; Temiyasathit, S.; Lenton, K.; Manu, A.; Longaker, M.T.; Jacobs, C.R.; Spilker, R.L.; Guo, H.; Brunski, J.B.; et al. Primary cilia act as mechanosensors during bone healing around an implant. *Med. Eng. Phys.* **2012**, *35*, 392–402. [CrossRef] [PubMed]
22. Li, J.; Yin, X.; Huang, L.; Mouraret, S.; Brunski, J.B.; Cordova, L.; Salmon, B.; Helms, J.A. Relationships among Bone Quality, Implant Osseointegration, and Wnt Signaling. *J. Dent. Res.* **2017**, *96*, 822–831. [CrossRef] [PubMed]
23. Pei, X.; Wang, L.; Chen, C.; Yuan, X.; Wan, Q.; Helms, J.A. Contribution of the PDL to Osteotomy Repair and Implant Osseointegration. *J. Dent. Res.* **2017**, *96*, 909–916. [CrossRef] [PubMed]
24. Meier, E. The Wood Database 2018-2019. Available online: http://www.wood-database.com/ (accessed on 26 January 2019).
25. Seong, W.J.; Kim, U.K.; Swift, J.Q.; Heo, Y.C.; Hodges, J.S.; Ko, C.C. Elastic properties and apparent density of human edentulous maxilla and mandible. *Int. J. Oral Maxillofac. Surg.* **2009**, *38*, 1088–1093. [CrossRef] [PubMed]
26. Baldi, D.; Lombardi, T.; Colombo, J.; Cervino, G.; Perinetti, G.; Di Lenarda, R.; Stacchi, C. Correlation between Insertion Torque and Implant Stability Quotient in Tapered Implants with Knife-Edge Thread Design. *BioMed Res. Int.* **2018**, *2018*, 7201093. [CrossRef] [PubMed]
27. Yin, X.; Li, J.; Salmon, B.; Huang, L.; Lim, W.H.; Liu, B.; Hunter, D.J.; Ransom, R.C.; Singh, G.; Gillette, M.; et al. Wnt Signaling and Its Contribution to Craniofacial Tissue Homeostasis. *J. Dent. Res.* **2015**, *94*, 1487–1494. [CrossRef]
28. Cicciu, M.; Cervino, G.; Milone, D.; Risitano, G. FEM Investigation of the Stress Distribution over Mandibular Bone Due to Screwed Overdenture Positioned on Dental Implants. *Materials* **2018**, *11*, 1512. [CrossRef]
29. Bouxsein, M.L.; Boyd, S.K.; Christiansen, B.A.; Guldberg, R.E.; Jepsen, K.J.; Muller, R. Guidelines for assessment of bone microstructure in rodents using micro-computed tomography. *J. Bone Min. Res.* **2010**, *25*, 1468–1486. [CrossRef]
30. Schropp, L.; Isidor, F. Timing of implant placement relative to tooth extraction. *J. Oral Rehabil.* **2008**, *35* (Suppl. 1), 33–43. [CrossRef] [PubMed]
31. Mouraret, S.; Hunter, D.J.; Bardet, C.; Brunski, J.B.; Bouchard, P.; Helms, J.A. A pre-clinical murine model of oral implant osseointegration. *Bone* **2014**, *58*, 177–184. [CrossRef]
32. Yin, X.; Li, J.; Chen, T.; Mouraret, S.; Dhamdhere, G.; Brunski, J.B.; Zou, S.; Helms, J.A. Rescuing failed oral implants via Wnt activation. *J. Clin. Periodontol.* **2016**, *43*, 180–192. [CrossRef] [PubMed]
33. Yuan, X.; Pei, X.; Zhao, Y.; Li, Z.; Chen, C.H.; Tulu, U.S.; Liu, B.; Van Brunt, L.A.; Brunski, J.B.; Helms, J.A. Biomechanics of Immediate Postextraction Implant Osseointegration. *J. Dent. Res.* **2018**, *97*, 987–994. [CrossRef] [PubMed]
34. Zhou, W.; Han, C.; Yunming, L.; Li, D.; Song, Y.; Zhao, Y. Is the osseointegration of immediately and delayed loaded implants the same?—Comparison of the implant stability during a 3-month healing period in a prospective study. *Clin. Oral Implants Res.* **2009**, *20*, 1360–1366. [CrossRef] [PubMed]
35. West, J.D.; Oates, T.W. Identification of stability changes for immediately placed dental implants. *Int. J. Oral Maxillofac. Implants* **2007**, *22*, 623–630. [PubMed]
36. Barewal, R.M.; Stanford, C.; Weesner, T.C. A randomized controlled clinical trial comparing the effects of three loading protocols on dental implant stability. *Int. J. Oral Maxillofac. Implants* **2012**, *27*, 945–956.
37. Friberg, B.; Sennerby, L.; Meredith, N.; Lekholm, U. A comparison between cutting torque and resonance frequency measurements of maxillary implants. A 20-month clinical study. *Int. J. Oral Maxillofac. Surg.* **1999**, *28*, 297–303. [CrossRef]
38. Friberg, B.; Sennerby, L.; Linden, B.; Grondahl, K.; Lekholm, U. Stability measurements of one-stage Branemark implants during healing in mandibles. A clinical resonance frequency analysis study. *Int. J. Oral Maxillofac. Surg.* **1999**, *28*, 266–272. [CrossRef]
39. Branemark, P.I.; Hansson, B.O.; Adell, R.; Breine, U.; Lindström, J.; Hallén, O.; Ohman, A. Osseointegrated implants in the treatment of the edentulous jaw. Experience from a 10-year period. *Scand. J. Plast. Reconstr. Surg. Suppl.* **1977**, *16*, 1–132.

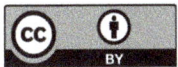

© 2019 by the authors. Licensee MDPI, Basel, Switzerland. This article is an open access article distributed under the terms and conditions of the Creative Commons Attribution (CC BY) license (http://creativecommons.org/licenses/by/4.0/).

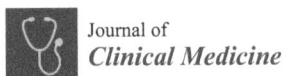

Article

Heat Generation at the Implant–Bone Interface by Insertion of Ceramic and Titanium Implants

Holger Zipprich [1,*,†], Paul Weigl [1,†], Eugenie König [2], Alexandra Toderas [3], Ümniye Balaban [4] and Christoph Ratka [1]

1 Department of Prosthodontics, Faculty of Oral and Dental Medicine at Goethe University, 60590 Frankfurt am Main, Germany; weigl@em.uni-frankfurt.de (P.W.); c.ratka@gmx.de (C.R.)
2 Private Practice, 60385 Frankfurt am Main, Germany; koenig-@hotmail.de
3 Private Practice, 60313 Frankfurt am Main, Germany; toderasalexandra@gmail.com
4 Institute of Biostatistics and Mathematical Modelling at Goethe University, 60590 Frankfurt am Main, Germany; balaban@med.uni-frankfurt.de
* Correspondence: zipprich@em.uni-frankfurt.de; Tel.: +49-69-63014714; Fax: +49-69-63013711
† Holger Zipprich and Paul Weigl contributed equally to this study.

Received: 30 August 2019; Accepted: 17 September 2019; Published: 25 September 2019

Abstract: Purpose: The aim of this study is to record material- and surface-dependent heat dissipation during the process of inserting implants into native animal bone. Materials and Methods: Implants made of titanium and zirconium that were identical in macrodesign were inserted under controlled conditions into a bovine rib tempered to 37 °C. The resulting surface temperature was measured on two bone windows by an infrared camera. The results of the six experimental groups, ceramic machined (1), sandblasted (2), and sandblasted and acid-etched surfaces (3) versus titanium implants with the corresponding surfaces (4, 5, and 6) were statistically tested. Results: The average temperature increase, 3 mm subcrestally at ceramic implants, differed with high statistical significance ($p = 7.163 \times 10^{-9}$, resulting from group-adjusted linear mixed-effects model) from titanium. The surface texture of ceramic implants shows a statistical difference between group 3 (15.44 ± 3.63 °C) and group 1 (19.94 ± 3.28 °C) or group 2 (19.39 ± 5.73 °C) surfaces. Within the titanium implants, the temperature changes were similar for all surfaces. Conclusion: Within the limits of an in vitro study, the high temperature rises at ceramic versus titanium implants should be limited by a very slow insertion velocity.

Keywords: zirconia; dental implant; insertion; bone–implant interface; heat; bone damage; early loss

1. Introduction

Although titanium and its alloys have been used successfully in dental implantology for more than five decades, there is increasing demand for a nonmetallic alternative.

The alternative material should, of course, retain the good properties of titanium and, if possible, even improve it and eliminate the disadvantages. These primarily include the color, which can cause a greyish discoloration of the peri-implant soft tissue in the esthetic area, leading to the patient's perception that the replaced tooth root is made of metal. Patients particularly prioritize high simulation quality for materials used to replace lost tissue. This has led to a similar development in restorative dentistry, although inlays and onlays made of gold alloy or crowns and bridges with a metal framework have had excellent long-term clinical results. Nevertheless, their importance is increasingly diminishing because they are being replaced by all-ceramic restorations, as patients perceive ceramic to simulate tooth hardness much better than metal. Even metal crowns and bridge frameworks that are nonvisible, because they are fully veneered, have increasingly been replaced by high-strength ceramic versions. This trend, which exists in restorative dentistry, now seems to be repeated in oral implantology:

an artificial tooth root made of ceramic simulates the replaced tissue better than titanium. In other words, in terms of the choice of materials, patients always opt for, or clinicians always tend to use, ceramics for replacing tooth tissue.

A major disadvantage of ceramic implants is their early loss that occurs in clinical trials and is observable in daily practice, which is usually associated with no clinically apparent inflammation. This phenomenon, described as aseptic loosening, is caused by a lack of osseointegration [1] or linked to reactivation of the inflammatory immune system [2]. Different forms of bone injury caused by osteotomy can be eliminated because identical osteotomy protocols are used clinically to create the bone cavity for titanium and ceramic implants. Only during implant insertion can it be assumed that there is a higher risk of overheating with ceramics than with titanium because of their different thermal conductivities. Overheating leads to increased damage or destruction of the bone directly on the implant surface.

The aim of this study is to record the material-dependent heat dissipation during the process of inserting implants into native animal bone in an in vitro setup. In addition, the influence of different implant surface treatments is evaluated. Implants made of titanium and zirconium that were identical in macrodesign were used for this purpose.

2. Materials and Methods

2.1. Implant Specimen and Surface Treatments

Y-TZP (Yttria–Tetragonal Zirconia Polycrystal) two-piece zirconia implants (5 × 14 mm) from the BPI system (BPI Biological and Physical GmbH & Co. KG, Sindelfingen, Germany) served in their packed original state as the specimen for machined ceramic implants. These cylindrical screw implants were designed with four apical cutting grooves and had a self-cutting property (Figure 1).

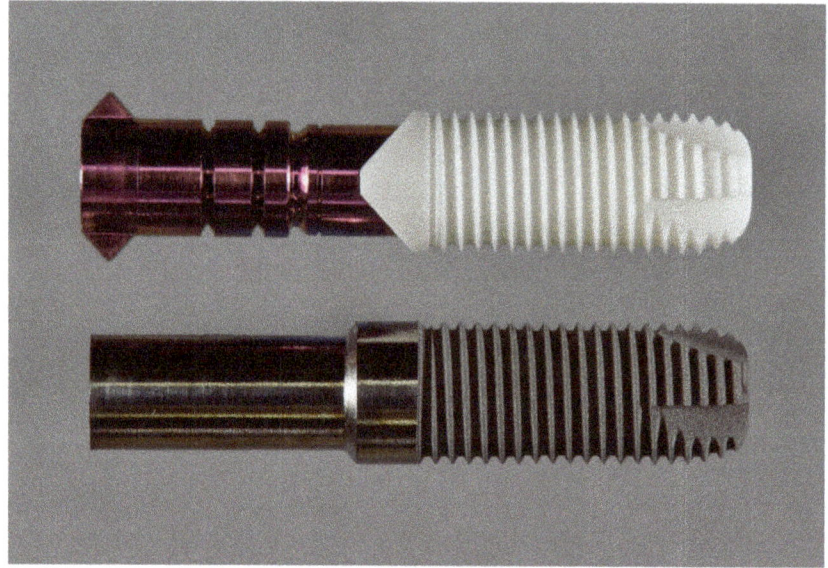

Figure 1. Implants made of zirconia and titanium with identical macrodesigns of the endosteal part coupled with the metallic insertion device.

However, the implants made of titanium from the same manufacturer differed in macrodesign from the above-mentioned ceramic implants. Therefore, the endosteal parts of the BPI ceramic implants were re-engineered to match endosteal titanium grade 4 machined parts. To simplify the re-engineering, the titanium implants were not manufactured as a two-piece (implant and abutment separable) but as a one-piece implant system (Figure 1).

In addition to the influence of the implant materials on heat generation at the implant–bone interface during the insertion process, the effect of an implant surface modification was also investigated. The topography of each surface type was scanned under a scanning electron microscope (SEM S-4500, Hitachi, Tokyo, Japan) (Figure 2). The roughness (Sa) of the implant surface in each group was measured according to ISO-25178 by a laser-scanning microscope (KEYENCE, VK-X100, Osaka, Japan).

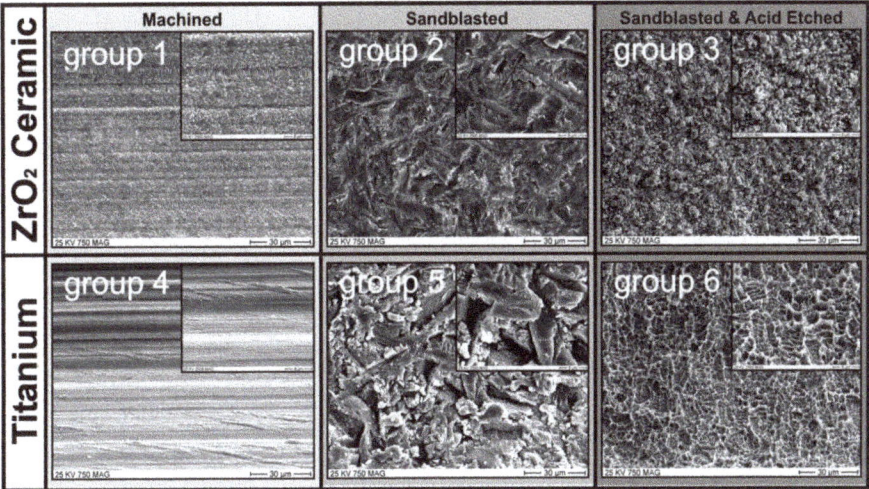

Figure 2. SEM images showing results of the different implant surface treatments. **Groups 1** and **4**: nontreated machined surfaces; **Groups 2** and **5**: sandblasted surfaces (corundum mesh size = 110 μm, working pressure = 6 bar); **Groups 3** and **6**: sandblasted and acid-etched surfaces (result: hydrophilic).

Based on two different methods of surface treatment, 6 groups of implant specimens were produced:

Groups 1 and 4: nontreated, machined, Y-TZP, two-piece zirconia (group 1) and one-piece titanium implants (group 4). The machined surface is shown in Figure 2 (Groups 1 and 4). The diameter of both implants was 5.00 mm.

Groups 2 and 5: once testing with group 1 and 4 implant specimens was finished, each implant was cleaned by water steam jet and 70% ethanol. The implant was additionally given a microstructure by sandblasting with corundum (mesh size = 110 μm, working pressure = 6 bar) at an automatic turning speed of 100 rpm until the diameter of the implants was reduced to 4.95 mm. The SEM images in Figure 2 (Groups 2 and 5) show the result of the surface treatment.

Groups 3 and 6: Once testing with group 2 and 5 implant specimens was finished, each implant was cleaned again by water steam jet and ethanol (70%). The sandblasted surface was then acid-etched to produce a nanostructure showing hydrophilic properties. The result of the acid-etching process is shown in Figure 2 (Groups 3 and 6). The diameter of the implants was further reduced to 4.90 mm.

2.2. Measurement of Heat Generation and Dissipation

The temperature at the bone–implant interface during insertion was dynamically measured by an infrared camera PI160 (PI16048T900, Optris, Berlin, Germany). The infrared camera took real-time images at a frequency of 120 Hz with an uncooled microbolometer focal plane array (FPA) detector with 160×120 pixels. The sensor had a spectral range from 7.5 to 13 μm and was equipped with a wide-angle lens with a field of view (FOV) of $48° \times 37°$. The thermal sensitivity with respect to the relative accuracy of the camera was 0.1 °C, and the minimum measuring distance was 20 mm. The absolute accuracy of the measurement was 2 °C. The temperature data from the camera were transmitted to the computer as thermal images, evaluated using Optris PI Connect software, and transferred to a spreadsheet for statistical analysis.

2.3. Bone Segments

It has been reported that the macroscopic structure of cortex and cancellous bone in the bovine rib is similar to that in the human jaw, and the bone density dependent on its position could be comparable to classes I–IV according to Lekholm & Zarb or D2–D4 according to the Mish classification in the human jaw [3–6]. The distal part of the bovine rib was used and classified as D2/D3 bone. Therefore, 14 ribs were used in this study to simulate the condition in the human jaw. Bone density measurements have not been made because the friction when inserting cylindrical implants arises mainly on the hard cortex bone [7,8] if a sufficiently high torque has been generated there (40 to 60 Ncm in this study). Therefore, when selecting the bone segments, particular care was taken to ensure that the cortical layer thickness was somewhat the same for all bovine bony ribs [7].

2.4. Experimental Settings

In each experiment, the implant was connected to the screwing unit, ensuring a stable rotational speed during insertion of the implant. In the screwing unit, the driving force was produced by a pneumatic cylinder (C85N10-75, ISO air cylinder series C85, SMC Pneumatik GmbH, Egelsbach, Germany). Then, the motor (DC-servo drive series 3564K024B CS, Faulhaber GmbH & Co KG, Schöneich, Germany) connected to a gearbox (series 30/1, 134:1, Faulhaber GmbH & Co KG, Schöneich, Germany) transmitted the force to the torque sensor (DR-20-2Nm; Lorenz Messtechnik GmbH, Alfdorf, Germany) and the collet holder. The implant was connected to the collet holder by a round-headed Allen key (3 mm) to allow rotation. The Allen key was loosely fitted to the mounting post of the implant so that insertion of the implant could remain centered in the prepared bone cavity guided by implant threads and a cone-shaped apex.

The screwing unit could be driven forward or backward axially, and its movement was recorded by a linear inductive distance sensor (LVP 100, Micro-Epsilon Messtechnik GmbH & Co. KG, Ortenburg, Germany). To simulate the environment of surrounding tissues, the bone segment and the implant were covered in a preheated polycarbonate thermo box (37 °C) to prevent heat dissipation. The infrared camera was fixed to the cover of the thermo box. The complete experimental settings are shown in Figure 3.

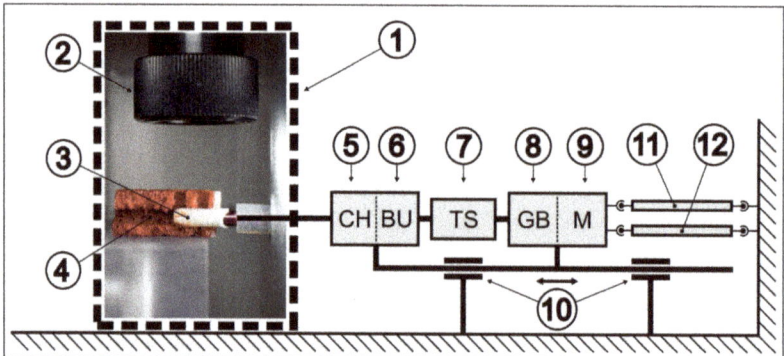

Figure 3. Diagram of the experimental setting. (**1**) Thermo box; (**2**) lens of infrared camera; (**3**) fully inserted ceramic implant; (**4**) transection of the rib segment; (**5**) collet holder (CH); (**6**) bearing unit (BU); (**7**) torque sensor (TS); (**8**) gearbox (GB); (**9**) motor (M); (**10**) linear bearing; (**11**) pneumatic cylinder; (**12**) distance sensor.

2.5. Experimental Protocol

Fourteen of the zirconia implants (groups 1–3) were included in the whole experiment, and each implant underwent 3 loops as a result of the surface treatments applied. After each implant had been assigned to one bovine rib, each bovine rib ($BR_{(1)}$–$BR_{(14)}$) was cut into 3 sequential rib segments ($RS1_{BR(1)}$–$RS3_{BR(1)}$ to $RS1_{BR(14)}$–$RS3_{BR(14)}$). Each implant (I1–I14) would undergo one type of surface modification (machined (m), sandblasted (sb), sandblasted and acid-etched (ae)) before each test program (TP1–TP3). The test sequence of the samples and the corresponding rib segments were organized as follows:

Each implant was inserted into one new rib segment after each surface modification. First, all machined implants ($I1_{(m)}$–$I14_{(m)}$) were inserted into 14 rib segments ($RS1_{BR(1)-BR(14)}$). Then, after sandblasting, implants ($I1_{(sb)}$–$I14_{(sb)}$) were inserted into rib segments ($RS2_{BR(1)-BR(14)}$). Finally, after acid-etched treatment, implants ($I1_{(ae)}$–$I14_{(ae)}$) were inserted into rib segments ($RS3_{BR(1)-BR(14)}$). Surface modification usually took several days. In order to maintain the bone in the same fresh condition in all the tests, bone segments were frozen beforehand in Ringer's solution at −10 °C and were defrosted immediately prior to the experiment.

The titanium implants underwent identical protocols. Since they were made especially for this study, a higher number of pieces was available at the beginning of the trial. Therefore, with torques outside the interval of 40 to 60 Ncm, new Ti implants were used to repeat the insertion test so that 15 measurements per group could be realized (Table 1). The selected torque window was clinically sufficient for immediate restoration of ceramic implants (>35 Ncm), which are often still used as one-piece implants. Furthermore, smaller torques do not produce sufficiently high temperatures by friction between the implant surface and the hard cortical bone [8] to be able to detect the effect of different thermal conductivities between titanium and ceramic at the bone–implant interface.

Contrary to Ti implants, for this study only 14 ceramic implants were available from the manufacturer. Therefore, when the torque was too low or too high, bone penetration tests with the respective surface structure were no longer repeated in order to mechanically protect the connection of the implant driver with the ceramic implant. In addition, cleaning the surfaces of bone remnants would have been a process in which, above all, the roughened ceramic surfaces could have been structurally changed; thus, the equality of specimens could no longer be ensured. Because of this limitation of available ceramic implants, only 8 measurements in group 1, 11 measurements in group 2, and 11 measurements in group 3 could be realized (Table 1).

When one test started, the selected bone segment would be defrosted in Ringer's solution at 37 °C and stored at the same temperature in the oven to simulate the human condition.

The implant bed was prepared using a twist drill (Type N, 118° DIN 338 R-N, Gühring KG, Albstadt, Germany) at the speed of 800 rpm. Since the bone was already wetted, additional water cooling was not necessary. To ensure a comparable insertion resistance in the three loops, the diameter of each implant site matched the implant diameter, that is, twist drills with diameters of 4.3, 4.25, and 4.20 mm were used in loops 1, 2, and 3, respectively.

To dynamically record temperature directly at the bone–implant interface, two bone windows perpendicular to the insertion path were made at 3 and 9 mm subcrestally by a twist drill (Figure 4).

Table 1. Temperature increase of the 6 groups.

Group	Analyzed (40–60 Ncm/Inserted)	Material	Surface Treatment	Surface Roughness Sa (µm)	Compacta Thickness (mm)	Insertion Torque (Ncm)	Temperature Increase BW-1 (°C)	ΔT > 10 °C BW-1 No.	Time (s)	ΔT > 13 °C BW-1 No.	Time (s)	ΔT > 18 °C BW-1 No.	Time (s)	Temperature Increase BW-2 (°C)
1	8/14	ZrO$_2$	M	0.93 ± 0.16	2.51 ± 0.25	52.61 ± 5.10	19.94 ± 3.28	8/8	39.06	8/8	25.10	5/8	11.36	7.50 ± 2.64 °C
2	11/14	ZrO$_2$	S	1.86 ± 0.38	2.75 ± 0.47	48.97 ± 6.43	19.39 ± 5.73	11/11	28.10	10/11	16.93	6/11	7.98	6.14 ± 2.40 °C
3	11/14	ZrO$_2$	SAE	2.14 ± 0.62	2.61 ± 0.39	48.79 ± 5.19	15.44 ± 3.63	10/11	20.37	8/11	10.19	3/11	0.43	6.07 ± 3.11 °C
4	15/22	Ti Grade 4	M	0.37 ± 0.04	2.46 ± 0.12	50.10 ± 8.69	9.33 ± 4.18	7/15	22.49	3/15	19.07	1/15	20.40	6.03 ± 3.69 °C
5	15/20	Ti Grade 4	S	2.15 ± 0.24	2.46 ± 0.12	50.99 ± 7.97	9.20 ± 3.31	6/15	23.05	2/15	15.65	-	-	4.33 ± 3.26 °C
6	15/21	Ti Grade 4	SAE	1.89 ± 0.18	2.42 ± 0.09	50.72 ± 7.22	7.68 ± 2.68	2/15	17.45	-	-	-	-	4.41 ± 2.47 °C

M = machined, S = sandblasted, SAE = sandblasted and acid etched, BW = bone window.

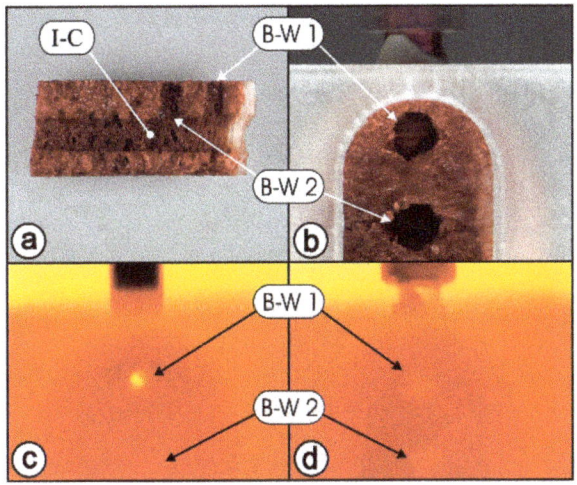

Figure 4. Dynamic temperature record at the bone–implant interface. (**a**) Transection of a rib segment; (**b**) overview of a rib segment; (**c**) infrared image at T3 in Figure 5; (**d**) infrared image at T7 in Figure 5. I-C = Implant Cavity 1; B-W 1 = Bone Window 1; B-W 2 = Bone Window 2.

A

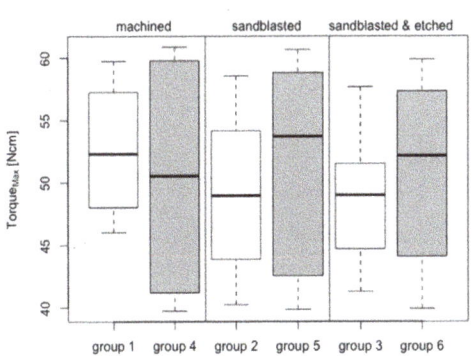

B

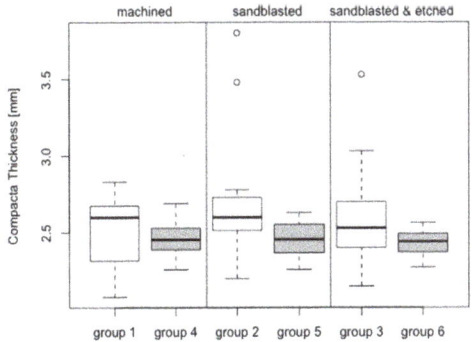

Figure 5. *Cont.*

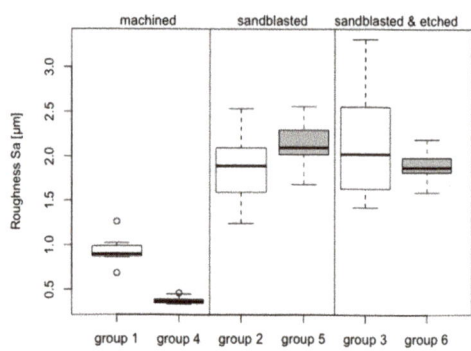

Figure 5. Box plots comparing (**A**) insertion torque, (**B**) cortical bone thickness, and (**C**) roughness.

Before each test, the bone was brought to a temperature of 37 °C inside an oven with saturated humidity. After the bone segment was immobilized, the implant was prewetted in Ringer's solution used to simulate human blood, and then it was driven with a starting pressure of 5 N and a constant rotational speed of 25 rpm to a depth of 12 mm inside the bone. Meanwhile, the infrared camera continuously recorded the temperature through each bone window (2b & T7 in Figure 5), and the difference between the maximum and the starting temperature (37 °C) during insertion would be calculated (ΔT). The change of torque was recorded by torque sensors (DR-20, Lorenz Messtechnik GmbH, Alfdorf, Germany) with the frequency of 100 Hz. Data from groups in which the insertion torque was above 60 Ncm or below 40 Ncm were excluded from the analysis.

After each experiment, the thickness of cortical bone at the insertion point was measured with a caliper gauge. When the temperature, measured at the position 3 mm subcrestally, exceeded 47 °C (ΔT >10 °C) [9], 50 °C (>13 °C) [10], or 55 °C (>18 °C) [11], the corresponding exposure time was calculated.

2.6. Statistical Analysis

Continuous variables are represented as mean ± standard deviation for each group. Comparisons were performed using the Mann–Whitney U test, t-test, or paired t-test. Comparisons with more than 2 groups were analyzed by ANOVA or the Kruskal–Wallis test, depending on Gaussian distribution. Additionally, comparisons using adjusted linear mixed-effects models (LMEs) were performed. Gaussian distributions of data were assessed with the Shapiro–Wilk test. The level of significance in post hoc tests was corrected for multiple testing. The level of significance was set at $\alpha = 0.05$, and all tests were two-sided. Statistical analysis was performed using R 3.6.1 with the packages multicomp 1.4-10, nlme 3.1-140, and plotrix 3.6-3. R, and the packages used are available from CRAN at http://CRAN.R-project.org/.

3. Results

3.1. Group-Related Parameters of Specimens and in Vitro Setup

To ensure that temperature change assessments were comparable with each other, only the implants with insertion torque between 40 and 60 Ncm were included in the analysis. Six machined and three sandblasted implants (groups 1 and 2, respectively) that exceeded an insertion torque of 60 Ncm, and three sandblasted etched implants (group 3) that had an insertion torque under 40 Ncm, were excluded from the analysis. From groups 4 to 6, all 15 specimens were analyzed. The resulting insertion torque was comparable for all 6 groups (group 1: 52.61 ± 5.10 Ncm; group 2: 48.97 ± 6.43

Ncm; group 3: 48.79 ± 5.19 Ncm; group 4: 50.10 ± 8.69 Ncm; group 5: 50.99 ± 7.97 Ncm; group 6: 50.72 ± 7.22 Ncm; $p > 0.05$; Figure 5a.).

The thickness of the cortical plate of the bovine bone rib was similar between the 6 groups (group 1: 2.51 ± 0.25 mm; group 2: 2.75 ± 0.47 mm; group 3: 2.61 ± 0.39 mm; group 4: 2.46 ± 0.12 mm; group 5: 2.46 ± 0.12 mm; group 6: 2.42 ± 0.09 mm; $p > 0.05$; Figure 5b).

The average roughness (Sa) of the machined implants (group 1: 0.93 ± 0.16 μm; group 4: 0.37 ± 0.04) was, as expected, significantly lower than that of sandblasted implants (group 2: 1.86 ± 0.38 μm; group 5: 2.15 ± 0.24 μm; all comparisons have p-values < 0.001) and sandblasted and acid-etched implants (group 3: 2.14 ± 0.62 μm; group 6: 1.89 ± 0.18 μm; all comparisons have p-values < 0.001; Figure 5c). The difference in surface roughness between ceramic and titanium implants after sandblasting (group 2 vs. group 5) and after sandblasting and acid-etching (groups 3 vs. 6) was not statistically significant ($p > 0.05$). The roughness between the machined surfaces (groups 1 and 4) was not statistically significant ($p > 0.05$). In paired comparisons of the surface treatments, the machined and the sandblasted groups showed significant differences (groups 1 and 4 $p = 1.213 \times 10^{-4}$; groups 2 and 5 $p = 0.025756$). The sandblasted and acid-etched groups (groups 3 and 6) showed no significant differences ($p > 0.05$).

3.2. Maximum Temperature Increase

3.2.1. Bone Window 1

In bone window 1 (located 3 mm subcrestally), the average temperature increase at the zirconia implants had a high statistically significant difference to that of titanium implants ($p = 7.163 \times 10^{-9}$, resulting from group-adjusted linear mixed-effects models).

Within the zirconia implants (groups 1: 19.94 °C ± 3.28 °C; 2: 19.39 °C ± 5.73 °C; 3: 15.44 °C ± 3.63 °C) there were significant differences between groups 2 and 3 ($p = 0.04426$) and groups 1 and 3 ($p = 0.007525$; Figure 6). By contrast, there was no significant difference between the comparison of groups 1 and 2 ($p > 0.05$).

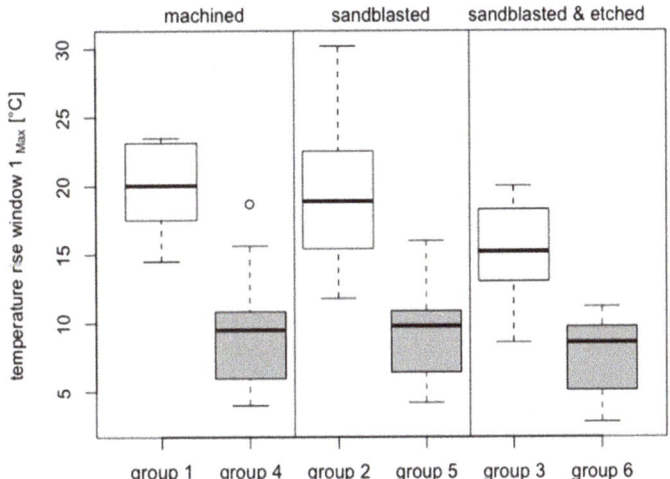

Figure 6. Box plots showing rise of temperature at bone window 1—results of all 6 groups.

Within the titanium implants (group 4: 9.33 °C ± 4.18 °C; group 5: 9.20 °C ± 3.31 °C; group 6: 7.68 °C ± 2.68 °C), the temperature changes were similar for all groups ($p > 0.05$).

In paired comparisons of the different materials with the identical surface treatments, all groups showed highly significant differences (groups 1 and 4 $p = 3.728 \times 10^{-11}$; groups 2 and 5 $p = 7.721 \times 10^{-6}$; groups 3 and 6 $p = 1.725 \times 10^{-6}$ Figure 6).

3.2.2. Bone Window 2

In bone window 2 (located 9 mm subcrestally), the average temperature increase at the zirconia implants had a high statistically significant difference than that of titanium implants ($p = 7.182 \times 10^{-12}$, resulting from group-adjusted linear mixed-effects models).

Within the zirconia implants (group 1: 7.50 °C ± 2.64 °C; group 2: 6.14 °C ± 2.40 °C; group 3: 6.07 °C ± 3.11 °C), the temperature changes were similar for all groups ($p > 0.05$).

Within the titanium implants (group 4: 6.03 °C ± 3.69 °C; group 5: 4.33 °C ± 3.26 °C; group 6: 4.41 °C ± 2.47 °C), the temperature changes were similar for all groups ($p > 0.05$).

3.3. Overheating Exposure Time

3.3.1. Bone Window 1

ΔT > 10 °C

In bone window 1, the average exposure times under ΔT > 10 °C at the zirconia implants were 39.06 s for machined (all 8 of 8 in group 1), 28.10 s for sandblasted (11 of 11 in group 2), and then decreased to 20.37 s for sandblasted etched implants (10 of 11 in group 3). The average exposure times under ΔT >10 °C at the titanium implants were 22.49 s for machined (7 of 15 in group 4), 23.05 s for sandblasted (6 of 15 in group 5), and then decreased to 17.45 s for sandblasted etched implants (2 of 15 in group 6). None of the tested implants experienced a temperature increase of more than 10 °C over a period of more than 60 s.

ΔT > 13 °C

The average exposure time under ΔT >13 °C for ceramic implants was 25.10 s in group 1, 16.93 s in group 2, and 10.19 s in group 3. Three machined implants (group 1: 42.2, 36.1, and 32.1 s) and two sandblasted implants (group 2: 34.6 and 33.2 s) experienced more than 30 s temperature increase of over 13 °C. No sandblasted and acid-etched implants (group 3) experienced such a temperature change for longer than 30 s.

The average exposure time under ΔT >13 °C for titanium implants was 19.03 s at 3 of 15 implants in group 4 (group 4: 19.8, 21.8, and 15.6 s). Two machined implants experienced more than 13 °C temperature increase (group 5: 13.9 and 17.4 s) No sandblasted and acid-etched implants (group 6) experienced a temperature increase of 13 °C or more.

ΔT > 18 °C

The average exposure time under ΔT > 18 °C for ceramic implants was 11.36 s at 5 of 8 implants in group 1, 7.98 s at 6 of 11 implants in group 2, and 0.43 s at 3 of 11 implants in group 3. Two machined ceramic implants (group 1: 25.4 and 14.2 s) and two sandblasted ceramic implants (group 2: 19.0 and 16.7 s) experienced a temperature increase of more than 18 °C for more than 14 s. No sandblasted and acid-etched implants (group 3) experienced a temperature change greater than 18 °C for more than 14 s.

Only one titanium implant (group 4) exceeded 18.70 °C and had an exposure time of 20.40 s for ΔT > 18 °C.

3.3.2. Bone Window 2

In bone window 2, the temperature increase never exceeded values > 10 °C.

3.4. Material-Dependent Thermal Energy Propagation

Figure 7 shows the image captured by the infrared camera during the process of inserting titanium and ceramic implants, both with sandblasted and acid-etched surfaces. Prior to the insertion process—meaning the implants were completely outside of the bone cavity—there was very little temperature difference between the titanium implant (33.2 °C) and the ceramic implant (31.2 °C). Bone window 1 shows the nearly regulated temperature of the thermo box (Figure 3) encapsulating the in vitro setup (37.5 °C; 37.2 °C).

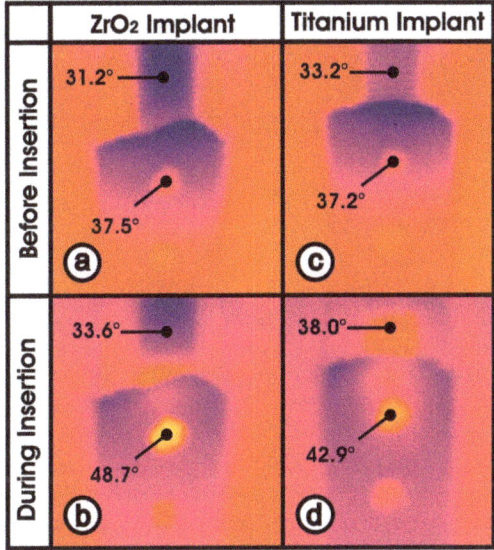

Figure 7. Material-dependent heat dissipation. (**a**) ceramic implant before insertion; (**b**) ceramic implant during insertion; (**c**) titanium implant before insertion; (**d**) titanium implant during insertion.

At the moment of maximum temperature development during implant insertion, the ceramic implant was heated to 48.7 °C below the cortical bone (bone window 1) and to 33.6 °C outside the bone. In contrast, the titanium implant showed 42.9 °C within bone window 1 and 38.0 °C outside the bone. Thus, at the same distance, the titanium implant had a 3 times lower temperature gradient than the ceramic implant during the insertion process ($\Delta T_{ceramic}$ = 15.1 °C vs. $\Delta T_{titanium}$ = 4.9 °C).

The summary of all results is shown in Table 1.

4. Discussion

The aim of the in vitro study was to dynamically detect heat development at the bone–implant interface during the entire process of inserting a cylindrical screw implant into bone. For this purpose, an in vitro setup was developed, which achieves the highest possible quality of simulation of the clinical conditions and uses of test specimens, which differ in only one parameter, as far as possible.

4.1. Identical Specimen

It was important for good reproducibility of the temperature values at the implant surface that the implant specimens had an identical endosteal macrodesign and were identically manufactured (Figures 1 and 2). The measured surface roughness (Figure 5b) did not differ significantly between the ceramic (ZrO_2) and titanium implant materials in the sandblasted and sandblasted-etched surfaces. Only on the machined implants was the titanium surface statistically significantly smoother.

Repetition of the test series with the same implants after each additional surface treatment allowed for a nearly identical macrodesign with a different microdesign. Only removal of material by subtractive surface treatment caused a reduction in implant diameter. However, this was recorded by measurement and taken into account in the osteotomy protocol. In other words, the last cutter for bone preparation was also correspondingly smaller in diameter.

4.2. In Vitro Setup

Several published articles reporting on heat development when screwing an implant into the bone cavity have used bovine bone [12], in particular the bovine rib [9,10,13–16]. Bone segments with a cortical thickness of around 2.5 mm were chosen in order to mimic the known thickness of the human mandible (1.0–2.5 mm) [17–19] and to ensure the almost same amount of friction between bone and implant surfaces [7,8]. The temperature rise was generated in the ceramic implant mainly in the cortex bone (see bone window No. 1). In cancellous bone, however, there were no statistically significant differences in the temperature increase. This reinforces the assumed mechanism of temperature generation: in the case of a sufficiently high torque (40–60 Nm) and a conventional screw thread, most of the friction is generated between hard bone and the implant surface. Only special aggressive threads—for example, in Nobel Active in spongy bone, a mechanism other than friction—can generate high torque or primary stability—compression of trabeculae. Therefore, in the selection of the bone ribs, particular attention was paid to a comparable layer thickness of the cortex [7]. Since the spongy part of the rib in the present macrodesign of the examined implants (cylindrical, conventional screw thread) hardly generates any friction or heating, determination of the bone mineral density was omitted. Therefore, a high variation in the bone density in the spongy region of the rib probably has no influence on the measurement results in bone window 2.

Although blood circulation was absent in this case, the remaining conditions such as the chemical composition, density, humidity, structure, as well as mechanical and thermal properties were similar to those of the human bone. By contrast, artificial bone models cannot properly simulate the human bone because there are huge differences in thermal conductivity and heat capacity [20].

The anatomical structure—cortical bone and the underlying cancellous bone—are suitable for simulation of a toothless, healed alveolar bone. In order to keep the high anatomical variance of bovine ribs reasonably small in this investigation, the ribs were frozen after a test run so that measurements could at least be done on the identical bovine rib after the respective surface treatment of the implants for the second and third test runs.

An infrared camera (Figure 3) measured the temperature during the insertion process. In contrast to this investigation, Markovic et al. [21] captured the temperature at the surface of a bone segment. The two bone windows in this study allowed temperature to be measured directly on the implant surface. As a result, system-related measurement distortions due to differently positioned temperature probes in peri-implant bone could be avoided [9,10,13–16].

The above factors resulted in a relatively small variation of the temperature values per experimental group (Figures 6 and 7). Thus, the goal of good reproducibility of the measurement conditions was achieved in the experimental setup used. In addition, the direct measurement of the surface temperature of the implants makes the nonsimulated, cooling effect of a well-perfused bone marrow smaller than with probes placed in the peri-implant bone [9,10,13–16]. Furthermore, the low thermal conductivity of bone (approximately 1/100 of titanium) can lead to thermal isolation of the sensors. The temperature-controlled thermo box (Figure 3(1)) additionally contributed to the good reproducibility of the measured temperature values (Figure 7).

In the selection of bovine ribs, care was taken to ensure that the layer thickness of the cortical bone did not differ a great deal (Figure 5b). It is apparent that, in a cylindrical implant, the heat generated by friction is primarily generated by the hard cortical bone and only slightly by the soft cancellous bone located below. The torques achieved during the insertion process were another indicator of identical experimental conditions: trial implants were hardly distinguishable in macro- and microdesigns and comparable layer thicknesses of the cortical bone (Figure 5a). In this study, the experimental parameters were chosen to simulate a high insertion torque (40–60 Ncm). It was above the average level suggested by most manufacturers (35 or 45 Ncm); nevertheless, this range was still below the maximum endurance for the ceramic implants.

In the case of rare outliers in insertion torques, the temperature readings were not included in the evaluation, but the complete measurement was repeated with the respective implant.

The remaining parameters (ambient temperature, rpm and feed at insertion, and dimension of the bone cavity) were kept reproducible and constant with conventional control circuits in the experimental setup (Figure 3).

4.3. Temperature Increase at Bone Window 1

The implant surface temperatures just below the cortical bone were highly significantly different between the ceramic and titanium implants. Statistical evaluation was performed using a group-adjusted linear mixed-effects model.

The increased temperature of the ceramic implant was due to its poor thermal conductivity. It was 2.5 W/mK and, thus, nearly ten times lower than titanium (22 W/mK). The thermal energy generated at the bone–implant interface during insertion dissipated poorly over the ceramic implant at locations further away. The thermal energy remained at the place of its formation and led to a higher temperature. This phenomenon is visible in Figure 7 from the infrared camera image. During the insertion process, the ceramic implant outside the bone (33.6 °C) heated up significantly less than the titanium implant (38.0 °C) under nearly identical experimental conditions. This means that much more heat (48.7 °C) was created in the bone at window 1 on the ceramic implant surface than in the titanium implant (42.9 °C). The increase in temperature, due to the greatly reduced thermal conductivity of ceramics, can hardly be reduced by intensive water cooling because the water has no access to the implant–bone interface during screwing-in of the implant [8], and the poor heat conduction of ceramics only cools the implant, which is not yet in the bone. It is obvious that only an extremely slow insertion of the implant can reduce the heating of the cortex bone [7,8,12,22].

Analysis of the temperature in bone window 1 (Figure 6) for all six experimental groups again showed a statistically significant increase in temperature at the ceramic implant compared to the titanium implant, regardless of the surface structure. However, the increase in temperature of ceramic implants with sandblasted and acid-etched surfaces (15.44 °C) was statistically significantly smaller than that with the machined (19.94 °C) or purely sandblasted (19.39 °C) ceramic surface. This effect of surface modification could possibly occur as a result of the high porosity of the sandblasted and acid-etched surface of ZrO_2 implants (Figure 2). In particular, it shows nanoscopic pores smaller than 500 nm. This type of pore is too small to be reflected in the roughness average (Sa) but can be filled with blood and other tissue fluids, which in turn can function as heat storage and a cooling fluid. In other words, the blood and tissue fluid on the surface are heated. The heat capacity of water is 4.182 kJ/kg/K, which is more than 10 times higher than that of zirconia at 0.4 kJ/kg/K, and the density of zirconia is 6.08 g/cm^3, which is 6 times higher than that of water. Thus, in order to increase the temperature of blood or tissue fluid on the blasted and acid-etched surface by 1 °C, a 1.72 times higher heat energy would be required than in the ZrO_2 surfaces without fluids captured in nanoscopic pores—like machined (group 1) or sandblasted surfaces (group 2), where the latter results in a higher temperature increase at the implant–bone interfaces (Figure 6).

Another explanation of the result is based on a tribological effect [23]. Improved lubrication by the fluid trapped in the nanoscopic pores produces reduced heat development as it rotates through the cortical bone.

However, the temperature increase in the titanium implants is independent of their surface condition (Figure 6). This result might be related to good thermal conductivity, which allows rapid cooling of the titanium surface in bone window 1. In the bone window itself, there is no friction caused by close-fitting peri-implant bone.

4.4. Temperature Increase at Bone Window 2

The temperatures at the implant surface occurring in cancellous bone were different between the ceramic and titanium implants. Statistical evaluation was performed using a group-adjusted linear mixed-effects model.

The inter-group comparison (Figure 8) shows no statistically significant differences in temperature increase with respect to the test parameters of implant material and surface texture. Owing to low rigidity and the tissue structure interspersed with fat, the cancellous bone causes considerably less friction at the implant–bone interface than at the stiff and hard cortical bone. Therefore, the different thermal conductivities of the ceramic and titanium implants probably play a minor role in the temperature increase in bone window 2.

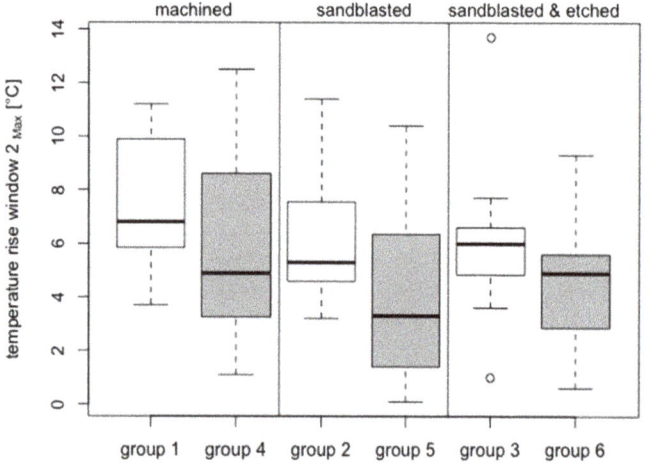

Figure 8. Box plots showing rise of temperature at bone window 2—results of all 6 groups.

4.5. Differences in Bone Window 1 versus Bone Window 2

In this study, the bone windows for heat measurement were prepared 3 and 9 mm subcrestally in order to measure the change of the bone–implant interfacial temperature during implant insertion at the positions near the cortex and inside the implant cavity, respectively. As expected, the interfacial increase of temperature near the cortex was higher than that deep in the cancellous bone, regardless of the surface modification. In the study by Sener et al., the highest temperature in the process of preparing the implant bed was also observed in the superficial part of the implant cavity, and the heat decreased in the direction of the implant apex [17].

The different structure of cortical and cancellous bone as well as the higher frictional coefficient of hard cortical bone can lead to different frictional effects on the bone–implant surface; furthermore, the bone region at window 1 is exposed to friction for a longer time than the region of window 2 near the apex of the implant cavity. These factors, combined with the different thermal conductivities of the cortical and cancellous bone, result in more heat energy produced and accumulated in the cortical part during implant insertion.

Previously published studies showed different temperature increases during insertion of a titanium implant (0.55–9.81 °C) [12,21,24,25]. This might be due to temperatures being measured at the outer surface of the bone segment [24] or at a distance of 0.5–1 mm from the implant [12,21,25]. In addition, Sumer et al. [9] found more heat was generated with ceramic drills than with stainless steel drills at the superficial part of the drilling cavity.

4.6. Heat Caused Damage to Peri-implant Bone

The damage to the bone caused by overheating is related to the time it is exposed to the heating [26–28]. The higher the bone–implant interfacial temperature, the shorter the time it takes for bone damage to appear [26]. Eriksson and Albrektsson claim that bone damage occurs when the bone–implant interfacial temperature reaches at least 47 °C for 1 min [27]. As a result, the primary stability of the implants would decrease, and implants might loosen shortly after loading [28]. Furthermore, it was shown by Lundskog [26] that osteocytes underwent necrosis as soon as the bone was exposed to 50 °C for more than 30 s. Schmelzeisen et al. [28] showed that a temperature between 50 and 60 °C caused irreversible damage to osteocytes for an exposure time of 8 to 20 s. Based on that study, the median values of 55 °C and 14 s were applied as critical parameters in the current study. The interfacial temperature of ceramic implants measured near the cortical plate (bone window 1) were 56.94 °C on machined, 56.39 °C on sandblasted, and 52.43 °C on sandblasted-etched implants, with the starting temperature of 37 °C. Thus, the potential for bone damage induced by overheating was present on each surface. However, the heat and the relative exposure time decreased with the sandblasted and acid-etched surfaces, suggesting that the risk of bone damage could be reduced with proper surface modification.

Nevertheless, the results of this in vitro study might not fully represent the reality under clinical conditions [11,29]. The difference resulting from blood circulation and the thermal conductivity between nonlive and live tissues can influence the change in interfacial temperature [26]. Since the blood flow is six times higher in cancellous bone than in cortical bone, and blood can absorb part of the heat produced during implant insertion, the interfacial temperature increase in the cancellous bone is supposed to be smaller than that in the cortical bone. In view of this fact, the authors did not expect a significant cooling effect inside a patient's cortical bone.

Based on this study, the heat produced during the implant insertion process mainly depends on the implant material and less on surface modification.

5. Conclusions

The results of this in vitro study show a temperature rise that is dangerous for the peri-implant cortical bone when a ceramic implant is inserted. Despite limited transferability to the clinical situation, the authors recommend a very slow insertion velocity for ceramic implants to avoid early implant losses.

Author Contributions: Conceptualization, H.Z., P.W. and E.K.; Data curation, H.Z.; Formal analysis, H.Z., E.K., U.B. and C.R.; Funding acquisition, H.Z.; Investigation, H.Z., E.K., A.T. and C.R.; Methodology, H.Z., E.K. and A.T.; Project administration, H.Z., P.W. and C.R.; Resources, H.Z.; Software, H.Z.; Supervision, H.Z., P.W. and C.R.; Validation, H.ZFig., P.W., E.K., A.T. and C.R.; Visualization, H.Z., P.W. and C.R.; Writing—original draft, H.Z., P.W., E.K. and C.R.; Writing—review & editing, H.Z., P.W., E.K., A.T., U.B. and C.R.

Acknowledgments: This research did not receive any specific grant from funding agencies in the public, commercial, or not-for-profit sectors.

Conflicts of Interest: The authors declare no conflicts of interest.

References

1. Cionca, N.; Müller, N.; Mombelli, A. Two-piece zirconia implants supporting all-ceramic crowns: A prospective clinical study. *Clin. Oral Implant. Res.* **2015**, *26*, 413–418. [CrossRef] [PubMed]
2. Albrektsson, T.; Jemt, T.; Mölne, J.; Tengvall, P.; Wennerberg, A. On inflammation-immunological balance theory-A critical apprehension of disease concepts around implants: Mucositis and marginal bone loss may represent normal conditions and not necessarily a state of disease. *Clin. Implant Dent. Relat. Res.* **2019**, *21*, 183–189. [CrossRef] [PubMed]
3. Lachmann, S.; Jager, B.; Axmann, D.; Gomez-Roman, G.; Groten, M.; Weber, H. Resonance frequency analysis and damping capacity assessment. Part I: An in vitro study on measurement reliability and a method of comparison in the determination of primary dental implant stability. *Clin. Oral Implant. Res.* **2006**, *17*, 75–79. [CrossRef]

4. Garcia-Vives, N.; Andres-Garcia, R.; Rios-Santos, V.; Fernandez-Palacin, A.; Bullon-Fernandez, P.; Herrero-Climent, M.; Herrero-Climent, F. In vitro evaluation of the type of implant bed preparation with osteotomes in bone type IV and its influence on the stability of two implant systems. *Med. Oral Patol. Oral Cir. Bucal* **2009**, *14*, 455–460.
5. Moon, S.H.; Um, H.S.; Lee, J.K.; Chang, B.S.; Lee, M.K. The effect of implant shape and bone preparation on primary stability. *J. Periodontal Implant Sci.* **2010**, *40*, 239–243. [CrossRef] [PubMed]
6. Baker, J.A.; Vora, S.; Bairam, L.; Kim, H.I.; Davis, E.L.; Andreana, S. Piezoelectric vs. conventional implant site preparation: Ex vivo implant primary stability. *Clin. Oral Implant. Res.* **2012**, *23*, 433–437. [CrossRef]
7. Matsuoka, M.; Motoyoshi, M.; Sakaguchi, M.; Shinohara, A.; Shigeede, T.; Saito, Y.; Matsuda, M.; Shimizu, N. Friction heat during self-drilling of an orthodontic miniscrew. *Int. J. Oral Maxillofac. Surg.* **2011**, *40*, 191–194. [CrossRef]
8. Aghvami, M.; Brunski, J.B.; Tulu, U.S.; Chen, C.H.; Helms, J.A. A Thermal and Biological Analysis of Bone Drilling. *J. Biomech. Eng.* **2018**, *140*, 101010. [CrossRef]
9. Sumer, M.; Misir, A.F.; Telcioglu, N.T.; Guler, A.U.; Yenisey, M. Comparison of heat generation during implant drilling using stainless steel and ceramic drills. *J. Oral Maxillofac. Surg.* **2011**, *69*, 1350–1354. [CrossRef]
10. Biyikli, S.; Modest, M.F.; Tarr, R. Measurements of thermal properties for human femora. *J. Biomed. Mater. Res.* **1986**, *20*, 1335–1345. [CrossRef] [PubMed]
11. Trisi, P.; Berardini, M.; Falco, A.; Vulpiani, M.P.; Masciotra, L. Effect of 50 to 60°C heating on osseointegration of dental implants in dense bone: An in vivo histological study. *Implant Dent.* **2014**, *23*, 516–521. [CrossRef] [PubMed]
12. Flanagan, D. Heat generated during seating of dental implant fixtures. *J. Oral Implantol.* **2014**, *40*, 174–181. [CrossRef] [PubMed]
13. Matthews, L.S.; Hirsch, C. Temperatures measured in human cortical bone when drilling. *J. Bone Jt. Surg.* **1972**, *54*, 297–308. [CrossRef] [PubMed]
14. Matthews, L.S.; Green, C.A.; Goldstein, S.A. The thermal effects of skeletal fixation-pin insertion in bone. *J. Bone Jt. Surg.* **1984**, *66*, 1077–1083. [CrossRef] [PubMed]
15. Bachus, K.N.; Rondina, M.T.; Hutchinson, D.T. The effects of drilling force on cortical temperatures and their duration: An in vitro study. *Med. Eng. Phys.* **2000**, *22*, 685–691. [CrossRef]
16. Oh, H.J.; Wikesjo, U.M.; Kang, H.S.; Ku, Y.; Eom, T.G.; Koo, K.T. Effect of implant drill characteristics on heat generation in osteotomy sites: A pilot study. *Clin. Oral Implant. Res.* **2011**, *22*, 722–726. [CrossRef]
17. Sener, B.C.; Dergin, G.; Gursoy, B.; Kelesoglu, E.; Slih, I. Effects of irrigation temperature on heat control in vitro at different drilling depths. *Clin. Oral Implant. Res.* **2009**, *20*, 294–298. [CrossRef] [PubMed]
18. Schmelzeisen, H. Thermische Schäden bei der Osteosynthese. *OP-Journal* **1992**, *8*, 26–29. (In German)
19. Eriksson, A.R.; Albrektsson, T.; Albrektsson, B. Heat caused by drilling cortical bone. Temperature measured in vivo in patients and animals. *Acta. Orthop. Scand.* **1984**, *55*, 629–631. [CrossRef]
20. Kunze, K.G.; Hofstetter, H.; Posalaky, I.; Winkler, B. Veränderung der Knochendurchblutung nach Osteotomien und Osteosynthesen. *Unfallchirurgie* **1981**, *7*, 169–180. (In German) [CrossRef]
21. Markovic, A.; Misic, T.; Milicic, B.; Calvo-Guirado, J.L.; Aleksic, Z.; Dinic, A. Heat generation during implant placement in low-density bone: Effect of surgical technique, insertion torque and implant macro design. *Clin. Oral Implant. Res.* **2013**, *24*, 798–805. [CrossRef]
22. Stocchero, M.; Jinno, Y.; Toia, M.; Ahmad, M.; Papia, E.; Yamaguchi, S.; Becktor, J.P. Intraosseous Temperature Change during Installation of Dental Implants with Two Different Surfaces and Different Drilling Protocols: An In Vivo Study in Sheep. *J. Clin. Med.* **2019**, *8*, 1198. [CrossRef] [PubMed]
23. Ludema, K.C.; Ajayi, L. *Friction, Wear, Lubrication: A Textbook in Tribology*, 2nd ed.; CRS Press: Boca Raton, FL, USA, 2018; ISBN 9781482210170.
24. Markovic, A.; Misic, T.; Mancic, D.; Jovanovic, I.; Scepanovic, M.; Jezdic, Z. Real-time thermographic analysis of low-density bone during implant placement: A randomized parallel-group clinical study comparing lateral condensation with bone drilling surgical technique. *Clin. Oral Implant. Res.* **2014**, *25*, 910–918. [CrossRef]
25. Sumer, M.; Keskiner, I.; Mercan, U.; Misir, F.; Cankaya, S. Assessment of heat generation during implant insertion. *J. Prosthet. Dent.* **2014**, *112*, 522–525. [CrossRef] [PubMed]
26. Lundskog, J. Heat and bone tissue. An experimental investigation of the thermal properties of bone and threshold levels for thermal injury. *Scand. J. Plast. Reconstr. Surg.* **1972**, *9*, 1–80. [PubMed]

27. Eriksson, A.R.; Albrektsson, T. Temperature threshold levels for heat-induced bone tissue injury: A vital-microscopic study in the rabbit. *J. Prosthet. Dent.* **1983**, *50*, 101–107. [CrossRef]
28. Schmelzeisen, H. *Der Bohrvorgang in der Kortikalis: Mechanik, Thermometrie, Morphologie*; Springer: Berlin/Heidelberg, Germany, 1990. (In German)
29. Trisi, P.; Berardini, M.; Falco, A.; Vulpiani, M.P. Effect of temperature on the dental implant osseointegration development in low-density bone: An in vivo histological evaluation. *Implant Dent.* **2015**, *24*, 96–100. [CrossRef] [PubMed]

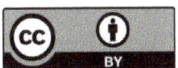

© 2019 by the authors. Licensee MDPI, Basel, Switzerland. This article is an open access article distributed under the terms and conditions of the Creative Commons Attribution (CC BY) license (http://creativecommons.org/licenses/by/4.0/).

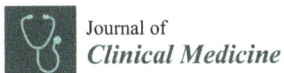

Article

Intraosseous Temperature Change during Installation of Dental Implants with Two Different Surfaces and Different Drilling Protocols: An In Vivo Study in Sheep

Michele Stocchero [1], Yohei Jinno [1,*], Marco Toia [1], Marianne Ahmad [1], Evaggelia Papia [2], Satoshi Yamaguchi [3] and Jonas P. Becktor [1]

1. Department of Oral & Maxillofacial Surgery and Oral Medicine, Faculty of Odontology, Malmö University, 20506 Malmö, Sweden
2. Department of Materials Science and Technology, Faculty of Odontology, Malmö University, 20506 Malmö, Sweden
3. Department of Biomaterials Science, Osaka University Graduate School of Dentistry, Osaka 565-0871, Japan
* Correspondence: yohei.jinno@mau.se; Tel.: +46-076-896-3758

Received: 25 July 2019; Accepted: 6 August 2019; Published: 11 August 2019

Abstract: Background: The intraosseous temperature during implant installation has never been evaluated in an in vivo controlled setup. The aims were to investigate the influence of a drilling protocol and implant surface on the intraosseous temperature during implant installation, to evaluate the influence of temperature increase on osseointegration and to calculate the heat distribution in cortical bone. Methods: Forty Brånemark implants were installed into the metatarsal bone of Finnish Dorset crossbred sheep according to two different drilling protocols (undersized/non-undersized) and two surfaces (moderately rough/turned). The intraosseous temperature was recorded, and Finite Element Model (FEM) was generated to understand the thermal behavior. Non-decalcified histology was carried out after five weeks of healing. The following osseointegration parameters were calculated: Bone-to-implant contact (BIC), Bone Area Fraction Occupancy (BAFO), and Bone Area Fraction Occupancy up to 1.5 mm (BA1.5). A multiple regression model was used to identify the influencing variables on the histomorphometric parameters. Results: The temperature was affected by the drilling protocol, while no influence was demonstrated by the implant surface. BIC was positively influenced by the undersized drilling protocol and rough surface, BAFO was negatively influenced by the temperature rise, and BA1.5 was negatively influenced by the undersized drilling protocol. FEM showed that the temperature at the implant interface might exceed the limit for bone necrosis. Conclusion: The intraosseous temperature is greatly increased by an undersized drilling protocol but not from the implant surface. The temperature increase negatively affects the bone healing in the proximity of the implant. The undersized drilling protocol for Brånemark implant systems increases the amount of bone at the interface, but it negatively impacts the bone far from the implant.

Keywords: oral implants; osseointegration; implant installation; anchorage technique; histology; osteotomy; intraosseous temperature; in vivo study; finite element model

1. Introduction

Despite the high success rate of dental implants [1,2], early and late implant failures are still encountered [3,4]. It is known that the surgical approach is one key-factor for successful implant treatment [5]. It was advocated that an optimal surgical technique should provide initial mechanical implant stability necessary for the initiation of the osseointegration process [6,7]. Simultaneously, implants should be installed with a gentle and atraumatic surgical technique, avoiding excessive biomechanical and thermal stresses to the bone [8].

Undersized drilling is one of the most common surgical techniques for increasing primary implant stability. With this technique, an implant is installed in a substantially smaller osteotomy than its diameter [9]. The rationale of such a procedure is to maximize the initial implant contact with the bone locally and, thus, secure the implant stability [10]. This approach increases the implant rotational resistance, measured as the insertion torque value (ITV) [11]. This condition is often considered desirable [12], especially when immediate or early loading protocols are applied [13].

However, there are some concerns among researchers and clinicians regarding the host bone reaction to increased lateral compression, especially when the cortical bone layer is involved [14]. Excessive stresses and strains beyond bone physiological limits can have disadvantageous effects on the local microcirculation and bone cellular responses, leading to so-called bone compression necrosis [15]. In vivo studies and clinical research reported an extensive area of apoptotic osteocytes, tissue damage, and ultimately peri-implant bone loss [16–18]. Moreover, previous consensus reports indicated compression necrosis as a possible risk factor for peri-implant tissues disease [19,20].

Besides the over-compression of the pristine bone, a thermal injury may be an additional factor inducing bone necrosis. When the bone is heated above 53 °C, irreversible tissue damage was observed [21], while 47 °C for 1 min is considered as the border condition for the occurrence of an injury [22]. Although the risk of bone overheating during the drilling procedure was extensively investigated [23], the increase of temperature during implant installation, was seldom reported [24]. During the seating into an osteotomy site, energy is supplied to the bone and part of it is transferred as frictional heat [25]. According to thermodynamics, thermal energy is partially absorbed and conducted by the implant itself, and by the bone, in the form of temperature increase [26].

It is unknown whether the frictional heat generated during implant installation can cause an increase in bone temperature exceeding the threshold of initiating irreversible tissue damage. The temperature may be influenced by several factors, including implant-osteotomy size discrepancy and implant micro-design. One could postulate that the installation of an implant in an undersized osteotomy and the use of a moderately rough surface would generate a greater temperature increase in the bone than a larger osteotomy and a turned surface.

However, the in vivo intraosseous temperature during implant installation was never previously evaluated in a controlled experimental setting. Besides that, the effect of such temperature on histomorphometric parameters is unknown.

The primary aim of this in vivo study was to investigate the influence of the drilling protocol and implant surface on the intraosseous temperature change during dental implant installation. The secondary aims were to evaluate the influence of the temperature on osseointegration and peri-implant bone healing and to calculate the heat distribution in cortical bone.

2. Materials and Methods

2.1. Study Design and Samples

This study was approved by the ethical committee of the Ecole Nationale Vétérinaire d'Alfort, Paris, France, (reference number: 02343.03) and it is reported according to the ARRIVE (Animal Research Reporting of in Vivo Experiments) guidelines [27]. Ten female Finnish Dorset crossbred sheep (average; years old and 54 kg) were used and housed together for one week before surgery. A total of forty 3.75 mm × 7 mm dental implants (Brånemark system® MKIII RP implant, Nobel Biocare AB, Göteborg, Sweden) were installed, including 20 implants with moderately rough oxidized titanium surface (TiUnite® surface) and 20 implants with a turned surface. The present implant surfaces, investigated by a broad variety of preclinical and clinical research [28–30], presents the following surface characteristics according to Wennerberg and Albrektsson with the parameters Sa (the arithmetic average height deviation from mean plane) and Sdr (the developed surface ratio): 1.1 μm and 0.9 μm (Sa); 37% and 34% (Sdr) for TiUnite® and turned surface, respectively [31].

2.2. Surgical Procedures

All surgeries were done under general anesthesia with ketamine (Imalgene 1000®, Merial, Villeurbanne, France), and diazepam (Valium, Roche, Boulogne-Billancourt, France) for injection, and with 2.5% isoflurane (Forane®/Forene®, Drägerverk AG, Lubeck, Germany) for inhalation. The surgical room had a controlled temperature set at 19 °C.

In each sheep, the metatarsal bone of one leg was shaved and disinfected with 40% ethanol and 0.5% chlorhexidine. After skin incision, the bone was exposed with periosteal elevator, and 4 implants were installed in the ventral metatarsal bone plate, consisting of approximately 1 mm of cortical bone, along the longitudinal direction.

Based on the drilling protocol and implant surface topography, four experimental groups were designed as showed in Table 1.

Table 1. Description of the experimental groups.

	Drilling Protocol	Implant Surface
Group A (n = 10)	Undersized	Moderately rough
Group B (n = 10)	Non-undersized	Moderately rough
Group C (n = 10)	Undersized	Turned
Group D (n = 10)	Non-undersized	Turned

Each metatarsal bone received one implant per group. The sequence of the implantation for each metatarsal bone, according to the experimental group (A, B, C, D) was randomized by a computer-generated method, Microsoft® excel (Version 15.30). The sequential implant osteotomies were free-hand prepared at approximately 20 mm inter-implant distance.

The surgical instrumentation sequence was performed following two different drilling protocols. In all groups, a 2.0 mm drill, 2.8 mm step drill, and 3.0 mm drill were used. Hereafter, the osteotomy was finalized based on the group (Figure 1a):

- Group A and C (undersized drilling protocol): 3.2 drill and tap drill were subsequently used for the preparation of the coronal 1.5 mm, in order to favor the engagement of the first threads during the implant installment.
- Group B and D (non-undersized drilling protocol): 3.2 drill and tap drill were subsequently used for the entire thickness of the cortical bone.

All drilling procedures were performed at 1200 rpm under abundant saline irrigation using a total of two new drill sets. Implant installation was carried out at 25 rpm without saline irrigation. Both the drilling procedure and implant installation were performed using a SA-310 W&H Elcomed implant unit (W&H, Burmoos, Austria). The insertion torque value (ITV) was recorded using the specific function and saved to a USB memory. Implants where ITV exceeded 80 Ncm during installation were manually installed by a manual torque wrench. Based on the ITV, three classes were distinguished: ITV ≤ 45 Ncm; 45 < ITV < 80 Ncm; ITV ≥ 80 Ncm. The flap was closed using a resorbable suture (Vicryl™, Ethicon®, Sommerville, NJ, USA) for the inner layer and non-absorbable suture for the external layer (Ethicon™, Ethicon®, Sommerville, NJ, USA). Morphine (0.1 mg/kg) was given intravenously every second hour during the operation and subcutaneously for the three first postoperative days.

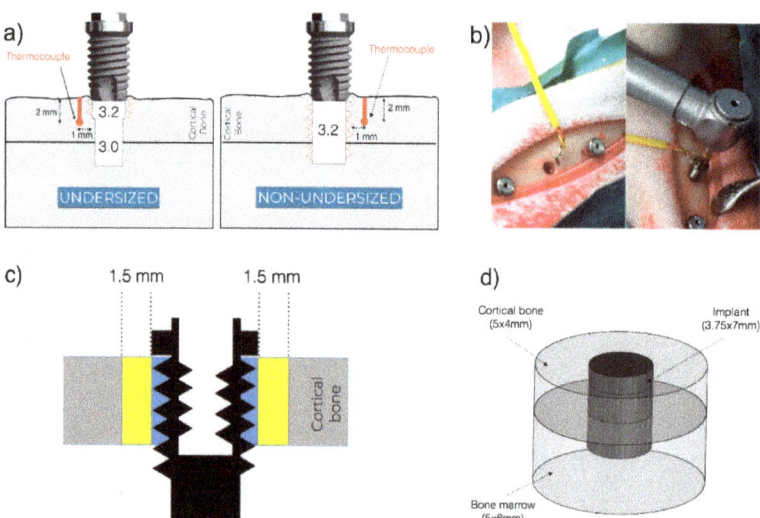

Figure 1. (**a**) Representation of the osteotomy preparation: the undersized drilling protocol on the left and non-undersized drilling protocol on the right. The osteotomy dimensions are depicted in the figures. The thermocouple site was prepared 2 mm deep into the cortical bone and 1 mm from the implant surface. (**b**) Overview of the surgical field with the thermocouple in position before implant installation (**left**) and during implant installation (**right**). (**c**) Representation of the regions of interest for histomorphometrical parameters. Bone-to-implant Contact (BIC) was calculated only for the cortical portion. Bone Area Fraction Occupancy (BAFO) was calculated in the blue part. Bone Area 1.5 (BA1.5) was calculated in the yellow part. (**d**) The Finite Element Model (FEM) was composed of three cylindrical elements: Cortical bone, bone marrow, and implant.

2.3. Temperature Measurement

Intraosseous temperature was measured using the type-K thermocouple (Omega Engineering Limited, Manchester, UK) with a 0.5 mm tip, coupled to a HH12C handheld thermometer (Omega Engineering Limited, Manchester, UK). This dual-channel meter device is able to record the lower and maximum temperature with 2.5 measurements per second and a resolution of 0.1 °C. The tip of the thermocouple was inserted in a prepared drilled hole in the proximity of the implant osteotomy. More in details, the thermocouple site was prepared in a predetermined position in a proximal or distal site at 1 mm from the implant surface (Figure 1a) with the aid of a metal surgical template. To prepare the site, which had a diameter of 0.5 mm and a depth of 2 mm, a lance drill (Precision Drill, Nobel Biocare AB, Göteborg, Sweden) was used. To ensure the reproducibility of the hole depth, the drill was inserted until the marked line met the upper border of the template. Once the osteotomy was prepared, the thermocouple was inserted and kept the position until the thermometer showed a stable value (basal temperature). The installation of the implants was carried out approximately 1 min after the finalization of the drilling procedure. During the implant installation, the temperature was measured, and the maximum value was recorded as the maximum value (Figure 1b). The difference between the maximum and basal temperature for each site was calculated as the temperature change.

2.4. Preparation of Samples

After a healing period of five weeks, all animals were euthanized with an intravenous injection of a combination of 4000 mg embutramide, 538.4 mg mebezonium, and 87.8 mg tetracaine (T61, Intervet International, Unterschleißheim, Germany) and metatarsal bone blocks containing the implants were retrieved. Blocks were fixed in 4% formalin for seven days before dehydration by ascending concentration of ethanol, and embedded in light-curing methylmethacrylate (Technovit 7200 VLC, Heraeus Kulzer, Wehrheim, Germany) for undecalcified ground section procedures. The embedded bone samples with implant were sectioned parallel to the long axis at the center position of the implant using a diamond saw cutting machine (EXAKT 300, EXAKT Advanced Technologies GmbH, Norderstedt, Germany), and grinded and polished until a final section thickness of 30 µm (EXAKT 400CS, EXAKT Advanced Technologies GmbH, Norderstedt, Germany). The non-decalcified sections were stained in toluidine blue and pyronin G, and photographed using light microscopy with a digital imaging system (NanoZoomer S210, HAMAMATSU, Shizuoka, Japan).

2.5. Histomorphometric Analysis

Quantitative histomorphometry was performed considering the cortical layer only. All measurements were carried out with an image analysis software (Image J v.1.43u, National Institute of Health). The following variables were calculated:

- Bone-to-implant contact (BIC): On each side of the implant, the percentage of the bone in direct contact with the implant surface in the entire length of the implant placed in the bone was calculated. The mean value of the two sides was used for each implant.
- Bone Area Fraction Occupancy (BAFO): On each side of the implant, the percentage of the area within the implant threads occupied by visibly distinguishable bone was calculated. The mean value of the two sides was used for each implant.
- Bone Area Fraction Occupancy up to 1.5 mm (BA1.5): On each side of the implant a region of interest up to 1.5 mm from the implant outer diameter line was considered (Figure 1c). The percentage of the area occupied by visibly distinguishable bone was calculated. The mean value of the two sides was used for each implant.

2.6. Finite Element Model

In order to have a deeper understanding of the thermal behavior at the peri-implant bone, a Finite Element Model (FEM) was generated (Figure 1d). The model was composed of three cylindrical elements: Cortical bone (dimensions: 5 mm × 4 mm), bone marrow (dimensions: 5 mm × 6 mm), and implant (dimensions: 3.75 mm × 7 mm) designed by the CAD software (Solidworks Simulation 2011, Dassault Systèmes Solidworks, Waltham, MA, USA). Two different calorific values were set to the upper and bottom surface of the fixture related to the drilling hole with different diameters.

Steady conduction analysis was conducted by voxel-based Finite Element Analysis (FEA) software (VOXELCON2015, Quint, Fuchu, Japan). The thermal conductivity of cortical bone, bone marrow, and implant were set to 0.6 W/mK, 0.3 W/mK, and 20 W/mK, respectively [32,33]. The air temperature around those models was set to 19 °C.

The temperature change in the location of the thermocouple (2 mm depth from cortical bone surface and 1 mm away from the fixture surface) was approximated to 8 °C and 4 °C for the undersized drilling protocol groups and non-undersized drilling protocol groups, respectively. Until converging the calorific value, the steady conduction analysis was repeatedly conducted.

2.7. Statistical Methods

Categorical variables were reported as relative frequency, while continuous variables were reported as mean ± standard deviation after checking the normality of the distribution. Wilcoxon rank-sum test was used to test the influence of the drilling protocol and implant surface on temperature change.

Multiple regression models were used to evaluate the effect of the drilling protocol, implant surface, temperature change on the histomorphometric parameters (BIC, BAFO, BA1.5). *p*-values < 0.05 were considered statistically significant. The R statistical software package was used for the statistical evaluation and modelling (available at www.r-project.org/).

3. Results

3.1. ITV, General Healing and Temperature

All animals survived during surgical procedures and the experimental period. No implant was lost during the healing period. Signs of minor periosteal reaction were noted in three metatarsal bone samples. Such a response did not undermine the peri-implant bone healing and was limited to the periosteal area, which was not considered in this study. All implants were included in the statistical analysis. The relative distribution of the ITV class among the groups is displayed in Figure 2a.

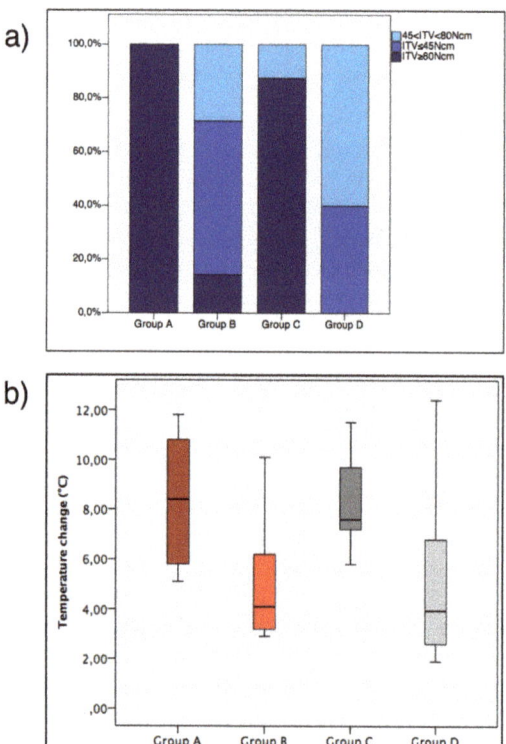

Figure 2. (**a**) Cumulative percentage of insertion torque value (ITV) classes divided per group. Note that all implants installed for group A had a ITV ≥ 80 Ncm. (**b**) Temperature change represented in box-plots.

The values for basal and maximum temperature are indicated in Table 2. Temperature change values are shown in Figure 2b. The temperature change was affected by the drilling protocol ($p < 0.001$), while it was not influenced by the surface topography ($p = 0.879$).

Table 2. Basal temperature and maximum temperature for the different groups are shown in °C. SD: Standard deviation; Max: maximum value; Min: minimum value.

	Basal Temperature				Maximum Temperature			
	Mean	SD	Max	Min	Mean	SD	Max	Min
Group A	31.3	2.3	34.5	28.4	39.6	3.3	45.3	34.7
Group B	31.0	3.4	34.7	23.7	36.0	3.4	41.5	28.6
Group C	31.0	3.3	34.0	23.6	39.1	3.7	44.0	33.4
Group D	31.3	2.3	34.2	27.5	36.4	1.8	39.9	33.6

3.2. Histomorphometric Parameters

Representation of the histologic sections are displayed in Figure 3.

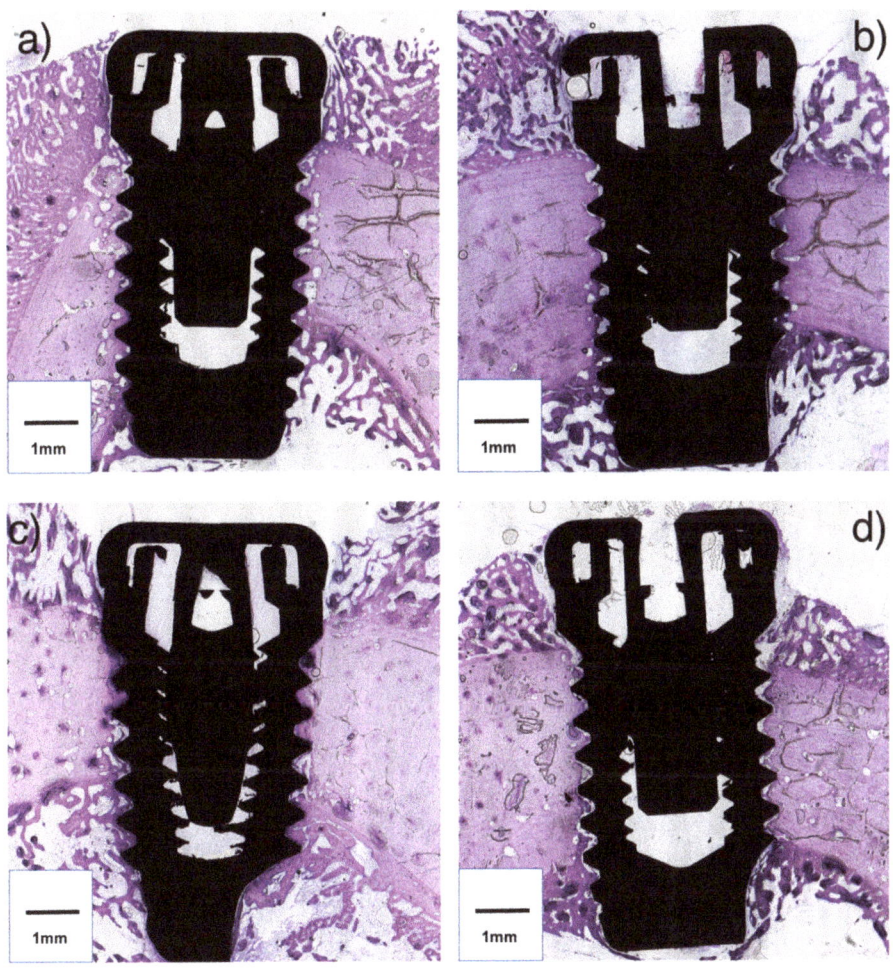

Figure 3. Histologic sections of the implant and peri-implant bone (original magnification 20×). Representations of group A, B, C, and D are depicted in (**a**), (**b**), (**c**), and (**d**), respectively.

Mean values and standard deviation for BIC, BAFO, and BA1.5 are presented in Figure 4.

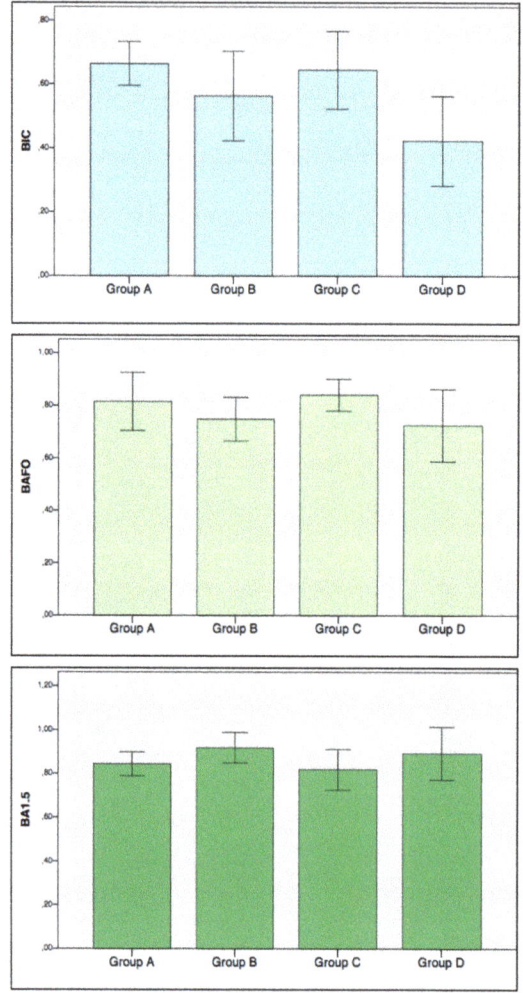

Figure 4. Bone to Implant Contact (**BIC**), Bone Area Fraction Occupancy (**BAFO**), and Bone Area Fraction Occupancy up to 1.5 mm (**BA1.5**) results represented as mean values. Error bars represent the standard deviation.

According to robust multiple regression analysis (Adjusted R^2: 0.37, $p = 0.0001$), BIC was statistically significantly influenced by the implant surface ($p = 0.01$) and the drilling protocol ($p = 0.0001$). More specifically, BIC was increased with a moderately rough surface and undersized drilling protocol. BAFO was negatively affected by temperature increase ($p = 0.01$). Moreover BAFO was positively affected by the undersized drilling protocol ($p = 0.0006$) (Adjusted R^2: 0.24, $p = 0.005$). BA1.5 was moderately affected by the undersized drilling protocol ($p < 0.001$) (Adjusted R^2: 0.11, $p = 0.06$ for the model). No significant influence on BA1.5 was noted for the temperature change.

3.3. Finite Element Model

Temperature distribution at the center section is shown in Figure 5. The calorific value of the normal model was 30.8 W/m^3. The calorific values of the upper fixture and bottom fixture were 30.8 W/m^3 and 60.4 W/m^3, respectively. The calorific value of fixture for the undersized drilling model showed 1.96 times greater than that for the non-undersized drilling model. The bone temperature at the interface with the implant surface was calculated for both models.

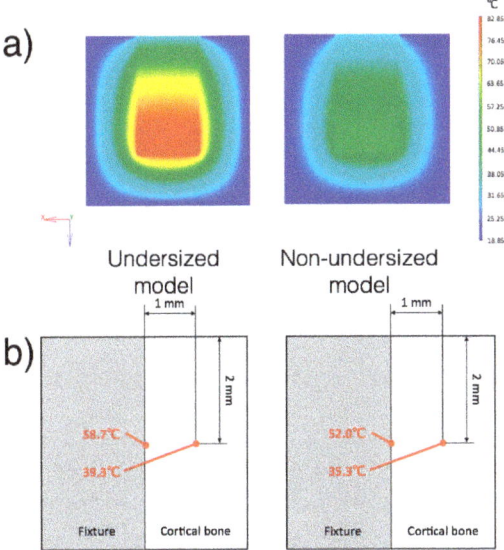

Figure 5. (**a**) The temperature distribution calculated on the Finite Element Model (FEM). The undersized drilling model and non-undersized model are displayed on the left and on the right, respectively. The temperature is displayed in °C. Note how the heat is poorly distributed around the implant surface. This means that the overheating risk is limited to the bone in the proximity to the implant. (**b**) Calculation of the bone temperature at the implant interface according to the FEM. This value was calculated by entering the value recorded with the thermocouple in the experimental part.

4. Discussion

In the present in vivo study, the intraosseous temperature was measured during dental implant installation into cortical bone, following two different drilling protocols and with two different implant surfaces. In addition, histomorphometric parameters of osseointegration were evaluated in relation to the bone temperature recorded during the implant installation and a computational model was created to examine the thermal distribution. To the knowledge of the authors, the current investigation represents the first in vivo experiment with this setup.

4.1. Bone Temperature

In the present study, it was discovered that the intraosseous temperature during implant installation was influenced by the drilling protocol. During implant installation, a certain amount of energy is also dissipated into heat [25]. As previous in vitro studies have observed, the rotational torque is positively related to bone heating during implant installation [24,34]. Accordingly, in this study, the installation of implants into undersized sites developed a great friction resistance, resulting in both in a higher ITV (Figure 3) and temperature increase, compared with non-undersized osteotomies. Specifically, the undersized drilling protocol groups resulted in a median increase of temperature of approximately 8 °C, while in the non-undersized drilling protocol groups, it was approximately 4 °C. The maximum recorded temperature of 45.3 °C exceeded the limit of cell damage, which is 45 °C according to Ludewig [35], but it was lower than the critical value for bone necrosis, which is 50 °C according to Lundskog [36]. In the early 1980s, Eriksson, whose doctoral thesis greatly contributed to the knowledge on bone tissue regeneration, stated that the threshold level for bone survival was 47 °C for 1 min [37]. However, the temperature recorded in the present study was detected at 1 mm from the implant surface. To have a better understanding of the temperature behavior in the proximity of the implant, a FEM was designed. It was estimated that the temperature at the bone-implant interface for the undersized groups and non-undersized groups reached 58.7 °C and 52.0 °C respectively (Figure 5). Thus, according to the FEM calculation, the installation of the implant caused a frictional heat over the critical temperature for bone injury at the bone-implant interface. One may expect that implants installed with an undersized drilling protocol would create a major extent of tissue damage. Still, such an overheating condition is restricted to the proximity of the implant, as shown by the model. Since the temperature change was affected by the drilling protocol ($p < 0.001$), but was not influenced by the surface topography ($p = 0.879$), the surface characteristics (parameters Sa and Sdr) were not included in the design of the FEM.

Such results are confirmed by histomorphometry. In effect, it was demonstrated that the temperature generated during implant installation has a tangible biologic impact, since the amount of bone between the threads, namely BAFO, is negatively affected by the temperature increase. This finding is in accordance with Eriksson's study, in which they observed a loss of 10% of bone tissue after 30 days when a rabbit tibia was heated to 47 °C for 1 min [22]. This study supports the conclusion that the portion of the bone in proximity with the implant surface might be the most sensitive to heating at the implant installation. Moreover, based on the FEM analysis and histomorphometric results, this heating might induce bone damage if the undersized drilling protocol is applied. The influence of the heat generated by the drilling procedures was likely to be excluded since one minute elapsed before the implant installation. Previous research indicated that the bone returned to baseline temperature after approximately 30 s [38].

Nevertheless, due to the low thermal conductivity properties of cortical bone, we could expect a low grade of heat distribution through the bone [39]. Thus, the risk of bone overheating is limited to the bone in the proximity to the bone-to-implant interface.

It has to be said that Eriksson observed how bone cells are susceptible to the exposure time, other than peak temperature [40]. In the present experiment, the maximum temperature endured for a few seconds, then it gradually descended. However, the actual temperature/time curve was not recorded, representing a limitation of the study.

4.2. Drilling Protocol

The present findings showed that an undersized drilling protocol per se might not be detrimental to osseointegration for the Brånemark implant. In a previous study by the authors, implants were inserted in sheep mandible according to two different drilling techniques [41]. The results showed that implants inserted into an undersized osteotomy caused tissue damage to the peri-implant bone. In particular, large remodeling cavities with resorption activity were noted, and a lower amount of bone was identified up to 1.5 mm distance from the implant, both from histomorphometric μ-CT analysis. In addition, the drilling protocol seemed not to influence the amount of total BIC. Such findings are partially confirmed by the present results, since the amount of bone up to 1.5 mm from implant surface (BA1.5), was negatively influenced by the undersized drilling protocol. An explanation could be that the bone compression during the implant installation in a tight osteotomy would trigger a remodeling process at a distance from the implant interface. On the other hand, the temperature change does not influence this parameter, since the thermal conductivity of the bone would prevent the heat from being transferred at such a distance from the implant.

Compared with the previous sheep study [41], a number of differences were noted. In the former study, an implant with a micro-threaded neck was used, while the Brånemark type implant was utilized in the present investigation. A previous FEA study on the press-fit phenomena at the implant insertion, [42] affirmed that the micro-thread portion, induced more relevant strains compared to the situation without microthreads. Thus, one could expect greater bone damage after undersized drilling in such a scenario. On the contrary, the undersized drilling protocol positively influenced the amount of bone in close proximity to the implant, i.e., BIC and BAFO, in the present study. It could be assumed that a large portion of the bone in contact with the implant might be the original bone that was forced to the implant surface during the implant installation and still not removed. This finding was observed in several previous studies, which used a similar implant design [5,43,44]. In normal conditions, such tissue will be gradually resorbed with time and eventually substituted with vital bone, according to the remodeling process [45].

4.3. Surface

An interesting finding of the present study was that the type of implant surface did not influence the bone temperature. It could be expected that a moderately rough surface could increase the friction and thereby the heat [46,47]. However, no differences were noticed in the temperature increase between moderately rough and turned surfaced implants. According to the results, a moderately rough surface had a positive effect on the amount of bone in contact with the implant. This finding confirms that such surface topography is able to promote the osteoconductive properties of the implant, compared to turned surfaced implants, as reported by animal and human histologic reports by Ivanoff et al. and Zechner et al. [28,48].

4.4. Clinical Applications and Limitations

The study represents one of the first attempts to study the implant insertion temperature in an in vivo setting. Results demonstrated that an undersized drilling protocol causes an increase of intraosseous temperature during implant seating. A temperature increase negatively affected the amount of peri-implant bone. Thus, it may be suggested to reduce the friction overheating during implant installation. This would include decreasing the rotational speed [49], the use of the self-tapping implant design [24], the use of irrigation during implant installation, and the selection of the proper drilling protocol based on the implant design and the bone quality.

Considering the limitations in the present study, the record of the temperature was limited to the peak value during each insertion. Further studies are needed to evaluate the exact duration of the heat. In addition, from the present study, we cannot confirm whether the increase of the temperature caused tissue necrosis, since no specific stain for cell metabolism and tissue turnover was used. Moreover, the relationship between the compression and the heat, following undersized drilling was not explored. Future studies should be designed in order to indicate whether there is a predominant factor in the generation of tissue damage in the proximity of the implant. Finally, it must be stated that the sheep model, which has been broadly used in dental implant research, presents similarities and differences compared to human bone [50]. The thickness and density of cortical bone may approximate clinical scenarios, such as encountered in the mandible. In addition, sheep bone turnover resembles bone processes in humans, even though it is slightly more rapid. The healing period of five weeks was selected according to our previous research [41], since the influence of the surgical protocol is more evident at this stage in the peri-implant bone. However, the metatarsal bone, while it represents an accessible and convenient substrate for orthopedic and dental implant research, presents quite large anatomical and physiological differences compared with the human jaw, and it may display slightly divergent thermal properties. Therefore the present findings must be taken with reasonable caution.

5. Conclusions

Within the limitations of the present study, it was shown that different drilling protocol for the Brånemark implant system affects both the intraosseous temperature during implant installation and the peri-implant bone healing. The undersized drilling protocol provokes a greater increase of bone temperature in the proximity of the implant compared with non-undersized drilling. The temperature at the bone-implant interface may exceed the critical value for thermal necrosis, and it may have negative effects on peri-implant bone healing. The present results indicate that undersized drilling increases the amount of bone in the proximity of the implant, but it has a negative impact on the bone area far from the implant surface. The moderately rough surface does not influence the bone temperature, while it increased the bone attached to the implant. Further studies are needed to confirm the present results and to deeply investigate the thermal behavior and the biologic effect of peri-implant bone overheating during implant installation and to provide guidelines on the clinical decisions for the proper drilling protocol, based on the bone quality and implant design.

Author Contributions: Conceptualization—M.S. and J.B.; Data curation—M.S., Y.J. and S.Y.; Formal analysis—M.S. and S.Y.; Funding acquisition—J.B.; Investigation—M.S., Y.J., M.T., M.A. and E.P.; Methodology—M.S., Y.J., M.A., E.P. and S.Y.; Project administration—E.P. and J.B.; Resources—Y.J., M.T. and M.A.; Software—S.Y.; Supervision—J.B.; Validation—Y.J., M.T., E.P. and J.B.; Visualization—M.T. and E.P.; Writing—Original draft—M.S., Y.J. and S.Y.; Writing—Review & Editing—M.T., M.A., E.P., S.Y. and J.B.

Funding: This research was supported by own budget in Department of Oral & Maxillofacial Surgery and Oral Medicine, Faculty of Odontology, Malmö University, Sweden.

Acknowledgments: The authors are grateful to Benoit Lecuelle and Thomas Lilin from Ecole Nationale Vétérinaire d'Alfort, Paris, France and Simone Selvaggio, Italy for their valuable help during the surgical procedures.

Conflicts of Interest: The authors declare no conflict of interest.

References

1. Chrcanovic, B.R.; Kisch, J.; Albrektsson, T.; Wennerberg, A. A retrospective study on clinical and radiological outcomes of oral implants in patients followed up for a minimum of 20 years. *Clin. Implant. Dent. Relat. Res.* **2018**, *20*, 199–207. [CrossRef] [PubMed]
2. Donati, M.; Ekestubbe, A.; Lindhe, J.; Wennstrom, J.L. Marginal bone loss at implants with different surface characteristics A 20-year follow-up of a randomized controlled clinical trial. *Clin. Oral Implants Res.* **2018**, *29*, 480–487. [CrossRef] [PubMed]
3. Chrcanovic, B.R.; Kisch, J.; Albrektsson, T.; Wennerberg, A. Factors Influencing Early Dental Implant Failures. *J. Dent. Res.* **2016**, *95*, 995–1002. [CrossRef] [PubMed]
4. Derks, J.; Hakansson, J.; Wennstrom, J.L.; Tomasi, C.; Larsson, M.; Berglundh, T. Effectiveness of implant therapy analyzed in a Swedish population: Early and late implant loss. *J. Dent. Res.* **2015**, *94*, 44s–51s. [CrossRef] [PubMed]
5. Albrektsson, T.; Branemark, P.I.; Hansson, H.A.; Lindstrom, J. Osseointegrated titanium implants. Requirements for ensuring a long-lasting, direct bone-to-implant anchorage in man. *Acta Orthop. Scand.* **1981**, *52*, 155–170. [CrossRef] [PubMed]
6. Esposito, M.; Hirsch, J.M.; Lekholm, U.; Thomsen, P. Biological factors contributing to failures of osseointegrated oral implants. Success criteria and epidemiology. *Eur. J. Oral Sci.* **1998**, *106*, 527–551. [CrossRef] [PubMed]
7. Szmukler-Moncler, S.; Salama, H.; Reingewirtz, Y.; Dubruille, J.H. Timing of loading and effect of micromotion on bone-dental implant interface: Review of experimental literature. *J. Biomed. Mater. Res.* **1998**, *43*, 192–203. [CrossRef]
8. Albrektsson, T.; Zarb, G.; Worthington, P.; Eriksson, A.R. The long-term efficacy of currently used dental implants: A review and proposed criteria of success. *Int. J. Oral Maxillofac. Implants* **1986**, *1*, 11–25.
9. Friberg, B.; Sennerby, L.; Grondahl, K.; Bergstrom, C.; Back, T.; Lekholm, U. On cutting torque measurements during implant placement: A 3-year clinical prospective study. *Clin. Implant. Dent. Relat. Res.* **1999**, *1*, 75–83. [CrossRef]
10. Bilhan, H.; Geckili, O.; Mumcu, E.; Bozdag, E.; Sunbuloglu, E.; Kutay, O. Influence of surgical technique, implant shape and diameter on the primary stability in cancellous bone. *J. Oral Rehabil.* **2010**, *37*, 900–907. [CrossRef]
11. Stocchero, M.; Toia, M.; Cecchinato, D.; Becktor, J.P.; Coelho, P.G.; Jimbo, R. Biomechanical, Biologic, and Clinical Outcomes of Undersized Implant Surgical Preparation: A Systematic Review. *Int. J. Oral Maxillofac. Implants* **2016**, *31*, 1247–1263. [CrossRef] [PubMed]
12. O'Sullivan, D.; Sennerby, L.; Meredith, N. Measurements comparing the initial stability of five designs of dental implants: A human cadaver study. *Clin. Implant. Dent. Relat. Res.* **2000**, *2*, 85–92. [CrossRef] [PubMed]

13. Esposito, M.; Grusovin, M.G.; Willings, M.; Coulthard, P.; Worthington, H.V. The effectiveness of immediate, early, and conventional loading of dental implants: A Cochrane systematic review of randomized controlled clinical trials. *Int. J. Oral Maxillofac. Implants* **2007**, *22*, 893–904. [PubMed]
14. Stocchero, M. *On Influence of Undersized Implant Site On Implant Stability and Osseointegration*; Malmö University: Malmö, Sverige, 2018.
15. Bashutski, J.D.; D'Silva, N.J.; Wang, H.L. Implant compression necrosis: Current understanding and case report. *J. Periodontol.* **2009**, *80*, 700–704. [CrossRef] [PubMed]
16. Duyck, J.; Corpas, L.; Vermeiren, S.; Ogawa, T.; Quirynen, M.; Vandamme, K.; Jacobs, R.; Naert, I. Histological, histomorphometrical, and radiological evaluation of an experimental implant design with a high insertion torque. *Clin. Oral Implants Res.* **2010**, *21*, 877–884. [CrossRef] [PubMed]
17. Cha, J.Y.; Pereira, M.D.; Smith, A.A.; Houschyar, K.S.; Yin, X.; Mouraret, S.; Brunski, J.B.; Helms, J.A. Multiscale analyses of the bone-implant interface. *J. Dent. Res.* **2015**, *94*, 482–490. [CrossRef]
18. Toia, M.; Stocchero, M.; Cecchinato, F.; Corra, E.; Jimbo, R.; Cecchinato, D. Clinical Considerations of Adapted Drilling Protocol by Bone Quality Perception. *Int. J. Oral Maxillofac. Implants* **2017**, *32*, 1288–1295. [CrossRef]
19. Berglundh, T.; Armitage, G.; Araujo, M.G.; Avila-Ortiz, G.; Blanco, J.; Camargo, P.M.; Chen, S.; Cochran, D.; Derks, J.; Figuero, E.; et al. Peri-implant diseases and conditions: Consensus report of workgroup 4 of the 2017 World Workshop on the Classification of Periodontal and Peri-Implant Diseases and Conditions. *J. Clin. Periodontol.* **2018**, *45*, S286–S291. [CrossRef]
20. Schwarz, F.; John, G.; Schmucker, A.; Sahm, N.; Becker, J. Combined surgical therapy of advanced peri-implantitis evaluating two methods of surface decontamination: A 7-year follow-up observation. *J. Clin. Periodontol.* **2017**, *44*, 337–342. [CrossRef]
21. Eriksson, A.; Albrektsson, T.; Grane, B.; McQueen, D. Thermal injury to bone. A vital-microscopic description of heat effects. *Int. J. Oral Surg.* **1982**, *11*, 115–121. [CrossRef]
22. Eriksson, A.R.; Albrektsson, T. Temperature threshold levels for heat-induced bone tissue injury: A vital-microscopic study in the rabbit. *J. Prosthet. Dent.* **1983**, *50*, 101–107. [CrossRef]
23. Augustin, G.; Zigman, T.; Davila, S.; Udilljak, T.; Staroveski, T.; Brezak, D.; Babic, S. Cortical bone drilling and thermal osteonecrosis. *Clin. Biomech. (Bristol, Avon)* **2012**, *27*, 313–325. [CrossRef]
24. Markovic, A.; Misic, T.; Milicic, B.; Calvo-Guirado, J.L.; Aleksic, Z.; Ethinic, A. Heat generation during implant placement in low-density bone: Effect of surgical technique, insertion torque and implant macro design. *Clin. Oral Implants Res.* **2013**, *24*, 798–805. [CrossRef] [PubMed]
25. Matsuoka, M.; Motoyoshi, M.; Sakaguchi, M.; Shinohara, A.; Shigeede, T.; Saito, Y.; Matsuda, M.; Shimizu, N. Friction heat during self-drilling of an orthodontic miniscrew. *Int. J. Oral Maxillofac. Surg.* **2011**, *40*, 191–194. [CrossRef] [PubMed]
26. Wong, K.; Boyde, A.; Howell, P.G. A model of temperature transients in dental implants. *Biomaterials* **2001**, *22*, 2795–2797. [CrossRef]
27. Berglundh, T.; Stavropoulos, A. Preclinical in vivo research in implant dentistry. Consensus of the eighth European workshop on periodontology. *J. Clin. Periodontol.* **2012**, *39*, 1–5. [CrossRef]
28. Ivanoff, C.J.; Widmark, G.; Johansson, C.; Wennerberg, A. Histologic evaluation of bone response to oxidized and turned titanium micro implants in human jawbone. *Int. J. Oral Maxillofac. Implants* **2003**, *18*, 341–348.
29. Karl, M.; Albrektsson, T. Clinical Performance of Dental Implants with a Moderately Rough (TiUnite) Surface: A Meta-Analysis of Prospective Clinical Studies. *Int. J. Oral Maxillofac. Implants* **2017**, *32*, 717–734. [CrossRef]
30. Wennerberg, A.; Albrektsson, T. Effects of titanium surface topography on bone integration: A systematic review. *Clin. Oral Implants Res.* **2009**, *20*, 172–184. [CrossRef]
31. Wennerberg, A.; Albrektsson, T. On implant surfaces: A review of current knowledge and opinions. *Int. J. Oral Maxillofac. Implants* **2010**, *25*, 63–74.
32. Davidson, S.R.; James, D.F. Measurement of thermal conductivity of bovine cortical bone. *Med. Eng. Phys.* **2000**, *22*, 741–747. [CrossRef]
33. Aghvami, M.; Brunski, J.B.; Serdar Tulu, U.; Chen, C.H.; Helms, J.A. A Thermal and Biological Analysis of Bone Drilling. *J. Biomech. Eng.* **2018**, *140*. [CrossRef]
34. Wikenheiser, M.A.; Markel, M.D.; Lewallen, D.G.; Chao, E.Y. Thermal response and torque resistance of five cortical half-pins under simulated insertion technique. *J. Orthop. Res.* **1995**, *13*, 615–619. [CrossRef]
35. Ludewig, R. *Temperaturmessungen Beim Knochensagen*; University of Gissen: Gissen, Germany, 1972.

36. Lundskog, J. Heat and bone tissue. An experimental investigation of the thermal properties of bone and threshold levels for thermal injury. *Scand. J. Plast. Reconstr. Surg.* **1972**, *9*, 72–74.
37. Eriksson, A.R. *Heat-Induced Bone Tissue Injury: An in Vivo Investigation of Heat Tolerance of Bone Tissue and Temperature Rise in the Drilling of Cortical Bone*; University of Göteborg: Gothenburg, Sweden, 1984.
38. Gurdan, Z.; Vajta, L.; Toth, A.; Lempel, E.; Joob-Fancsaly, A.; Szalma, J. Effect of pre-drilling on intraosseous temperature during self-drilling mini-implant placement in a porcine mandible model. *J. Oral Sci.* **2017**, *59*, 47–53. [CrossRef]
39. Flanagan, D. Heat generated during seating of dental implant fixtures. *J. Oral Implantol.* **2014**, *40*, 174–181. [CrossRef]
40. Eriksson, R.A.; Albrektsson, T. The effect of heat on bone regeneration: An experimental study in the rabbit using the bone growth chamber. *J. Oral Maxillofac. Surg.* **1984**, *42*, 705–711. [CrossRef]
41. Stocchero, M.; Toia, M.; Jinno, Y.; Cecchinato, F.; Becktor, J.P.; Naito, Y.; Halldin, A.; Jimbo, R. Influence of different drilling preparation on cortical bone: A biomechanical, histological, and micro-CT study on sheep. *Clin. Oral Implants Res.* **2018**. [CrossRef]
42. Natali, A.N.; Carniel, E.L.; Pavan, P.G. Dental implants press fit phenomena: Biomechanical analysis considering bone inelastic response. *Dent. Mater.* **2009**, *25*, 573–581. [CrossRef]
43. Roberts, W.E. Bone tissue interface. *J. Dent. Educ.* **1988**, *52*, 804–809.
44. Roberts, W.E.; Garetto, L.P.; DeCastro, R.A. Remodeling of devitalized bone threatens periosteal margin integrity of endosseous titanium implants with threaded or smooth surfaces: Indications for provisional loading and axially directed occlusion. *J. Indiana Dent. Assoc.* **1989**, *68*, 19–24.
45. Osborn, J.F. Dynamic aspects of the implant-bone-interface. In *Dental implants. Materials and systems*; Heimke, G., Ed.; Carl Hanser Verlag: Munchen, Germany, 1980; pp. 111–123.
46. Shalabi, M.M.; Wolke, J.G.; Jansen, J.A. The effects of implant surface roughness and surgical technique on implant fixation in an in vitro model. *Clin. Oral Implants Res.* **2006**, *17*, 172–178. [CrossRef]
47. Dos Santos, M.V.; Elias, C.N.; Lima, C.J.H. The effects of superficial roughness and design on the primary stability of dental implants. *Clin. Implant. Dent. Relat. Res.* **2011**, *13*, 215–223. [CrossRef]
48. Zechner, W.; Tangl, S.; Furst, G.; Tepper, G.; Thams, U.; Mailath, G.; Watzek, G. Osseous healing characteristics of three different implant types. *Clin. Oral Implants Res.* **2003**, *14*, 150–157. [CrossRef]
49. Sumer, M.; Keskiner, I.; Mercan, U.; Misir, F.; Cankaya, S. Assessment of heat generation during implant insertion. *J. Prosthet. Dent.* **2014**, *112*, 522–525. [CrossRef]
50. Pearce, A.I.; Richards, R.G.; Milz, S.; Schneider, E.; Pearce, S.G. Animal models for implant biomaterial research in bone: A review. *Eur. Cell Mater.* **2007**, *13*, 1–10. [CrossRef]

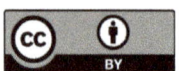

© 2019 by the authors. Licensee MDPI, Basel, Switzerland. This article is an open access article distributed under the terms and conditions of the Creative Commons Attribution (CC BY) license (http://creativecommons.org/licenses/by/4.0/).

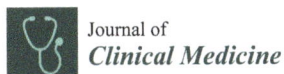

Article

On the Cleanliness of Different Oral Implant Systems: A Pilot Study

Dirk U. Duddeck [1,2,*], Tomas Albrektsson [3], Ann Wennerberg [4], Christel Larsson [5] and Florian Beuer [5]

1. Department of Prosthodontics, Geriatric Dentistry and Craniomandibular Disorders, University Charité Berlin, 14197 Berlin, Germany
2. CleanImplant Foundation, Research Department, 10117 Berlin, Germany
3. Department of Biomaterials, Institute for Clinical Sciences, Sahlgrenska Academy, University of Gothenburg, 40530 Gothenburg, Sweden
4. Department of Prosthodontics, Institute of Odontology, The Sahlgrenska Academy, University of Gothenburg, 40530 Gothenburg, Sweden
5. Department of Prosthodontics, Faculty of Odontology, Malmö University, 20506 Malmö, Sweden
* Correspondence: dirk.duddeck@gmx.de; Tel.: +49-171-5477991

Received: 16 July 2019; Accepted: 19 August 2019; Published: 22 August 2019

Abstract: (1) Background: This paper aimed to compare the cleanliness of clinically well-documented implant systems with implants providing very similar designs. The hypothesis was that three well-established implant systems from Dentsply Implants, Straumann, and Nobel Biocare were not only produced with a higher level of surface cleanliness but also provided significantly more comprehensive published clinical documentation than their correspondent look-alike implants from Cumdente, Bioconcept, and Biodenta, which show similar geometry and surface structure. (2) Methods: Implants were analyzed using SEM imaging and energy-dispersive X-ray spectroscopy to determine the elemental composition of potential impurities. A search for clinical trials was carried out in the PubMed database and by reaching out to the corresponding manufacturer. (3) Results: In comparison to their corresponding look-alikes, all implants of the original manufacturers showed—within the scope of this analysis—a surface free of foreign materials and reliable clinical documentation, while the SEM analysis revealed significant impurities on all look-alike implants such as organic residues and unintended metal particles of iron or aluminum. Other than case reports, the look-alike implant manufacturers provided no reports of clinical documentation. (4) Conclusions: In contrast to the original implants of market-leading manufacturers, the analyzed look-alike implants showed significant impurities, underlining the need for periodic reviews of sterile packaged medical devices and their clinical documentation.

Keywords: dental implants; surface properties; titanium; materials testing; implant contamination; implant surface; scanning electron microscopy; energy-dispersive X-ray spectrometry

1. Introduction

The advent of osseointegration has led to a clinical breakthrough in oral implants. Minimally rough, turned implants were the first osseointegrated oral implants used, with the first patient treated in 1965 [1]. These turned screws remain the most clinically documented implants of all with 75% of all studies in long-term reports [2]. Over time, other clinically documented oral implant systems have increasingly begun to be used. Those systems may have preferred slightly different surfaces; moderately rough implants have been the treatment of choice since the turn of the millennium, since they have demonstrated improved clinical results [3]. The surface of moderately rough implant systems may be manufactured in different ways, by subtractive methods such as the combination of blasting and acid etching or anodization and by additive techniques, such as hydroxyapatite coating. Products from what are regarded as the three largest oral implant companies in the world including Osseo Speed implants from Dentsply–Sirona, SLA-implants from Straumann and TiUnite implants from Nobel Biocare, have been clinically documented in numerous papers spanning a period of over 5 to over 10 years of follow up with very high levels of survival and success [4–6].

Since some osseointegrated oral implant systems have been duly documented with a very good clinical outcome, numerous new implant manufacturers have tried to mimic the surfaces and geometries presented by the leading companies. These are so called copy-cat or at least "look-alike" implant systems which usually lack clinical documentation of their own but claim to be as good as the original implants they are trying to mimic. However, in clinical reality these implants lack the scientific evidence of similar performance.

One surface characteristic of sterile packaged oral implants is their cleanliness. Oral implants may display different surface of an inorganic or organic nature. These impurities may derive from the manufacturing handling and packaging processes and may remain on the commercially available implant. We are presently lacking in knowledge of the precise clinical risks of implant impurities. However, contaminations are technically avoidable and, generally speaking, the authors assume all of us would prefer clean implants to avoid potential problems from surface impurities.

The aim of the present paper was to compare the cleanliness of proper clinically documented implant systems with implants that are very similar in design and surface; OsseoSpeed from Dentsply Implants was compared to a German look-alike implant called Cumdente; Standard Plus Implant SLA from Straumann was compared to a Chinese look-alike implant called Bioconcept (claiming to be 100% compatible with Straumann); and a TiUnite-surfaced implant NobelActive from Nobel Biocare was compared to a Swiss/Taiwanese implant system called Biodenta. Our hypothesis was that the three major and well-established implant systems have significantly comprehensive clinical documentation and have their implants produced in a significantly cleaner manner than would the respective look-alike systems.

Every single dental implant has to be clean, as this is a medical device that could harm patients—even if we found one single implant with impurities, this implant was intentionally sold for the therapy of one real patient. This paper was not intended to show a statistically relevant number of average contaminations for specific implant types. All implants in this study were randomly purchased and labeled for clinical use. Each sample of these medical devices was produced using a certain regime of quality management. If the quality management of a manufacturer cannot ensure a certain level of cleanliness, a single implant with significant impurities, which are technically avoidable, is proof of a lack of quality.

2. Experimental Section

Implant types used for this analysis were the following: Astra Tech–Dentsply Implants (OsseoSpeed EV, Mölndal, Sweden), Straumann (Standard Plus SLA Implant, Zürich, Switzerland), Nobel Biocare (NobelActive Internal RP, Zürich, Switzerland), Cumdente (AS Implant, Tübingen, Germany), Bioconcept (Tissue Level Implant, Jiangsu, China), Biodenta (Dental Implant, Bernek, Switzerland). The three implants from market-leading manufacturers and the correspondent three look-alike implants were purchased in the period between March 2018 and May 2019, either by ghost-shopping, where the ordering practice was reimbursed from the research fund or by direct order. In all six cases, the manufacturers or the respective distributors were not informed about the purpose of the implant order. None of the samples were provided free of charge. Prices varied from 191 euro to 322 euro for the samples of market-leading brands and from 78 euro to 276 euro for the look-alike products.

All of the six samples collected were carefully unpacked, mounted on the sample holder on carbon tabs without touching the implant surface, and analyzed with a scanning electron microscope (SEM) in a particle-free clean room environment (according Class 100 US Federal Standard 209E, Class 5 DIN EN ISO 14644-1) to avoid artifacts from the ambient air (Figure 1).

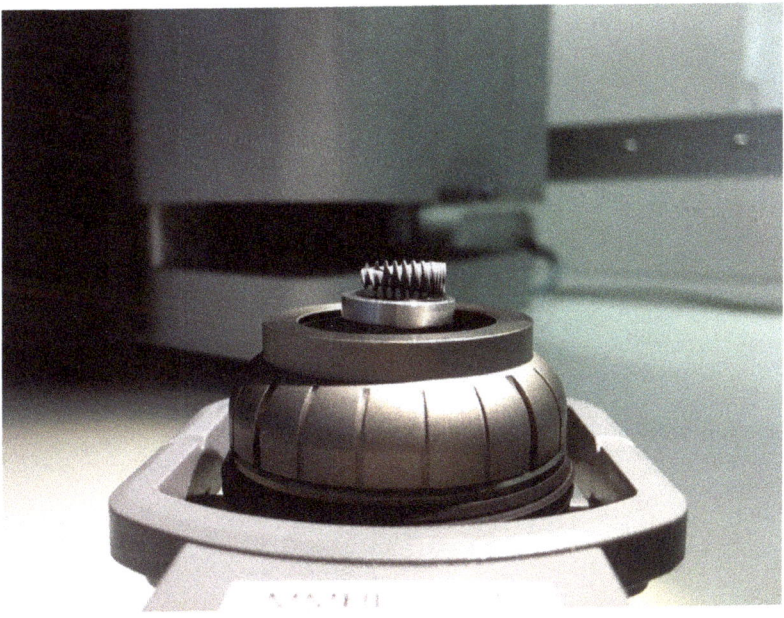

Figure 1. Implant sample with a length of 10 mm mounted on the SEM sample holder.

The scientific workstation used was a Phenom proX Scanning Electron Microscope (Eindhoven, Netherlands), equipped with a high-sensitivity backscattered electron (BSE) detector. The detector for the energy-dispersive X-ray spectroscopy (EDS) and elemental analysis was a thermoelectrically cooled silicon drift detector (SDD) type, with an active detector area of 25 mm^2.

The high-sensitivity BSE detector allows a magnification of up to 100,000× with a resolution down to 15 nm. This study used material-contrast images from 500× to a magnification of 5000×. Material-contrast imaging gave additional information about the chemical nature and allocation of different remnants or contaminations on the sample material.

In order to achieve a complete overview of the horizontally mounted implant sample and comprehensive surface quality information in high resolution, implants were scanned at a magnification of 500× in the "Image-Mapping" mode prior to the detailed analysis of potential impurities. This technique produces up to 600 single high-resolution SEM images of the implant surface that were digitally composed into one large image, with an extremely high resolution. The composed SEM image, showing the full size of the implant from shoulder to apex, made it possible to count particles in the visible field (viewing angle of approximately 120°) and to identify areas of interest for a subsequent EDS spot analysis. After the mapping process, SEM images of impurities and other regions of interest were produced with 500×, 1000× 2500×, and 5000× magnification. In the next step, the elemental composition of particles was determined and, where possible, the differential spectra of particles were achieved to subtract signals from the core material and such focus on signals from the superficial contamination (Figure 2).

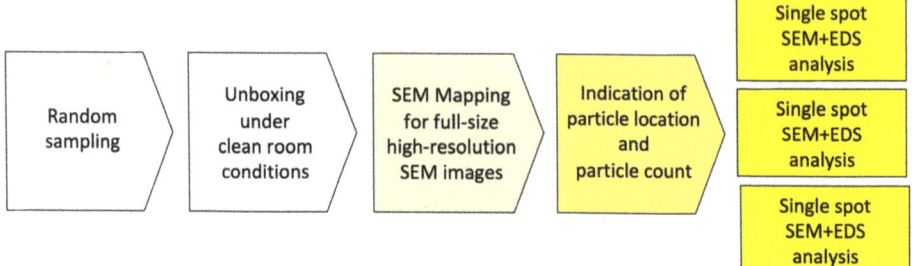

Figure 2. Workflow of the SEM/EDS analysis.

All of the analyses, as well as the complete setup, as described above were performed at the Medical Materials Research Institute, Berlin, Germany, which is an officially accredited (Deutsche Akkreditierungsstelle–DAkkS) and externally audited testing laboratory according to the international standards DIN EN ISO 9001:2015, ISO 22309:2015 and DIN EN ISO/IEC 17025. These standards were chosen as a precondition in order to assure testing procedures at the highest level of accuracy.

In addition to the SEM/EDS analysis, all of the implants in this study were provisionally evaluated from a surface topographical point of view by interferometry. All implants seemed to be in the moderately rough surface range, i.e., with Sa (Sa = arithmetical mean height of the surface) values of between 1 and 2 micrometers.

2.1. Clinical Documentation of Analyzed "Look-Alike" Implant Systems

A search for available clinical trial regarding the dental implant systems was carried out. Initially the website of each dental implant manufacturer was searched (www.biodenta.com, www.bioconcept.cn, www.cumdente.com). In addition, the manufacturers were contacted via their respective contact e-mail address on their websites, requesting any scientific documentation regarding clinical performance such as published papers or summaries of ongoing projects. If no response was received within one week, a reminder was sent.

Furthermore, a search for clinical trials was performed in the PubMed database (PubMed.gov, US National Library of Medicine, National Institutes of Health). The search terms "dental implants" (MeSH) and "dental implants" (free text) were used in combination with the product name "Biodenta", "Bioconcept", and "Cumdente". No limits were set. (("dental implants" [MeSH Terms] OR ("dental" [All Fields] AND "implants" [All Fields]) OR "dental implants" [All Fields]) AND biodenta [All Fields]), (("dental implants" [MeSH Terms] OR ("dental" [All Fields] AND "implants" [All Fields]) OR "dental implants" [All Fields]) AND bioconcept [All Fields], (("dental implants" [MeSH Terms] OR ("dental" [All Fields] AND "implants" [All Fields]) OR "dental implants" [All Fields]) AND cumdente [All Fields])).

2.2. Clinical Documentation of OsseoSpeed, SLA, and TiUnite Implant Systems

With respect to the implant systems OsseoSpeed from Dentsply-Sirona, SLA from Straumann, and TiUnite from Nobel Biocare, these belong to the most clinically documented oral implant systems in the world [2]. To remain brief, we decided to only quote five papers for each system as the total number of clinical reports on these devices amounts to several hundred scientific papers.

3. Results

3.1. SEM Imaging and Elemental Analysis

Implants were analyzed in three groups. In the first group, the implant from Astra Tech–Dentsply Implants (OsseoSpeed) and the implant from Cumdente (AS Implant) were compared. The full-size

SEM image of the Astra Tech implant—digitally composed of 455 single SEM images (tiles)—showed a homogenous surface with no foreign material (Figure 3).

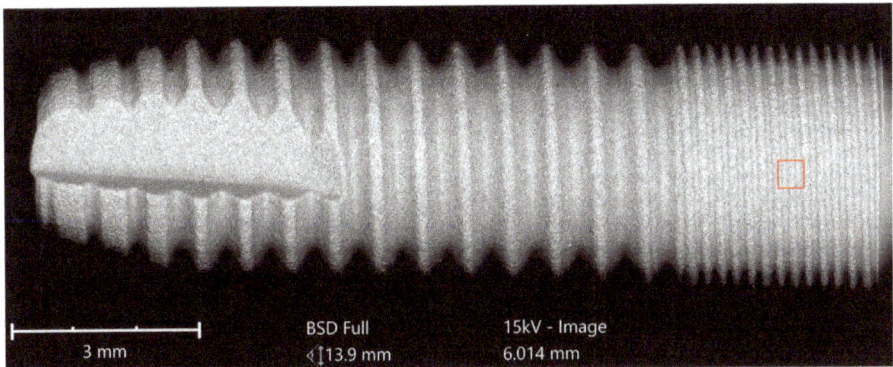

Figure 3. SEM mapping of OsseoSpeed implant (Astra Tech–Dentsply Implants). Magnification of the red marked area is shown in Figure 4.

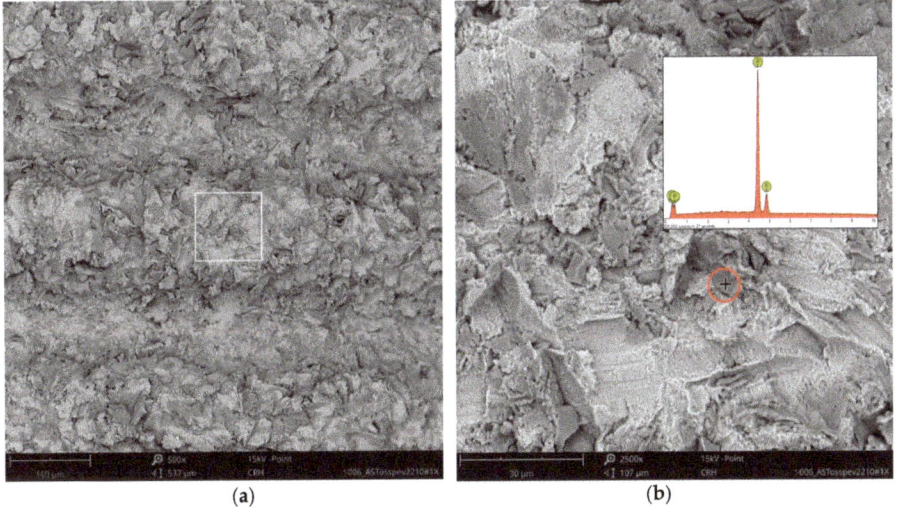

Figure 4. OsseoSpeed surface: (**a**) the red marked area in Figure 3 magnified 500×; (**b**) higher magnification (2500×) of the white marked area in the left image with EDS spot analysis of an embedded TiO_2-particle (spot is marked with "+" in the red circle) showing only signals of the blasting material.

Higher magnification could identify the TiO_2 particles from the blasting process seen as sharp-edged particles of 5–10 mm embedded in the titanium surface. Elemental analysis of these particles only displayed signals of titanium and oxygen (Figure 4).

The Cumdente implant showed several anomalies in the correspondent full-size image, composed of 422 tiles (Figure 5).

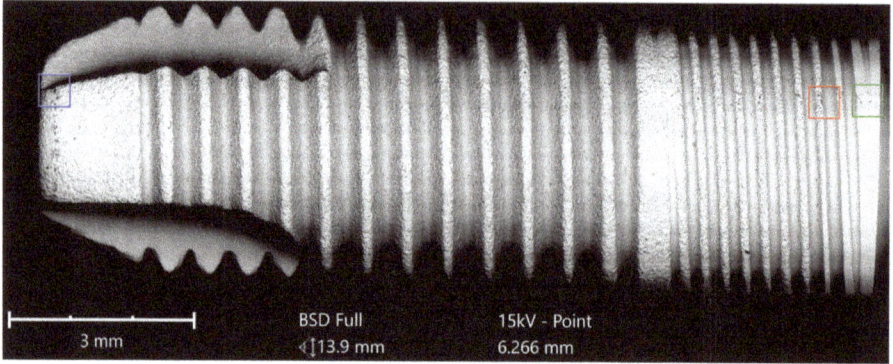

Figure 5. SEM mapping of the AS Implant (Cumdente); Red marked area—see magnification in Figure 6, blue marked area—see magnification in Figure 7, green marked area—see magnification in Figure 8.

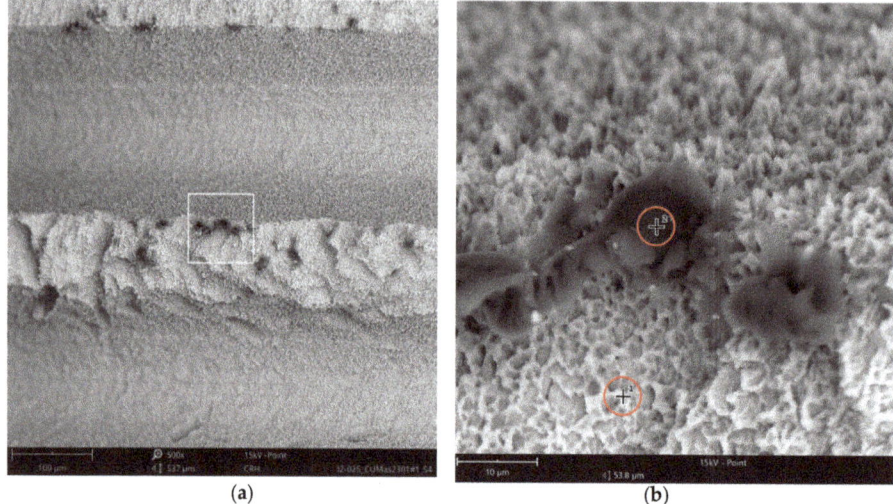

Figure 6. AS Implant (Cumdente) with organic particles (10–50 μm) at the implant shoulder: (**a**) systematic contamination of exposed threads, red marked area of Figure 5 in 500×; (**b**) magnification (5000×) of white marked area in the left image. The EDS differential measurement of the marked spots was identical to the particles in Figure 7.

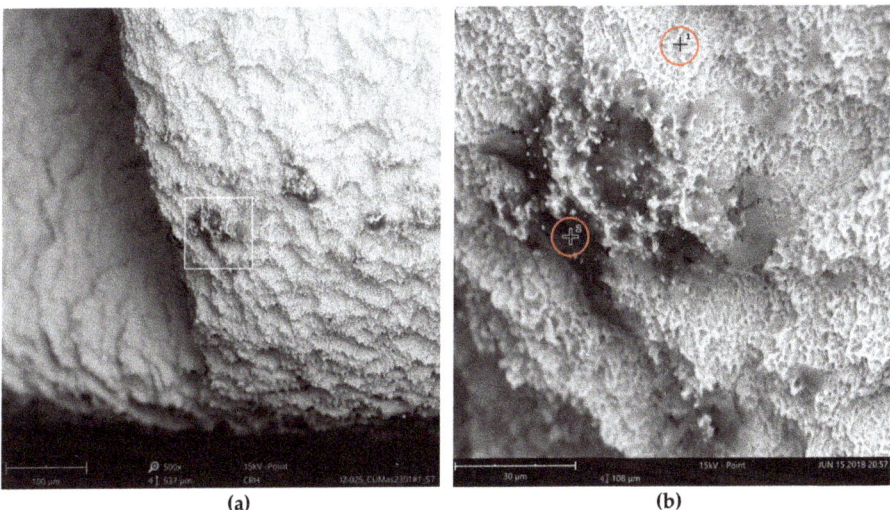

Figure 7. AS Implant (Cumdente) with organic particles (5–70 µm) at the implant's apex: (**a**) blue marked area of Figure 5 in 500×; (**b**) magnification (5000×) of white marked area in Figure 7a; EDS differential measurement of marked spots is shown in Figure 8.

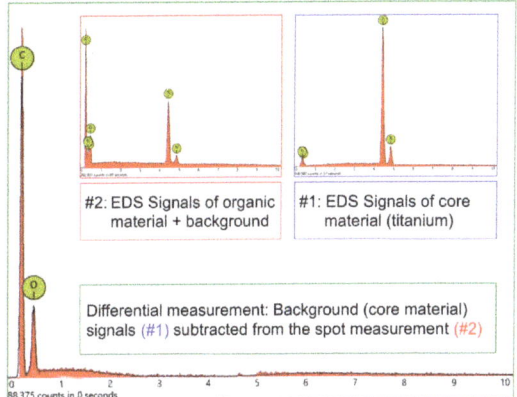

Figure 8. EDS differential measurement of the organic particle in Figure 7. Graph #1 shows titanium as the core material of this implant, with characteristic peaks at 0.452 KeV (La), 4.508 KeV (Lb), and 4.932 KeV (Kb). Graph #2 shows the spectrum of the particle with additional signals of the titanium background. The subtraction of X-ray quanta from the background material reveals the elemental composition of the impurity, which is carbon (characteristic Ka peak at 0.277 KeV) and oxygen (Ka peak at 0.523 KeV).

The SEM images with higher magnification revealed systematic contamination with multiple (>100) organic particles (5–60 µm) on exposed parts of the implant, as seen on the micro-threads next to the implant shoulder (Figure 6) and near the implant's apex (Figure 7).

In order to receive information about the particles' elemental composition, EDS measurement was performed with a spot focused on the foreign material, where background material was always detected as well, and another spot focused in direct proximity, where only the implant's core material was detected (spot #1 and #2 in Figures 6b and 7b, respectively). Using a software application, it was possible to subtract the signals of the core material so that the differential measurement revealed more precise information about the elemental composition of the foreign material. Figure 8 shows the differential EDS measurement of the particle in Figure 7, with a clear signal of carbon as the major element in this impurity.

One larger area at the implant shoulder showed numerous particles (5–40 µm) (Figure 9) with significant signals, not only of carbon but also of fluorine, as seen in the differential EDS analysis (Figure 10). The texture and elemental composition of the foreign material suggest that these particles are most likely remnants of polytetrafluoroethylene (PTFE), used at different implant production stages.

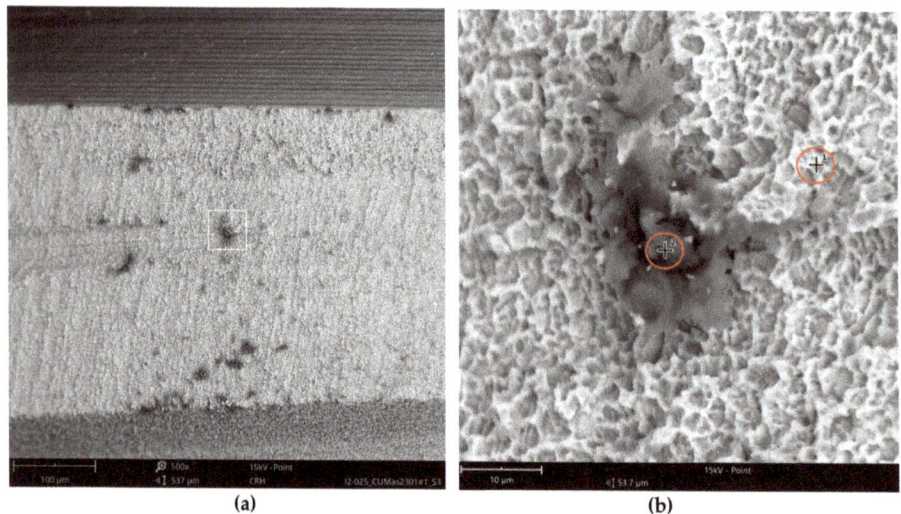

Figure 9. Possible remnants of polytetrafluoroethylene (PTFE), AS Implant (Cumdente); (**a**) green marked area of Figure 5 in 500× shows a larger area of impurities; (**b**) magnification (5000×) of white marked area in the left image; EDS differential measurement of the marked spots is shown in Figure 10.

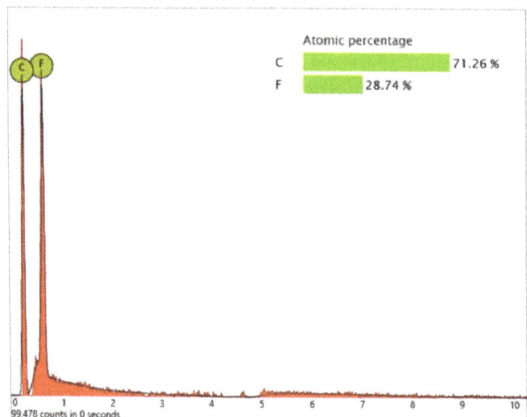

Figure 10. EDS differential measurement of the particles in Figure 9 with significant X-ray quanta of carbon and fluorine. Note that the quantitative information provided by the EDS analysis does not always reflect the precise stoichiometric relationship of the particle's chemical elements.

The second group compared the Straumann Standard Plus SLA Tissue Level Implant with an implant of the same geometry from Bioconcept, both made of commercially pure grade 4 titanium, which is a composition of 99% titanium, 0.50% iron (maximum), oxygen 0.40% (maximum), carbon 0.085 (maximum), hydrogen 0.015% (maximum), and nitrogen 0.05% (maximum), according to the ASTM F67 specification. The SEM imaging of the Straumann implant could not detect any organic or inorganic contaminants (Figures 11 and 12).

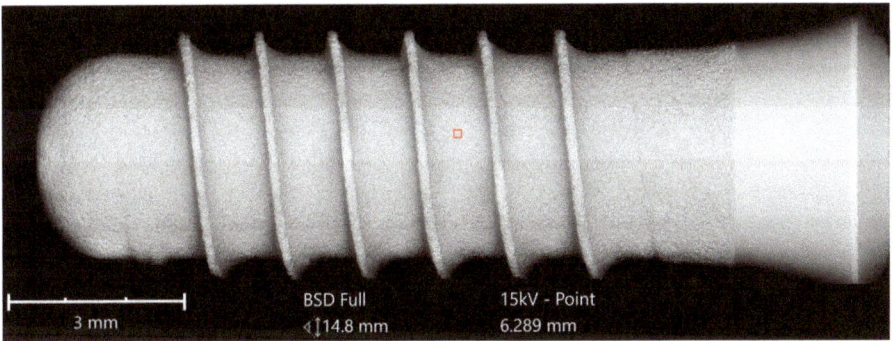

Figure 11. SEM mapping, Standard Plus SLA implant (Straumann); Magnification of red marked area is shown in Figure 12.

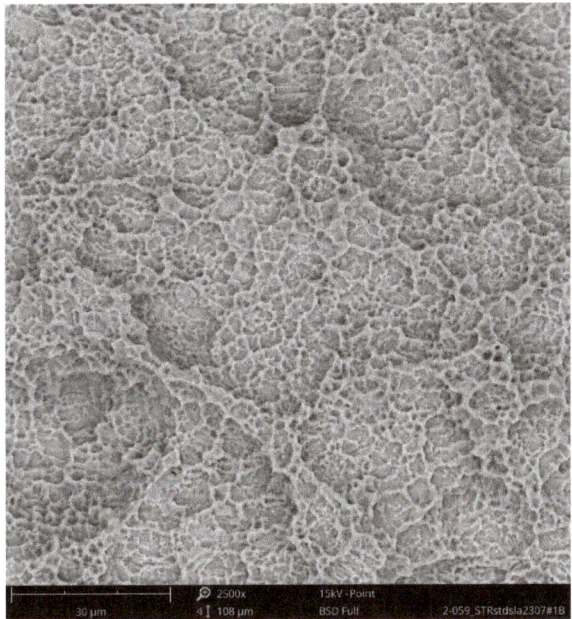

Figure 12. Surface of Standard Plus SLA implant (SEM 2500×); red marked area in Figure 11 with the typical texture of a sandblasted and acid-etched titanium surface, free of foreign materials.

While the Straumann implant can be rated as clean at the micron level, the analysis of the Bioconcept implant revealed several impurities, although the full-size image showed no systematic larger contamination (Figure 13). With higher magnification, approximately 20 small organic particles (10–20 µm) were found on the implant's surface, one particle showing additional signals of sulfur (Figure 15).

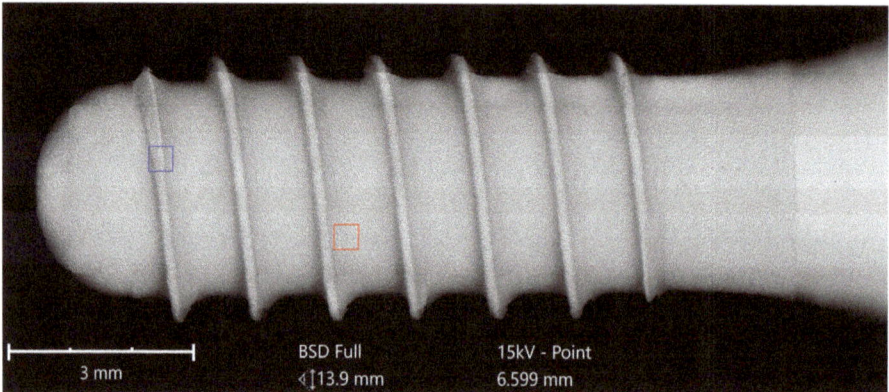

Figure 13. SEM mapping, Tissue Level Implant (Bioconcept); red marked area—see magnification in Figure 15, blue marked area—see magnification in Figure 14.

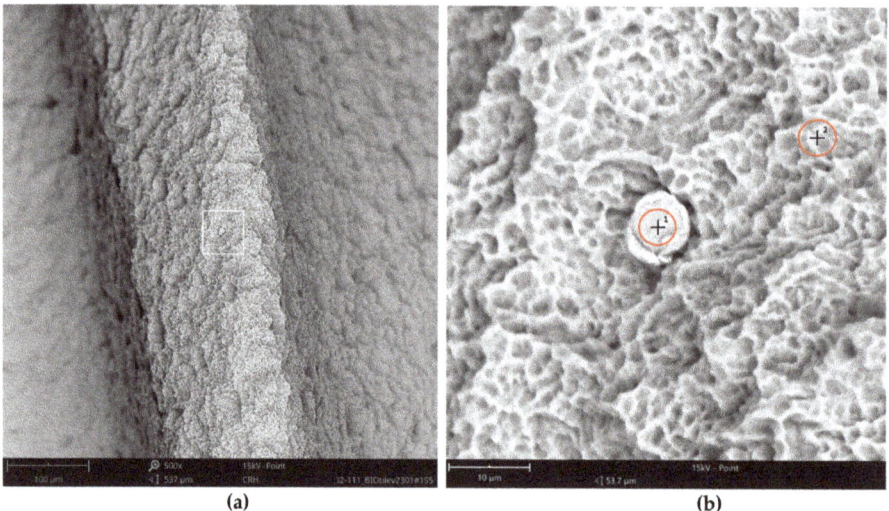

Figure 14. Metal particle on the surface of the Bioconcept implant; (**a**) blue marked area in Figure 13, SEM 500×; (**b**) magnification (5000×) of white marked area in the left image (**a**) showing bright metal impurity (8 μm) and 2 points of EDS spot measurement (#1 = metal particle, #2 = core material).

Surprisingly, one metal particle of 8 μm was found on the Bioconcept implant, seemingly entirely composed of iron, as the qualitative and quantitative elemental analysis and differential measurement of this particle revealed (Figures 14 and 16).

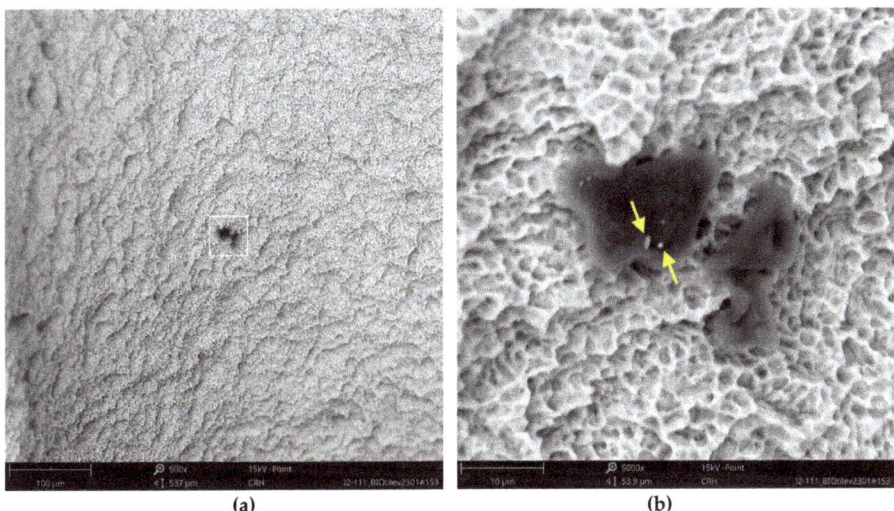

Figure 15. Bioconcept implant with organic particles (10–15 µm); (**a**) red marked area in Figure 13, SEM 500×; (**b**) magnification (5000×) of white marked area in the left image (**a**); arrows indicate two embedded metal particles (0.5–1 µm) showing significant iron signals in the subsequent EDS differential measurement.

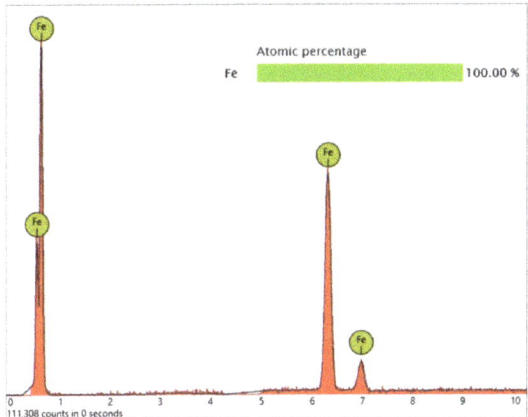

Figure 16. EDS differential measurement of the metal particle in Figure 14, revealing iron as the major element of the impurity.

The third group compared the NobelActive implant from Nobel Biocare with the Dental Implant from Biodenta. Both implants have an anodized surface with a characteristic titanium oxide layer. The area analysis of the NobelActive implant showed calcium and phosphorous signals in addition to titanium and oxygen. Within the scope of this analysis, neither inorganic nor organic particles were detected on the Nobel Biocare implant (Figures 17 and 18).

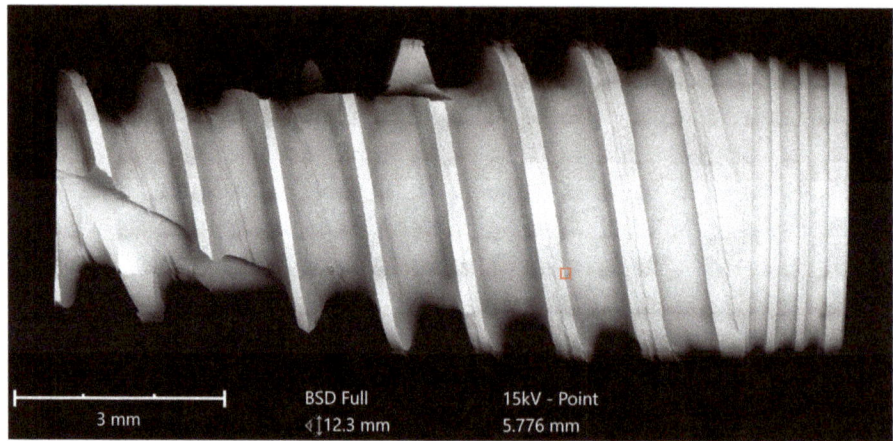

Figure 17. SEM mapping: NobelActive Internal RP implant (Nobel Biocare); red marked area—see magnification in Figure 18.

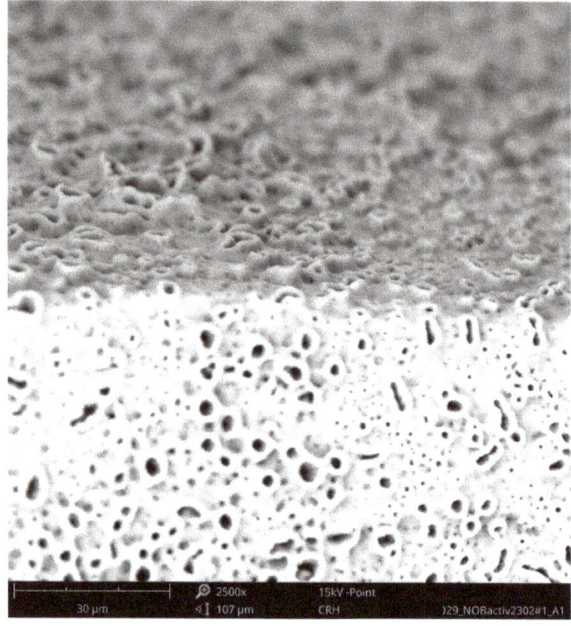

Figure 18. Surface of the NobelActive Internal RP implant (2500×); magnification of red marked area in Figure 17 with the typical texture of an anodized titanium surface, free of foreign materials.

While the full-size SEM image of the Biodenta implant exposed no significant organic contamination (Figure 19), the area analysis of the core material showed, in addition to calcium, phosphorous, titanium, and oxygen, high levels of magnesium in the EDS (Figure 20) that were not seen on the Nobel Biocare implant.

Significant traces of aluminum were detected in three areas of exposed threads and can be seen as bright particles (5–10 µm) in Figure 21. The graph in Figure 22 shows the correspondent EDS differential measurement of metal particles in Figure 20a.

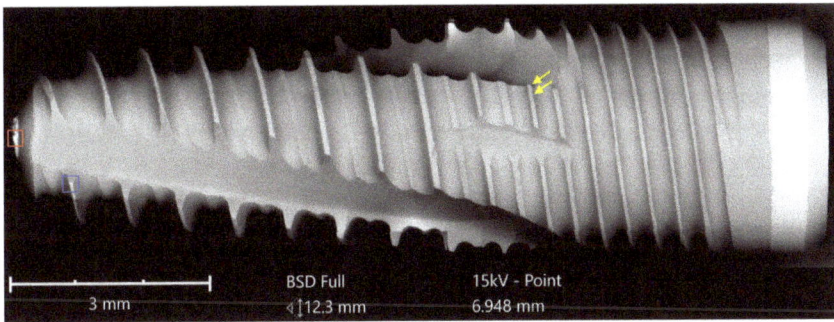

Figure 19. SEM mapping: Dental Implant (Biodenta); yellow arrows indicate spots with aluminum as shown in Figure 21. Magnifications of the blue and red marked areas are shown in Figure 23.

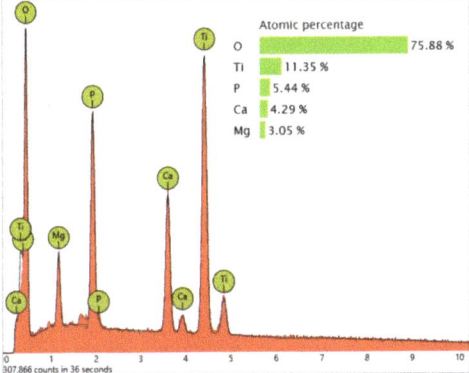

Figure 20. EDS area analysis of the implant's core material (Biodenta).

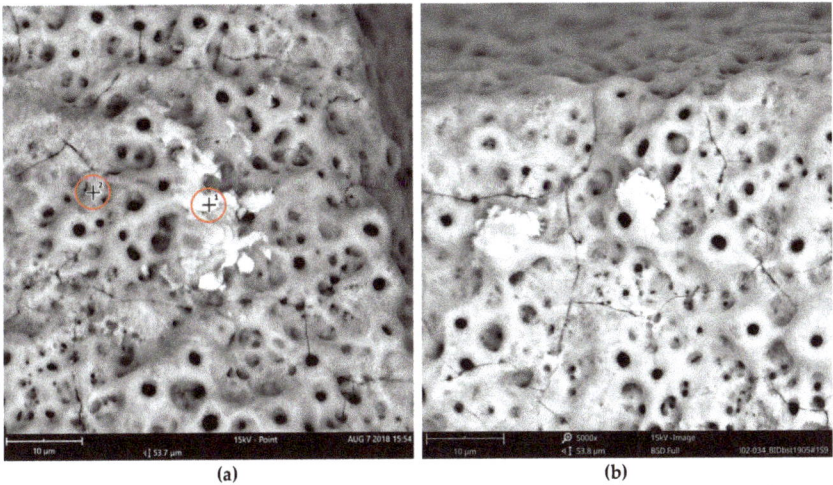

Figure 21. Aluminum-containing particles (5–10 µm) on the surface of the Biodenta implant; location shown using yellow arrows in Figure 19; (**a**) SEM 5000× with 2 points of EDS spot measurement shown in Figure 22; (**b**) impurities with similar size in close proximity to particles shown in the left image (**a**).

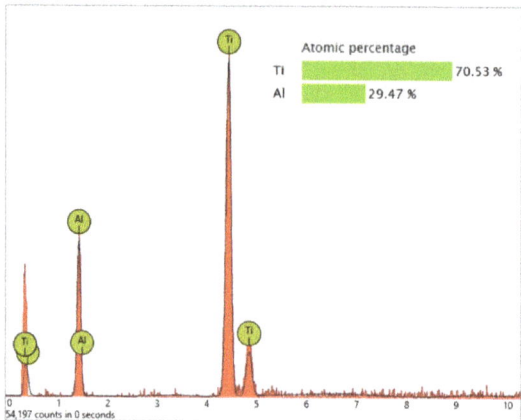

Figure 22. EDS differential measurement of the metal particle in Figure 20 (**a**), showing significant X-ray quanta of aluminum. The lack of oxygen signals indicates that these particles were not made of aluminum oxide.

These aluminum-containing particles must be rated as inorganic impurities as they are not comparable with sharp-edged aluminum oxide particles, used for blasting procedures of other implants. Apart from this, it is noticeable that the approximately 3 µm thick oxide layer was damaged at several exposed locations of the Biodenta implant (Figure 23).

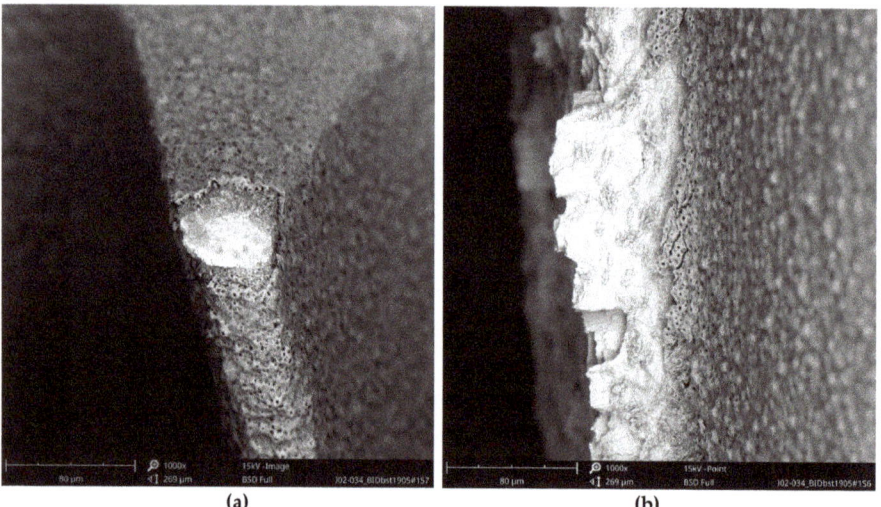

Figure 23. Damaged oxide layer of the Biodenta implant, SEM 1000×: (**a**) magnification of the blue marked area in Figure 19 showing the damage at the exposed implant thread; (**b**) magnification of the red marked area in Figure 19 demonstrates the large-area irregularity of the oxide layer at the implant apex.

3.2. Documentation of Clinical Results

None of the copy-cat manufacturers' websites contained any information regarding published clinical trials of the implant systems. No manufacturers responded to the email requesting scientific documentation regarding clinical performance. No manufacturers presented such documentation. The PubMed database search identified no papers regarding the Bioconcept or Cumdente system, but two papers for the Biodenta system. The two Biodenta papers were, however, in vitro trials that evaluated the company's CAD/CAM (computer-aided design/computer-aided manufacturing) system, not the clinical outcome of the implants [7,8]. Broadening the search by deleting "dental implants" and only using the respective company name did not identify any publications for the Cumdente system but one additional paper for the Biodenta system [9]. However, this paper did not report on the clinical outcome of implants. No clinical documentation of implant outcome was noticed for the Bioconcept system.

The OsseoSpeed implant has a very solid clinical documentation verifying excellent clinical results for up to 7 years in clinical function [10–14]. Similar excellent clinical results apply to the SLA implants from Straumann [4,15–18] and the TiUnite implants from Nobel Biocare [5,19–22], where these two implant systems have been documented for more than 10 years in numerous studies.

4. Discussion

In general, the implants OsseoSpeed (Astra Tech–Dentsply Implants), Standard Plus SLA Implant (Straumann), and NobelActive (Nobel Biocare) showed—within the scope of this analysis—a surface free of foreign materials in the SEM. The Cumdente AS Implant with a similar geometry compared to the Astra Tech OsseoSpeed implant demonstrated a surface with substantial organic contaminants and most likely remnants of Teflon. The Straumann look-alike implant from Bioconcept exposed numerous organic particles and two small particles containing significant amounts of iron. The Nobel Biocare look-alike implant from Biodenta showed high levels of magnesium and small particles with aluminum on the surface. These particles, with a diameter of 5 to 10 µm, and organic contaminants with a similar size, are small enough for phagocytosis by macrophages that would be theoretically possible for particles without a chemical bonding to the implant surface.

It may, therefore, be said that the original implants were cleaner than the correspondent look-alike devices. The price range for the look-alike implants indicated that the definition of a copy-cat product or look-alike implant is not necessarily based on a low price.

To the knowledge of the present authors, no defined thresholds have been published in peer reviewed journals until now, with respect to what may represent "acceptable" levels of impurities and what must be regarded as "unacceptable impurities". However, the non-profit CleanImplant Foundation (www.cleanimplant.org) has presented a consensus statement on surface impurities signed by Luigi Canullo (Rome, Italy), Jaafar Mouhyi (Marrakesh, Morroco), Michael Norton (London, UK), and four of the authors of this paper Tomas Albrektsson, Florian Beuer, Dirk Duddeck, and Ann Wennerberg [23]. In this consensus statement, surface anomalies and remnants of blasting materials were not considered clinically relevant, in contrast to the metal particles of tungsten, nickel, iron, chromium, copper, tin or antimony found on the surfaces of some implants. Single organic particles smaller than 50 µm in diameter were considered less vicious than numerous particles, with a maximum of 30 particles along the circumference of the implant. Major plaque-like organic contaminants exceeding the size of 50 µm and PTFE particles, presumably originating from Teflon baskets used during implant production, were considered unacceptable.

Other foreign bodies routinely seen adjacent to implants such as titanium particles [24–26] or the accidental presence of cement in the bone-to-implant interface that, according to some investigators, may be found in 59% of cemented implants [27], may combine to cause peri-implantitis [28].

Impurities on sterile packaged implants—caused by metal particles and contaminations with organic substances such as thermoplastic materials, synthetic polymers, or polysiloxanes—are technically avoidable, as this paper demonstrated. The academic discussion as to what extent implant pollution is acceptable normally ends quickly when dental professionals know about such contamination of an implant system and the next patient for an implant therapy is their partner or child. We should avoid using sterile packaged implants with verifiable impurities and therewith follow the well-established "precautionary principle" as an evolution of the ancient medical principle of "primum non nocere".

From a clinical point of view, it is obvious that Astra Tech–Dentsply Implants, Straumann, and Nobel Biocare have solidly documented clinical results reported in hundreds of scientific papers. On the other hand, a long history of clinical documentation representing high-quality efforts in the past is no guarantee for a high level of production quality and a clean surface at present, accentuating the need for periodic reviews by independent institutions. With respect to the look-alike systems, none of them had any properly documented clinical reports available. The absence of clinical documentation of look-alike systems may indicate either that they see themselves as identical to the implants they have copied or that they see implants as commodity products where all implant systems will work well clinically. The possibility first mentioned was critically analyzed in this paper comparing the cleanliness of different implant systems. The second possibility that implants are commodity products may be criticized against the knowledge of numerous implant systems that have been withdrawn from the market due to the unforeseen clinical problems over longer times of follow-up [29].

In essence, our hypothesis was verified in that the major implant systems displayed cleaner surfaces than those of their respective look-alike implants. However, whether the relative lack of cleanliness of look-alike implants indicates that they have an impaired clinical function in comparison to the major systems remains uncertain. Having said this, oral implants are placed in human beings and, therefore, it seems strongly advisable to present clinical results in peer-reviewed journals for every oral implant system to be used clinically. In this regard, the look-alike implants are clearly inferior to the major documented oral implant systems and none of the look-alike systems investigated had any clinical documentation of their own, which must be regarded as a major shortcoming. Since differences obviously exist between the major systems and the respective look-alike implants, clinicians using the latter devices must inform their patients of this fact and that the implants placed are totally un-documented with respect to clinical outcome.

5. Conclusions

In contrast to the original implants of market-leading manufacturers, the analyzed look-alike implants showed significantly more impurities, underlining the need for periodic reviews of the production quality by independent institutions. Multiple organic particles and remnants of PTFE (Cumdente), organic particles containing sulfur, particles containing iron (Bioconcept) or impurities with aluminum (Biodenta)—all particles small enough for possible phagocytosis—expose patients to unknown risks. In addition to the results of SEM/EDS analysis, the lack of clinical documentation of the analyzed look-alike implants raises concerns.

Author Contributions: Conceptualization, D.U.D., A.W., and T.A.; Investigation, D.U.D., C.L., and A.W.; Resources, D.U.D.; Writing—Original Draft Preparation, D.U.D., T.A., A.W., and C.L., Writing—Review and Editing, A.W., C.L., and F.B.; Supervision, D.U.D.; Project Administration, D.U.D.

Funding: This research received no external funding.

Acknowledgments: SEM images and elemental analyses for this paper were performed with technical support from the Medical Materials Research Institute–mmri.berlin, Max-Planck-Str. 3, Zentrum für Mikrosysteme und Materialien (ZMM), 12489 Berlin–Adlershof, Germany.

Conflicts of Interest: Tomas Albrektsson is a scientific consultant to Nobel Biocare. All other authors declare no conflict of interest.

References

1. Branemark, P.I.; Hansson, B.O.; Adell, R.; Breine, U.; Lindström, J.; Hallén, O.; Ohman, A. Osseointegrated implants in the treatment of the edentulous jaw. Experience from a 10-year period. *Scand. J. Plast. Reconstr. Surg. Suppl.* **1977**, *16*, 1–132. [PubMed]
2. Jimbo, R.; Albrektsson, T. Long-term clinical success of minimally and moderately rough oral implants: A review of 71 studies with 5 years or more of follow-up. *Implant Dent.* **2015**, *24*, 62–69. [CrossRef] [PubMed]

3. Wennerberg, A.; Albrektsson, T.; Chrcanovic, B. Long-term clinical outcome of implants with different surface modifications. *Eur. J. Oral Implantol.* **2018**, *11* (Suppl. 1), S123–S136. [PubMed]
4. Buser, D.; Janner, S.F.; Wittneben, J.G.; Bragger, U.; Ramseier, C.A.; Salvi, G.E. 10-year survival and success rates of 511 titanium implants with a sandblasted and acid-etched surface: A retrospective study in 303 partially edentulous patients. *Clin. Implant Dent. Relat. Res.* **2012**, *14*, 839–851. [CrossRef] [PubMed]
5. Glauser, R. Implants with an Oxidized Surface Placed Predominantly in Soft Bone Quality and Subjected to Immediate Occlusal Loading: Results from an 11-Year Clinical Follow-Up. *Clin. Implant Dent. Relat. Res.* **2016**, *18*, 429–438. [CrossRef] [PubMed]
6. Toljanic, J.A.; Ekstrand, K.; Baer, R.A.; Thor, A. Immediate Loading of Implants in the Edentulous Maxilla with a Fixed Provisional Restoration without Bone Augmentation: A Report on 5-Year Outcomes Data Obtained from a Prospective Clinical Trial. *Int. J. Oral Maxillofac. Implant.* **2016**, *31*, 1164–1170. [CrossRef] [PubMed]
7. Katsoulis, J.; Muller, P.; Mericske-Stern, R.; Blatz, M.B. CAD/CAM fabrication accuracy of long- vs. short-span implant-supported FDPs. *Clin. Oral Implant. Res.* **2015**, *26*, 245–249. [CrossRef]
8. Rismanchian, M.; Shafiei, S.; Nourbakhshian, F.; Davoudi, A. Flexural strengths of implant-supported zirconia based bridges in posterior regions. *J. Adv. Prosthodont.* **2014**, *6*, 346–350. [CrossRef]
9. Rismanchian, M.; Shafiei, S.; Askari, N.; Khodaeian, N. Comparison of shear bond strength of two veneering ceramics to zirconia. *Dent. Res. J.* **2012**, *9*, 628–633. [CrossRef]
10. Boven, G.C.; Slot, J.W.A.; Raghoebar, G.M.; Vissink, A.; Meijer, H.J.A. Maxillary implant-supported overdentures opposed by (partial) natural dentitions: A 5-year prospective case series study. *J. Oral Rehabil.* **2017**, *44*, 988–995. [CrossRef]
11. Cooper, L.F.; Reside, G.; Raes, F.; Garriga, J.; Tarrida, L.; Wiltfang, J.; Kern, M.; Bruyn, H. Immediate provisionalization of dental implants in grafted alveolar ridges in the esthetic zone: A 5-year evaluation. *Int. J. Periodontics Restor. Dent.* **2014**, *34*, 477–486. [CrossRef]
12. Mertens, C.; Steveling, H.G. Early and immediate loading of titanium implants with fluoride-modified surfaces: Results of 5-year prospective study. *Clin. Oral Implant. Res.* **2011**, *22*, 1354–1360. [CrossRef]
13. Noelken, R.; Moergel, M.; Kunkel, M.; Wagner, W. Immediate and flapless implant insertion and provisionalization using autogenous bone grafts in the esthetic zone: 5-year results. *Clin. Oral Implant. Res.* **2018**, *29*, 320–327. [CrossRef]
14. Raes, S.; Raes, F.; Cooper, L.; Giner Tarrida, L.; Vervaeke, S.; Cosyn, J.; De Bruyn, H. Oral health-related quality of life changes after placement of immediately loaded single implants in healed alveolar ridges or extraction sockets: A 5-year prospective follow-up study. *Clin. Oral Implant. Res.* **2017**, *28*, 662–667. [CrossRef]
15. Fischer, K.; Stenberg, T. Prospective 10-year cohort study based on a randomized controlled trial (RCT) on implant-supported full-arch maxillary prostheses. Part 1: Sandblasted and acid-etched implants and mucosal tissue. *Clin. Implant Dent. Relat. Res.* **2012**, *14*, 808–815. [CrossRef]
16. French, D.; Larjava, H.; Ofec, R. Retrospective cohort study of 4591 Straumann implants in private practice setting, with up to 10-year follow-up. Part 1: Multivariate survival analysis. *Clin. Oral Implant. Res.* **2015**, *26*, 1345–1354. [CrossRef]
17. Roccuzzo, M.; Grasso, G.; Dalmasso, P. Keratinized mucosa around implants in partially edentulous posterior mandible: 10-year results of a prospective comparative study. *Clin. Oral Implant. Res.* **2016**, *27*, 491–496. [CrossRef]
18. Zhang, X.X.; Shi, J.Y.; Gu, Y.X.; Lai, H. Long-Term Outcomes of Early Loading of Straumann Implant-Supported Fixed Segmented Bridgeworks in Edentulous Maxillae: A 10-Year Prospective Study. *Clin. Implant Dent. Relat. Res.* **2016**, *18*, 1227–1237. [CrossRef]
19. Degidi, M.; Nardi, D.; Piattelli, A. 10-year follow-up of immediately loaded implants with TiUnite porous anodized surface. *Clin. Implant Dent. Relat. Res.* **2012**, *14*, 828–838. [CrossRef]
20. Imburgia, M.; Del Fabbro, M. Long-Term Retrospective Clinical and Radiographic Follow-up of 205 Branemark System Mk III TiUnite Implants Submitted to Either Immediate or Delayed Loading. *Implant Dent.* **2015**, *24*, 533–540. [CrossRef]
21. Karl, M.; Albrektsson, T. Clinical Performance of Dental Implants with a Moderately Rough (TiUnite) Surface: A Meta-Analysis of Prospective Clinical Studies. *Int. J. Oral. Maxillofac. Implant.* **2017**, *32*, 717–734. [CrossRef]

22. Ostman, P.O.; Hellman, M.; Sennerby, L. Ten years later. Results from a prospective single-centre clinical study on 121 oxidized (TiUnite) Branemark implants in 46 patients. *Clin. Implant Dent. Relat. Res.* **2012**, *14*, 852–860. [CrossRef]
23. Duddeck, D.; Albrektsson, T.; Wennerberg, A.; Mouhyi, J.; Norton, M.; Canullo, L.; Beuer, F. CleanImplant Trusted Quality Mark 2017–2018—Guideline and Consensus Paper. Available online: www.cleanimplant.org (accessed on 26 June 2019).
24. Albrektsson, T.; Becker, W.; Coli, P.; Jemt, T.; Mölne, J.; Sennerby, L. Bone loss around oral and orthopedic implants: An immunologically based condition. *Clin. Implant Dent. Relat. Res.* **2019**, *21*, 786–795. [CrossRef]
25. Tawse-Smith, A.; Ma, S.; Siddiqi, A.; Duncan, W.J.; Girvan, L.; Hussaini, H.M. Titanium Particles in the Peri-Implant Tissues: Surface Analysis and Histological Response. *Clin. Adv. Periodontics* **2012**, *2*, 232–238. [CrossRef]
26. Wennerberg, A.; Ide-Ektessabi, A.; Hatkamata, S.; Sawase, T.; Johansson, C.; Albrektsson, T.; Martinelli, A.; Södervall, U.; Odelius, H. Titanium release from implants prepared with different surface roughness. *Clin. Oral Implant. Res.* **2004**, *15*, 505–512. [CrossRef]
27. Korsch, M.; Obst, U.; Walther, W. Cement-associated peri-implantitis: A retrospective clinical observational study of fixed implant-supported restorations using a methacrylate cement. *Clin. Oral Implant. Res.* **2014**, *25*, 797–802. [CrossRef]
28. Wilson, T.G., Jr.; Valderrama, P.; Burbano, M.; Blansett, J.; Levine, R.; Kessler, H.; Rodrigues, D.C. Foreign bodies associated with peri-implantitis human biopsies. *J. Periodontol.* **2015**, *86*, 9–15. [CrossRef]
29. Qian, J.; Wennerberg, A.; Albrektsson, T. Reasons for marginal bone loss around oral implants. *Clin. Implant Dent. Relat. Res.* **2012**, *14*, 792–807. [CrossRef]

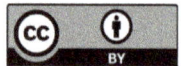

© 2019 by the authors. Licensee MDPI, Basel, Switzerland. This article is an open access article distributed under the terms and conditions of the Creative Commons Attribution (CC BY) license (http://creativecommons.org/licenses/by/4.0/).

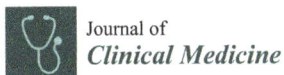

Article

The Effect of In Vitro Electrolytic Cleaning on Biofilm-Contaminated Implant Surfaces

Christoph Ratka [1,†], Paul Weigl [1,†], Dirk Henrich [2], Felix Koch [3], Markus Schlee [3] and Holger Zipprich [1,*]

1. Department of Prosthodontics, Goethe University, 60590 Frankfurt am Main, Germany
2. Department of Trauma, Hand & Reconstructive Surgery, Goethe University, 60590 Frankfurt am Main, Germany
3. Private Practice, and Department of Maxillofacial Surgery, Goethe University, 60590 Frankfurt am Main, Germany
* Correspondence: zipprich@em.uni-frankfurt.de; Tel.: +49-69-6301-4714; Fax: +49-69-6301-3711
† These authors contributed equally to this work.

Received: 15 August 2019; Accepted: 3 September 2019; Published: 6 September 2019

Abstract: Purpose: Bacterial biofilms are a major problem in the treatment of infected dental and orthopedic implants. The purpose of this study is to investigate the cleaning effect of an electrolytic approach (EC) compared to a powder-spray system (PSS) on titanium surfaces. Materials and Methods: The tested implants (different surfaces and alloys) were collated into six groups and treated ether with EC or PSS. After a mature biofilm was established, the implants were treated, immersed in a nutritional solution, and streaked on Columbia agar. Colony-forming units (CFUs) were counted after breeding and testing (EC), and control (PSS) groups were compared using a paired sample t-test. Results: No bacterial growth was observed in the EC groups. After thinning to 1:1,000,000, 258.1 ± 19.9 (group 2), 264.4 ± 36.5 (group 4), and 245.3 ± 40.7 (group 6) CFUs could be counted in the PSS groups. The difference between the electrolytic approach (test groups 1, 3, and 5) and PSS (control groups 2, 4, and 6) was statistically extremely significant (p-value $< 2.2 \times 10^{-16}$). Conclusion: Only EC inactivated the bacterial biofilm, and PSS left reproducible bacteria behind. Within the limits of this in vitro test, clinical relevance could be demonstrated.

Keywords: dental implant; biofilm; infection; perio-prosthetic joint infection; periimplantitis; electrolytic cleaning

1. Introduction

Growing numbers of inserted dental implants correlate to an increasing number of infected implants [1]. Periimplantitis (PI) is defined as an inflammatory process affecting both periimplant soft and hard tissue. Craterlike bone defects, ongoing bone loss, pus, and bleeding on probing (BoP) are clinical parameters that have to be present to justify the diagnosis of PI [2,3]. PI correlates to bacterial biofilms growing on implants or abutments [4]. In view of the various definitions of PI and the lack of agreement in the dental community about an acceptable threshold of bone loss, there is no consensus on when pathology starts and how PI can be diagnosed precisely. Hence, there is no consensus about prevalence data [5–7]. A proper treatment modality is lacking [8]. Whether the bacterial biofilm is the single causal factor or only correlates to PI [9] is still a matter of discussion. This debate about etiology is not merely an academic question, but may influence the success rate of therapy, because of possible differences in specimen susceptibility and uncorrectable surgical or mechanical obstacles. In any event, biofilm needs to be removed to prevent progression of disease, or to treat PI successfully. As implant surfaces exposed to the oral cavity are immediately colonized by bacteria, the surfaces need to be re-osseointegrated for good long-term results [10].

Infection of plates or other orthopedic devices, or endoprostheses caused by polymicrobial biofilms, is a major challenge. The average infection rate of implants in the shoulder, knee, and hip is less than 2% in most treatment centers [11,12]. A recent meta-analysis demonstrates an overall cumulative incidence of endoprosthetic joint infection across all studies of 0.78% [13]. It has been reported that, in the United States, more than 1 million implants placed in shoulders, knees, and hips need to be replaced every year due to infections [14]. A systematic review showed a reinfection rate of 7.6% (95% CI 3.4–13.1) of hip and knee replacements [15]. Polymicrobial biofilm on orthopedic implants shows high resistance to immune defense, and will result in local inhibition of granulocyte activity around the implant. This effect is referred to as frustrated phagocytosis, which leads to degranulation, reduced ingestion ability, and production of oxygen radicals in the granulocytes [16]. The standard treatment protocol for infected orthopedic implants is replacement in a one- or two-stage procedure, with a success rate of 80–90% [17,18]. Even early infections within the first 30 days after implantation that are treated by aggressive debridement and long-time antibiotics yield success rates of only 71% [19,20].

In most cases, all treatment modalities fail to cure infected implants, requiring replacement of the implant or causing at least an inadequate failure rate and immense costs. Therefore, it is necessary to search for another approach to decontaminate infected implants.

Several ablative methods to remove biofilms, such as mechanical debridement with curettes, brushes, lasers, cotton pellets, cold plasma, or air-powder sprays, combined or not combined with disinfecting or antibiotic agents, have been discussed. Re-osseointegration of formerly infected dental implant surfaces was reported in animal studies for between 39% and 46% of the surface [21]. There is no evidence of whether and to what percentage re-osseointegration occurs clinically. A recent review of the literature demonstrated the equality of all published methods, and no method seemed able to achieve stable results over time [22]. Follow-up revealed recurrence of the disease in up to 100% for some methods after one year [8]. A powder-spray system (PSS) is commonly used to clean implant surfaces. Erythritol (size 14 µm) or glycine (size 25 µm) particles are accelerated by air pressure (2 bar). When the particles impact at an angle of 30–60° at an ideal working distance of 3–5 mm, the kinetic energy of the powder removes biofilm, according to the manufacturer's manual. Several animal studies investigating re-osseointegration after cleaning with a PSS proved incomplete re-osseointegration [21]. Improvement of periimplant parameters, such as BoP, probing depth, and pus was clinically proven after the PSS, but re-osseointegration was not proven. Furthermore, the PSS failed to demonstrate superiority over any other treatment modality [23–25]. Possible reasons for this incomplete cleaning efficacy might be craterlike bone defects, with limited access and thus an improper working angle and distance of the device, the macro- and micro-design of implant surface, and oversized particles for much smaller bacteria hidden in the microstructure of textured implants. In an in vitro test, implants contaminated with *E. coli* were treated with a continuous current of 0–10 mA. Two implants were loaded as either cathode or anode, resulting in reduced numbers of bacteria on both implants. On anodic implants, a current of more than 75 mA caused complete killing of the bacteria [26]. Zipprich et al. loaded the implant as a cathode, and a platinum-coated titanium acted as the anode [27]. In this in vitro trial, the implants were exposed to a sodium-iodine solution buffered by lactic acid to avoid alkalization of the salt solution [27]. Hydrolytic splitting of water produces hydrogen cations as long as the implants are loaded. These hydrogen cations penetrate the biofilm, and after an electron has been taken from the implant surface, hydrogen forms between the implant surface and the biofilm. The hydrogen bubbles remove the biofilm. While all the other discussed methods for removing a biofilm are ablative, the electrolytic approach presented here works under the biofilm, directly on the implant surface, regardless of surface characteristics or alloy. Our results support the finding that the potassium iodine solution allows a higher current than the previously published sodium chloride solution [27]. This results in higher hydrogen production and a possible direct bactericidal effect. A cooperating working group examined the exact working mode of this method and proved its effectiveness in killing bacteria [28]. The current gold standard in dentistry is to remove biofilm with a PSS. These positive preliminary results for an electrolytic approach (EC) encouraged the authors to compare the cleaning effect of air-powder-water spray as an accepted method of cleaning contaminated implant surfaces with the new electrolytic approach in vitro.

2. Materials and Methods

2.1. Null Hypothesis

The null hypothesis is that the electrolytic approach works equally as well as PSS cleaning.

2.2. Preparation of Test Implant and Grouping

For the study, test implants were designed and produced by the authors to be as close as possible to clinical reality in implant and orthopedic surgery. The test specimens were made of grade 4 and 5 titanium, and consisted of a test and a carrier part (Figure 1). The design of the test part was similar to a standard, parallel-threaded dental implant (∅ 4.0 mm/L = 11.0 mm pitch = 0.6 mm) with different surface modifications. The carrier part was machined to serve as the electricity conductor and to fix the test specimen in the experimental set-up without influencing the area of interest of the test area. Furthermore, the test and carrier part could be separated at a predetermined breaking point to avoid bacterial contamination of the test area during handling.

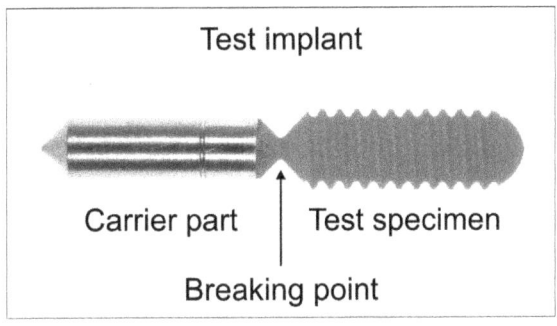

Figure 1. The structure of test implants.

Six groups of implants ($n = 12$ per group, 72 in total) were investigated. Ten per group were treated (60 in total), while two served as negative controls and were not treated (12 in total):

Group 1: titanium grade 4 + sandblasting and acid-etching + electrolytic cleaning;
Group 2: titanium grade 4 + sandblasting and acid-etching + air-powder-water spray cleaning;
Group 3: titanium grade 5 + sandblasting and acid-etching + electrolytic cleaning;
Group 4: titanium grade 5 + sandblasting and acid-etching + air-powder-water spray cleaning;
Group 5: titanium grade 4 + anodic oxidation + electrolytic cleaning;
Group 6: titanium grade 4 + anodic oxidation + air-powder-water spray cleaning.

Groups 1, 3, and 5 (test group) were treated with an electrolytic treatment, and groups 2, 4, and 6 (control group) were treated with a PSS.

2.3. Saliva Collection

In order to ensure a diversity of microorganisms, saliva was collected from three volunteers (different ages, 2 male, 1 female, healthy, no medication or drugs). The collected saliva (3 mL) was pooled, centrifuged to spin down any large debris and cells (2600 g for 10 min), and the liquid supernatant was mixed with 0.5 L nutrition solution culture (Bacto Tryptic Soy Broth, Becton Dickenson, Heidelberg, Germany), and incubated under 37 °C on the rocking device for 48 h, as previously described [29]. The solution was then filled into tubes (1.5 mL, Eppendorf Safe-Lock Tubes, Eppendorf, Hamburg, Germany) and frozen at −18 °C to provide identical samples for all further tests.

2.4. Establishing the Biofilm

To breed the biofilm on the implants, the required bacterial samples were thawed and bred with 300 mL nutrition solution in a beaker at 37 °C for 24 h. The carrier parts of the sterilized implants were masked to reduce bacterial contamination and fixed on a base plate. The experimental set-up was then immersed in the beaker with the culture medium to initiate formation of the biofilm. The beaker was placed in the rocking incubator for 14 days at a temperature of 37 °C. Previous tests with daily checks with a scanning electron micrograph (SEM) had demonstrated that 14 days were necessary to achieve a mature, multilayer biofilm (Figure 2). Every two days, the bacterial culture medium was replaced with freshly prepared nutritional solution.

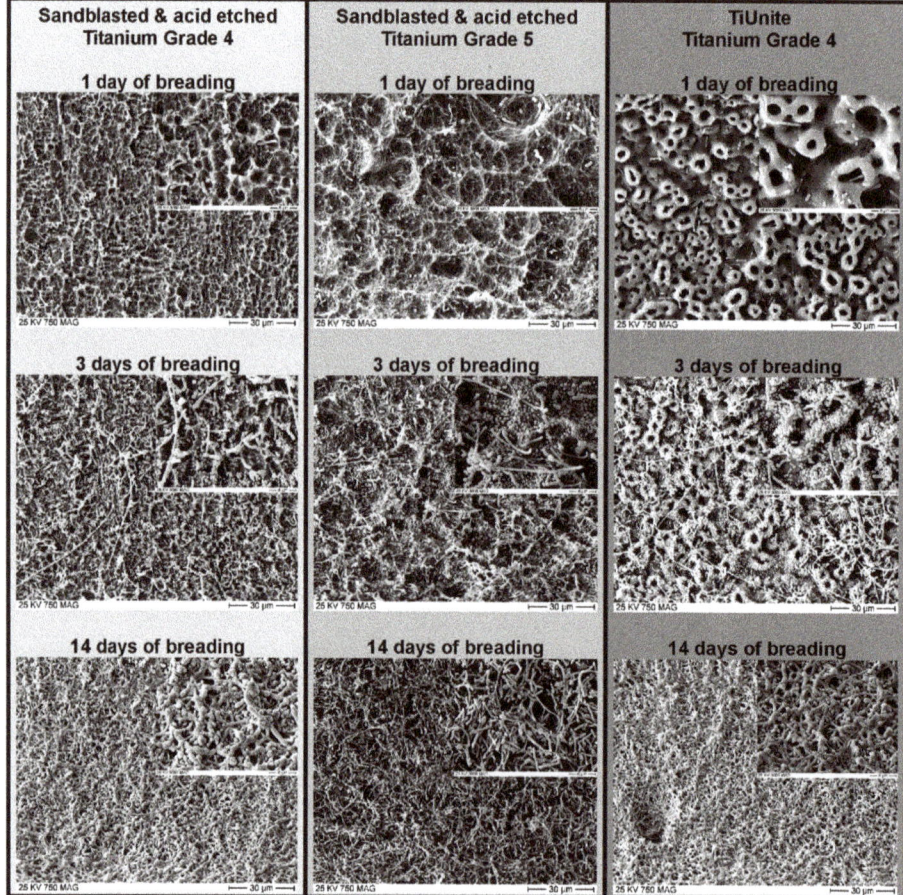

Figure 2. Progredient formation of biofilms on different surfaces.

2.5. Electrolytic Cleaning (Test Group)

The implants in groups 1, 3, and 5 were cleaned by an electrolytic process. Figure 3 shows the construction of the electrolytic chamber. After demasking of the biofilm-coated test implant with a customized ejector, the implant was mounted on the bottom of the electrolytic chamber with a customized connector. The test implant served as the cathode. The connector had an inner titanium sleeve (titanium grade 4) covered by an insulating polyetheretherketone (PEEK) carrier. The inner titanium sleeve was connected to the electric source, and the PEEK carrier masked the carrier part of the test implant for only three quarters. This design was chosen to guarantee that it was possible to separate the test specimen using a customized tool, without touching the PEEK carrier, which was not been cleaned during the electrolytic procedure. The connector was mounted in a polytetrafluoroethylene (PTFE) socket to ensure stability of the electrolytic chamber.

After the cathode was fixed, the glass cylinder of the chamber was mounted, and 35 mL of electrolyte (sodium iodide (200 g/L), potassium iodide (200 g/L), L(+)-lactic acid (20 g/L), and water (800 g/L)) was poured into the chamber. Fresh electrolyte was used for each test.

The anode (titanium grade 4) was coated with platinum to prevent passivation of its surface. The anode was fixed in a hollow PTFE tube to ensure direct contact of the platinum-plated part with the electrolyte (∅ 5.0 mm/L = 4.0 mm). After the other end of the PTFE tube had been mounted in the cap of the chamber, the anode and cathode were connected to a voltage source (PeakTech 6060, PeakTech, Ahrensburg, Germany).

A voltage of 6 V was applied for 5 minutes, resulting in a current of up to 1100 mA.

After the cleaning process was finished, the cap of the chamber was removed, and the used electrolyte was poured into a beaker. The biofilm floated as a visible layer on the fluid in the beaker, and was pipetted with some fluid to prove the vitality of the collected bacteria (waste from electrolytic cleaning).

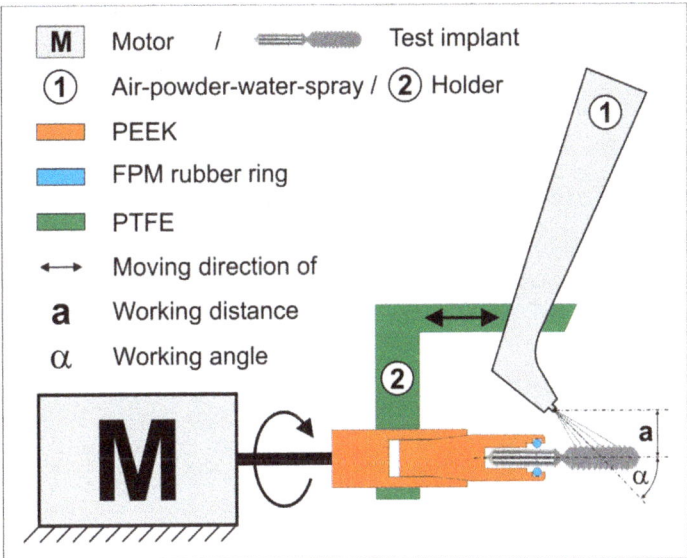

Figure 3. The assembly of the powder-water spray device. PEEK = polyetheretherketone, FPM = fluorine rubber, PTFE = polytetrafluorothgylene.

2.6. Air-Powder-Water Spray (PSS) Cleaning (Control Group)

The implants in groups 2, 4, and 6 were treated by a PSS (BA 8000, Mectron GmbH, Cologne, Germany). To ensure a reproducible and comparable cleaning effect, a test apparatus was assembled, as shown in Figure 4. The aim was to reproduce the working angle and distance according to the manufacturer´s operating manual (45° and 10 mm). The test implants were mounted on a sterile PEEK carrier (Figure 4, in orange), which masked three quarters of the carrier part and was then fixed in a PTFE connecting bar (Figure 4). The holder provided the same working angle and distance for all the tested implants. The holder and its fixed handpiece were moved manually along the implant axis while the test implant rotated, being driven by a motor around its axis (40 rpm) to ensure proper and repeatable cleaning of the implants (Figure 4). Sterile water (Aqua ad injectabilia, Braun, Melsungen, Germany) and aminoacetic acid powder (glycine powder, Mectron GmbH, Cologne, Germany) were used with an air pressure of 2 bar being applied for 60 s. The waste liquid produced during the cleaning process was collected in a beaker to prove the vitality of the removed biofilm (waste from air-powder-water cleaning).

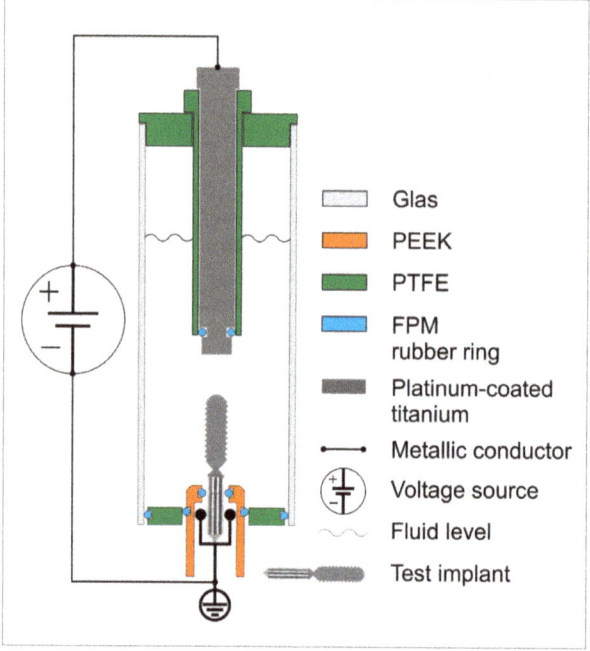

Figure 4. The structure of the electrolytic chamber.

2.7. Rinsing and Test Sample Incubation

After cleaning, the test and control implants were rinsed with air-water spray for 5 seconds (distance of 5 cm) and dried with oil-free air. The test parts were then broken off at the predetermined breaking point in a sterile manner, transferred to Eppendorf tubes filled with 1.5 mL nutritional solution, and incubated at 37 °C for 24 h. Ehrensberger et al. demonstrated that no additional colonies grew when incubation time was extended 18 h. [30]

2.8. Analysis of the Bacterial Growth

The solution in each Eppendorf tube was pipetted, transferred and streaked with an L-spatula on blood agar (Columbia Blood Agar-VWR, BDH Chemicals, Leuven, Belgium). The plate was incubated at 37 °C for 24 h.

The rest of the contents of the Eppendorf tube was gradually diluted in six steps to 1:1,000,000. Each step was also spread on a blood agar plate and treated as described above. In total, seven dilution steps were bred (210 in test group, 210 in control group, 420 in total).

The change in the plate condition was photographed after 24 h. The number of colony-forming units (CFUs) were counted using the software ImageJ (version 1.51u, National Institutes of Health,

Bethesda, MD, USA). The difference between the two Poisson rates has been applied to evaluate the difference in bacterial growth.

2.9. Sterility of the Experimental Set-Up (Positive Control)

To prove the sterility of the different experimental set-ups, the air-powder-water spray was directed to blood agar plates (two per group, six in total). The sterility of the nutritional solution was proved by breeding it at 37 °C for 24 h, and then spreading it on a blood agar plate. The agar plates were incubated at 37 °C for 24 h, and then CFUs were counted.

2.10. Quality of Biofilm (Negative Control)

To prove the quality of the biofilm, two test implants from each group (12 in total) served as the negative control and were not cleaned. After biofilm formation, the nutritional solution was rinsed away with sterile water. One implant per group (six in total) was rinsed with sterile water (Aqua ad injectabilia, Braun, Melsungen, Germany) and dried in air for 24 h. The usual fixation in ethanol was not done, to avoid washing-out of the matrix. The samples were gold-coated and examined using a Philips SE XL30 (LaB6 cathode) scanning electron micrograph (SEM) with 20 kV power and a spot size 4 to check biofilm formation and quality. One implant per group (six in total) was incubated in an Eppendorf tube with 1.5 mL nutritional solution and bred at 37 °C for 24 h. In anticipation of floating bacteria, the nutritional solution was spread on blood agar and bred at 37 °C for 24 h. Colony forming units (CFUs) were then counted (Figure 5).

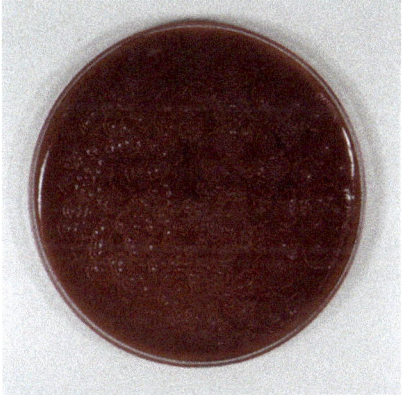

Figure 5. Bacterial growth with the nutritional solution of the negative control (not treated). Dilution grade 1:1,000,000.

2.11. Vitality of Bacteria after Cleaning

To prove the vitality, the waste from both cleaning methods (electrolytic and PSS) was spread on blood agar and bred at 37 °C for 24 h. Then CFUs were counted.

2.12. Counting Colonies

The number of colonies that had grown on the blood agar plates were manually counted using the ImageJ (version 1.51u) software.

2.13. Statistics

The number of colonies that had grown on the blood agar plates after a dilution to 1:1,000,000 where manually counted and processed by the ImageJ (version 1.51u) software.

Continuous variables are reported as mean ± standard deviation. All groups were tested for normality by the Shapiro-Wilk test. Comparisons between the two cleaning methods were performed with the paired sample *t*-test. Comparisons between the surface and material groups for AirFlow were performed with the Kruskal-Wallis test.

A two-sided *p*-value of ≤0.05 was considered statistically significant. Statistical analysis was performed with R (R Foundation for Statistical Computing, Vienna, Austria).

3. Results

3.1. Quality of Biofilm (Negative Control)

The formation of a mature layer of biofilm completely covering the surface of all six tested implants was demonstrated upon checking by scanning electron micrograph (SEM). Six implants were not treated, but were incubated as described. CFUs could not be counted because the blood agar plate was totally covered with a closed layer of bacteria.

3.2. Colony-Forming Unit Count

In groups 1, 3, and 5 (test groups, electrolytic cleaning), 210 blood agar plates were evaluated. Not a single CFU could be counted on any blood agar plate. Neither dilution (Figure 6) nor alloy nor surface had any influence on this observation.

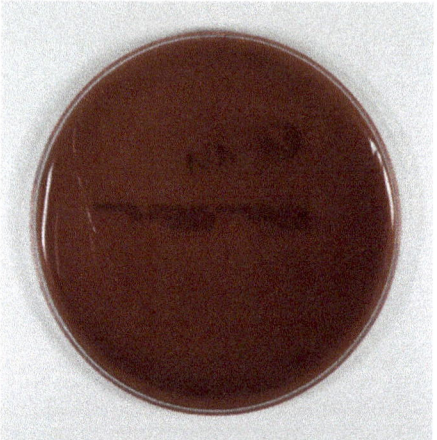

Figure 6. Bacterial growth after electrolytic cleaning. Dilution grade 1:1.

The cultivation of the waste liquid collected from the electrolytic cleaning process also showed no bacterial growth.

In the control groups (2, 4, and 6; PSS; 210 agar plates), the growth of bacteria was observed on every agar plate with any dilution grade (Figure 7), irrespective of dilution, alloy, or surface. CFU counting was not possible in the first five steps of dilution (from 1:1 to 1:100,000), because the bacteria grew over the whole agar plate. CFU counting was possible at a dilution of 1:1,000,000. In all PSS groups, more than 200 CFUs were documented (group 2 = 258.1 ± 19.9, group 4 = 264.4 ± 36.5, group 6 = 245.3 ± 40.7) (Table 1). The cultivation of the collected waste liquid always showed bacterial growth.

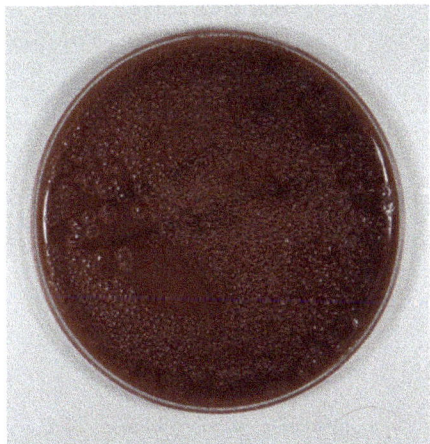

Figure 7. Bacterial growth after air-powder-water spray cleaning. Dilution grade 1: 1,000,000.

Table 1. Colony-forming unit (CFU) counts per grade of titanium, surface, dilution, and cleaning method.

Cleaning Method	Electrolytic	PPS	Electrolytic	PPS	Electrolytic	PPS
Material & Surface	Group 1: Ti Grade 4 + SAE	Group 2: Ti Grade 4 + SAE	Group 3: Ti Grade 5 + SAE	Group 4: Ti Grade 5 + SAE	Group 5: Ti Grade 4 + AO	Group 6: Ti Grade 4 + AO
Dilution	∅ CFU	∅ CFU	∅ CFU	∅ CFU	∅ CFU	∅ CFU
1:1	0	na	0	na	0	na
1:10	0	na	0	na	0	na
1:100	0	na	0	na	0	na
1:1000	0	na	0	na	0	na
1:10,000	0	na	0	na	0	na
1:100,000	0	na	0	na	0	na
1:1,000,000	0	258.1 ± 19.9	0	264.4 ± 36.5	0	245.3 ± 40.7

The difference between the electrolytic approach (test groups 1, 3, and 5) and PSS (control groups 2, 4, and 6) was statistically extremely significant (p-value $< 2.2 \times 10^{-16}$). In control groups 2, 4, and 6 (PSS), no difference in cleaning efficacy could be detected (p-value = 0.3465) when comparing the different implant materials and surfaces. In test groups 1, 3, and 5 (electrolytic approach), no colony-forming units (CFUs) were detected. Therefore, there were no differences between the different implant materials and surfaces.

3.3. Sterility of Experimental Set-Up (Positive Control)

No sign of bacterial growth was observed on the blood agar after PSS was sprayed directly onto blood agar plates. No sign of bacterial growth was observed on the blood agar after the nutritional solution was bred. This indicates that the air-powder-water spray system and the prepared nutritional solution were free from bacterial contamination.

4. Discussion

The application of voltage to reduce bacterial load has been described several times in the literature. Ehrensberger et al. [30] evaluated the influence of cathodic voltage-controlled electrical stimulation (CVCES) to eradicate methicillin-resistant *S. aureus* (MRSA) from titanium surfaces in vitro and in Long-Evans rats. The application of −1.8 V for 1 h reduced MRSA CFU counts by 87% in bone and 88% in titanium, compared to the open-circuit potential in vitro, and by 97% in titanium in vivo. No histological changes were detected in the rat model. CVCES increased the interfacial capacitance (from 18.93 to 98.25 µF/cm^2) and decreased the polarization resistance (from 868.25 to 108 Ω/cm^2). Because of the negative charge of the titanium surface and the negative surface charge of *S. aureus*, attachment of the biofilm may be influenced. Furthermore, it has been discussed that the electric field on polarized electrodes generates anions by electrolytic splitting, which disrupts and pushes away the biofilm [24,31,32]. The major reaction at the cathode is the reduction of water or the reduction of oxygen:

Reaction 1: $2H_2O + 2e^- \rightarrow H_2 + OH^-$
Reaction 2: $O_2 + 4^- + 2H_2O \rightarrow 4 OH^-$

Blenkinsopp et al. proposed an altered transport of ions within the biofilm [33]. Portinga et al. demonstrated an extended attachment of bacteria to the biofilm after donation of their free electrons to the matrix. Free electrons on the cathode might disturb this adherence [31,34], To summarize, the antimicrobial effects seem to be related to voltage-dependent surface properties of the titanium.

Several authors [26,35,36] have reported that loading two contaminated dental implants (one as anode and the other as cathode) in NaCl as electrolyte significantly reduces the number of bacteria. The downside of the published method is that toxic chloric and hypochlorous acid are reaction products, and the pH in the periimplant area decreased or increased significantly.

Zipprich et al. [27] introduced an electrolytic approach to remove biofilm from explanted implants by using a mixture of sodium iodide, potassium iodide, and water buffered by L(+)-lactic acid. Schneider et al. [28] investigated the underlying mechanism of this method of electrolytic cleaning. Several disinfecting agents, such as triiodide and hydrogen peroxide, were generated on the implant surface loaded as the cathode. The authors proved in an in vitro test that the major effect in removing the biofilm was the generation of hydrogen on the implant surface, which pushed away the biofilm mechanically. Based on these findings, the authors decided to prove the effectiveness and efficiency of this approach in this in vitro test. It is very difficult to perform a controlled in vitro study on a "real" biofilm in real periimplantitis cases, because its three-dimensional structure is destroyed while the implant is removed, and anaerobic bacteria would not survive this process. The nutritional and biological conditions of an in vivo biofilm will differ from biofilms used in this in vitro test. Such samples may harbor different mixtures of bacteria. This pitfall compromises all in vitro studies done on periimplant biofilms. On the other hand, it was demonstrated that microbiota associated with periimplantitis are quite variable and inconsistent [4].

Different methods of growing biofilms have been published. Most of the articles used single-species biofilms with very little relation to real periimplant biofilms. *S. aureus* is a colony-forming bacterium associated with infected dental or orthopedic implants, and was bred for several days on titanium surfaces [30,37]. Mohn used *E. coli*, which is not associated with periimplantitis [26]. Other authors harvested intraoral subgingival plaque and exposed titanium plates in a nutritional solution for seven days [38]. John et al. cultivated biofilms by exposing titanium plates fixed on splints for 48 hours in the oral cavity of two specimens [39]. In preparation for this study, we were not able to reproduce the claims of these authors to achieve a mature biofilm covering the complete implant surface in the published timeline, when using a model with intraoral bacteria. It took 14 days to achieve a multilayer mature biofilm covering the whole implant surface (Figure 2).

To imitate micro- and macrostructure, we decided to use lifelike test implants. To carry such implants in the mouth for several days to accumulate bacteria would be unacceptable for humans. Consequently, we had to develop a realistic extraoral model to breed a biofilm. A single-species model was used, and did not form a complete monolayer of bacteria nor a multilayer biofilm. To achieve the most realistic diversity of microorganisms, the saliva was collected and pooled from three volunteers, bred extra-orally, and frozen to ensure the same biota for all the tests. In preparation for this study, we found out that it takes 14 days to achieve the expected quality and thickness of biofilm. In vitro, it could have been demonstrated that a cold plasma device can clean heling abutments more effectively than conventional cleaning [40].

No published method was able to remove all bacteria from implant surfaces in the clinical setting. Moreover, bacteria will re-colonize implant surfaces exposed to the oral cavity within a matter of hours [10]. The theory that elimination of the biofilm will cure periimplantitis is an attractive one [4]. Clinically, it may be necessary to remove the bacteria and extracellular matrix in a way that will allow re-osseointegration of formerly infected surfaces.

We were able to demonstrate that no bacteria could be cultivated in the nutritional solution and powder used for a PSS, thus proving the sterility of the experimental set-up. The vitality of the bred biofilm was proved visually by SEM and by CFU counting after its cultivation on blood agar plates. As different titanium alloys and surface modifications are used in dental and orthopedic surgery, we tested titanium grades 4 and 5, as well as acid-etched, sandblasted, and anodized implant surfaces. Their effectiveness in the removal of bacteria was compared to a standard method (PSS).

The results were unequivocally clear. It was not possible to breed bacteria after the implants had been cleaned by the electrolytic approach. Every implant cleaned by the air-powder-water spray contained so many bacteria that all the blood agar plates were totally overgrown with a lawn of bacteria. A single CFU could only be counted after dilution to 1:1,000,000. The waste collected while using the PSS contained vital bacteria, and breeding them on blood agar plates demonstrated their vitality.

In conclusion, the air-powder-water spray does not sufficiently remove the biofilm. This might explain why, in a recent review, a re-osseointegration rate of only 39%–46% was possible in animal models [21]. Considering the angle of threads, the micro-texture of the implants combined with oversized particles, and craterlike bone defects, it is more possible to follow the manufacturer´s manual (working distance of 3–5 mm and an angle of 30–60°) and to clean the microstructure properly. The electrolytic approach sterilized all the tested implants, irrespective of alloy or surface. No vital bacteria were detectable. For this reason, the null hypothesis had to be rejected.

The electrolytic approach seems to be a promising method for treating infected dental and orthopedic implants.

5. Conclusions

In this study, it was proven that electrolytic cleaning of lifelike dental implants contaminated with vital oral biofilms sterilizes the implant surfaces. One of the gold-standard methods of cleaning by air-powder-water spray failed to achieve an adequate result. Clinical testing is necessary to prove the clinical impact of these findings in dentistry and orthopedic surgery.

Author Contributions: Conceptualization, C.R., P.W., D.H., F.K. and H.Z.; methodology, C.R., P.W., D.H., F.K., M.S and H.Z.; software, C.R.; validation, C.R., P.W., D.H., F.K., M.S. and H.Z.; formal analysis, C.R., M.S. and H.Z.; investigation, C.R., D.H. and H.Z.; resources, H.Z.; data curation, C.R., P.W., M.S. and H.Z.; writing—original draft preparation, C.R., M.S. and H.Z.; writing—review and editing, C.R., P.W., D.H., F.K., M.S. and H.Z.; visualization, C.R., P.W., M.S. and H.Z.; supervision, C.R. and H.Z.; project administration, C.R and H.Z.; funding acquisition, M.S., H.Z.

Funding: This research was funded by by Zyfoma GmbH, Welterstadt, Germany.

Acknowledgments: The authors Schlee and Zipprich declare themselves as holding patents on the described technology, and to have financial interests. We appreciate Ümniye Balaban from the Institute for Biostatistics and Mathematical Modeling Center of Health Sciences, Hospital and Department of Medicine of the Goethe University for her support with the statistics. We appreciate Charlotte zur Megede and Jana Weiler for support in collecting the data.

Conflicts of Interest: The authors M.S. and H.Z. declare themselves as holding patents on the described technology, and to have financial interests. M.S. was involved in the design of the study, analysis and interpretation of the data, writing and the decision to publish this data.

References

1. Sendyk, D.I.; Chrcanovic, B.R.; Albrektsson, T.; Wennerberg, A.; Zindel Deboni, M.C. Does Surgical Experience Influence Implant Survival Rate? A Systematic Review and Meta-Analysis. *Int. J. Prosthodont.* **2017**, *30*, 341–347. [CrossRef]

2. Lang, N.P.; Berglundh, T. Periimplant diseases: Where are we now?—Consensus of the Seventh European Workshop on Periodontology. *J. Clin. Periodontol.* **2011**, *38*, 178–181. [CrossRef]
3. Berglundh, T.; Armitage, G.; Araújo, M.G.; Avila-Ortiz, G.; Blanco, J.; Camargo, P.M.; Chen, S.; Cochran, D.; Derks, J.; Figuero, E.; et al. Peri-implant diseases and conditions: Consensus report of workgroup 4 of the 2017 World Workshop on the Classification of Periodontal and Peri-Implant Diseases and Conditions. *J. Periodontol.* **2018**, *89*, S313–S318. [CrossRef]
4. Mombelli, A.; Décaillet, F. The characteristics of biofilms in peri-implant disease. *J. Clin. Periodontol.* **2011**, *38*, 203–213. [CrossRef]
5. Mombelli, A.; Müller, N.; Cionca, N. The epidemiology of peri-implantitis. *Clin. Oral Implants Res.* **2012**, *23*, 67–76. [CrossRef]
6. Derks, J.; Tomasi, C. Peri-implant health and disease. A systematic review of current epidemiology. *J. Clin. Periodontol.* **2015**, *42*, S158–S171. [CrossRef]
7. Coli, P.; Christiaens, V.; Sennerby, L.; de Bruyn, H. Reliability of periodontal diagnostic tools for monitoring peri-implant health and disease. *Periodontology 2000* **2017**, *73*, 203–217. [CrossRef]
8. Esposito, M.; Grusovin, M.G.; Worthington, H.V. Treatment of peri-implantitis: What interventions are effective? A Cochrane systematic review. *Eur. J. Oral Implant.* **2012**, *5*, S21–S41.
9. Canullo, L.; Montegrotto Group for the Study of Peri-implant Disease; Schlee, M.; Wagner, W.; Covani, U. International Brainstorming Meeting on Etiologic and Risk Factors of Peri-implantitis, Montegrotto (Padua, Italy), August 2014. *Int. J. Oral Maxillofac. Implants* **2015**, *30*, 1093–1104. [CrossRef]
10. Fürst, M.M.; Salvi, G.E.; Lang, N.P.; Persson, G.R. Bacterial colonization immediately after installation on oral titanium implants. *Clin. Oral Implants Res.* **2007**, *18*, 501–508. [CrossRef]
11. Zoubos, A.B.; Galanakos, S.P.; Soucacos, P.N. Orthopedics and biofilm—What do we know? A review. *Med. Sci. Monit.* **2012**, *18*, RA89–RA96. [CrossRef]
12. Cargill, J.S.; Upton, M. Low concentrations of vancomycin stimulate biofilm formation in some clinical isolates of Staphylococcus epidermidis. *J. Clin. Pathol.* **2009**, *62*, 1112–1116. [CrossRef]
13. Hexter, A.T.; Hislop, S.M.; Blunn, G.W.; Liddle, A.D. The effect of bearing surface on risk of periprosthetic joint infection in total hip arthroplasty: A systematic review and meta-analysis. *Bone Joint J.* **2018**, *100-B*, 134–142. [CrossRef]
14. Gilson, M.; Gossec, L.; Mariette, X.; Gherissi, D.; Guyot, M.H.; Berthelot, J.M.; et al. NIH consensus conference: Total hip replacement. NIH Consensus Development Panel on Total Hip Replacement. *JAMA* **1995**, *273*, 1950–1956.
15. Rowan, F.E.; Donaldson, M.J.; Pietrzak, J.R.; Haddad, F.S. The Role of One-Stage Exchange for Prosthetic Joint Infection. *Curr. Rev. Musculoskelet. Med.* **2018**, *11*, 370–379. [CrossRef]
16. Zimmerli, W.; Sendi, P. Pathogenesis of implant-associated infection: the role of the host. *Semin. Immunopathol.* **2011**, *33*, 295–306. [CrossRef]
17. Biring, G.S.; Kostamo, T.; Garbuz, D.S.; Masri, B.A.; Duncan, C.P. Two-stage revision arthroplasty of the hip for infection using an interim articulated Prostalac hip spacer: A 10- to 15-year follow-up study. *J. Bone Joint Surg. Br.* **2009**, *91*, 1431–1437. [CrossRef]
18. Sia, I.G.; Berbari, E.F.; Karchmer, A.W. Prosthetic Joint Infections. *Infect. Dis. Clin. North Am.* **2005**, *19*, 885–914. [CrossRef]
19. Byren, I.; Bejon, P.; Atkins, B.L.; Angus, B.; Masters, S.; McLardy-Smith, P.; Gundle, R.; Berendt, A. One hundred and twelve infected arthroplasties treated with 'DAIR' (debridement, antibiotics and implant retention): antibiotic duration and outcome. *J. Antimicrob. Chemother.* **2009**, *63*, 1264–1271. [CrossRef]
20. Helou, O.C.; Berbari, E.F.; Lahr, B.D.; Eckel-Passow, J.E.; Razonable, R.R.; Sia, I.G.; Virk, A.; Walker, R.C.; Steckelberg, J.M.; Wilson, W.R.; et al. Efficacy and safety of rifampin containing regimen for staphylococcal prosthetic joint infections treated with debridement and retention. *Eur. J. Clin. Microbiol. Infect. Dis.* **2010**, *29*, 961–967. [CrossRef]
21. Tastepe, C.S.; Van Waas, R.; Liu, Y.; Wismeijer, D. Air powder abrasive treatment as an implant surface cleaning method: A literature review. *Int. J. Oral Maxillofac. Implants* **2012**, *27*, 1461–1473.
22. Claffey, N.; Clarke, E.; Polyzois, I.; Renvert, S. Surgical treatment of peri-implantitis. *J. Clin. Periodontol.* **2008**, *35*, 316–332. [CrossRef]

23. De Almeida, J.M.; Matheus, H.R.; Rodrigues Gusman, D.J.; Faleiros, P.L.; Januário de Araújo, N.; Noronha Novaes, V.C. Effectiveness of Mechanical Debridement Combined With Adjunctive Therapies for Nonsurgical Treatment of Periimplantitis: A Systematic Review. *Implant Dent.* **2017**, *26*, 137–144. [CrossRef]
24. Del Pozo, J.L.; Rouse, M.S.; Mandrekar, J.N.; Steckelberg, J.M.; Patel, R. The electricidal effect: Reduction of Staphylococcus and pseudomonas biofilms by prolonged exposure to low-intensity electrical current. *Antimicrob. Agents Chemother.* **2009**, *53*, 41–45. [CrossRef]
25. Schwarz, F.; Becker, K.; Sager, M. Efficacy of professionally administered plaque removal with or without adjunctive measures for the treatment of peri-implant mucositis. A systematic review and meta-analysis. *J. Clin. Periodontol.* **2015**, *42*, 202–213. [CrossRef]
26. Mohn, D.; Zehnder, M.; Stark, W.J.; Imfeld, T. Electrochemical Disinfection of Dental Implants—A Proof of Concept. *PLoS ONE* **2011**, *6*, e16157. [CrossRef]
27. Zipprich, H.; Ratka, C.; Schlee, M.; Brodbeck, U.; Lauer, H.C.; Seitz, O. Periimplantitistherapie: Durchbruch mit neuer Reinigungsmethode. *Dentalmagazin* **2013**, *31*, 14–17.
28. Schneider, S.; Rudolph, M.; Bause, V.; Terfort, A. Electrochemical removal of biofilms from titanium dental implant surfaces. *Bioelectrochemistry* **2018**, *121*, 84–94. [CrossRef]
29. Tian, Y.; He, X.; Torralba, M.; Yooseph, S.; Nelson, K.E.; Lux, R.; McLean, J.S.; Yu, G.; Shi, W. Using DGGE profiling ro develop a novel culture medium suitable for oral microbial communities. *Mol. Oral Microbiol.* **2010**, *25*, 357–367. [CrossRef]
30. Ehrensberger, M.T.; Tobias, M.E.; Nodzo, S.R.; Hansen, L.A.; Luke-Marshall, N.R.; Cole, R.F.; Wild, L.M.; Campagnari, A.A. Cathodic voltage-controlled electrical stimulation of titanium implants as treatment for methicillin-resistant Staphylococcus aureus periprosthetic infections. *Biomaterials* **2015**, *41*, 97–105. [CrossRef]
31. Poortinga, A.T.; Smit, J.; Van Der Mei, H.C.; Busscher, H.J. Electric field induced desorption of bacteria from a conditioning film covered substratum. *Biotechnol. Bioeng.* **2001**, *76*, 395–399. [CrossRef]
32. Van Der Borden, A.; Van Der Mei, H.; Busscher, H. Electric block current induced detachment from surgical stainless steel and decreased viability of Staphylococcus epidermidis. *Biomaterials* **2005**, *26*, 6731–6735. [CrossRef]
33. A Blenkinsopp, S.; Khoury, A.E.; Costerton, J.W. Electrical enhancement of biocide efficacy against Pseudomonas aeruginosa biofilms. *Appl. Environ. Microbiol.* **1992**, *58*, 3770–3773.
34. Poortinga, A.; Bos, R.; Busscher, H. Measurement of charge transfer during bacterial adhesion to an indium tin oxide surface in a parallel plate flow chamber. *J. Microbiol. Methods* **1999**, *38*, 183–189. [CrossRef]
35. Sahrmann, P.; Zehnder, M.; Mohn, D.; Meier, A.; Imfeld, T.; Thurnheer, T. Effect of low direct current on anaerobic multispecies biofilm adhering to a titanium implant surface. *Clin. Implant Dent. Relat. Res.* **2014**, *16*, 552–556. [CrossRef]
36. Sandvik, E.L.; McLeod, B.R.; Parker, A.E.; Stewart, P.S. Direct Electric Current Treatment under Physiologic Saline Conditions Kills Staphylococcus epidermidis Biofilms via Electrolytic Generation of Hypochlorous Acid. *PLoS ONE* **2013**, *8*, e55118. [CrossRef]
37. Salvi, G.E.; Fürst, M.M.; Lang, N.P.; Persson, G.R. One-year bacterial colonization patterns of Staphylococcus aureus and other bacteria at implants and adjacent teeth. *Clin. Oral Implants Res.* **2008**, *19*, 242–248. [CrossRef]
38. Koban, I.; Holtfreter, B.; Hübner, N.-O.; Matthes, R.; Sietmann, R.; Kindel, E.; Weltmann, K.-D.; Welk, A.; Kramer, A.; Kocher, T. Antimicrobial efficacy of non-thermal plasma in comparison to chlorhexidine against dental biofilms on titanium discs in vitro - proof of principle experiment. *J. Clin. Periodontol.* **2011**, *38*, 956–965. [CrossRef]
39. John, G.; Schwarz, F.; Becker, J. Taurolidine as an effective and biocompatible additive for plaque-removing techniques on implant surfaces. *Clin. Oral Investig.* **2015**, *19*, 1069–1077. [CrossRef]
40. Stacchi, C.; Berton, F.; Porrelli, D.; Lombardi, T. Reuse of Implant Healing Abutments: Comparative Evaluation of the Efficacy of Two Cleaning Procedures. *Int. J. Prosthodont.* **2018**, *31*, 161–162. [CrossRef]

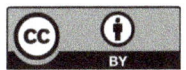 © 2019 by the authors. Licensee MDPI, Basel, Switzerland. This article is an open access article distributed under the terms and conditions of the Creative Commons Attribution (CC BY) license (http://creativecommons.org/licenses/by/4.0/).

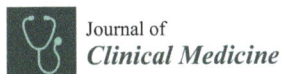

Communication

Is Complete Re-Osseointegration of an Infected Dental Implant Possible? Histologic Results of a Dog Study: A Short Communication

Markus Schlee [1,2], Loubna Naili [3], Florian Rathe [1,4], Urs Brodbeck [5] and Holger Zipprich [6,*]

1. Private Practice, Forchheim, Germany; markus.schlee@32schoenezaehne.de (M.S.); florian.rathe@32schoenezaehne.de (F.R.)
2. Department of Maxillofacial Surgery, Goethe University, 60590 Frankfurt am Main, Germany
3. Private Practice, Kirchbachstraße 186, 28211 Bremen, Germany; lnaili@students.uni-mainz.de
4. Private Practice and Department of Prosthodontics, Danube University, 3500 Krems, Austria
5. Private Practice, 8051 Zürich, Switzerland; ursbrodbeck@bluewin.ch
6. Department of Prosthodontics, Goethe University, 60590 Frankfurt am Main, Germany
* Correspondence: zipprich@em.uni-frankfurt.de; Tel.: +49-69-6301-4714; Fax: +49-69-6301-3711

Received: 6 November 2019; Accepted: 9 January 2020; Published: 16 January 2020

Abstract: Complete reosseointegration after treatment of periimplantitis was never published yet. This short scientific communication reports about results of a randomized controlled preclinical study. An electrolytic approach was compared to a classical modality (ablative, cotton pellets soaked with sodium chloride solution and H_2O_2. For electrolytic cleaning a complete reosseointegration was achieved in several cases serving as a proof of concept.

Keywords: periimplantitis; electrolytic cleaning; augmentation; air flow; re-osseointegration; dog study

1. Introduction

Ligature-induced inflammation and bone loss in a dog model was introduced to imitate periimplantitis in humans and preclinically study different treatment approaches. Schwarz et al. [1] compared bone defects in 24 patients with advanced periimplantitis to ligature-induced bone defects at 30 implants in five beagle dogs. Defect morphology was similar in both entities. The authors concluded that the dog model would be an appropriate model for simulating periimplantitis in humans. Seong at al. reported the possibility of spontaneous healing after ligature removal in dogs [2]. The authors claimed that further clarification of differences between the forced acute bone loss induced by ligatures and the chronic process in clinical periimplantitis would be necessary. Nevertheless, the dog model provided valuable insights into the etiology and pathogenesis of periimplantitis [3] and may be a reasonable model for studying whether re-osseointegration of implant surfaces covered by bacterial biofilms is possible. Based on animal studies, re-osseointegration is feasible, although unpredictable, as it varies between studies and depends on implant surface characteristics and defect morphology [4,5].

In this preclinical randomized and controlled trial, electrolytic cleaning (EC) versus classical cleaning (CC, rubbing a gauze strip soaked in H_2O_2 (3%), followed by a strip soaked in saline (0.9%)) was employed to prove whether complete re-osseointegration is possible in a dog model. This approach was chosen on the basis of previous studies [5]. A custom-made pilot series device and the pilot electrolyte (sodium and potassium iodine) of the in vitro study of Ratka et al. [6] were used in this study. The aim of this short scientific communication is to share histologic results and to prove whether complete re-osseointegration is possible when EC has been used as a decontamination technique.

2. Experimental Section

The study was approved by the Internal Review Board of the University of São Paulo (2013.1.1193.58.3 by CEUA (Comissão de Ética no Uso de Animais)). No sample size calculation could be done because this was the first in vivo trial and no data were available. To have a high chance of achieving significance, we used a large number of dogs compared to existing literature (8 dogs). Two months after extraction (T1) of all premolars and the first molars in the left and right mandible, 4 implants per quadrant were placed (Figure 1). It was planned to place two different brands of implants: 48 BL implants (BL SLA® 3.3 × 8.0 mm, Straumann, Basel, Switzerland) and 16 Nobel Active implants (NA TiUnite® 3.5 × 8.5mm, Nobel Biocare, Kloten, Switzerland). In view of the expected bone defects, the inter-implant distance was at least 6 mm (Figure 1). In addition to the study implants, extra implants were placed, provided there was sufficient space and the study implants would not be impeded. Ligatures were pushed into the sulcus at T2 (4 months) and removed at T3 (7 months). A hygiene program was set up, and the implants were treated at T4 (8 months) by either CC or EC in a randomized manner with the use of sealed envelopes. The mode of action of EC has been described before [6,7]. In summary, the implants were negatively loaded with a current of around 5 V, and rinsed with an electrolyte which passed an anode inside a spray-head (Figure 4c). Sodium iodine (200 g/L), potassium iodine (200 g/L), and L (+)-lactic acid (20 g/L) were used as the electrolyte [6] and an early prototype of a spray-head (Figure 4c) as the source of current (5 min, 400 mA) in the present study. The current directs anions and cations to the electric field. While the anions at the anode form an iodine disinfecting solution, the cations penetrate the biofilm, take an electron from the implant surface, and the emerging hydrogen bubbles (H_2) lift off the bacterial biofilm. The CC implants were treated by rubbing a gauze strip soaked in H_2O_2 (3%), followed by a strip soaked in saline (0.9%, Braun Melsungen, Germany). All sites were augmented with autogenous bone harvested from the ramus area of the lateral mandible (Micross Safescraper, Zantomed, Duisburg, Germany), covered with a collagen membrane (Bio-Gide, Geistlich, Wohlhusen, Switzerland), and the flap was coronally advanced to cover the augmented area without tension. One implant per dog (2 Nobel, 4 Straumann) was randomly selected and not treated to serve as a negative control. The animals were sacrificed for histologic evaluation at T5 (11 months). Standardized x-rays were taken at T1, 2, 4, and 5. Bleeding on probing (BoP) as well as an assessment of pocket depth (PD) at T2, 4, and 5 (Figure 2) were performed. Preparation of samples followed the technique introduced by Donath [8], and staining was done with Stevenel's blue or Toluidine blue. Bone gain was assessed using a digital tool (NDP.view 2.5.19, (Hamamatsu Photonics KK, Shizuoka, Japan)) and analyzed histomorphometrically.

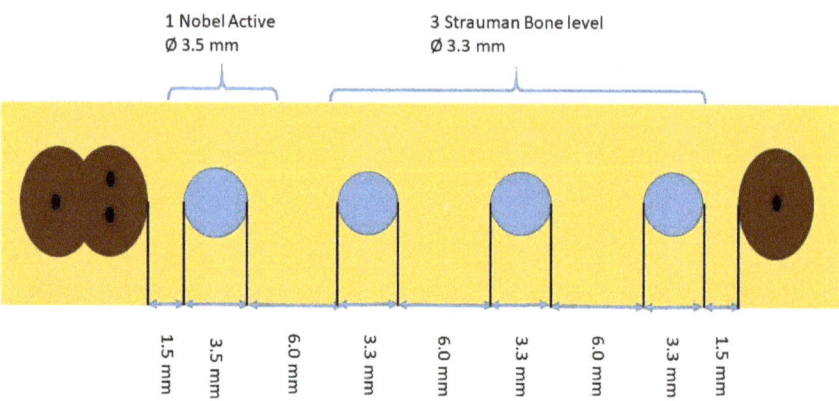

Figure 1. Allocation of implant positions.

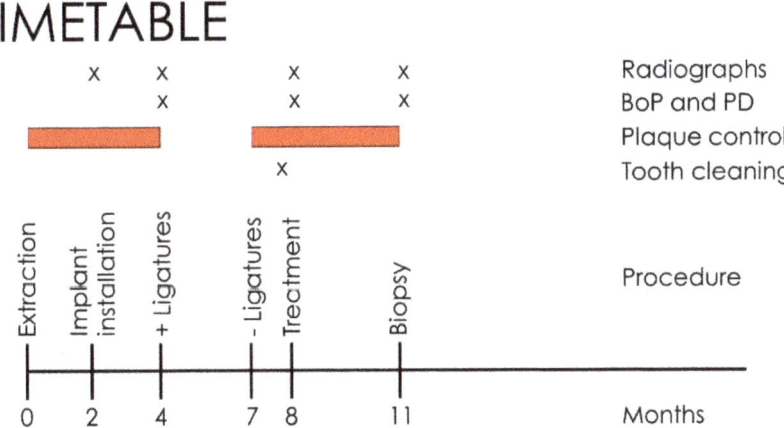

Figure 2. Timetable of the dog study.

3. Results

Sixty-five implants were finally placed (Table 1). Fourteen TiUnite® implants and 43 SLA® implants were treated (EC & CC) and eight implants (2 TiUnite® and 6 SLA®) were left untreated. Two implants could not be placed due to the required distances (Figure 1). All implants displayed massive horizontal bone loss before treatment, in most cases merging with neighboring defects (Figures 3 and 4), which left a site that was difficult to augment. Forty-eight implants were exposed during healing whereas nine EC (5 TiUnite® and 4 SLA®) and eight CC (3 TiUnite® and 5 SLA®) implants stayed covered until T5. Complete re-osseointegration could be demonstrated for implants treated by CC in one implant and for four TiUnite® and six SLA® implants treated by EC (Figures 5–8). The median bone gain for implants which healed submerged was 1.58 ± 0.76 in the case of EC and 1.19 ± 0.29 in the case of CC. The boxplot appears in Figure 9.

Table 1. Allocation of implant positions.

Dog	Quadrant	Straumann	Nobel	Straumann Not Treated	Nobel Not Treated	Total	Not Placed
1	right	2	1			3	1
	left	3	1	1		5	
2	right	3	1			4	
	left	3	1	1		5	
3	right	3	1			4	
	left	2	1	1		4	
4	right	3	0		1	4	
	left	3	1			4	
5	right	3	1			4	
	left	3	0		1	4	
6	right	3	1	1		5	
	left	3	1			4	
7	right	2	1			3	1
	left	2	1	1		4	
8	right	3	1			4	
	left	2	1	1		4	
total		43	14	6	2	65	2
Straumann						49	
Nobel						16	

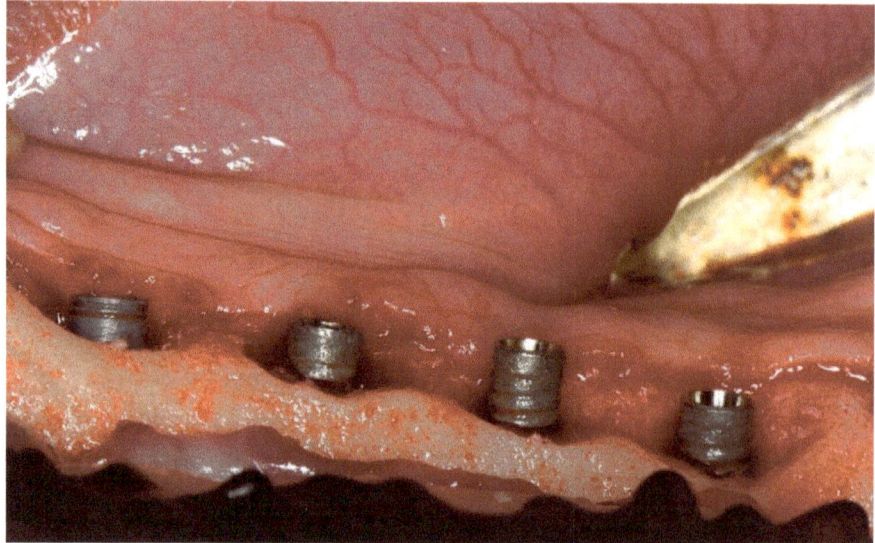

Figure 3. Massive horizontal bone loss results in merging bone defects and massive resorption of the whole ridge.

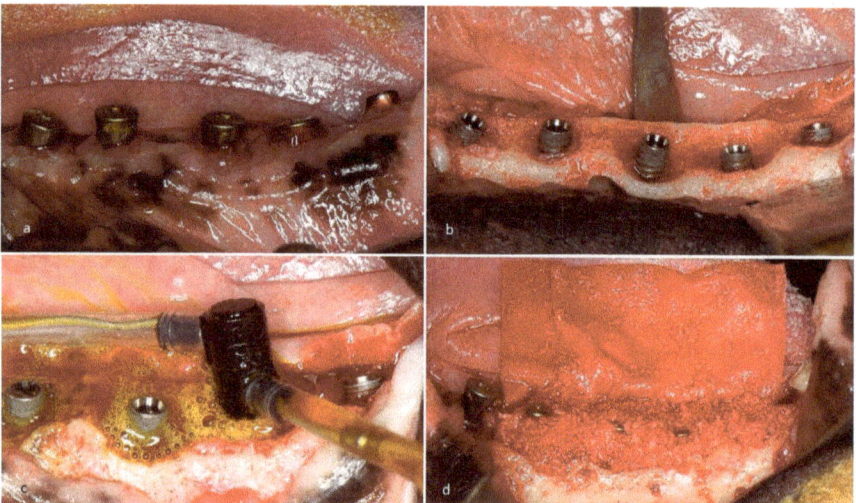

Figure 4. (**a**) Infected site prior to treatment, (**b**) reflected flap indicates a complex merged defect morphology, (**c**) electrolytic cleaning with a spray-head, (**d**) augmented site before collagen membrane was applied.

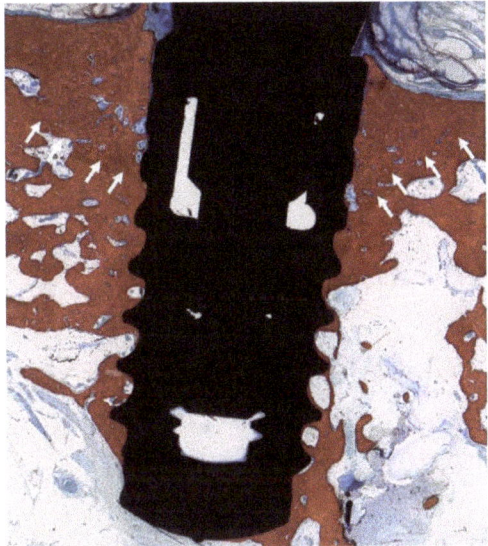

Figure 5. Histologic evaluation of healing after electrolytic cleaning (EC) (SLA® surface). The arrows indicate the bony crest before treatment. Complete coverage of the formerly exposed implant surface was achieved.

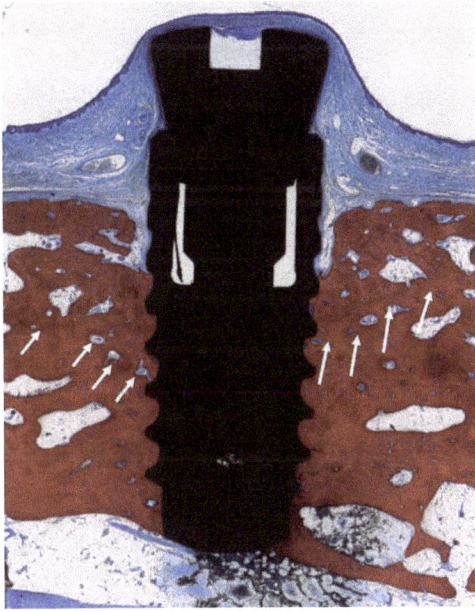

Figure 6. Histologic evaluation of healing after classical cleaning (CC) (SLA® surface). The arrows indicate the bony crest before treatment. Bone-to-implant contact was achieved but full regeneration could not be achieved in any implant.

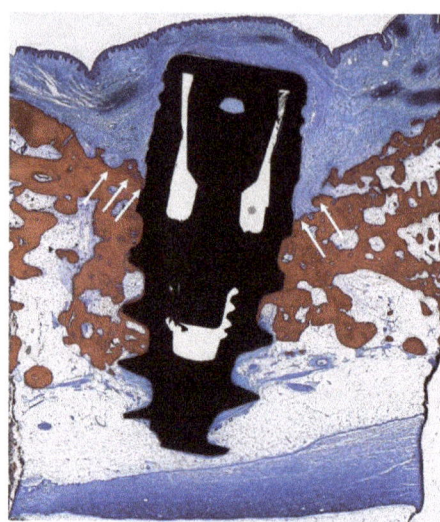

Figure 7. Histologic evaluation of healing after CC (TiUnite® surface). The arrows indicate the bony crest before treatment. A small amount of new bone-to-implant contact was achieved. No re-osseointegration could be achieved on major parts of the implant surface.

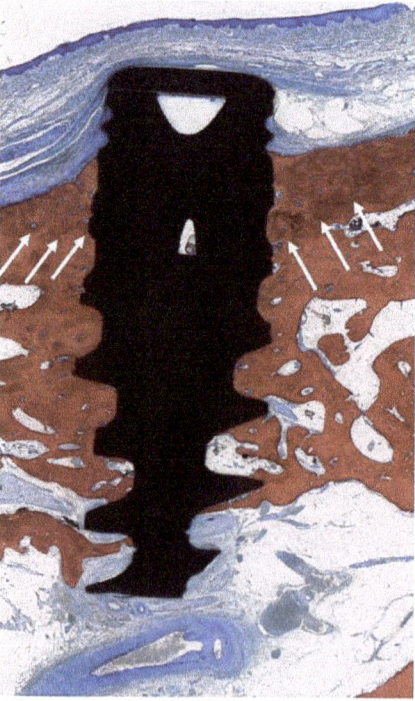

Figure 8. Histologic evaluation of healing after EC (TiUnite® surface). The arrows indicate the bony crest before treatment. Bone-to-implant contact was achieved as more crestal than the neighboring bone level.

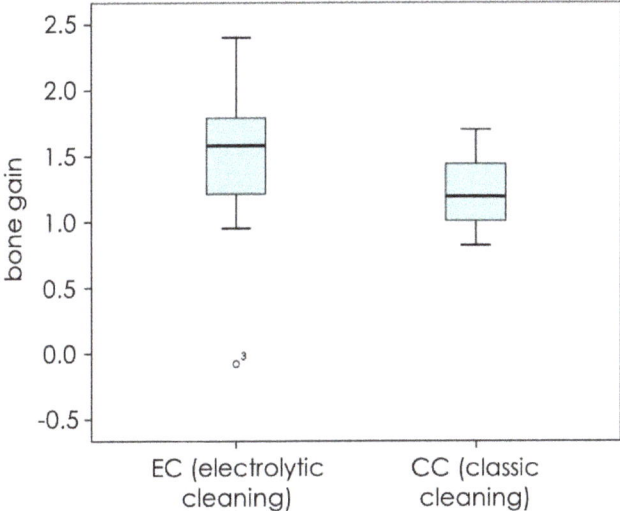

Figure 9. Bone gain for submerged implants at T5 in CC (8 implants) and EC (9 implants) groups display higher bone gain for the EC group.

4. Discussion

The results of this preclinical study may differ from results gained with the final devices used for this technique. Nevertheless, they may serve as proof of principle. As submerged healing was sought, the high number of exposures was an undesirable result. This may correlate with the fact that most of the defects were horizontal and required vertical augmentation. Furthermore, uneventful healing was not possible because of dogs biting on the surgical sites. Implants exposed to the platform cannot regenerate completely and were therefore excluded from statistical evaluation. This limits the meaningfulness of the study. Consequently, we were not able to prove the superiority of one of the treatment modalities in regenerating bone in contact with the implant surface because of the sample size.

Nevertheless, 17 implants were not exposed. When comparing bone regeneration in EC and CC in these cases, EC tended to be superior based on median, without reaching significance. Eight implants in the EC group achieved complete re-osseointegration, but none in the CC group. To the best of the authors' knowledge, complete regeneration has never before been described in the literature. This paper does not investigate the reasons for this observation. In the context of previous literature, it may be assumed that EC in contrast to CC removes the bacterial biofilm and other remnants to an extent that makes complete re-osseointegration possible [6,7]. The latter was proven through histology (Figures 5–8). Re-osseointegration is defined as new bone in direct contact with the formerly infected implant surface. Soft tissue thickness correlates to bone level. Thus bone regeneration to the platform cannot be expected in the case of exposure if the shoulder of the implant was visible [9]. If chewing forces were applied to the implant, complete regeneration also cannot be expected, even if the site stayed covered. Interestingly, complete regeneration was only possible in the EC group—even under these circumstances.

The regenerative potential of horizontal bone defects with no walls is worse than for contained, multi-walled defects [4,7]. In this animal study we observed massive horizontal bone loss and merging defects resulting in a severely resorbed ridge (Figure 3). In humans, an inter-implant distance of 3 mm is usually sufficient to maintain an interdental bone peak in the case of bone loss around implants [10]. We used an inter-implant distance of 6 mm and yet the defects still merged. This might be an indication that ligature-induced periimplantitis in a dog model behaves differently to periimplantitis in humans.

Considering our findings, dog models might be inappropriate for investigating the amount of bone generation. Fewer implants per ridge are suggested for future dog studies.

5. Conclusions

As a proof of concept, complete re-osseointegration was proven after electrolytic cleaning and augmentation.

Author Contributions: Conceptualization, M.S. and H.Z.; Data curation, M.S.; Formal analysis, M.S., L.N. and H.Z.; Funding acquisition M.S., U.B. and H.Z.; Investigation, M.S., L.N. and H.Z.; Methodology, M.S., U.B., F.R. and H.Z.; Project administration, M.S. and H.Z.; Resources, M.S. and H.Z.; Supervision, M.S. and H.Z.; Validation, M.S., L.N. and H.Z.; Visualization, M.S., L.N. and H.Z.; Writing—original draft, M.S.; Writing—review & editing, M.S., U.B., L.N., F.R., and H.Z. All authors have read and agreed to the published version of the manuscript.

Funding: The study was financed by Schlee, Zipprich and Brodbeck privately.

Conflicts of Interest: The authors Schlee, Zipprich and Brodbeck declare that they own shares in GalvoSurge Dental AG and hold patents. The other authors declare to have no conflict of interest.

References

1. Schwarz, F.; Herten, M.; Sager, M.; Bieling, K.; Sculean, A.; Becker, J. Comparison of naturally occurring and ligature-induced peri-implantitis bone defects in humans and dogs. *Clin. Oral Implants Res.* **2007**, *18*, 161–170. [CrossRef] [PubMed]
2. Seong, W.J.; Kotsakis, G.; Huh, J.-K.; Jeong, S.C.; Nam, K.Y.; Kim, J.R.; Heo, Y.C.; Kim, H.-C.; Zhang, L.; Evans, M.D.; et al. Clinical and microbiologic investigation of an expedited peri-implantitis dog model: An animal study. *BMC Oral Health* **2019**, *19*, 150. [CrossRef] [PubMed]
3. Schwarz, F.; Sculean, A.; Engebretson, S.P.; Becker, J.; Sager, M. Animal models for peri-implant mucositis and peri-implantitis. *Periodontol. 2000* **2015**, *68*, 168–181. [CrossRef] [PubMed]
4. Schwarz, F.; Sahm, N.; Schwarz, K.; Becker, J. Impact of defect configuration on the clinical outcome following surgical regenerative therapy of peri-implantitis. *J. Clin. Periodontol.* **2010**, *37*, 449–455. [CrossRef] [PubMed]
5. Renvert, S.; Polyzois, I.; Maguire, R. Re-osseointegration on previously contaminated surfaces: A systematic review. *Clin. Oral Implants Res.* **2009**, *20* (Suppl. 4), 216–227. [CrossRef] [PubMed]
6. Ratka, C.; Weigl, P.; Henrich, D.; Koch, F.; Schlee, M.; Zipprich, H. The Effect of In Vitro Electrolytic Cleaning on Biofilm-Contaminated Implant Surfaces. *J. Clin. Med.* **2019**, *8*, 1397. [CrossRef] [PubMed]
7. Schlee, M.; Rathe, F.; Brodbeck, U.; Ratka, C.; Zipprich, H. Treatment of periimplantitis-electrolytic cleaning versus mechanical and electrolytic cleaning—A randomized controlled clinical trial—6 month results. *J. Clin. Med.* **2019**, *8*, 1909. [CrossRef] [PubMed]
8. Jovanovic, S.A.; Kenney, E.B.; Carranza, F.A.; Donath, K. The regenerative potential of plaque-induced peri-implant bone defects treated by a submerged membrane technique: An experimental study. *Int. J. Oral Maxillofac Implants* **1993**, *8*, 13–18. [PubMed]
9. Linkevicius, T.; Puisys, A.; Linkeviciene, L.; Peciuliene, V.; Schlee, M. Crestal Bone Stability around Implants with Horizontally Matching Connection after Soft Tissue Thickening: A Prospective Clinical Trial. *Clin. Implant Dent. Relat. Res.* **2015**, *17*, 497–508. [CrossRef] [PubMed]
10. Tarnow, D.P.; Cho, S.C.; Wallace, S.S. The effect of inter-implant distance on the height of inter-implant bone crest. *J. Periodontol.* **2000**, *71*, 546–549. [CrossRef] [PubMed]

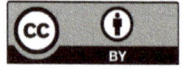

© 2020 by the authors. Licensee MDPI, Basel, Switzerland. This article is an open access article distributed under the terms and conditions of the Creative Commons Attribution (CC BY) license (http://creativecommons.org/licenses/by/4.0/).

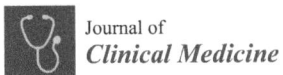

Article

Factors Influencing Early Marginal Bone Loss around Dental Implants Positioned Subcrestally: A Multicenter Prospective Clinical Study

Teresa Lombardi [1], Federico Berton [2], Stefano Salgarello [3], Erika Barbalonga [4], Antonio Rapani [2], Francesca Piovesana [2], Caterina Gregorio [5], Giulia Barbati [2], Roberto Di Lenarda [2] and Claudio Stacchi [2,*]

1. Private Practice, 87011 Cassano allo Ionio, Italy
2. Department of Medical, Surgical and Health Sciences, University of Trieste, 34129 Trieste, Italy
3. Department of Medical and Surgical Specialties, Radiological Sciences and Public Health, University of Brescia, 25123 Brescia, Italy
4. Private Practice, 6600 Locarno, Switzerland
5. Department of Statistics, University of Padova, 35121 Padova, Italy
* Correspondence: claudio@stacchi.it; Tel.: +39-0481-531229

Received: 17 July 2019; Accepted: 2 August 2019; Published: 4 August 2019

Abstract: Early marginal bone loss (MBL) is a non-infective remodeling process of variable entity occurring within the first year after implant placement. It has a multifactorial etiology, being influenced by both surgical and prosthetic factors. Their impact remains a matter of debate, and controversial information is available, particularly regarding implants placed subcrestally. The present multicenter prospective clinical study aimed to correlate marginal bone loss around platform-switched implants with conical connection inserted subcrestally to general and local factors. Fifty-five patients were enrolled according to strict inclusion/exclusion criteria by four clinical centers. Single or multiple implants (AnyRidge, MegaGen, South Korea) were inserted in the posterior mandible with a one-stage protocol. Impressions were taken after two months of healing (T1), screwed metal-ceramic restorations were delivered three months after implant insertion (T2), and patients were recalled after six months (T3) and twelve months (T4) of prosthetic loading. Periapical radiographs were acquired at each time point. Bone levels were measured at each time point on both mesial and distal aspects of implants. Linear mixed models were fitted to the data to identify predictors associated with MBL. Fifty patients (25 male, 25 female; mean age 58.0 ± 12.8) with a total of 83 implants were included in the final analysis. The mean subcrestal position of the implant shoulder at baseline was 1.24 ± 0.57 mm, while at T4, it was 0.46 ± 0.59 mm under the bone level. Early marginal bone remodeling was significantly influenced by implant insertion depth and factors related to biological width establishment (vertical mucosal thickness, healing, and prosthetic abutment height). Deep implant insertion, thin peri-implant mucosa, and short abutments were associated with greater marginal bone loss up to six months after prosthetic loading. Peri-implant bone levels tended to stabilize after this time, and no further marginal bone resorption was recorded at twelve months after implant loading.

Keywords: abutment height; subcrestal implants; marginal bone loss; implant insertion depth; vertical mucosal thickness; biological width

1. Introduction

A complex cascade of biological events occurs after implant insertion. In this type of surgery, wound healing response after surgical trauma is conditioned by the presence of foreign material in the host bone. According to studies by Donath [1,2], a foreign material inside the human body may elicit four types of host response: rejection, dissolution, resorption, or demarcation. Demarcation, which represents a protective reaction aiming to separate a foreign body impossible to dissolute or resorb from healthy tissue, usually results in fibrous encapsulation. However, when biocompatible material is surrounded by bone in a protected environment (with neither infection nor micromovements), bone encapsulation usually occurs, forming a robust bone-to-implant interface, which can be used for clinical purposes: the osseointegration phenomenon [3]. The majority of osseointegrated implants show successful long-term clinical outcomes due to the establishment of steady-state bone remodeling activity. However, the condition of foreign-body equilibrium may be compromised by various factors at different times. The main clinical sign of imbalance between bone apposition and resorption is a marginal bone loss (MBL) [4]. Marginal bone stability around dental implants has always been considered one of the main criteria for defining implant success [5].

Early MBL is a non-infective remodeling process of variable entity occurring within the first year after implant placement. It has a multifactorial etiology, being influenced by both surgical factors (insufficient crestal width and/or implant malpositioning, bone overheating during implant site preparation, implant crest module characteristics, excessive cortical compression) and prosthetic variables (type of implant/abutment connection, entity and location of implant/abutment microgap, number of abutment disconnections, abutment height, residual cement, early loading) [6–9]. Early MBL represents an adaptive response of peri-implant marginal bone to the combined effect of these factors and has been considered to have an important prognostic value for predicting long-term implant success. A recent study on implants positioned at the crestal level suggested that early MBL >0.44 mm in the first six months after prosthetic loading is a risk indicator for peri-implant bone loss progression [10].

Modifications of horizontal and vertical relationships between implant-abutment junction (IAJ) and bone crest have been suggested to influence the entity of early MBL. The horizontal displacement of the microgap location far from the bone crest using an abutment narrower than the implant neck (platform switching) has been demonstrated to be effective in reducing early MBL [11,12]. Conversely, controversial information is available regarding implants placed subcrestally. Some authors recommended placement of the implant platform 1 or 2 mm below the alveolar crest to better maintain marginal bone levels [13,14]. However, other studies reported an increased extension of inflammatory infiltrate due to deep positioning of the IAJ, resulting in greater MBL compared to implants placed equicrestally [15,16].

Therefore, the primary aim of the present multicenter prospective clinical study was to analyze factors potentially influencing early MBL around platform-switched implants with conical connection inserted subcrestally, up to 15 months after implant placement.

2. Material and Methods

2.1. Study Protocol

This multicenter prospective clinical study was reported in strict adherence to the criteria of the STROBE (Strengthening the Reporting of Observational Studies in Epidemiology) checklist. All procedures were performed per the recommendations of the Declaration of Helsinki, as revised in Fortaleza (2013), for investigations with human subjects. The study protocol was approved by the relevant Ethical Committee (Regione Calabria, Sezione Area Nord, No. 46/2016), and was recorded in a public register of clinical trials (www.clinicaltrials.gov-NCT03077880). All eligible patients were thoroughly informed of the study protocol (including surgical and prosthetic procedures, follow-up visits, potential risks involved, and possible therapeutic alternatives), and signed an informed consent form. Patients authorized the use of their data for research purposes.

2.2. Selection Criteria

Any partially edentulous patient requiring implant therapy for fixed prosthetic rehabilitation in the posterior mandible was eligible for this study, subject to the following inclusion and exclusion criteria.

General inclusion criteria were: (I) age >18 years; (II) good general health; (III) patient willing and fully capable to comply with the study protocol; (IV) written informed consent given.

Local inclusion criteria were: (I) presence of keratinized mucosa with a minimum buccolingual width of 4 mm; (II) bone crest with at least 6 mm width and 8 mm height above the mandibular canal in the site when the implant was planned; (III) healed bone crest (at least 6 months elapsed from tooth extraction); (IV) no grafted bone; (V) full mouth plaque score (FMPS) <25% and full mouth bleeding score (FMBS) <20%; (VI) implant insertion torque (IT) >20 Ncm; (VII) presence of the opposing dentition; (VIII) subcrestal positioning. Exclusion criteria were: (I) history of head or neck radiation therapy; (II) uncontrolled diabetes (hemoglobinA1c >7.5%); (III) immunocompromised patients (HIV infection or chemotherapy within the past 5 years); (IV) present or past treatment with intravenous bisphosphonates; (V) patient pregnancy or lactating at any time during the study; (VI) psychological or psychiatric problems; (VII) alcohol or drugs abuse; (VIII) participating in other studies, if the present protocol could not be properly followed.

All patients, selected consecutively between April 2016 and October 2017, were treated independently by four operators (T.L., S.S., E.B., and C.S.) in four private offices. Data collection was performed by a single independent examiner (F.B.).

All patients received oral hygiene instructions and underwent deplaquing 1 week before surgery. Cone beam computed tomography (CBCT) was performed to analyze available bone volume and to plan implant insertion.

2.3. Surgical and Restorative Procedures

All patients were administered with antibiotic prophylaxis (amoxicillin 2 g) one hour before surgery. A mid-crestal incision was performed under local anesthesia, preserving an adequate quantity of keratinized tissue on both buccal and lingual sides. A full-thickness buccal flap was elevated, and vertical mucosal thickness of the undetached lingual flap was measured with a periodontal probe at the center of the programmed implant site, as described elsewhere [17]. The lingual flap was subsequently elevated, and implant site preparation was performed under abundant irrigation of cold saline solution following the manufacturer's recommendations for subcrestal placement. Platform-switched implants with conical connection (AnyRidge, MegaGen, Gyeongbuk, South Korea) were inserted under bone level, and peak IT values were recorded by the surgical motor (Implantmed, W&H, Burmoos, Austria). Implants were immediately connected to healing or transepithelial abutments (Octa, MegaGen, Gyeongbuk, South Korea), adapting their length to the site-specific soft tissue vertical thickness. Flaps were sutured with single stitches and Sentineri technique using synthetic monofilament [18]. Patients were prescribed post-surgical antibiotic therapy (amoxicillin 1 g twice a day) for six days, and nonsteroidal anti-inflammatory drugs (ibuprofen 600 mg), when necessary. Sutures were removed 10–14 days after surgery. Patients were instructed not to use removable prostheses during the entire healing period.

After two months of healing, implants were clinically and radiographically evaluated, and final impressions were taken. Prosthetic abutments height was chosen, adapting their length to the site-specific soft tissue vertical thickness. After functional and aesthetic try-in, screw-retained metal-ceramic rehabilitations were delivered.

Periodontal status was assessed using the modified plaque index (mPI) and modified sulcus bleeding index (mSBI) at prosthesis delivery and after 6 and 12 months of functional loading [19]. The mean of the four values recorded for each implant (mesial, distal, buccal, and lingual) was subsequently analyzed.

2.4. Radiographic Measurements

Digital radiographs were taken using a long-cone paralleling technique with a Rinn-type film holder at the time of implant placement (baseline—T0), at impression taking (2 months after implant placement—T1), at prosthetic restoration delivery (3 months after implant placement—T2), and after 6 and 12 months of prosthetic loading (T3 and T4, respectively) (Figure 1).

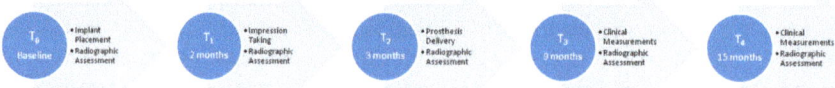

Figure 1. Summary of the visits.

The distance between IAJ and bone crest was measured at each time interval, on both mesial and distal aspects of the implant. A positive value was assigned when the bone crest was coronal to the IAJ, whereas a negative value was assigned when the bone crest was apical to the IAJ.

Any radiograph showing signs of deformation or poor image quality was immediately repeated. All measurements were taken by a single calibrated examiner (F.P.), on a 30-inch led-backlit color diagnostic display, using measuring software (Image J 1.52a, National Institutes of Health, USA) (Figure 2). Each measurement was repeated three times at three different time points, as proposed by Gomez-Roman and Launer [20]. Examiner calibration was performed by assessing ten radiographs, with a different author (F.B.) serving as a reference examiner. Intra-examiner and inter-examiner concordances were 91.9% and 85.2%, respectively, for linear measurements within ±0.1 mm.

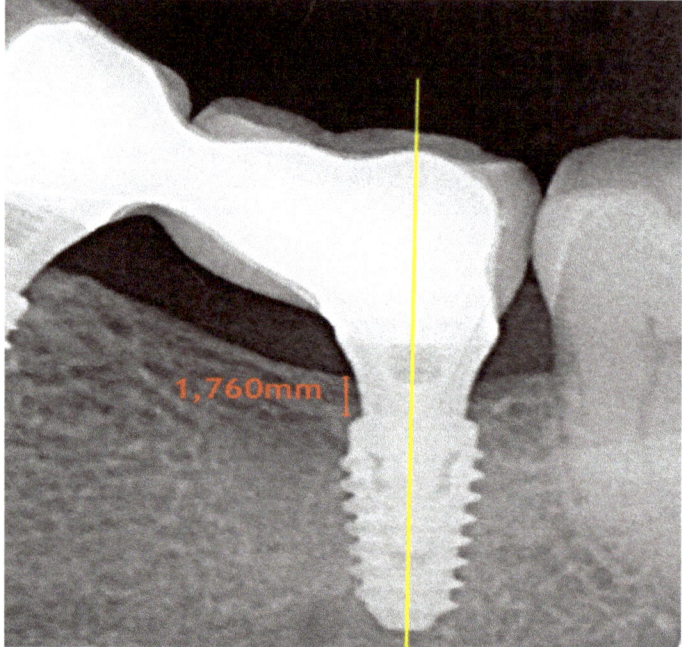

Figure 2. Bone level measurement.

2.5. Predictor and Outcome Variables

Primary predictor variables and their respective period of activity were evaluated as follows: (i) vertical mucosal thickness (thick >2 mm vs. thin ≤2 mm; from T0 to T4); (ii) implant insertion torque (>50 Ncm vs. ≤50 Ncm; from T0 to T1); (iii) depth of implant insertion (mm; from T0 to T4); (iv) healing abutment height (long ≥3 mm vs. short <3 mm; from T0 to T2); (v) number of abutment disconnections (zero vs. multiple; from T0 to T4); (vi) prosthetic abutment height (long ≥3 mm vs. short <3 mm; from T2 to T4); (vii) type of prosthetic restoration (single crown vs. short-span bridge; from T2 to T4). The influence of the following patient-related variables, possibly correlated with the predictor and outcome variables, were also evaluated from T0 to T4: (i) age; (ii) gender; (iii) smoking status (smoker vs. no smoker); (iv) periodontal status (periodontal health vs. chronic periodontitis).

Primary outcome (dependent variable):

- early MBL (up to 12 months from prosthetic loading).

Secondary outcomes:

- implant failure: implant mobility or implant removal due to progressive marginal bone loss. Implant stability was tested by tightening abutment screws (35 N/cm) at prosthesis delivery.
- any complication or adverse event.

2.6. Statistical Analysis

Statistical analysis was performed using R software version 3.5.3 (nlme package; version 3.1.140). Early MBL at each time point was defined as the difference between the depth of implant insertion at the time and depth of implant insertion at baseline.

The means of mesial and distal early MBL at each follow-up were compared using a t-test for paired data. No significant differences were found (T1: Toss = 0.413, d.f. (degrees of freedom) = 82, p = 0.68; T2: Toss = 0.002, d.f. = 82, p = 1; T3: Toss = −0.143, d.f. = 82, p = 0.89; T4: Toss = −0.027, d.f. = 82, p = 0.98), hence the mean between mesial and distal MBL was used as a primary outcome in subsequent analysis.

Linear mixed models were fitted to the data to identify predictors associated with MBL. Since not all variables were active at all time-points, four different models were estimated. First, a global model (Model A) was built, considering all four follow-up time points. Preliminary models with only one covariate at a time, plus time and peri-implant bone level at T0, were estimated to select the covariates to be included in the final multivariable model. Only covariates with p < 0.05 entered the final model. Covariates taken into account were those that might have affected the primary outcome over the whole follow-up period: age, gender, smoking status, periodontal status, vertical mucosal thickness, and multiple abutment disconnections. Time was considered a continuous variable measured in months, and was modeled using a linear spline function with one knot at T3, as indicated by graphical preliminary exploratory analyses. Subsequently, models considering different follow-up times were estimated:

- Model B: T1
- Model C: T1, T2
- Model D: T2, T3, T4

In these models, in addition to the covariates used in Model A, other independent variables active only at specific time points were added (implant insertion torque in Model B; healing abutment height in Model C; prosthetic abutment height and type of prosthetic restoration in Model D).

In models C and D, time was used as a categorical variable. Time was not included in Model B as only one MBL measurement was involved. Covariate selection was performed using preliminary models, as explained above.

The random-effects structure of each model was evaluated using the Likelihood Ratio Test. For all models, the most suitable structure was random intercept on the subject and random intercept on the operator, except for Model B, in which only random intercept on the operator was included.

3. Results

3.1. Demographics and Clinical Outcomes

Of a total of 228 patients evaluated for eligibility, 55 consecutive patients (T.L. 20; S.S. 9; E.B. 6; C.S. 20) fulfilled all inclusion/exclusion requirements and were enrolled in the present study. Included patients (27 male, 28 female; mean age 57.3 ± 12.6, age-range 32–85) were treated between June 2016 and March 2017 with the insertion of a total of 91 implants in the posterior mandible. Two implants in two patients were not placed subcrestally (negative value of the mean between mesial and distal measurements). Three implants in three patients failed to osseointegrate and were removed before taking impressions (primary failure rate of 3.3%). Two patients (three implants) were lost at 6-month follow-up (one patient of T.L. was jailed, and one patient of C.S. moved abroad). Finally, fifty patients (25 male, 25 female; mean age 58.0 ± 12.8, age-range 32–85), with a total of 83 implants that received single or short-span screwed metal-ceramic restorations, completed all phases of the study and were included in the final analysis. The final sample was balanced in terms of age and gender distribution. Complete demographics and characteristics of the included patients are summarized in Table 1.

Table 1. Characteristics of the included patients.

	Total	%
Age		
Male	56.2 ± 13.8	-
Female	59.2 ± 12.3	-
Gender		
Male	25	50
Female	25	50
Smoking Status		
Smoker	7	14
Non Smoker	43	86
Periodontal Status		
Periodontal Health	37	74
Chronic Periodontitis	13	26

No complications or adverse effects were recorded, and no additional implants were lost. All 83 implants were functioning satisfactorily 6 months and 12 months after prosthetic loading. Although slight increases in mPI and mSBI values were recorded at 15-month follow up, no significant differences were recorded between T3 and T4.

3.2. Marginal Bone Level Changes

The mean subcrestal position of the implant shoulder at T0 was 1.24 ± 0.57 mm under bone level, while at T4, it was 0.46 ± 0.59 mm. At the end of the follow-up period, out of a total of 83 implants, the platform of 63 implants remained subcrestal (75.9%), four resulted in equicrestal (4.8%), and 16 resulted in supracrestal (19.3%).

The pattern of marginal bone resorption over time was the following: mean MBL at T1 was 0.5 ± 0.34 mm. An additional mean MBL of 0.18 ± 0.22 mm was registered at T2. A further increase in mean MBL of 0.11 ± 0.20 mm occurred at T3, while complete marginal bone stabilization was observed at T4 (mean MBL compared to T3 = 0.00 ± 0.19 mm). Marginal bone levels at the different time-points are represented in Figure 3.

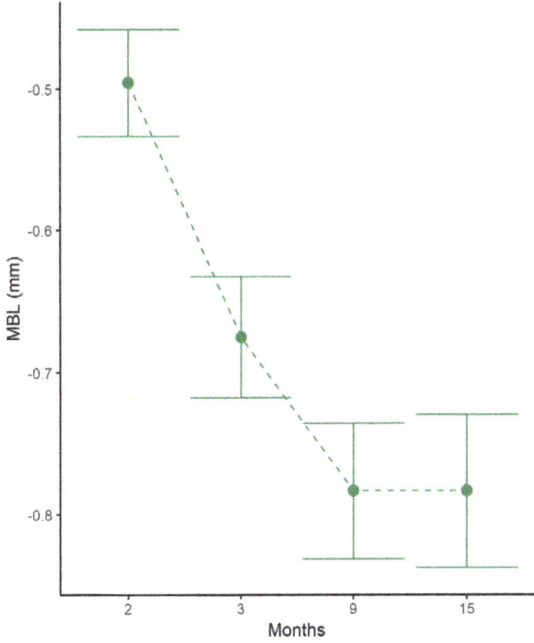

Figure 3. Marginal bone variations at different time points. MBL: marginal bone loss.

Results of preliminary linear mixed models analyzing factors possibly influencing MBL from T0 and T4 are reported in Table 2. From T0 to T4, no significant relationships between early MBL and patient age, gender, smoking status, periodontal status, and multiple abutment disconnections were demonstrated. By contrast, implant insertion depth and presence of thin peri-implant mucosa demonstrated significant negative influence upon early MBL from T0 to T4 ($p < 0.01$ and $p = 0.01$, respectively). Complete results of the multivariable analysis are reported in Table 3.

Table 2. Preliminary univariable linear mixed models, analyzing factors possibly influencing marginal bone loss from implant insertion to 12-months after prosthetic loading.

	MBL (mm)	Std. Error	d.f.	t-Value	p-Value
Age	0.00	0.00	49	−0.49	0.63
Gender	−0.02	0.08	49	−0.21	0.83
Smoking Status	0.12	0.10	49	1.15	0.26
Periodontal Status	−0.02	0.09	49	−0.25	0.80
Multiple Abutment Disconnections	0.03	0.08	30	0.43	0.67

MBL: marginal bone loss; Std: standard; DF: degrees of freedom. Adjusted for time effect and depth of implant insertion.

Table 3. Multivariable linear mixed models, analyzing factors influencing marginal bone loss from implant insertion to 12-months after prosthetic loading.

	MBL (mm)	Std. Error	d.f.	t-Value	p-Value	95% CI
Vertical Mucosal Thickness	0.24	0.08	30	2.91	0.01	0.07; 0.41
Depth of Implant Insertion	−0.23	0.07	30	−3.37	<0.01	−0.37; −0.09

MBL: marginal bone loss; Std: standard; DF: degrees of freedom; CI: confidence interval. Adjusted for time effect.

MBL variability within patients and operators was evaluated by a random-effects model and, from T0 to T1, was observed to be 0.25 mm (0.19; 0.34) and 0.21 mm (0.13; 0.35), respectively.

Preliminary linear mixed models analyzing factors possibly influencing MBL within specific time frames showed no significant associations between implant insertion torque and MBL (from T0 to T1; $p = 0.62$) or between type of prosthetic restoration (single crown vs. short-span bridge) and marginal bone levels (from T2 to T4; $p = 0.92$). Conversely, healing abutment height (from T0 to T2) and prosthetic abutment height (from T2 to T4) had a significant influence on early MBL. In particular, short healing and prosthetic abutments (<3 mm height) were correlated with greater MBL ($p < 0.01$ for both variables). Results of multivariable analysis analyzing factors influencing MBL within specific time frames are reported in Table 4.

Table 4. Multivariable linear mixed models, analyzing factors influencing marginal bone loss within specific time frames.

	Time Interval	MBL (mm)	Std. Error	d.f.	t-Value	p-Value	95% CI
Healing Abutment Height Short (vs. Long)	T0–T2	−0.27	0.07	29	−3.83	<0.01	−0.41; −0.13
Prosthetic Abutment Height Short (vs. Long)	T2–T4	−0.44	0.07	29	−6.42	<0.01	−0.58; −0.3

MBL: marginal bone loss; Std: standard; DF: degrees of freedom; CI: confidence interval; T0: baseline; T1: 2-month visit; T2: 3-month visit; T4: 15-month visit. Adjusted for time effect, depth of implant insertion, and vertical mucosal thickness.

4. Discussion

The present multicenter prospective clinical study showed that platform-switched implants with internal conical connection placed subcrestally presented a reduction in marginal bone levels during the first year of function. Thoroughly analyzing this result, early MBL occurred in the first six months after prosthetic loading. At 15-month follow-up, peri-implant marginal bone levels remained unaltered (difference T4–T3: 0.00 ± 0.19 mm). This finding is in accordance with previous studies on subcrestal implants, showing that MBL mainly occurs in the first period of function [14,21], followed by stabilization of marginal bone levels or even slight marginal bone gain [22].

In the present investigation, a statistically significant positive correlation was demonstrated between the depth of implant insertion and early MBL ($p < 0.01$), confirming a tendency shown in previous studies [22,23]. To be exact, our statistical model suggested that a 1-mm depth increase below the mean implant position at T0 (1.24 mm subcrestal) led to a greater MBL of 0.23 mm at T4. However, from a clinical point of view, it should be underlined that implants with deeper apico-coronal positioning at T0 (>1.5 mm under bone level) resulted in a more subcrestal position at T4, when compared with implants placed more superficially at baseline (<1.5 mm under bone level) (Table 5). Further studies are needed to establish the ideal insertion depth for subcrestal implants, balancing the amount of MBL with the biological shield offered by the presence of bone coronal to the implant shoulder.

Table 5. Bone loss variations in groups with different implant insertion depth.

Insertion Depth	N° Of Implants	Mean Depth At T0	Mean Depth At T4
>1.5 mm	20	2.01 ± 0.48 mm	0.94 ± 0.76 mm
<1.5 mm	63	1.00 ± 0.34 mm	0.31 ± 0.42 mm

T0: baseline; T4: 15-month visit.

General variables, such as age, gender, periodontal status, and smoking habits, appeared not to play a significant role in influencing MBL during the first months of healing. Even if smoking and history of periodontitis are well-known risk factors for the long-term success of implant therapy, their action is time-dependent and often is not predictive for early bone loss after 1-year follow-up [24,25]. Additionally, the one abutment-one time protocol did not have a significant protective action on MBL in comparison to multiple abutment disconnections (three times, in the present study), in agreement with a recent prospective study [26]. This outcome is also consistent with a recent meta-analysis concluding that favorable changes in peri-implant marginal bone level associated with the one abutment-one time protocol should be viewed with caution as its clinical significance remains uncertain [27].

In the present study, the greatest MBL occurred within two months after implant insertion (mean 0.5 ± 0.34 mm), likely due to bone remodeling following surgical trauma and biological width establishment around one-stage implants.

In our sample, variations in implant insertion torque (>50 Ncm vs. ≤50 Ncm) did not influence MBL during the early healing period. This finding is in accordance with some previous clinical trials [28,29] and is in contrast with other studies, showing a negative impact of high torques on marginal bone stability [30–32]. However, the relationship between insertion torque and cortical compression, possibly leading to marginal bone resorption, is strictly dependent upon some crucial factors, which were not always adequately controlled in the aforementioned studies: implant crest module design, implant diameter, and cortical bone thickness around implants [6,33,34]. In the present investigation, detrimental distribution of compressive forces to cortical bone following implant insertion was reduced by the subcrestal positioning of implants (not compressing the most coronal part of the cortical bone) and by the crest module design of the fixture used in this study, the platform of which was significantly narrower than the wider part of the implant body (3.3 mm vs. 4.3 mm).

Conversely, all investigated variables involved in biological width establishment (vertical mucosal thickness, healing abutment height, and prosthetic abutment height) had a significant influence on marginal bone remodeling. Biological width is the three-dimensional space necessary for the establishment of a soft tissue barrier around dental implants once they become exposed to the oral cavity [35]. Peri-implant soft tissue can be divided into two main zones: a coronal epithelial portion and a more apical fiber-rich connective tissue [35,36]. Recently, the biological width around two-piece dental implants placed at the crestal level has been measured in human histologic studies. Vertical dimensions varied from 3.26 to 3.6 mm, representing the minimum space required to create an optimal seal and protect the underlying tissue from external agents [37,38]. When vertical space is insufficient for biological width establishment, the healing process includes marginal bone resorption.

In the present study, thin vertical mucosal thickness (≤2 mm), short healing abutments (<3 mm), and short prosthetic abutments (<3 mm) were significantly associated with greater marginal bone resorption (Figure 4). These data are in accordance with numerous clinical trials and a meta-analysis conducted with implants placed at crestal level [17,39–43], even if this matter has been widely debated. In clinical practice and also in the present study, abutment height is adapted to site-specific soft tissue thickness, with the consequence that short abutments have usually been selected in the presence of thin peri-implant mucosa. This condition could represent a confounding factor when analyzing the real influence of both factors on MBL. Recent studies conducted on separate groups (thick mucosa with long and short abutments; thin mucosa with long and short abutments) indicate that MBL during biological width establishment around dental implants placed at crestal level is influenced by abutment height irrespective of vertical mucosal thickness [9,44].

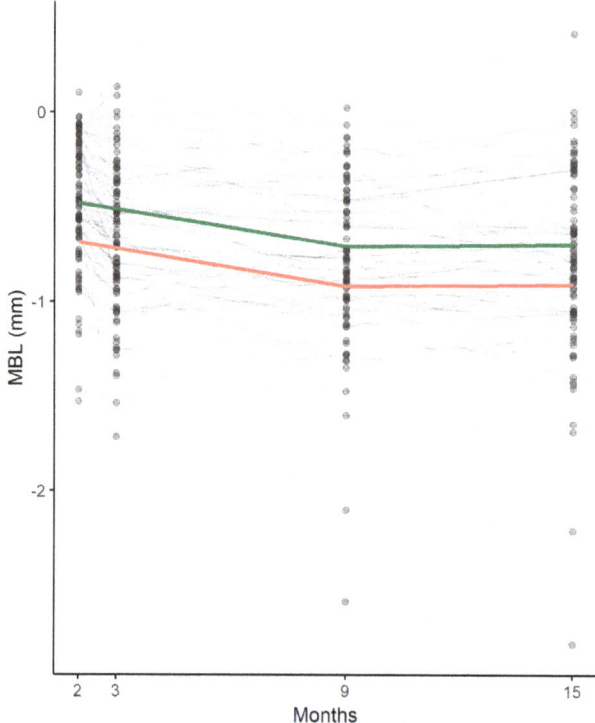

Figure 4. Marginal bone remodeling at different time points estimated by the statistical model: pattern of thick (green) and thin (pink) peri-implant mucosa in the entire sample. MBL: marginal bone loss.

Very few data on these topics are present in literature for subcrestal implants. Some authors suggested adapting the vertical position of implants in relation to soft tissue thickness in order to prevent early MBL [45,46]. The rationale behind this proposal is that subcrestal implant placement could provide additional space for biologic width formation, from the bone crest to the implant platform, resulting in reduced marginal bone remodeling in the presence of thin peri-implant mucosa. However, further clinical and histological studies are necessary to confirm this hypothesis.

Some limitations must be considered when interpreting the outcomes of the present study. These results are not to be generalized for all types of implants: fixtures with a flat-to-flat connection placed subcrestally showed persistent acute inflammation at the microgap between implant and abutment, resulting in increased MBL [15]. The platform-switched conical connection is currently to be considered the pattern of choice to minimize marginal bone remodeling when planning subcrestal implant placement [47].

Another limitation is the use of periapical radiographs to assess marginal bone levels: this method, allowing evaluation of only mesial and distal aspects of peri-implant bone, reduces sensitivity in detecting marginal bone changes.

Moreover, thresholds adopted in the present study to define an abutment as short or long (long: ≥3 mm height; short: <3 mm height) were arbitrary. Future studies should confirm the suitability of these values to define abutment length for implants placed subcrestally.

Finally, the present study collected data from a limited pool of patients in a specific site (posterior mandible): therefore, further trials are needed to generalize these results to a broader population and different areas of the mouth.

5. Conclusions

Early marginal bone remodeling around platform-switched implants with conical connection inserted subcrestally was significantly influenced by implant insertion depth and factors related to biological width establishment (vertical mucosal thickness, healing, and prosthetic abutment height). Deep implant insertion, thin peri-implant mucosa, and short abutments were associated with greater marginal bone loss up to six months after prosthetic loading. Peri-implant bone levels tended to stabilize after this time, and no further marginal bone resorption was recorded at twelve months after implant loading.

The outcomes of this study should be confirmed and generalized by further clinical trials with greater numerosity and conducted in different areas of the mouth.

Finally, further investigations are needed to establish the ideal insertion depth for subcrestal implants, balancing the amount of MBL with the biological shield offered by the presence of bone coronal to the implant shoulder.

Author Contributions: Conceptualization, T.L. and C.S.; Data curation, F.B., A.R., and F.P.; Formal analysis, C.G., G.B., and C.S. Investigation, T.L., S.S., E.B., and C.S.; Methodology, C.G., G.B., and R.D.L.; Project administration, R.D.L.; Resources, T.L. and R.D.L.; Software, F.P.; Supervision, G.B. and C.S.; Validation, F.B. and E.B.; Visualization, S.S.; Writing—original draft, T.L. and C.S.; Writing—review and editing, F.B., S.S., E.B., and A.R.

Funding: This research received no external funding. The APC was funded by MegaGen Implant Co., Ltd.

Acknowledgments: The authors wish to thank Sergio Spinato and Richard de Roeck for their help in reviewing and editing the final manuscript.

Conflicts of Interest: The authors have no conflict of interest related to this study.

References

1. Donath, K. Pathogenesis of bony pocket formation around dental implants. *J. Dent. Assoc. S. Afr.* **1992**, *47*, 204–208. [PubMed]
2. Donath, K.; Laass, M.; Günzl, H.J. The histopathology of different foreign body reactions in oral soft tissue and bone tissue. *Virchows Arch. A Pathol. Anat. Histopathol.* **1992**, *420*, 131–137. [CrossRef] [PubMed]
3. Albrektsson, T.; Chrcanovic, B.; Jacobsson, M.; Wennerberg, A. Osseointegration of implants—A biological and clinical overview. *JSM Dent. Surg.* **2017**, *2*, 1022–1027.
4. Trindade, R.; Albrektsson, T.; Tengvall, P.; Wennerberg, A. Foreign body reaction to biomaterials: On mechanisms for buildup and breakdown of osseointegration. *Clin. Implant Dent. Relat. Res.* **2016**, *18*, 192–203. [CrossRef] [PubMed]
5. Albrektsson, T.; Zarb, G.; Worthington, P.; Eriksson, A.R. The long-term efficacy of currently used dental implants: A review and proposed criteria of success. *Int. J. Oral Maxillofac. Implant.* **1986**, *1*, 11–25.
6. Oh, T.J.; Yoon, J.; Misch, C.E.; Wang, H.-L. The causes of early implant bone loss: Myth or science? *J. Periodontol.* **2002**, *73*, 322–333. [CrossRef] [PubMed]
7. Tatarakis, N.; Bashutski, J.; Wang, H.-L.; Oh, T.J. Early implant bone loss: Preventable or inevitable? *Implant Dent.* **2012**, *21*, 379–386. [CrossRef]
8. Qian, J.; Wennerberg, A.; Albrektsson, T. Reasons for marginal bone loss around oral implants. *Clin. Implant Dent. Relat. Res.* **2012**, *14*, 792–807. [CrossRef]
9. Spinato, S.; Stacchi, C.; Lombardi, T.; Bernardello, F.; Messina, M.; Zaffe, D. Biological width establishment around dental implants is influenced by abutment height irrespective of vertical mucosal thickness: A cluster randomized controlled trial. *Clin. Oral Implant. Res.* **2019**, *30*, 649–659. [CrossRef]
10. Galindo-Moreno, P.; León-Cano, A.; Ortega-Oller, I.; Monje, A.; O'Valle, F.; Catena, A. Marginal bone loss as success criterion in implant dentistry: Beyond 2 mm. *Clin. Oral Implant. Res.* **2015**, *26*, e28–e34. [CrossRef]
11. Santiago, J.F., Jr.; Batista, V.E.; Verri, F.R.; Honório, H.M.; de Mello, C.C.; Almeida, D.A.; Pellizzer, E.P. Platform-switching implants and bone preservation: A systematic review and meta-analysis. *Int. J. Oral Maxillofac. Surg.* **2016**, *45*, 332–345. [CrossRef] [PubMed]
12. Hsu, Y.T.; Lin, G.H.; Wang, H.L. Effects of platform-switching on peri-implant soft and hard tissue outcomes: A systematic review and meta-analysis. *Int. J. Oral Maxillofac. Implant.* **2017**, *32*, e9–e24. [CrossRef] [PubMed]

13. Donovan, R.; Fetner, A.; Koutouzis, T.; Lundgren, T. Crestal bone changes around implants with reduced abutment diameter placed non-submerged and at subcrestal positions: A 1-year radiographic evaluation. *J. Periodontol.* **2010**, *81*, 428–434. [CrossRef] [PubMed]
14. Aimetti, M.; Ferrarotti, F.; Mariani, G.M.; Ghelardoni, C.; Romano, F. Soft tissue and crestal bone changes around implants with platform-switched abutments placed nonsubmerged at subcrestal position: A 2-year clinical and radiographic evaluation. *Int. J. Oral Maxillofac. Implant.* **2015**, *30*, 1369–1377. [CrossRef] [PubMed]
15. Broggini, N.; McManus, L.M.; Hermann, J.S. Periimplant inflammation defined by the implant-abutment interface. *J. Dent. Res.* **2006**, *85*, 473–478. [CrossRef] [PubMed]
16. Gatti, C.; Gatti, F.; Silvestri, M.; Mintrone, F.; Rossi, R.; Tridondani, G.; Piacentini, G.; Borrelli, P. A prospective multicenter study on radiographic crestal bone changes around dental implants placed at crestal or subcrestal level: One-year findings. *Int. J. Oral Maxillofac. Implant.* **2018**, *33*, 913–918. [CrossRef] [PubMed]
17. Linkevicius, T.; Apse, P.; Grybauskas, S.; Puisys, A. The influence of soft tissue thickness on crestal bone changes around implants: A 1-year prospective controlled clinical trial. *Int. J. Oral Maxillofac. Implant.* **2009**, *24*, 712–719.
18. Sentineri, R.; Lombardi, T.; Berton, F.; Stacchi, C. Laurell-Gottlow suture modified by Sentineri for tight closure of a wound with a single line of sutures. *Br. J. Oral Maxillofac. Surg.* **2016**, *54*, e18–e19. [CrossRef]
19. Mombelli, A.; van Oosten, M.A.; Schurch, E.; Lang, N. The microbiota associated with successful or failing implants. *Oral Microbiol. Immunol.* **1987**, *2*, 145–151. [CrossRef]
20. Gomez-Roman, G.; Launer, S. Peri-implant bone changes in immediate and non-immediate root-analog stepped implants-a matched comparative prospective study up to 10 years. *Int. J. Implant Dent.* **2016**, *2*, 15. [CrossRef]
21. Fickl, S.; Zuhr, O.; Stein, J.M.; Hurzeler, M.B. Peri-implant bone level around implants with platform-switched abutments. *Int. J. Oral Maxillofac. Implant.* **2010**, *25*, 577–581.
22. Froum, S.J.; Cho, S.C.; Suzuki, T.; Yu, P.; Corby, P.; Khouly, I. Epicrestal and subcrestal placement of platform-switched implants: 18 month-result of a randomized, controlled, split-mouth, prospective clinical trial. *Clin. Oral Implant. Res.* **2018**, *29*, 353–366. [CrossRef] [PubMed]
23. Koutouzis, T.; Neiva, R.; Nonhoff, J.; Lundgren, T. Placement of implants with platform-switched Morse taper connections with the implant-abutment interface at different levels in relation to the alveolar crest: A short-term (1-year) randomized prospective controlled clinical trial. *Int. J. Oral Maxillofac. Implant.* **2013**, *28*, 1553–1563. [CrossRef] [PubMed]
24. Collaert, B.; De Bruyn, H. Immediate functional loading of TiOblast dental implants in full-arch edentulous maxillae: A 3-year prospective study. *Clin. Oral Implant. Res.* **2008**, *19*, 1254–1260. [CrossRef] [PubMed]
25. Vervaeke, S.; Collaert, B.; Cosyn, J.; De Bruyn, H. A 9-year prospective case series using multivariate analyses to identify predictors of early and late peri-implant bone loss. *Clin. Implant Dent. Relat. Res.* **2016**, *18*, 30–39. [CrossRef] [PubMed]
26. Borges, T.; Leitão, B.; Pereira, M.; Carvalho, Á.; Galindo-Moreno, P. Influence of the abutment height and connection timing in early peri-implant marginal bone changes: A prospective randomized clinical trial. *Clin. Oral Implant. Res.* **2018**, *29*, 907–914. [CrossRef]
27. Atieh, M.A.; Tawse-Smith, A.; Alsabeeha, N.H.M.; Ma, S.; Duncan, W.J. The one abutment-one time protocol: A systematic review and meta-analysis. *J. Periodontol.* **2017**, *88*, 1173–1185. [CrossRef]
28. Khayat, P.G.; Arnal, H.M.; Tourbah, B.I.; Sennerby, L. Clinical outcome of dental implants placed with high insertion torques (up to 176 Ncm). *Clin. Implant Dent. Relat. Res.* **2013**, *15*, 227–233. [CrossRef]
29. Grandi, T.; Guazzi, P.; Samarani, R.; Grandi, G. Clinical outcome and bone healing of implants placed with high insertion torque: 12-month results from a multicenter controlled cohort study. *Int. J. Oral Maxillofac. Surg.* **2013**, *42*, 516–520. [CrossRef]
30. Duyck, J.; Roesems, R.; Cardoso, M.V.; Ogawa, T.; De Villa Camargos, G.; Vandamme, K. Effect of insertion torque on titanium implant osseointegration: An animal experimental study. *Clin. Oral Implant. Res.* **2015**, *26*, 191–196. [CrossRef]
31. Barone, A.; Alfonsi, F.; Derchi, G.; Tonelli, P.; Toti, P.; Marchionni, S.; Covani, U. The effect of insertion torque on the clinical outcome of single implants: A randomized clinical trial. *Clin. Implant Dent. Relat. Res.* **2016**, *18*, 588–600. [CrossRef] [PubMed]

32. Marconcini, S.; Giammarinaro, E.; Toti, P.; Alfonsi, F.; Covani, U.; Barone, A. Longitudinal analysis on the effect of insertion torque on delayed single implants: A 3-year randomized clinical study. *Clin. Implant Dent. Relat. Res.* **2018**, *20*, 322–332. [CrossRef] [PubMed]
33. Norton, M. Primary stability versus viable constraint—A need to redefine. *Int. J. Oral Maxillofac. Implant.* **2013**, *28*, 19–21.
34. Spray, J.R.; Black, C.G.; Morris, H.F.; Ochi, S. The influence of bone thickness on facial marginal bone response: Stage 1 placement through stage 2 uncovering. *Ann. Periodontol.* **2000**, *5*, 119–128. [CrossRef] [PubMed]
35. Berglundh, T.; Lindhe, J.; Ericsson, I.; Marinello, C.P.; Liljenberg, B.; Thomsen, P. The soft tissue barrier at implants and teeth. *Clin. Oral Implant. Res.* **1991**, *2*, 81–90. [CrossRef]
36. Abrahamsson, I.; Berglundh, T.; Wennström, J.; Lindhe, J. The peri-implant hard and soft tissues at different implant systems. A comparative study in the dog. *Clin. Oral Implant. Res.* **1996**, *7*, 212–219. [CrossRef]
37. Judgar, R.; Giro, G.; Zenobio, E.; Coelho, P.G.; Feres, M.; Rodrigues, J.A.; Mangano, C.; Iezzi, G.; Piattelli, A.; Shibli, J.A. Biological width around one-and two-piece implants retrieved from human jaws. *BioMed Res. Int.* **2014**, *2014*, 850120. [CrossRef]
38. Tomasi, C.; Tessarolo, F.; Caola, I.; Wennström, J.; Nollo, G.; Berglundh, T. Morphogenesis of peri-implant mucosa revisited: An experimental study in humans. *Clin. Oral Implant. Res.* **2014**, *25*, 997–1003. [CrossRef]
39. Galindo-Moreno, P.; León-Cano, A.; Ortega-Oller, I.; Monje, A.; Suárez, F.; O'Valle, F.; Spinato, S.; Catena, A. Prosthetic abutment height is a key factor in peri-implant marginal bone loss. *J. Dent. Res.* **2014**, *93*, 80S–85S. [CrossRef]
40. Vervaeke, S.; Dierens, M.; Besseler, J.; De Bruyn, H. The influence of initial soft tissue thickness on peri-implant bone remodeling. *Clin. Implant Dent. Relat. Res.* **2014**, *16*, 238–247. [CrossRef]
41. Galindo-Moreno, P.; León-Cano, A.; Monje, A.; Ortega-Oller, I.; O'Valle, F.; Catena, A. Abutment height influences the effect of platform switching on peri-implant marginal bone loss. *Clin. Oral Implant. Res.* **2016**, *27*, 167–173. [CrossRef] [PubMed]
42. Spinato, S.; Galindo-Moreno, P.; Bernardello, F.; Zaffe, D. Minimum abutment height to eliminate bone loss: Influence of implant neck design and platform switching. *Int. J. Oral Maxillofac. Implant.* **2018**, *33*, 405–411. [CrossRef] [PubMed]
43. Chen, Z.; Lin, C.Y.; Li, J.; Wang, H.L.; Yu, H. Influence of abutment height on peri-implant marginal bone loss: A systematic review and meta-analysis. *J. Prosthet. Dent.* **2019**, *122*, 14–21.e2. [CrossRef] [PubMed]
44. Blanco, J.; Pico, A.; Caneiro, L.; Nóvoa, L.; Batalla, P.; Martín-Lancharro, P. Effect of abutment height on interproximal implant bone level in the early healing: A randomized clinical trial. *Clin. Oral Implant. Res.* **2018**, *29*, 108–117. [CrossRef] [PubMed]
45. Vervaeke, S.; Matthys, C.; Nassar, R.; Christiaens, V.; Cosyn, J.; De Bruyn, H. Adapting the vertical position of implants with a conical connection in relation to soft tissue thickness prevents early implant surface exposure: A 2-year prospective intra-subject comparison. *J. Clin. Periodontol.* **2018**, *45*, 605–612. [CrossRef] [PubMed]
46. Pico, A.; Martín-Lancharro, P.; Caneiro, L.; Nóvoa, L.; Batalla, P.; Blanco, J. Influence of abutment height and implant depth position on interproximal peri-implant bone in sites with thin mucosa: A 1-year randomized clinical trial. *Clin. Oral Implant. Res.* **2019**, *30*, 595–602. [CrossRef] [PubMed]
47. Palaska, I.; Tsaousoglou, P.; Vouros, I.; Konstantinidis, A.; Menexes, G. Influence of placement depth and abutment connection pattern on bone remodeling around 1-stage implants: A prospective randomized controlled clinical trial. *Clin. Oral Implant. Res.* **2016**, *27*, e47–e56. [CrossRef] [PubMed]

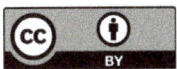

© 2019 by the authors. Licensee MDPI, Basel, Switzerland. This article is an open access article distributed under the terms and conditions of the Creative Commons Attribution (CC BY) license (http://creativecommons.org/licenses/by/4.0/).

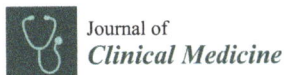

Article

The Effect of Tapered Abutments on Marginal Bone Level: A Retrospective Cohort Study

Simone Marconcini [1,*], Enrica Giammarinaro [2], Ugo Covani [1], Eitan Mijiritsky [3], Xavier Vela [4] and Xavier Rodríguez [5]

1 Department of Surgical, Medical, Molecular and Critical Area Pathology, University of Pisa, 56124 Pisa, Italy
2 Tuscan Dental Institute, Versilia General Hospital, 55041 Lido di Camaiore, Italy
3 Department of Otolaryngology Head and Neck Surgery and Maxillofacial Surgery, Tel-Aviv Sourasky Medical Center, Sackler School of Medicine, 61503 Tel Aviv, Israel
4 Department of Maxillofacial Surgery and Implantology, International University of Catalunya, 08001 Barcelona, Spain
5 Department of Oral Implantology, European University of Madrid, 28001 Madrid, Spain
* Correspondence: simosurg@gmail.com

Received: 8 July 2019; Accepted: 20 August 2019; Published: 24 August 2019

Abstract: Background: Early peri-implant bone loss has been associated to long-term implant-prosthetic failure. Different technical, surgical, and prosthetic techniques have been introduced to enhance the clinical outcome of dental implants in terms of crestal bone preservation. The aim of the present cohort study was to observe the mean marginal bone level around two-part implants with gingivally tapered abutments one year after loading. Methods: Mean marginal bone levels and change were computed following radiological calibration and linear measurement on standardized radiographs. Results: Twenty patients who met the inclusion criterion of having at least one implant with the tapered prosthetic connection were included in the study. The cumulative implant success rate was 100%, the average bone loss was −0.18 ± 0.72 mm, with the final bone level sitting above the implant platform most of the time (+1.16 ± 0.91 mm). Conclusion: The results of this cohort study suggested that implants with tapered abutments perform successfully one year after loading and that they are associated with excellent marginal bone preservation, thus suggesting that implant-connection macro-geometry might have a crucial role in dictating peri-implant bone levels.

Keywords: bone loss; convergence; clinical study

1. Introduction

Long-term dental implant survival has been extensively documented under different conditions, so that contemporary clinical dentistry has been focusing on means to achieve predictable implant success. Most of the authors agree on the fact that minimal marginal bone loss should be observed one year within the implant loading, as this quantity is a predictor of the long-term implant survival and success [1]. The extent of post-loading bone remodeling has been mainly related to two different phenomena: (1) The microbial infiltration at the implant-abutment (IA) micro-gap—with consequent inflammation and bone demineralization [2]; (2) the implant-abutment (IA) design [3].

The most accounted risk factor for marginal bone loss has been long considered the inflammatory infiltrate at the IA gap [4]. The understanding of the complex biological events impacting the cervical bone surrounding submerged implants begun with the fundamental animal histometric study by Ericsson [5] who typified the inflammatory infiltrate as a consistent finding in matching IA interfaces. This circumscribed inflammation resulted in a round connective demarcation wall that ultimately leads to bone demineralization and resorption [2,6,7]. Different studies indicated less marginal bone resorption around mis-matching implants (implants with a platform switching connection—PS)—when compared to matching implants—as well as a different organization of the connective tissue fibers [8]. Several theories have been proposed to explain this clinical manifestation, such as the shifting of the inflammatory infiltrate away from the bone, the additional room for protective connective tissue proliferation, or, best, the creation of a geometrical stop for biological width apical establishment. In fact, in matching implants, the fixture first thread is also the first topographic point where the rehabilitation turns from a smaller to a wider diameter, creating a mechanical retention for connective tissues. In short, marginal bone loss should be inevitable, at least to this extent [9]. In PS implants, the implant-abutment discrepancy acts equally, but at a more coronal level—at the platform level—where the connective fibers are retained. It could be hypothesized that the rehabilitation macro-geometry dictates soft and hard tissue position, independent of the effect of the inflammatory infiltrate produced by the gap [10,11].

The gingivally convergent abutment was developed with the idea of maximizing the available space for soft tissues, which is occupied by the bulky metal shoulder in divergent abutments [12]. The sloping profile of gingival convergent abutments would allow tissue to slide coronally in the early phases of healing, creating a thick connective seal above the IA gap.

What is really bearing the brunt of preserving marginal bone levels? Is it either the relative location of the implant-abutment (IA) junction or is it the connection macro-geometry?

The specific aim of this cohort study was to investigate the clinical and radiological outcome of implants with a convergent implant-abutment connection one year after loading.

2. Materials and Methods

This study was a retrospective, non-interventional analysis of consecutive patients treated with dental implants with a gingivally convergent abutment connection (Shelta XA, Sweden & Martina, Via Veneto 19, 35020, Due Carrare, Padova, Italy). This study was based on patients consecutively treated on a routine basis at one specialistic center (BORG, Carrer de la Mare de Déu de Sales, 67 08840 Viladecans, Barcelona, Spain) during the period from 2016 to 2018.

2.1. Inclusion and Exclusion Criteria

The medical records of patients who had at least one two-part implant rehabilitated with a convergent abutment with a one-year follow-up were reviewed. Patients were included if presenting a complete set of follow-up radiographs and intra-oral digital photographs. All implants were placed at a slightly sub-crestal level. Patient records were excluded if they did not present for bi-annual follow-up visits, if they had been rehabilitated with overdentures or full-arch prosthesis or if the implants had been placed with simultaneous guided bone regeneration.

2.2. Data Collection and Analysis

Data were directly entered into an Excel spreadsheet and then converted to a .csv file format in order to be read by the software for statistical analysis. The following population describing the variables were collected: Age, gender, implant characteristics (diameter, length), implant location (tooth number and anterior/posterior, maxillary/mandibular), type of implant-supported prosthetic restoration (single crown or partial bridge), and follow-up time.

2.3. Radiologic Marginal Bone Level Evaluation

Routine peri-apical radiographs obtained via the long-cone paralleling technique with a loop film holder (Rinn, Dentsply Australia Pty Ltd, Pacific Hwy, St Leonards NSW 2065, Australia) were used to measure the marginal bone levels. Radiographs were standardized by means of individual resin bites. The distance between the implant–abutment connection and the first bone-to-implant contact (fBIC) on mesial and distal surfaces was recorded. The scale was calibrated by the width of the dental implant achieving a unique pixel/mm ratio (Figure 1). Radiographic bone levels were calculated at the moment of prosthetic transfer connection (impression taking), at loading, and every six months after loading.

The mean marginal bone level for each implant was computed merging mesial and distal variations. The marginal bone change was defined as the difference between the last follow-up and the baseline MBL value, with negative values denoting a loss in bone height.

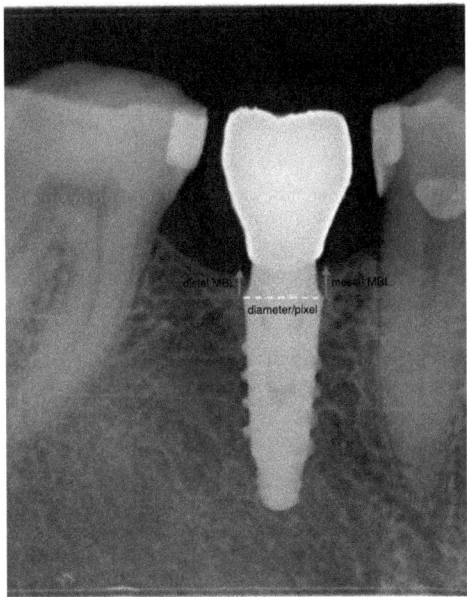

Figure 1. The picture is a schematic representation of the calibration performed on the software to achieve bone level linear measurements. The scale was set and calibrated by the width of the dental implant.

All measurements were performed by a single examiner (SM). The intra-examiner reproducibility was evaluated using the intraclass correlation analysis from the measurements in 10 patients, which revealed a strong correlation coefficient of 0.982 for MBL radiological measurements. Measurements were performed via the OsirisX software (Pixmeo SARL, 266 Rue de Bernex, CH-1233 Bernex, Switzerland).

2.4. Dichotomous Outcomes

- Implant failure was identified with eventual implant mobility or persistent infection, and whenever the implant presented signs and symptoms that led to the implant removal.
- Survival and success rates (SRs and CSRs, respectively) for implants, were calculated according to the criteria defined by Buser et al. in 1997 [13]. Successful implants were those showing a mean radiological peri-implant bone resorption within 1.5 mm during the first year of loading, and less than 0.2 mm/year during the following years.

2.5. Statistical Analysis

Descriptive and longitudinal statistics was performed on the R free software version 3.5.1 (02-07-2018). The longitudinal nonparametric analysis on marginal bone levels was implemented on the ld.f1 function within the package nparLD. This non-parametric method exhibits a competitive performance for small sample sizes and outliers. In the per-implant analysis, the ANOVA-type statistic (ATS) was calculated for the global alternatives with 'time' as the fixed su-plot factor. A p value < 0.05 has been used as a cut-off for significance and a robust analysis of variance and a Spearman's correlation coefficient has been performed. A further mixed effect model (function lmer within package lme4) was used to control for crossed random effects posed by patients contributing with more than one implant. This formula expects that there is going to be multiple responses per patient, and these responses will depend on each subject's baseline level. This effectively resolved the non-independence that stemmed from having multiple responses by the same subject.

3. Results

3.1. Study Population

In total, 20 patients received 36 implants. The mean age at the implant insertion was 56.2 ± 10.2 years (Table 1). Of the 20 patients, 65.0% were female and 35.0% were male. Of the 36 implants, 24 (66.6%) were placed in the maxilla and 12 (33.3%) were placed in the mandible. Implant diameters ranged from 3.8 mm to 5.0 mm—the mode being 4.2 mm diameter (70%)—and implant lengths ranged from 8.5 mm to 15 mm. Sixteen implants (44.4%) were splinted. Implants were more frequently placed in upper premolar positions (60%). Abutment heights ranged from 4 mm to 6 mm.

Table 1. Demographic data and clinical characteristics.

	Male	Female	Total
Number of Patients	7	13	20
Number of Implants	9	27	36
Mean Age			56.2 ± 10.2
Age Range			39–76

3.2. Survival and Adverse Events

At the last follow up, all 36 implants were healthy, stable and there were no reported failures; thus, the implant had a cumulative survival rate of 100%. No failure, defined as signs and symptoms that led to the implant removal, could be recorded. Therefore, the cumulative success rate was 100%. The average follow-up period was 1.5 years after loading.

3.3. Bone Levels

All the implants were radiographically examined by one author alien to the treatment procedure (SM) with the OsiriX DICOM viewer (Pixmeo SARL, 266 Rue de Bernex, CH-1233 Bernex, Switzerland).

The mean marginal bone level was +1.39 ± 0.91 mm at the moment of the prosthetic-transfer connection for definitive impression-taking (considered as the study baseline, Figure 2). One year after loading, the mean marginal bone level reached +1.16 ± 0.911 mm (Figure 2) with an average overall change of −0.18 ± 0.72 mm, occurring above the platform level at large (Figure 3). The change over time was significant (p value = 0.01) when the implant was modeled as the first cluster of analysis and the time was set as the only sub-plot factor (Table 2). The fitness of the model has been confirmed also with the mixed-effects model considering the random effect posed by patients contributing with more than one implant. The mean amount of bone resorption to be expected one year after loading was normally distributed (Figure 4).

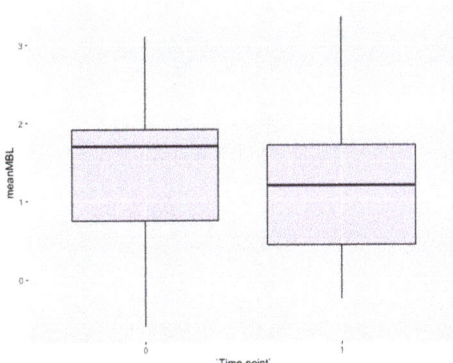

Figure 2. Box-plot of the mean marginal bone levels at the baseline and one year after loading.

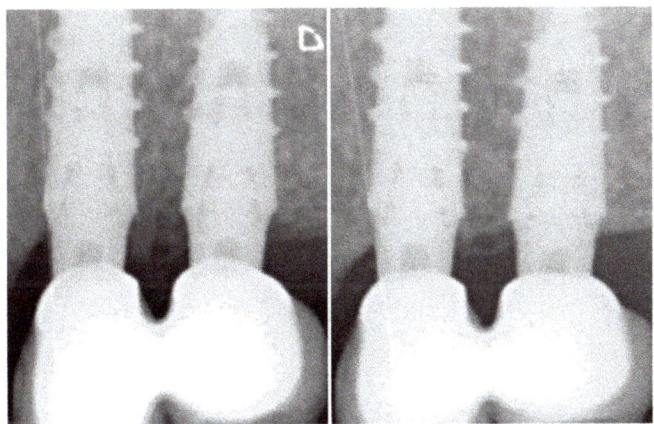

Figure 3. Radiographic appearance of the marginal bone levels at adjacent implants loaded with tapered abutment at loading (left) and one year after (right).

Table 2. Mean marginal bone level (MBL) in function by year, mm (per implant analysis) and statistical significance of time-effect according to the Behrens-Fisher test and the ANOVA results for implant-related factors.

Time-point	Mesial MBL	Distal MBL	Mean MBL	Delta MBL	p-value
Mean MBL in function by year, mm (per implant analysis) and statistical significance of time-effect.					
Overall					
Baseline	1.47 ± 0.87	1.30 ± 1.01	1.39 ± 0.91		
1-year	1.28 ± 0.98	1.04 ± 0.92	1.16 ± 0.91	−0.18 ± 0.72	0.01
Mandible					
Baseline	0.90 ± 0.76	0.55 ± 0.87	0.72 ± 0.77		
1-year	0.76 ± 0.67	0.47 ± 0.61	0.61 ± 0.60	−0.10 ± 0.29	0.19
Sub-plot factor analysis for "*Mandible* vs. *Maxilla* relative *treatment effect*" <MBL ~ jaw p-value 6.58 × 10^{-7}					
Maxilla					
Baseline	1.72 ± 0.81	1.63 ± 0.89	1.68 ± 0.72		
1-year	1.51 ± 1.02	1.29 ± 0.92	1.40 ± 0.93	−0.22 ± 0.84	0.06

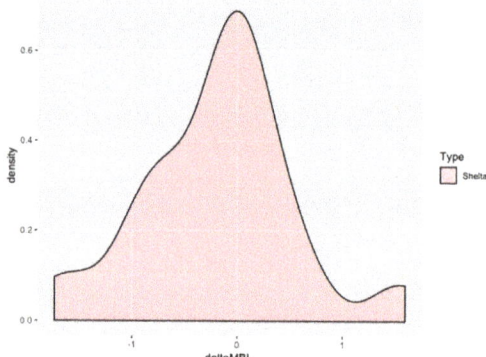

Figure 4. Density plot of the mean marginal bone change frequency distribution one year after loading in the entire cohort. The plot exquisitely shows a bell-shaped curve denoting a predictable amount of marginal bone resorption for the implant-abutment studied: most of the observations converged around zero.

The categorical data describing the implant-related factors and position (diameter, length, abutment height, jaw) were modeled on the multiway test. The implant diameter and length did not appear to affect the marginal bone, however, there was a relative significant effect given by the abutment height (p value < 0.05) in the mixed model: Longer abutments showed better marginal bone preservation at a one-year evaluation (Table 3). To investigate the question about which of the three abutment height categories differed, multiple comparisons with the Bonferroni adjustment were applied. The relationship held only for abutments longer than 5 mm; still, the linearity could not be confirmed.

Implants placed in the mandible and in the maxilla did not differ in terms of 1-year marginal bone loss, however, the first bone-to-implant contact at implants placed in the mandible was significantly lower than that of the maxilla most of the times (p value < 0.001).

Table 3. Mean marginal bone level (MBL) by implant abutment-height by year.

Sub-plot factor analysis for "Abutment Height treatment effect" <MBL ~ abutment height p-value 0.05					
Time-point	mesial MBL	distal MBL	mean MBL	delta MBL	*p*-value
4 mm					
Baseline	1.31 ± 0.96	0.97 ± 0.98	1.15 ± 0.94		
1-year	1.08 ± 0.91	0.77 ± 1.03	0.93 ± 0.93	−0.20 ± 0.83	0.36
5 mm					
Baseline	1.54 ± 0.86	1.52 ± 1.03	1.53 ± 0.92		
1-year	1.34 ± 1.08	1.16 ± 0.86	1.25 ± 0.94	−0.20 ± 0.70	0.17
6 mm					
Baseline	1.80 ± 0.69	1.43 ± 0.80	1.62 ± 0.70		
1-year	1.87 ± 0.35	1.53 ± 0.56	1.70 ± 0.43	0.08 ± 0.34	0.05

3.4. Secondary Outcomes: Soft Tissues

Peri-implant soft tissues appeared healthy and thick at each visit after loading (Figure 5). At the provisional prosthesis loading, 96% and 95% of the 36 implants had a papilla index >2 for the mesial and distal side, respectively. At the last follow up, 97% and 94% of the implants had a papilla index >2 for the mesial and distal side, respectively.

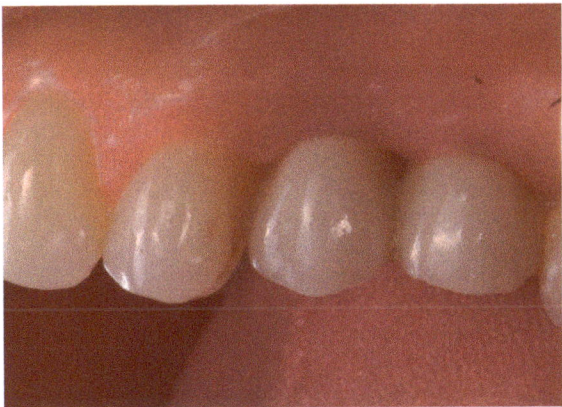

Figure 5. Clinical appearance of vestibular and inter-proximal soft tissues around adjacent implants loaded with tapered abutment.

4. Discussion

In the present study, the one-year healing around two-part implants with a gingival convergent abutment profile was evaluated. In 90% of the implants analyzed, the radiological bone level extended coronal to the IA border, at the abutment level. It is suggested that bone preservation may occur coronal to the IA connection of two-part implants loaded with convergent abutment profile as a consequence of advantageous macro-geometry, independent of the effect of the inflammatory infiltrate at the gap, and of the establishment of biologic width after prosthesis connection.

Results derived from animal studies showed that marginal bone resorption of about 2 mm occurred around two-part implants [14,15]. However, Welander et al. [16] suggested that osseointegration could occur coronal to the IA junction of two-part implants when the fixture was placed 2 mm sub-crestally.

A number of factors, according to prevalent literature, might influence the first-year marginal bone loss, such as neck configuration, surgical trauma, occlusal overload, mucositis, micro-gap colonization, biologic width formation, and flapless or flapped procedures [17–19]. The stability of the marginal bone levels might be determined by other factors, different from those acting during the healing phase. One of these factors is represented by the apico-coronal location of the implant head in respect to the bone crest [20]. In a recent systematic review, it was assessed that the effect of the sub-crestal implant positioning compared with equi-crestal position on the bone and soft tissues around dental implants with platform switching design: The authors reported that platform switch implants placed in a sub-crestal position had shown less marginal bone resorption when compared to implants placed with their head at the crest level [21].

The radiographic observation of post-loading bone remodeling generally coincided with the level of the first thread, and some authors suggested that this would be a consequence of the soft tissue's attempt to sit on top of the dental implant creating a mechanical protective seal [22].

Davarpanah [23] also observed that bone resorption around the implants placed at the supra-crestal level was less than that of the implants placed at the crestal level. However, it is true that when the thread is moved in a coronal direction, the implant platform is moved upward as well. For this reason, it would be impossible to demonstrate the relative influence of each contributing factor on bone resorption. Flores-Guillen et al. [24] compared submerged and trans mucosal platform switch implants and found that there were no differences at a five-year evaluation in terms of marginal bone loss achieving a mean value of −0.73 ± 0.81 mm. Therefore, the cumulative screening literature suggested that platform switching or, more in general, connection macro-geometry is more critical than the relative position of the platform crest module in determining early bone remodeling.

The recent systematic review by Messias et al. suggested that reporting the marginal bone change is insufficient for the correct evaluation of the implant performance: The authors recommended to report the crestal bone levels, in particular where no data is provided relative to the healing period [25]. Furthermore, reporting at which level the crestal bone is in an intimate contact with the implant seemed reasonable and more convenient for describing the effect of the IA macro-geometry on the marginal bone. In the present study, the overall bone change was −0.18 ± 0.72 mm one year after loading, occurring above the platform level, in any case. In fact, the one-year mean bone level was +1.16 ± 0.91 mm with a significant difference between the lower and upper jaw. The mean bone gain from the baseline to the last follow-up occurred in 33.0% of the implants analyzed, which is twice the frequency observed by Flores-Guillen et al. in the platform switch implants in the same given period [24].

Few studies evaluated the tissue response around the tapered convergent abutments [26]. The use of the tapered abutments, not only could improve the peri-implant bone level, but also diminish the sulcus length. In fact, it has been suggested that the biological phenomenon of the peri-implant bone preservation would be related with the circular connective tissue fibers stabilization around the abutment and the presence of a shallow sulcus [27]. In the present study, the cumulative implant success rate was 100%, with no implant showing any sign or symptom of mucositis or prosthetic complication. Peri-implant mucosa appeared healthy-pink, thick, and firm at each visit after loading. The plausible biologic explanation should be sought in the wound healing process that starts after the abutment connection: The convergent abutment would create a housing effect that protects the surrounding biological structures maintaining tissue stability over time.

The multiway analysis conducted on this study displayed a significant relative effect of the abutment height on the marginal bone loss: Implants with longer abutments (>5 mm) appeared to have minimal bone resorption. It has been hypothesized that an abutment with a height <2 mm does not provide sufficient soft tissue for establishing the peri-implant biologic width [28]. The establishment of the peri-implant biologic width follows the implant placement and connective tissue attachment to the abutment. Long abutments might be associated with a thicker gingival biotype, which in turn would be more effective at preventing inflammatory infiltration.

The present cohort study has different limitations that should be taken into account. First, the study design was retrospective, and a single-cohort, thus reducing the meaningfulness and external validity of the results. The implant was chosen as the first cluster of analysis which does not guarantee independence between implants, however the mixed effect model applied took the random effect posed by patients into account, not revealing any significant discrepancy with the fixed effect model. It must be remarked that the radiographic artifact of a stable first bone-to-implant contact does not necessarily imply histologic osseo-integration. However, the imaging accuracy of digital radiography is high with a precision of 0.1 mm or less. Still, the clinical relevance of such small entities is questionable and difficult to repeat among different operators [29]. Furthermore, the present study is a single cohort study without an internal control group.

5. Conclusions

Overall, the present study showed that implants rehabilitated with tapered abutments yielded excellent hard- and soft-tissue outcomes. In particular, after one year of loading, marginal bone levels consistently appeared above the implant platform, at the abutment level, with minimal bone change. It was suggested that the implant-connection macro-geometry might dictate peri-implant bone levels. Therefore, further prospective randomized trials are strongly recommended to support the present findings.

Author Contributions: All of the authors contributed with the investigation, supervision, writing, review, and editing of the study. The study conceptualization must be acknowledged to S.M., U.C., E.M., X.V., and X.R. Data curation, data visualization, and analysis must be acknowledged to S.M., E.G., X.V., and X.R.

Conflicts of Interest: The authors declare no conflict of interest.

References

1. Oh, T.J.; Yoon, J.; Misch, C.E.; Wang, H.L. The causes of early implant bone loss: Myth or science? *J. Periodontol.* **2002**, *73*, 322–333. [CrossRef] [PubMed]
2. Piattelli, A.; Vrespa, G.; Petrone, G.; Iezzi, G.; Annibali, S.; Scarano, A. Role of the micro-gap between implant and abutment: A retrospective histologic evaluation in monkeys. *J. Periodontol.* **2003**, *74*, 346–352. [CrossRef] [PubMed]
3. Jung, Y.C.; Han, C.H.; Lee, K.W. A 1-year radiographic evaluation of marginal bone around dental implants. *Int. J. Oral Maxillofac. Implants* **1996**, *11*, 811–818. [PubMed]
4. Astrand, P.; Engquist, B.; Dahlgren, S.; Gröndahl, K.; Engquist, E.; Feldmann, H. Astra Tech and Brånemark system implants: A 5-year prospective study of marginal bone reactions. *Clin. Oral Implant. Res.* **2004**, *15*, 413–420. [CrossRef] [PubMed]
5. Ericsson, I.; Persson, L.G.; Berglundh, T.; Marinello, C.P.; Lindhe, J.; Klinge, B. Different types of inflammatory reactions in peri-implant soft tissues. *J. Clin. Periodontol.* **1995**, *22*, 255–261. [CrossRef] [PubMed]
6. Canullo, L.; Quaranta, A.; Teles, R.P. The microbiota associated with implants restored with platform switching: A preliminary report. *J. Periodontol.* **2010**, *81*, 403–411. [CrossRef] [PubMed]
7. Canullo, L.; Pellegrini, G.; Allievi, C.; Trombelli, L.; Annibali, S.; Dellavia, C. Soft tissues around long-term platform switching implant restorations: A histological human evaluation. Preliminary results. *J. Clin. Periodontol.* **2011**, *38*, 86–94. [CrossRef]
8. Buser, D.; Wittneben, J.; Bornstein, M.M.; Grütter, L.; Chappuis, V.; Belser, U.C. Stability of contour augmentation and esthetic outcomes of implant-supported single crowns in the esthetic zone: 3-year results of a prospective study with early implant placement postextraction. *J. Periodontol.* **2011**, *82*, 342–349. [CrossRef]
9. Östman, P.O.; Hellman, M.; Sennerby, L. Ten years later. Results from a prospective single-centre clinical study on 121 oxidized (TiUnite™) Brånemark implants in 46 patients. *Clin. Implant Dent. Relat. Res.* **2012**, *14*, 852–860. [CrossRef]
10. Finelle, G.; Papadimitriou, D.E.V.; Souza, A.B.; Katebi, N.; Gallucci, G.O.; Araújo, M.G. Peri-implant soft tissue and marginal bone adaptation on implant with non-matching healing abutments: Micro-CT analysis. *Clin. Oral Implant. Res.* **2015**, *26*, e42–e46. [CrossRef]
11. Rodríguez, X.; Navajas, A.; Vela, X.; Fortuño, A.; Jimenez, J.; Nevins, M. Arrangement of Peri-implant Connective Tissue Fibers Around Platform-Switching Implants with Conical Abutments and Its Relationship to the Underlying Bone: A Human Histologic Study. *Int. J. Periodontics Restor. Dent.* **2016**, *36*, 533–540.
12. Canullo, L.; Tallarico, M.; Pradies, G.; Marinotti, F.; Loi, I.; Cocchetto, R. Soft and hard tissue response to an implant with a convergent collar in the esthetic area: Preliminary report at 18 months. *Int. J. Esthet. Dent.* **2017**, *12*, 306–323. [PubMed]
13. Buser, D.; Mericske-Stern, R.; Bernard, J.P.; Behneke, A.; Behneke, N.; Hirt, H.P.; Belser, U.C.; Lang, N.P. Long-term evaluation of non-submerged ITI implants. Part 1: 8-year life table analysis of a prospective multi-center study with 2359 implants. *Clin. Oral Implant. Res.* **1997**, *8*, 161–172. [CrossRef]
14. Hermann, J.S.; Cochran, D.L.; Nummikoski, P.V.; Buser, D. Crestal bone changes around titanium implants. A radiographic evaluation of unloaded nonsubmerged and submerged implants in the canine mandible. *J. Periodontol.* **1997**, *68*, 1117–1130. [CrossRef] [PubMed]
15. Hermann, J.S.; Schoolfield, J.D.; Schenk, R.K.; Buser, D.; Cochran, D.L. Influence of the size of the microgap on crestal bone changes around titanium implants. A histometric evaluation of unloaded non-submerged implants in the canine mandible. *J. Periodontol.* **2001**, *72*, 1372–1383. [CrossRef] [PubMed]
16. Welander, M.; Abrahamsson, I.; Berglundh, T. The mucosal barrier at implant abutments of different materials. *Clin. Oral Implant. Res.* **2008**, *19*, 635–641.
17. Qian, J.; Wennerberg, A.; Albrektsson, T. Reasons for marginal bone loss around oral implants. *Clin. Implant. Dent. Relat. Res.* **2012**, *14*, 792–807. [CrossRef]
18. Sanz-Sánchez, I.; Sanz-Martín, I.; Carrillo de Albornoz, A.; Figuero, E.; Sanz, M. Biological effect of the abutment material on the stability of peri-implant marginal bone levels: A systematic review and meta-analysis. *Clin. Oral Implant. Res.* **2018**, *29* (Suppl. 18), 124–144. [CrossRef]
19. Albrektsson, T.; Buser, D.; Sennerby, L. Crestal bone loss and oral implants. *Clin. Implant. Dent. Relat. Res.* **2012**, *14*, 783–791. [CrossRef]

20. Schwarz, F.; Hegewald, A.; Becker, J. Impact of implant-abutment connection and positioning of the machined collar/microgap on crestal bone level changes: A systematic review. *Clin. Oral Implant. Res.* **2014**, *225*, 417–425. [CrossRef]
21. Valles, C.; Rodríguez-Ciurana, X.; Clementini, M.; Baglivo, M.; Paniagua, B.; Nart, J. Influence of subcrestal implant placement compared with equicrestal position on the peri-implant hard and soft tissues around platform-switched implants: A systematic review and meta-analysis. *Clin. Oral Investig.* **2018**, *22*, 555–570. [CrossRef] [PubMed]
22. Khayat, P.G.; Hallage, P.G.; Toledo, R.A. An investigation of 131 consecutively placed wide screw-vent implants. *Int. J. Oral Maxillofac. Implant.* **2001**, *16*, 827–832.
23. Davarpanah, M.; Martinez, H.; Tecucianu, J.F. Apical-coronal implant position: Recent surgical proposals. Technical note. *Int. J. Oral Maxillofac. Implant.* **2000**, *15*, 865–872.
24. Flores-Guillen, J.; Álvarez-Novoa, C.; Barbieri, G.; Martín, C.; Sanz, M. Five-year outcomes of a randomized clinical trial comparing bone-level implants with either submerged or transmucosal healing. *J. Clin. Periodontol.* **2018**, *45*, 125–135. [CrossRef] [PubMed]
25. Messias, A.; Nicolau, P.; Guerra, F. Titanium dental implants with different collar design and surface modifications: A systematic review on survival rates and marginal bone levels. *Clin. Oral Implant. Res.* **2019**, *30*, 20–48. [CrossRef] [PubMed]
26. Cocchetto, R.; Canullo, L. The "hybrid abutment": A new design for implant cemented restorations in the esthetic zones. *Int. J. Esthet. Dent.* **2015**, *10*, 186–208. [PubMed]
27. Rodríguez-Ciurana, X.; Vela-Nebot, X.; Segalà-Torres, M.; Calvo-Guirado, J.L.; Cambra, J.; Méndez-Blanco, V.; Tarnow, D.P. The effect of interimplant distance on the height of the interimplant bone crest when using platform-switched implants. *Int. J. Periodontics Restor. Dent.* **2008**, *29*, 141–151.
28. Galindo-Moreno, P.; León-Cano, A.; Ortega-Oller, I.; Monje, A.; Suárez, F.; ÓValle, F.; Spinato, S.; Catena, A. Prosthetic Abutment Height is a Key Factor in Peri-implant Marginal Bone Loss. *J. Dent. Res.* **2014**, *93*, 80S–85S. [CrossRef]
29. De Bruyn, H.; Vandeweghe, S.; Ruyffelaert, C.; Cosyn, J.; Sennerby, L. Radiographic evaluation of modern oral implants with emphasis on crestal bone level and relevance to peri-implant health. *Periodontol 2000* **2000**, *62*, 256–270. [CrossRef]

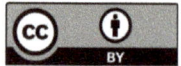

© 2019 by the authors. Licensee MDPI, Basel, Switzerland. This article is an open access article distributed under the terms and conditions of the Creative Commons Attribution (CC BY) license (http://creativecommons.org/licenses/by/4.0/).

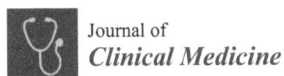

Article

Improvement of Quality of Life with Implant-Supported Mandibular Overdentures and the Effect of Implant Type and Surgical Procedure on Bone and Soft Tissue Stability: A Three-Year Prospective Split-Mouth Trial

Ron Doornewaard [1,*], Maarten Glibert [1], Carine Matthys [1], Stijn Vervaeke [1], Ewald Bronkhorst [2] and Hugo de Bruyn [1,2,*]

1. Department Periodontology & Oral Implantology, Dental School, Faculty Medicine and Health Sciences, Ghent University, De Pintelaan 185, 9000 Ghent, Belgium; maarten.glibert@ugent.be (M.G.); carine.matthys@ugent.be (C.M.); stijn.vervaeke@ugent.be (S.V.)
2. Section Implantology & Periodontology, Department of Dentistry, Radboudumc, Philips van Leydenlaan 25, 6525 EX Nijmegen, The Netherlands; ewald.bronkhorst@radboudumc.nl
* Correspondence: ron.doornewaard@ugent.be (R.D.); hugo.debruyn@radboudumc.nl (H.d.B.)

Received: 13 May 2019; Accepted: 28 May 2019; Published: 31 May 2019

Abstract: In fully edentulous patients, the support of a lower dental prosthesis by two implants could improve the chewing ability, retention, and stability of the prosthesis. Despite high success rates of dental implants, complications, such as peri-implantitis, do occur. The latter is a consequence of crestal bone loss and might be related to the implant surface and peri-implant soft tissue thickness. The aim of this paper is to describe the effect of implant surface roughness and soft tissue thickness on crestal bone remodeling, peri-implant health, and patient-centered outcomes. The mandibular overdenture supported by two implants is used as a split-mouth model to scrutinize these aims. The first study compared implants placed equicrestal to implants placed biologically (i.e., dependent on site-specific soft tissue thickness). The second clinical trial compared implants with a minimally to a moderately rough implant neck. Both studies reported an improvement in oral health-related quality of life and a stable peri-implant health after three years follow-up. Only equicrestal implant placement yielded significantly higher implant surface exposure, due to the establishment of the biologic width. Within the limitations of this study, it can be concluded that an implant supported mandibular overdenture significantly improves the quality of life, with limited biologic complications and high survival rates of the implants.

Keywords: bone loss; dental implant; overdenture; implant survival; peri-implantitis; implant surface; soft tissue; split-mouth design; oral health-related quality of life; patient-reported outcome measures

1. Introduction

Edentulousness is widely spread worldwide. According to the WHO the prevalence in the elderly population is 26% in the USA and between 15% and 78% in European countries. Among the edentulous population, a strong negative impact of poor oral conditions on daily life has been described. Edentulism could lead to diet changes where food rich in saturated fats and cholesterol are preferred. Besides diet changes, edentulousness is an independent risk factor for weight loss and could lead to social handicaps related to communication [1].

The support of a dental prosthesis by two implants could improve the chewing ability, retention, and stability of the prosthesis, which could lead to higher satisfaction and health-related quality of life.

Dental implants have been used since the early sixties to replace missing teeth by fixed or removable prostheses. Nowadays, this yields a predictable treatment outcome with success over 95% after 10 years of function [2].

To measure the improvement in health-related quality of life, the Oral Health Impact Profile (OHIP) is a widely used tool to assess currently applied dental procedures. It has also been used for evaluating the quality of life in more invasive surgical interventions in oral surgery [3]. The tool consists of a questionnaire to measure the impact of medical care on functional and social wellbeing [4]. Allen and McMillan reported significant improvement in satisfaction and health-related quality of life for patients who received implant-retained prostheses compared to those who received conventional dentures [5]. A panel of experts published a consensus statement where they described overwhelming evidence for a 2-implant supported overdenture as the first choice of treatment for the edentulous mandible instead of a conventional denture [6].

A recent review focusing on the Patient-Reported Outcome Measures (PROMs) showed compelling evidence to support that the fully edentulous patients experience higher satisfaction with an implant-supported overdenture in the mandible compared to a conventional denture [7]. These findings were confirmed by several other recent systematic reviews and meta-analyses [8–10].

De Bruyn and co-workers also concluded that patient satisfaction is highly individual and satisfaction with an implant-supported overdenture is never guaranteed. Hence, the decision to propose an implant-supported overdenture should be based on proper individual assessment [7].

Despite the improvement of the patient's quality of life and high survival and success rates of dental implants in patients with overdentures, dental implants are not free of complications. The most common complications following implant therapy are peri-implant mucositis (bleeding on probing and inflammation of the peri-implant soft tissues), and peri-implantitis (clinical and radiographic bone loss with or without suppuration). To detect inflammatory changes around the implant, several biologic parameters (plaque, bleeding, and suppuration) must be monitored during the patient's follow-up visits [11].

According to the latest consensus report of the "World Workshop on the Classification of Periodontal and Peri-implant Diseases and Conditions", the main clinical characteristic of peri-implant mucositis is bleeding on gently probing [12]. Erythema, swelling, and/or suppuration may also be present [13]. There is strong evidence from animal and human experimental studies that plaque is the etiological factor for peri-implant mucositis [11,14–18]. Peri-implantitis is described as a plaque-associated pathologic condition occurring in tissues around dental implants, characterized by inflammation in the peri-implant mucosa and subsequent progressive loss of supporting bone. Peri-implantitis sites exhibit clinical signs of inflammation, bleeding on probing, and/or suppuration, increased probing depths and/or recession of the mucosal margin in addition to radiographic bone loss [19]. Peri-implantitis is a consequence of crestal bone loss. Two recent consensus meetings highlighted the influence of implant material, shape and surface characteristics on the occurrence and progression of peri-implantitis. However, evidence for these suggestions is weak and future long-term studies are necessary to analyze these potential risk factors [20,21]. Beside these implant factors also other important factors like surgical, prosthetic, patient-related factors and foreign body reactions may contribute to crestal bone loss [21].

The composition and the topography of the implant surface have been a matter of debate during the last decades. Both composition and topography have their influence on implant surface roughness. The implant surface roughness is expressed in a Sa value. This three-dimensional value expresses an absolute difference in the height of each point compared to the arithmetical mean of the surface [22]. In the early years of implant dentistry two types of implant surfaces were used, the machined/turned surface (Sa = 0.5–1 µm) and the microporous titanium plasma-sprayed surface (Sa > 2 µm). The first one is smooth and the latter could be described as a rough implant surface. Surface modification was done to enlarge the surface, resulting in a greater bone-to-implant contact area. Implant surface modifications were done by sandblasting, acid-etching, anodic oxidation or hydroxyapatite coating.

These techniques resulted in a moderately rough implant surface (Sa = 1–2 µm), which is nowadays the most used surface roughness. Beside the higher bone-to-implant contact [23], a lower clinical failure rate [24] and a higher removal torque was observed compared to the smooth implant surfaces [25]. Hence, the surface modification made it possible to load the implant earlier or even immediately after the surgery. The resulting surface enlargement allowed shorter implants to be used, without jeopardizing the prognosis and with a reduced necessity for bone grafting procedures [2]. Beside the aforementioned benefits, related to faster integration, rough implant systems have been linked to increased bacterial adhesion [26]. The applied model in the latter study does not always mimic the clinical reality. However, A Cochrane systematic review suggested limited evidence that smooth surfaces had a 20% reduced risk of being affected by peri-implantitis over a three-year period [27,28]. This finding led to the commercial production of hybrid dental implants, combining the best of both systems. Hybrid dental implants have a minimally rough coronal part to decrease biofilm formation in the soft tissue crevice and a moderately rough implant body to enhance bone healing and speed up the osseointegration. These hybrid surfaces combine the effect of both surface roughnesses in the same implant. A short-term study indicated that the moderately rough and smooth coronal part showed the same crestal bone remodeling in the initial healing phase [29]. However, long-term studies to describe clinical parameters and peri-implant health are not yet available.

Some patient-related factors, such as certain metabolic syndrome components, medical conditions and/or the use of medication are known to have an effect on implant treatment outcome. Systematic reviews reveal that hyperglycemia has an increased risk for peri-implantitis [30,31], although the risk for more implant failures is comparable with the one observed in healthy patients. [32]. There is inconsistent and controversial evidence about the association with cardiovascular diseases [31]. Another meta-analysis revealed that there was no difference in implant survival rate between patients with and without osteoporosis. However, increased peri-implant bone loss was observed [33]. The intake of bisphosphonates, related to the treatment of osteoporosis, was not associated with an increased implant failure rate [34]. On the other hand, the same systematic review revealed an increased risk for implant failure with the intake of certain selective serotonin reuptake inhibitors and proton pump inhibitors [34]. Patients that are periodontally compromised are at higher risk for implant failure and crestal bone loss when compared with periodontally healthy subjects [35].

Another patient factor related to the failure of integrated implants is smoking. De Bruyn and Collaert described in a large retrospective study significantly higher failure rates of dental implants in smokers compared to non-smokers, both before and after functional loading, especially in the maxilla [36]. These findings are in agreement with a large meta-analysis of 18 studies showing an odds-ratio of 2.17 for implant failures in smokers were compared to non-smokers [37]. Besides implant failure smokers are more prone to peri-implant bone loss [38,39].

Also, biologic variances between patients could influence crestal bone loss around dental implants. Especially, soft tissue dimensions could play an important role in bone remodeling. The effect of peri-implant mucosal tissue thickness on the crestal bone loss was described in an animal study suggesting a certain minimal width of peri-implant mucosa may be required, and that bone resorption may take place allowing a stable soft tissue attachment [40]. The latter was confirmed in a human clinical trial, when there was a soft tissue thickness of 2 mm or less, crestal bone loss up to 1.45 mm may occur [41].

More recently Vervaeke and co-workers concluded that the initial bone remodeling was affected by the thickness of the peri-implant soft tissue [42]. They suggested that bone loss directly after implant placement, due to crestal bone remodeling, precludes the biologic width re-establishment and can be controlled by adapting the vertical depth position of the implant in the bone in relation to the soft tissue thickness at the time of implant placement. Hence, in thin tissues, a deeper subcrestal position in the bone may prevent partial exposure of the crestal part of the implant. Although crestal bone remodeling is a given fact after implant placement, related to the surgical trauma from periosteal elevation, as well as the drilling procedure, it is from a preventive point of view important to have the bone covering the implant as much as possible. Initial crestal bone loss, resulting in the absence of bone contact, can predict a future bone loss in patients prior to the disease. Galindo-Moreno and co-workers concluded that 96% of implants with a marginal bone loss above 2 mm at 18 months had lost 0.44 mm or more at six months post loading [43]. A critical long-term study where implants were placed in the partially edentulous mandible, indicated that bone loss in patients with thin (<2 mm) and a thick mucosa (>2 mm) was identical, when the implants were installed subcrestally to anticipate on the biologic width re-establishment [44].

Another subject of debate is the predictive value of biologic parameters around dental implants. Bleeding on probing, suppuration, plaque formation and probing pocket depth are the most widely used clinical parameters to describe health and/or disease around dental implants. These biologic parameters are most of the times included in the definition of peri-implantitis. However, a largely critical review showed the absence of a correlation between bone loss and the biologic parameters mean probing pocket depth and mean bleeding on probing. The authors also reported inconsistency and incompleteness in reporting on these parameters in the literature, which could affect decision-making in clinical practice [45].

Hence, the aim of this paper is to describe, by means of two prospective clinical split-mouth cohort studies, the effect of implant surface roughness and surgical implant depth positioning on crestal bone remodeling, peri-implant health, and patient-centered outcomes. The mandibular overdenture supported by two dental implants is used as a split-mouth model to scrutinize these aims.

2. Experimental Section

2.1. Patient Population and Surgical/Prosthetic Procedures

This paper includes two prospective split-mouth studies. Both studies included edentulous patients in need of a two-implant supported overdenture in the lower jaw. The same inclusion and exclusion were used for both studies. Inclusion criteria include: (1) Total complete edentulism for at least four months and (2) presence of sufficient residual bone volume to install two implants of 3.5 to 4.0 mm diameter and 8 to 11 mm length. Patients were excluded if they were: (1) Younger than 21, (2) suffered from systemic diseases, (3) current smokers and (4) had general contraindications for oral surgery (full dose head and neck radiation, intravenous administrated bisphosphonates, and ongoing chemotherapy). All patients were treated at the Ghent University Hospital by the same surgeon between January 2013 and September 2014. Twenty-six patients (study 1) received two moderately rough dental implants (Astra Tech Osseospeed TX™, Dentsply implants, York, PA, USA). The control implant was installed equicrestally (group 1), according to the manufacturer's guidelines with the rough implant surface completely surrounded by bone. The vertical position of the test implant (group 2) was adapted to the soft tissue thickness, allowing at least 3 mm space for biologic width establishment [42].

Another 23 patients (study 2) received two dental implants with a difference in implant surface roughness of the coronal part of the implant (Figure 1). All 46 implants were biologically guided taking the soft tissue thickness into account whereby care was taken to ensure a 3 mm soft tissue seal in contact with the abutment. All patients received one moderately rough implant (group 3) (Sa = 1.3 µm) (DCC, Southern implants, Irene, South Africa) and one test implant (group 4). The latter was a hybrid dental implant with a minimally rough coronal neck of 3 mm (Sa = 0.9 µm) combined with a moderately rough body (Sa = 1.3 µm) (MSC, Southern implants, Irene, South Africa).

Although two different brands were used in both studies, all 98 implants installed in the 49 patients were identical at the level of the abutment-implant connection. Implants had the same integrated platform-shift with a smooth implant bevel, the same internal deep conical connection and a similar macro design of the micro-threads on the implant neck.

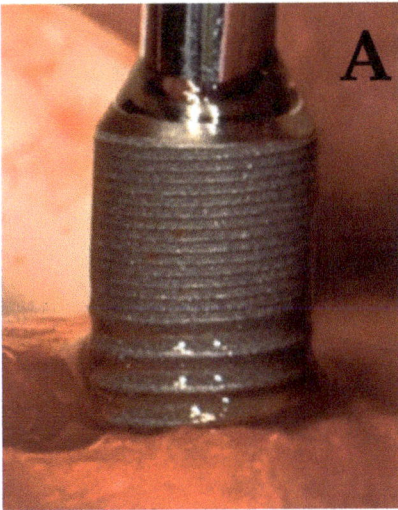 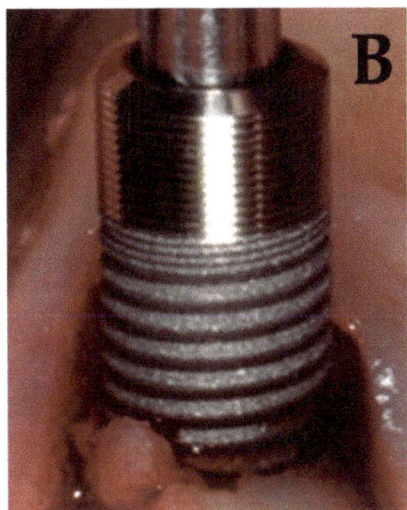

Figure 1. Placement of an implant with a moderately rough surface (**A**) and a hybrid implant with a minimally rough coronal neck (**B**).

Implants were immediately restored if primary stability was achieved (insertion-torque > 25 Ncm). Implants were restored either with locator abutments (study 1) or definitive titanium abutments (Compact Conical Abutments; Southern Implants, Irene, South Africa) and a healing cap with a standard abutment height of 4 mm (study 2).

Before surgery, all patients received new removable dentures in the mandible and maxilla to achieve a correct occlusion, appropriate teeth position, and appropriate smile line. The removable dentures were adapted after surgery to connect with the implants by one experienced prosthodontist. The surgical and prosthetic procedures have been described previously by Vervaeke and co-workers [46] and Glibert and co-workers [29].

The clinical trial has been conducted in full accordance with the Helsinki Decleration (1975) as revised in 2000. All patients were thoroughly informed and signed written informed consent. The study protocol was approved by the ethical committee of the Ghent University Hospital.

2.2. Clinical and Radiographic Examination

Follow-up visits were planned at 1 week, 1, 3, 6, 12, 24, and 36 months after surgery. After soft tissue healing was fully established, three months after surgery, peri-implant health was monitored and probing pocket depths, bleeding on probing and plaque scores were assessed on four implants sites: Midmesial, middistal, midbuccal, and midlingual. The bleeding- and plaque scores were measured on a dichotomous scale (0 = absence of bleeding on probing/absence of plaque; 1 = bleeding on probing/plaque). From the site level scores both for bleeding and plaque mean scores on implant level were calculated.

Digital peri-apical radiographs were taken at baseline (implant placement), at 3, 6, 12, 24, and 36 months using a guiding system in order to obtain the X-rays perpendicular to the film. The radiographic measurements were calibrated using the length of the implant, the distance between the threads or the diameter of the implant. Bone levels were determined as the distance from a reference point, which corresponds with the lower edge of the smooth implant bevel at the implant-abutment interface, to the most crestal bone-to-implant contact point. The baseline bone-to-implant contact levels are assessed from the implant-abutment interface. The baseline from the four experimental groups was logically comparable. Bone loss was determined by the difference of the bone level directly after implant placement and the bone level at the follow-up visit.

If necessary, calculus and plaque were removed and oral hygiene was reinforced during follow-up visits. Instructions with a (electric) toothbrush and interdental brushes were given based on the need, preferences and dexterity or motoric skills of the patient.

To measure the change in oral health-related quality of life the Oral Health Impact Profile-14 questionnaire (OHIP-14) is assessed before surgery, 3, and 12 months after connection of the prosthesis with the implants (Table 1). The questionnaire is based on 14 questions capturing seven domains: Functional limitation, physical pain, psychological discomfort, physical disability, psychological disability, social disability, and handicap. Of these seven domains, two questions need to be answered on a Likert scale. Score 4 is indicating a highly negative answer to the question and 0 means that there is no discomfort at all. The total score of the 14 questions can balance between 56 (maximally negative) to 0 (maximally positive).

Table 1. OHIP-14 questionnaire divided per domain.

Domain 1: Functional Limitation	
1	Have you had trouble pronouncing any words because of problems with your teeth, mouth, or denture?
2	Have you felt that your sense of taste has worsened because of problems with your teeth, mouth, or denture?
Domain 2: Physical Pain	
3	Have you had painful aching in your mouth?
4	Have you found it uncomfortable to eat any foods because of problems with your teeth, mouth, or denture?
Domain 3: Psychological Discomfort	
5	Have you been self-conscious because of your teeth, mouth, or denture?
6	Have you felt tense because of problems with your teeth, mouth, or denture?
Domain 4: Physical Disability	
7	Has been your diet been unsatisfactory because of problems with your teeth, mouth, or denture?
8	Have you interrupt meals because of problems with your teeth, mouth, or denture?
Domain 5: Psychological Disability	
9	Have you found it difficult to relax because of problems with your teeth, mouth or denture?
10	Have you been a bit embarrassed because of problems with your teeth, mouth, or denture?
Domain 6: Social Disability	
11	Have you been a bit irritable with other people because of problems with your teeth, mouth, or denture?
12	Have you had difficulty doing your usual jobs because of problems with your teeth, mouth, or denture?
Domain 7: Handicap	
13	Have you felt that life, in general, was less satisfying because of problems with your teeth, mouth, or denture?
14	Have you been totally unable to function because of problems with your teeth, mouth, or denture?

2.3. Statistics

Outcomes are reported with descriptive statistics (mean, SD, median, range, and 95% CI) and boxplots. All analyses concern pair-wise comparisons within patients. For continuous variables paired *t*-tests were applied, for dichotomous variables the McNemar test was used. The 95% confidence intervals are given to show the precision of an estimate of a certain effect.

The sample size for both studies was calculated using SAS Power and Sample size calculator for related samples based on an effect size of 1 mm and a standard deviation of 0.60, with the level of significance set at 0.05 and $\beta = 0.80$. The effect estimation was based on findings Vervaeke et al., 2014 [42].

For the OHIP-14 outcome, the impact of the change was assessed by calculating the "effect size" with the following formula:

((mean-OHIP before surgery) − (mean-OHIP three months after connection))/SD before surgery

As proposed by Cohen 1977 an "effect size" of 0.2 could be interpreted as a small change, 0.6 as a moderate change and > 0.8 as a large change.

3. Results

3.1. Study Population

A sample size of 14 patients for each study was calculated. Hence, minimums of 20 patients (= 40 implants) were consequently included to anticipate future dropouts.

Twenty-six patients in study I were initially treated with one equicrestally (group 1) and one subcrestally (group 2) placed implant. In study II, 23 patients were initially treated with one implant with a moderately rough implant neck (group 3) and one implant with a minimally rough implant neck (group 4). In total four experimental treatment groups were assessed. After a follow-up of at least three years, one patient was excluded, due to anatomical constraints requiring deviation of the surgical protocol. Two patients were excluded after starting smoking and one did not respond to the follow-up invitation. Hence, 45 patients with two implants each were available after a follow-up of three years and none of the implants had failed (survival 100%). A flowchart of the patients' distribution is shown in Figure 2. The study population consisted of 24 men and 21 women with a mean age at implant placement of 64 years (SD = 9.25, range = 43–85).

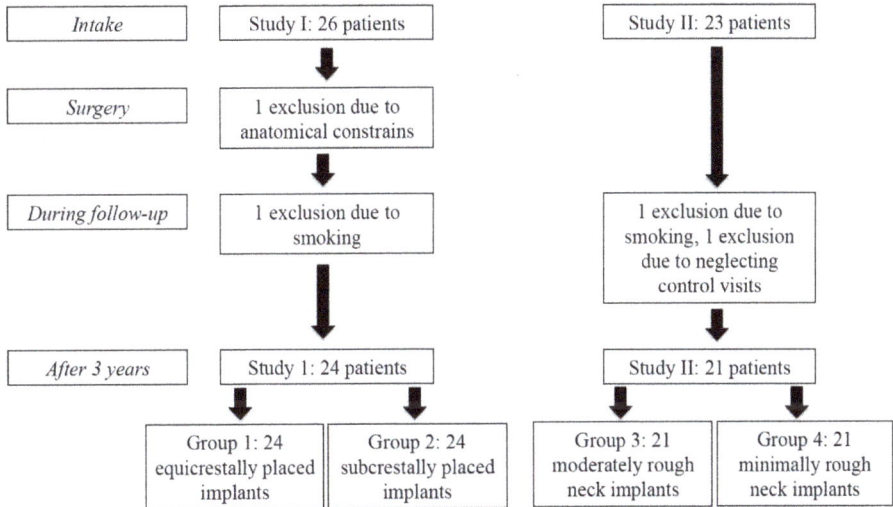

Figure 2. Flowchart of both study populations.

3.2. Mean Bone Level Difference

Table 2 shows the mean bone level and the corresponding changes of the four treatment groups at baseline and after 6, 12, 24, and 36 months. Initially, the bone level of the implants in the four groups is comparable and basically located at the implant crest. In the first six months bone remodeling was 0.7 mm for equicrestally placed implants and ranging from 0–0.3 mm in the other three subcrestally placed groups. Over time no further statistically significant bone level changes occurred in all groups (Figures 3–6). Figures 5 and 6 gives a schematic view of the bone remodeling over time, with the visible implant surface exposure in the equicrestally placed implant group (group 1).

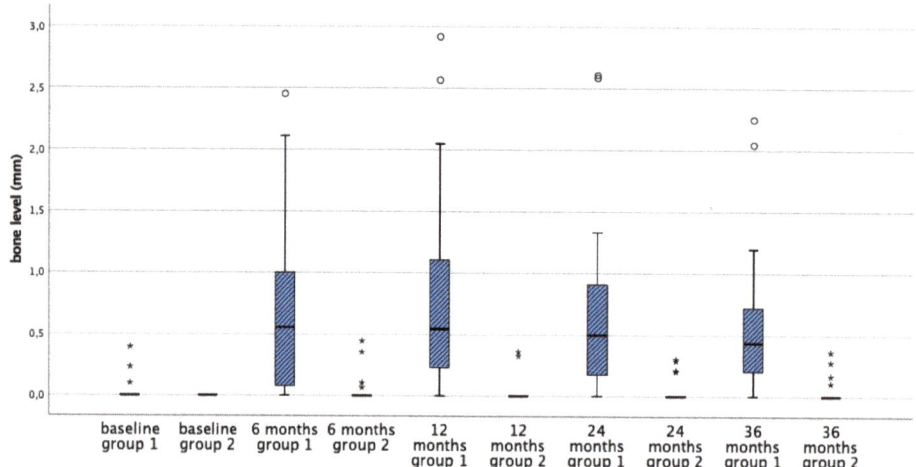

Figure 3. Boxplots representing the bone level at subsequent time points for the equicrestally (group 1) and subcrestally placed implants (group 2). * Outliers (≥3 × IQR above third quartile), ° suspected outliers (between 1.5 × IQR and 3 × IQR above third quartile).

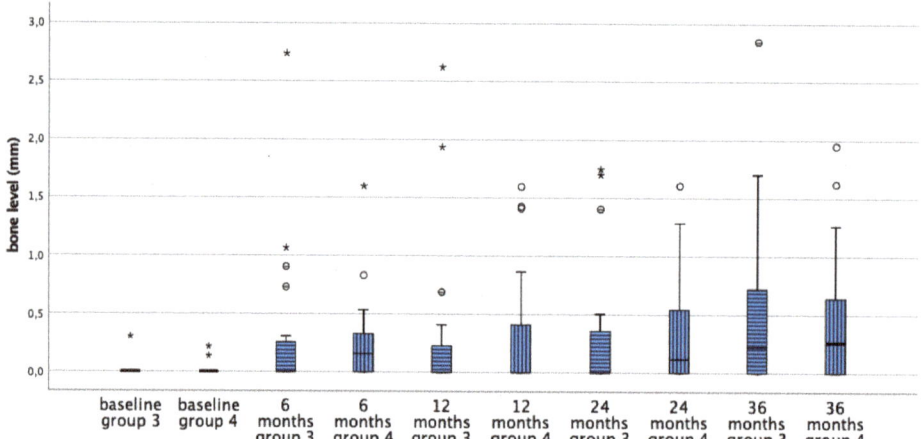

Figure 4. Boxplots representing the bone level at subsequent time points for the implants with a moderately rough neck (group 3) and minimally rough neck (group 4). * Outliers (≥3 × IQR above third quartile), ° suspected outliers (between 1.5 × IQR and 3 × IQR above third quartile).

Between groups the subcrestally placed implants of group 2 lost no bone at all. Groups 3 and 4 showed comparable bone remodeling. Hence, implant surface roughness did not affect initial nor long-term bone remodeling (Figures 4 and 6).

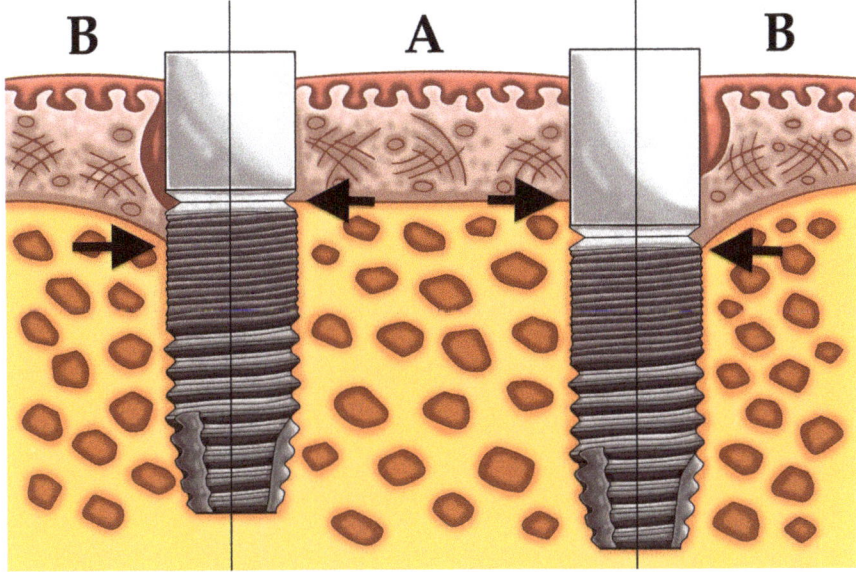

Figure 5. Schematic illustration of study 1, left equicrestally placed implant (group 1) and right subcrestally placed implant (group 2); showing the bone level at baseline (A) and bone level after bone remodeling (B).

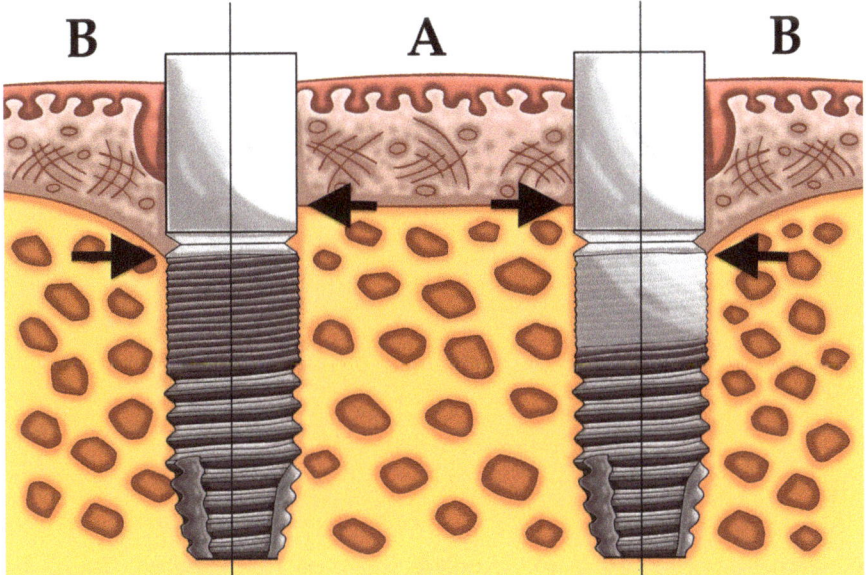

Figure 6. Schematic illustration of study 2, left implant with a moderately rough neck (group 3) and right implant with a minimally rough neck (group 4); showing the bone level at baseline (A) and bone level after bone remodeling (B).

Table 2. Mean bone level for each study group and the bone level difference between respectively equicrestally versus subcrestally placed implants and implants with moderately rough versus minimally rough neck; $p < 0.05$ indicates a statistically significant difference (paired t-test).

	Bone Level										
	Group 1: Equicrestal				Group 2: Subcrestal				Paired Difference		
	Mean (SD)	Median	Min	Max	Mean (SD)	Median	Min	Max	Mean dif	95% CI	p
Baseline	0.03 (0.09)	0.00	0.00	0.40	0.00 (0.00)	0.00	0.00	0.00	0.030	(−0.009,0.070)	0.123
6 months	0.72 (0.74)	0.59	0.00	2.45	0.04 (0.11)	0.00	0.00	0.45	0.678	(0.360,0.996)	<0.001
12 months	0.78 (0.81)	0.54	0.00	2.92	0.03 (0.10)	0.00	0.00	0.36	0.746	(0.397,1.096)	<0.001
24 months	0.69 (0.70)	0.51	0.00	2.61	0.04 (0.10)	0.00	0.00	0.30	0.644	(0.337,0.951)	<0.001
36 months	0.59 (0.59)	0.44	0.00	2.25	0.04 (0.10)	0.00	0.00	0.36	0.549	(0.297,0.802)	<0.001
	Group 3: Moderately Rough Neck				Group 4: Minimally Rough Neck				Paired Difference		
	Mean (SD)	Median	Min	Max	Mean (SD)	Median	Min	Max	Mean dif	95% CI	p
Baseline	0.01 (0.07)	0.00	0.00	0.30	0.02 (0.05)	0.00	0.00	0.22	−0.002	(−0.424,0.037)	0.902
6 months	0.33 (0.64)	0.00	0.00	2.74	0.27 (0.38)	0.18	0.00	1.60	0.064	(−0.118,0.245)	0.474
12 months	0.34 (0.68)	0.00	0.00	2.62	0.34 (0.53)	0.00	0.00	1.61	0.009	(−0.191,0.209)	0.926
24 months	0.36 (0.58)	0.00	0.00	1.75	0.37 (0.49)	0.23	0.00	1.60	−0.014	(−0.170,0.142)	0.853
36 months	0.51 (0.74)	0.22	0.00	2.84	0.45 (0.58)	0.26	0.00	1.95	0.066	(−0.114,0.246)	0.453

3.3. Biologic Parameters

On implant level only a statistically significant difference could be measured for the plaque score at 24 months ($p = 0.042$), with significantly less plaque for the equicrestally placed compared with subcrestally placed implants. However, at all other time points the plaque–and bleeding scores were not statistically significantly different, indicative of peri-implant health (Table 3).

Table 3. Mean plaque and bleeding on probing on implant level at 6, 12, 24 and 36 month for each study group and mean difference between respectively equicrestally versus subcrestally placed implants and implants with moderately rough versus minimally rough neck; $p < 0.05$ indicates a statistically significant difference (paired t-test).

	Plaque				
	Group 1: Equicrestal	Group 2: Subcrestal	Paired Difference		
	Mean (SD)	Mean (SD)	Mean dif	95% CI	p
6 months	0.44 (0.47)	0.52 (0.45)	−0.083	(−0.221,0.055)	0.224
12 months	0.45 (0.39)	0.56 (0.44)	−0.115	(−0.285,0.056)	0.178
24 months	0.42 (0.40)	0.51 (0.40)	−0.091	(−0.178,−0.003)	0.042
36 months	0.39 (0.43)	0.41 (0.42)	−0.022	(−0.148,0.104)	0.724
	Group 3: Moderately Rough Neck	Group 4: Minimally Rough Neck	Paired Difference		
	Mean (SD)	Mean (SD)	Mean dif	95% CI	p
6 months	0.38 (0.33)	0.40 (0.31)	−0.025	(−0.144,0.094)	0.666
12 months	0.37 (0.31)	0.35 (0.31)	0.017	(−0.136,0.169)	0.818
24 months	0.57 (0.36)	0.52 (0.36)	0.054	(−0.030,0.137)	0.189
36 months	0.39 (0.41)	0.43 (0.38)	−0.038	(−0.147,0.072)	0.481
	Bleeding on Probing				
	Group 1: Equicrestal	Group 2: Subcrestal	Paired Difference		
	Mean (SD)	Mean (SD)	Mean dif	95% CI	p
6 months	0.15 (0.22)	0.15 (0.22)	0.000	(−0.093,0.0933)	1.000
12 months	0.19 (0.18)	0.19 (0.18)	0.000	(−0.125,0.125)	1.000
24 months	0.23 (0.30)	0.20 (0.28)	0.023	(−0.090,0.136)	0.680
36 months	0.30 (0.33)	0.23 (0.25)	0.076	(−0.048,0.200)	0.216
	Group 3: Moderately Rough Neck	Group 4: Minimally Rough Neck	Paired Difference		
	Mean (SD)	Mean (SD)	Mean dif	95% CI	p
6 months	0.24 (0.31)	0.23 (0.24)	0.013	(−0.110,0.135)	0.834
12 months	0.20 (0.32)	0.23 (0.24)	−0.033	(−0.189,0.122)	0.653
24 months	0.25 (0.29)	0.30 (0.37)	−0.054	(−0.243,0.136)	0.551
36 months	0.08 (0.14)	0.07 (0.12)	0.013	(−0.084,0.109)	0.789

For the probing pocket depth at implant level only at 24 months a statistically significant difference between equicrestally placed compared to subcrestally placed implants could be observed (Table 4). After three years all groups are comparable indicative of peri-implant health.

Table 4. Mean probing pocket depth on implant level at 6, 12, 24 and 36 months for each study group and the mean difference between respectively equicrestally versus subcrestally placed implants and implants with a moderately rough versus minimally rough neck; $p < 0.05$ indicates a statistically significant difference (paired t-test).

	Probing Pocket Depth								
	Group 1: Equicrestal			Group 2: Subcrestal			Paired Difference		
	Mean (SD)	Min	Max	Mean (SD)	Min	Max	Mean dif	95% CI	p
6 months	1.88 (0.53)	1.00	3.25	2.01 (0.66)	1.00	3.75	−0.135	(−0.311,0.041)	0.125
12 months	1.70 (0.44)	1.00	2.50	1.83 (0.53)	1.00	2.75	−0.130	(−0.312,0.051)	0.149
24 months	2.30 (0.66)	1.50	4.50	2.57 (0.84)	1.25	4.50	−0.261	(−0.473,−0.048)	0.018
36 months	2.42 (0.69)	1.00	4.00	2.59 (0.71)	1.00	3.75	−0.163	(−0.0378,0.052)	0.130
	Group 3: Moderately Rough Neck			Group 4: Minimally Rough Neck			Paired Difference		
	Mean (SD)	Min	Max	Mean (SD)	Min	Max	Mean dif	95% CI	p
6 months	2.93 (0.71)	1.75	5.25	2.88 (0.65)	1.75	4.75	0.050	(−0.142,0.242)	0.592
12 months	2.65 (0.72)	1.75	4.75	2.68 (0.68)	1.75	4.50	−0.033	(−0.221,0.154)	0.709
24 months	2.48 (0.58)	1.25	3.50	2.34 (0.60)	1.00	3,25	0.143	(−0.114,0.401)	0.252
36 months	2.10 (0.68)	1.25	4.25	2.01 (0.58)	1.00	3.00	0.088	(−0.259,0.434)	0.603

3.4. Oral Health-Related Quality of Life

Based on 45 edentulous patients, receiving an implant-supported overdenture, the OHIP-14 index reduced from 13.37/56 (SD 9.97) at baseline to 4.42/56 (SD 4.94) after three months of functional loading. This result in a large effect size of 0.90, suggesting a strong improvement in oral health related quality of life. Between 3 and 12 months, no further changes were observed, resulting in small effect size (0.04), indicative of a very stable result over time (Figure 7). The reduction was statistically significant for all seven domains after three months (Table 5). For functional limitation, physical disability and handicap the effect size was moderate. For the other four domains, a large effect size was observed and most expressed for physical pain with an effect size of 1.04. The latter is logically given the fact that improved denture retention results in less mucosal irritation and consequently fewer complaints related to pain suffering.

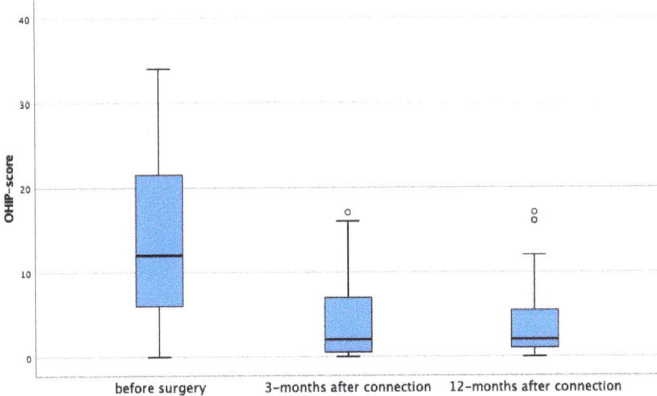

Figure 7. Boxplots representing the Oral Health Impact Profile-14 (OHIP-14) total score before surgery, 3 and 12 months after connection of the prosthesis with the implants. A score of 56 represents a maximal negative appreciation. ° Suspected outliers (between 1.5 × IQR and 3 × IQR above third quartile).

Table 5. Mean OHIP score and the mean difference for each of the seven domains before surgery and three months after connection with the calculated effect-size.

Domain	Mean-OHIP (SD)		Paired Difference			Effect-Size
	Before Surgery	Three Months after Connection	Mean Dif	95% CI	p	
functional limitation	2.30 (1.85)	1.14 (1.42)	1.16	(0.540,1.785)	0.001	0.63
physical pain	3.37 (2.06)	1.21 (1.55)	2.16	(1.440,2.886)	<0.001	1.04
psychological discomfort	2.52 (2.35)	0.65 (1.43)	1.87	(1.034,2.687)	<0.001	0.80
physical disability	2.12 (2.16)	0.44 (0.85)	1.68	(0.971,2.378)	<0.001	0.78
psychological disability	2.21 (1.91)	0.58 (0.93)	1.63	(0.930,2.326)	<0.001	0.85
social disability	1.67 (1.49)	0.16 (0.49)	1.51	(1.007,2.016)	<0.001	1.01
handicap	1.42 (1.48)	0.26 (0.66)	1.16	(0.683,1.642)	<0.001	0.78

4. Discussion

The current paper focuses on implant treatment outcome in patients, which were completely edentulous in both jaws. Retention of the lower denture is a typical problem in this category of patients, especially in the mandible as compared to the maxillary denture. The denture in the mandible is less retentive because of a smaller crestal bone support, a more expressed degree of bone resorption, and unfavorable distribution of occluding forces, as well as additional pressure of the tongue yielding dislocating forces. Often this results in functional discomfort and pain, the latter because of the absence of keratinized mucosa. In the maxilla, the denture is supported on the crest and on the hard structure of the palate, which is covered by keratinized tissue. A vacuum present during mastication, between the palatal coverage of the denture and the underlying tissues, improves the retention. Consequently, fully edentulous patients have more complaints with mandibular dentures and an overdenture retained on two implants has therefore been suggested as of minimal care in order to provide functional comfort [6]. Implant treatment in denture wearing patients can be used for split mouth studies as was the case in the two clinical studies presented in the present paper. The focus was on implant type and surgical procedure, defined as implant survival, crestal bone loss and biologic peri-implant health. The latter is an important aspect because peri-implant diseases may jeopardize treatment outcome in the long run and are often related to aesthetic appreciation. Additionally, the patient-centered outcome was assessed by using a validated Oral Health Related Quality of Life questionnaire.

After three years of follow-up, no implant failures could be recorded in the present study and all remaining patients remained fully functional. This 100% implant survival is in line with current literature on implant overdenture therapy [47].

Initial bone remodeling is a healing phenomenon related to the surgical procedure mainly the exposure of bone and periosteum during implant placement, as well as the depth placement in the bone. Given the fact that implant survival with currently available dental implant systems is successful and quite predictable, the research focuses on implant success. Implant treatment is considered a success when high implant survival is combined with bone stability over time, because the latter reflects the health of the peri-implant tissues. Indeed, worldwide consensus defined that peri implantitis, a disease condition of the implant resulting in pocket formation between the implant and soft tissue, is always preceded by the bone loss [12]. Additionally, soft tissue health also affects the aesthetic outcome, especially in the partially edentulous patient. Although aesthetics was not the key issue in the present paper, the study conditions tested may provide clinical guidelines that do affect aesthetics, as well as peri-implant health outcomes.

In the present paper, minimal initial bone remodeling ranging from 0–0.7 mm was assessed. After the physiological initial bone remodeling, no further bone loss could be observed up to three years of function. The effect of soft tissue thickness and implant surface roughness on the crestal bone loss was evaluated. The applied split-mouth study design corrects for inter-individual variability from the estimates of the treatment effect [48]. The results showed that the initial bone remodeling was affected by the originally present soft tissue thickness, but not by the implant surface roughness. After implant installation, a minimum of 3 mm soft tissue dimensions seems to be necessary for the re-establishment of the so-called "biologic width", indicative of the importance of the biologically guided implant placement. These findings are in accordance with an earlier published systematic review, including meta-analysis. There it is stated that implants placed with an initially thicker peri-implant soft tissue have less radiographic marginal bone loss in the short term [49]. Additionally, an increased early bone remodeling leads to implant surface exposure in patients with thin soft tissues, which increases the risk of on-going bone loss as shown by Vervaeke and colleagues in a nine year follow-up. A greater implant surface exposure increases the bacterial colonization of the implant surface, which could enlarge the chance to induce peri-implantitis [50]. From a clinical point of view, it is highly suggested that the surgeon adapts the surgical position of the implant in relation to the available pre-operative soft-tissue thickness.

It is generally accepted that osseointegration of moderately rough implants is enhanced as compared to minimally rough implants. This resulted in faster treatment protocols and reduced early failures. More recently, it was suggested that a minimally rough implant surface yields less crestal bone loss and less peri-implantitis on the long-term. A recent systematic review, including studies up to 10 years, reported on the survival rate and marginal bone loss of implants with different surface roughness. Implant survival was higher for moderately rough surfaces, but minimally rough surfaces showed the least marginal bone loss [51]. This outcome is in contrast to the outcome presented in another systematic review with meta-analysis. The latter evaluated the influence of the implant collar surface on marginal bone loss and revealed less bone loss for the rougher implant systems. However, 10 out of the 12 included studies showed results with less than five years of function. The only study with 10 years of follow-up showed less bone loss for the implants with a smooth collar compared to the implants with a rough collar. Yet, the authors stated that the results of their systematic review needed to be interpreted cautiously, due to several confounding factors [52]. Another systematic review with meta-analysis, which included only studies with at least, a five-year follow-up showed significantly less bone loss around smooth implant surfaces compared to moderately rough and rough implant surfaces [38]. Recently Donati and co-workers published the results of a 20-year follow-up RCT to evaluate the effect of a modified implant surface. In 51 patients at least one implant with a minimally rough surface and one with a modified surface was installed. The difference in mean bone level change between the two implant-systems was not statistically significant, and the moderate increase of implant surface roughness has no beneficial effect on long-term preservation of the peri-implant marginal bone level. A more detailed analysis of the paper revealed, however, that none of the 32 evaluated smooth implants showed more than 3 mm bone loss, whereas 3 out of the 32 modified implants showed bone loss between 3 and 6 mm. Only two smooth surface implants were diagnosed with peri-implantitis compared with five implants with a modified surface [53].

The findings of our paper are in accordance with the paper of Donati and co-workers, concluding that the surface roughness of the implant neck has no effect on bone level up to three years. The hybrid implant system used in our study combines the benefits of faster osseointegration, due to the moderately rough implant body, and the minimally rough surface around the implant neck suggests it is less prone to develop peri-implantitis [54]. Additionally, several studies conclude the beneficial effect of a smoother surface with a lower incidence of peri-implantitis and less bone loss on the long term. A further long-term follow-up of the current study population will elucidate the latter.

Besides implant survival and bone level stability, also peri-implant health is considered a perquisite for treatment success. Peri-implant health is defined on two levels. Plaque accumulation yields minor inflammation of the soft tissue surrounding the implant- restorative interface, coined as mucositis. It is diagnosed with bleeding of the tissues after probing the crevice between implant and mucosa. In a recent consensus report, the diagnosis of peri-implantitis has been redefined as a combination of probing pocket depths of at least 6 mm in combination with bleeding on probing or a bone level of at least 3 mm apical of the most coronal portion of the intraosseous part of the implant [12]. In our study, no patients showed ongoing bone-loss in combination with bleeding and increasing probing pocket depths. Hence, the incidence of peri-implantitis was 0.0%.

The absence of peri-implantitis was found despite a high plaque level. This could be explained by the elderly, fully edentulous patient population. De Waal and colleagues revealed that edentulous patients restored with implants showed more plaque compared to partially edentulous patients restored with implants. However, the plaque in the fully edentulous patients harbours a potentially less pathogenic peri-implant micro-flora [55,56].

Another explanation for the relatively high plaque scores could be the dexterity problems inducing imperfect cleaning abilities in elderly patients. On the other hand, plaque is screened at a given moment in time during the clinical inspection and this may be several hours after cleaning and not necessarily reflects the overall hygiene of the patient over time.

This is the reason why the bleeding index is considered more useful. It reflects the degree of inflammation as a result of the long-term plaque control and is less momentarily. The current study revealed that high plaque score did not result in high bleeding scores.

The support of a mandibular overdenture by two implants has a significant positive effect on the quality of life. The OHIP-14 score was calculated irrespective of the implant group because it is a patient-related outcome variable. On all the seven domains measured with the OHIP-14 questionnaire a statistically significant difference was measured, all in favor of the support of a mandible overdenture by two implants. These findings are in accordance with a clinical trial reporting a significant improvement in satisfaction and health-related quality of life when subjects who received two implants are compared with subjects requesting a new conventional denture. Besides the improvement in the quality of life, they reported that patients requesting implants reported that tooth loss and denture wearing problems had a much greater impact in their quality of life than patients seeking conventional dentures [5].

5. Conclusions

Within the limitations of this study, it can be concluded that an implant supported mandibular overdenture significantly improves the quality of life, with limited biologic complications and a high survival rate of the implants. All seven domains of the OHIP-14 questionnaire significantly reduced when the mandible overdenture is supported by two implants. No differences were observed in crestal bone remodeling between minimally rough and moderately rough implant surfaces. However, initial bone remodeling was affected by initial soft tissue thickness. Anticipating biologic width re-establishment by adapting the vertical position of the implant in relation to the available soft tissue thickness may avoid peri-implant bone loss. The biologic variance of the patient might be more important compared to the configuration of the implant surface. Long-term follow-up of the study is necessary to determine the influence of early implant surface exposure and implant surface roughness on crestal bone loss, biologic parameters, mechanical complication, and implant survival.

Author Contributions: Conceptualization, R.D. and H.d.B.; methodology, R.D. and E.B.; software, R.D. and E.B.; validation, R.D., H.d.B. and E.B.; formal analysis, R.D., H.d.B. and E.B.; investigation, R.D., M.G., S.V. and C.M.; resources, R.D., H.d.B.; data curation, E.B.; writing—original draft preparation, R.D.; writing—review and editing, H.d.B., M.G. and S.V.; visualization, R.D.; supervision, H.d.B.; project administration, R.D.

Acknowledgments: Special thanks to Mario de Timmerman for the illustrations.

Conflicts of Interest: The authors declare no conflict of interest.

References

1. Petersen, P.E.; Yamamoto, T. Improving the oral health of older people: the approach of the WHO Global Oral Health Programme. *Community Dent. Oral Epidemiol.* **2005**, *33*, 81–92. [CrossRef] [PubMed]
2. Buser, D.; Sennerby, L.; De Bruyn, H. Modern implant dentistry based on osseointegration: 50 years of progress, current trends and open questions. *Periodontology 2000* **2017**, *73*, 7–21. [CrossRef] [PubMed]

3. Pelo, S.; Saponaro, G.; Patini, R.; Staderini, E.; Giordano, A.; Gasparini, G.; Garagiola, U.; Azzuni, C.; Cordaro, M.; Foresta, E.; et al. Risks in surgery-first orthognathic approach: complications of segmental osteotomies of the jaws. A systematic review. *Eur. Rev. Med. Pharmacol. Sci.* **2017**, *21*, 4–12.
4. Slade, G.D.; Spencer, A.J. Development and evaluation of the Oral Health Impact Profile. *Community Dent. Health* **1994**, *11*, 3–11.
5. Allen, P.F.; McMillan, A.S. A longitudinal study of quality of life outcomes in older adults requesting implant prostheses and complete removable dentures. *Clin. Oral Implant. Res.* **2003**, *14*, 173–179. [CrossRef]
6. Feine, J.S.; Carlsson, G.E.; Awad, M.A.; Chehade, A.; Duncan, W.J.; Gizani, S.; Head, T.; Lund, J.P.; MacEntee, M.; Mericske-Stern, R.; et al. The McGill consensus statement on overdentures. Mandibular two-implant overdentures as first choice standard of care for edentulous patients. Montreal, Quebec, 24–25 May, 2002. *Int. J. Oral Maxillofac. Implant.* **2002**, *17*, 601–602.
7. De Bruyn, H.; Raes, S.; Matthys, C.; Cosyn, J. The current use of patient-centered/reported outcomes in implant dentistry: a systematic review. *Clin. Oral Implant. Res.* **2015**, *26* (Suppl. 11), 45–56. [CrossRef]
8. Zhang, L.; Lyu, C.; Shang, Z.; Niu, A.; Liang, X. Quality of Life of Implant-Supported Overdenture and Conventional Complete Denture in Restoring the Edentulous Mandible: A Systematic Review. *Implant Dent.* **2017**, *26*, 945–950. [CrossRef]
9. Kutkut, A.; Bertoli, E.; Frazer, R.; Pinto-Sinai, G.; Fuentealba Hidalgo, R.; Studts, J. A systematic review of studies comparing conventional complete denture and implant retained overdenture. *J. Prosthodont. Res.* **2018**, *62*, 1–9. [CrossRef]
10. Sivaramakrishnan, G.; Sridharan, K. Comparison of implant supported mandibular overdentures and conventional dentures on quality of life: A systematic review and meta-analysis of randomized controlled studies. *Aust. Dent. J.* **2016**, *61*, 482–488. [CrossRef]
11. Renvert, S.; Persson, G.R.; Pirih, F.Q.; Camargo, P.M. Peri-implant health, peri-implant mucositis, and peri-implantitis: Case definitions and diagnostic considerations. *J. Periodontol.* **2018**, *89* (Suppl. 1), S304–S312. [CrossRef]
12. Peri-implant diseases and conditions: Consensus report of workgroup 4 of the 2017 World Workshop on the Classification of Periodontal and Peri-Implant Diseases and Conditions. *Br. Dent. J.* **2018**, *225*, 141. [CrossRef]
13. Heitz-Mayfield, L.J.A.; Salvi, G.E. Peri-implant mucositis. *J. Periodontol.* **2018**, *89* (Suppl. 1), S257–S266. [CrossRef]
14. Pontoriero, R.; Tonelli, M.P.; Carnevale, G.; Mombelli, A.; Nyman, S.R.; Lang, N.P. Experimentally induced peri-implant mucositis. A clinical study in humans. *Clin. Oral Implant. Res.* **1994**, *5*, 254–259. [CrossRef]
15. Zitzmann, N.U.; Berglundh, T.; Marinello, C.P.; Lindhe, J. Experimental peri-implant mucositis in man. *J. Clin. Periodontol.* **2001**, *28*, 517–523. [CrossRef] [PubMed]
16. Salvi, G.E.; Aglietta, M.; Eick, S.; Sculean, A.; Lang, N.P.; Ramseier, C.A. Reversibility of experimental peri-implant mucositis compared with experimental gingivitis in humans. *Clin. Oral Implant. Res.* **2012**, *23*, 182–190. [CrossRef] [PubMed]
17. Meyer, S.; Giannopoulou, C.; Courvoisier, D.; Schimmel, M.; Muller, F.; Mombelli, A. Experimental mucositis and experimental gingivitis in persons aged 70 or over. Clinical and biological responses. *Clin. Oral Implant. Res.* **2017**, *28*, 1005–1012. [CrossRef] [PubMed]
18. Araujo, M.G.; Lindhe, J. Peri-implant health. *J. Periodontol.* **2018**, *89* (Suppl. 1), S249–S256. [CrossRef]
19. Schwarz, F.; Derks, J.; Monje, A.; Wang, H.L. Peri-implantitis. *J. Periodontol.* **2018**, *89* (Suppl. 1), S267–S290. [CrossRef]
20. Canullo, L.; Schlee, M.; Wagner, W.; Covani, U.; Montegrotto Group for the Study of Peri-implant Disease. International Brainstorming Meeting on Etiologic and Risk Factors of Peri-implantitis, Montegrotto (Padua, Italy), August 2014. *Int. J. Oral Maxillofac. Implant.* **2015**, *30*, 1093–1104. [CrossRef]
21. Albrektsson, T.; Buser, D.; Chen, S.T.; Cochran, D.; DeBruyn, H.; Jemt, T.; Koka, S.; Nevins, M.; Sennerby, L.; Simion, M.; et al. Statements from the Estepona consensus meeting on peri-implantitis, 2–4 February 2012. *Clin. Implant Dent. Relat. Res.* **2012**, *14*, 781–782. [CrossRef] [PubMed]
22. De Bruyn, H.; Christiaens, V.; Doornewaard, R.; Jacobsson, M.; Cosyn, J.; Jacquet, W.; Vervaeke, S. Implant surface roughness and patient factors on long-term peri-implant bone loss. *Periodontology 2000* **2017**, *73*, 218–227. [CrossRef] [PubMed]

23. Wennerberg, A.; Hallgren, C.; Johansson, C.; Danelli, S. A histomorphometric evaluation of screw-shaped implants each prepared with two surface roughnesses. *Clin. Oral Implant. Res.* **1998**, *9*, 11–19. [CrossRef]
24. Cochran, D.L. A comparison of endosseous dental implant surfaces. *J. Periodontol.* **1999**, *70*, 1523–1539. [CrossRef]
25. Lazzara, R.J.; Testori, T.; Trisi, P.; Porter, S.S.; Weinstein, R.L. A human histologic analysis of osseotite and machined surfaces using implants with 2 opposing surfaces. *Int. J. Periodontics Restor. Dent.* **1999**, *19*, 117–129.
26. Teughels, W.; Van Assche, N.; Sliepen, I.; Quirynen, M. Effect of material characteristics and/or surface topography on biofilm development. *Clin. Oral Implant. Res.* **2006**, *17* (Suppl. 2), 68–81. [CrossRef]
27. Esposito, M.; Coulthard, P.; Thomsen, P.; Worthington, H.V. The role of implant surface modifications, shape and material on the success of osseointegrated dental implants. A Cochrane systematic review. *Eur. J. Prosthodontics Restor. Dent.* **2005**, *13*, 15–31.
28. Esposito, M.; Ardebili, Y.; Worthington, H.V. Interventions for replacing missing teeth: different types of dental implants. *Cochrane Database Syst. Rev.* **2014**, CD003815. [CrossRef]
29. Glibert, M.; Matthys, C.; Maat, R.J.; De Bruyn, H.; Vervaeke, S. A randomized controlled clinical trial assessing initial crestal bone remodeling of implants with a different surface roughness. *Clin. Implant Dent. Relat. Res.* **2018**, *20*, 824–828. [CrossRef]
30. Monje, A.; Catena, A.; Borgnakke, W.S. Association between diabetes mellitus/hyperglycaemia and peri-implant diseases: Systematic review and meta-analysis. *J. Clin. Periodontol.* **2017**, *44*, 636–648. [CrossRef]
31. Papi, P.; Letizia, C.; Pilloni, A.; Petramala, L.; Saracino, V.; Rosella, D.; Pompa, G. Peri-implant diseases and metabolic syndrome components: a systematic review. *Eur. Rev. Med. Pharmacol. Sci.* **2018**, *22*, 866–875. [CrossRef]
32. Moraschini, V.; Barboza, E.S.; Peixoto, G.A. The impact of diabetes on dental implant failure: a systematic review and meta-analysis. *Int. J. Oral Maxillofac. Surg.* **2016**, *45*, 1237–1245. [CrossRef] [PubMed]
33. de Medeiros, F.; Kudo, G.A.H.; Leme, B.G.; Saraiva, P.P.; Verri, F.R.; Honorio, H.M.; Pellizzer, E.P.; Santiago Junior, J.F. Dental implants in patients with osteoporosis: A systematic review with meta-analysis. *Int. J. Oral Maxillofac. Surg.* **2018**, *47*, 480–491. [CrossRef]
34. Jung, R.E.; Al-Nawas, B.; Araujo, M.; Avila-Ortiz, G.; Barter, S.; Brodala, N.; Chappuis, V.; Chen, B.; De Souza, A.; Almeida, R.F.; et al. Group 1 ITI Consensus Report: The influence of implant length and design and medications on clinical and patient-reported outcomes. *Clin. Oral Implant. Res.* **2018**, *29* (Suppl. 16), 69–77. [CrossRef] [PubMed]
35. Safii, S.H.; Palmer, R.M.; Wilson, R.F. Risk of implant failure and marginal bone loss in subjects with a history of periodontitis: a systematic review and meta-analysis. *Clin. Implant Dent. Relat. Res.* **2010**, *12*, 165–174. [CrossRef] [PubMed]
36. De Bruyn, H.; Collaert, B. The effect of smoking on early implant failure. *Clin. Oral Implant. Res.* **1994**, *5*, 260–264. [CrossRef]
37. Hinode, D.; Tanabe, S.; Yokoyama, M.; Fujisawa, K.; Yamauchi, E.; Miyamoto, Y. Influence of smoking on osseointegrated implant failure: a meta-analysis. *Clin. Oral Implant. Res.* **2006**, *17*, 473–478. [CrossRef]
38. Doornewaard, R.; Christiaens, V.; De Bruyn, H.; Jacobsson, M.; Cosyn, J.; Vervaeke, S.; Jacquet, W. Long-Term Effect of Surface Roughness and Patients' Factors on Crestal Bone Loss at Dental Implants. A Systematic Review and Meta-Analysis. *Clin. Implant Dent. Relat. Res.* **2017**, *19*, 372–399. [CrossRef]
39. Vervaeke, S.; Collaert, B.; Cosyn, J.; De Bruyn, H. A 9-Year Prospective Case Series Using Multivariate Analyses to Identify Predictors of Early and Late Peri-Implant Bone Loss. *Clin. Implant Dent. Relat. Res.* **2016**, *18*, 30–39. [CrossRef]
40. Berglundh, T.; Lindhe, J. Dimension of the periimplant mucosa. Biological width revisited. *J. Clin. Periodontol.* **1996**, *23*, 971–973. [CrossRef]
41. Linkevicius, T.; Apse, P.; Grybauskas, S.; Puisys, A. The influence of soft tissue thickness on crestal bone changes around implants: a 1-year prospective controlled clinical trial. *Int. J. Oral Maxillofac. Implant.* **2009**, *24*, 712–719.
42. Vervaeke, S.; Dierens, M.; Besseler, J.; De Bruyn, H. The influence of initial soft tissue thickness on peri-implant bone remodeling. *Clin. Implant Dent. Relat. Res.* **2014**, *16*, 238–247. [CrossRef] [PubMed]
43. Galindo-Moreno, P.; Leon-Cano, A.; Ortega-Oller, I.; Monje, A.; F, O.V.; Catena, A. Marginal bone loss as success criterion in implant dentistry: Beyond 2 mm. *Clin. Oral Implant. Res.* **2015**, *26*, e28–e34. [CrossRef]

44. Canullo, L.; Camacho-Alonso, F.; Tallarico, M.; Meloni, S.M.; Xhanari, E.; Penarrocha-Oltra, D. Mucosa Thickness and Peri-implant Crestal Bone Stability: A Clinical and Histologic Prospective Cohort Trial. *Int. J. Oral Maxillofac. Implant.* **2017**, *32*, 675–681. [CrossRef]
45. Doornewaard, R.; Jacquet, W.; Cosyn, J.; De Bruyn, H. How do peri-implant biologic parameters correspond with implant survival and peri-implantitis? A critical review. *Clin. Oral Implant. Res.* **2018**, *29* (Suppl. 18), 100–123. [CrossRef]
46. Vervaeke, S.; Matthys, C.; Nassar, R.; Christiaens, V.; Cosyn, J.; De Bruyn, H. Adapting the vertical position of implants with a conical connection in relation to soft tissue thickness prevents early implant surface exposure: A 2-year prospective intra-subject comparison. *J. Clin. Periodontol.* **2018**, *45*, 605–612. [CrossRef] [PubMed]
47. Srinivasan, M.; Meyer, S.; Mombelli, A.; Muller, F. Dental implants in the elderly population: A systematic review and meta-analysis. *Clin. Oral Implant. Res.* **2017**, *28*, 920–930. [CrossRef]
48. Lesaffre, E.; Philstrom, B.; Needleman, I.; Worthington, H. The design and analysis of split-mouth studies: what statisticians and clinicians should know. *Stat. Med.* **2009**, *28*, 3470–3482. [CrossRef]
49. Suarez-Lopez Del Amo, F.; Lin, G.H.; Monje, A.; Galindo-Moreno, P.; Wang, H.L. Influence of Soft Tissue Thickness on Peri-Implant Marginal Bone Loss: A Systematic Review and Meta-Analysis. *J. Periodontol.* **2016**, *87*, 690–699. [CrossRef]
50. Quirynen, M.; Abarca, M.; Van Assche, N.; Nevins, M.; van Steenberghe, D. Impact of supportive periodontal therapy and implant surface roughness on implant outcome in patients with a history of periodontitis. *J. Clin. Periodontol.* **2007**, *34*, 805–815. [CrossRef]
51. Wennerberg, A.; Albrektsson, T.; Chrcanovic, B. Long-term clinical outcome of implants with different surface modifications. *Eur. J. Oral Implantol.* **2018**, *11* (Suppl. 1), S123–S136.
52. Koodaryan, R.; Hafezeqoran, A. Evaluation of Implant Collar Surfaces for Marginal Bone Loss: A Systematic Review and Meta-Analysis. *BioMed Res. Int.* **2016**, *2016*, 4987526. [CrossRef] [PubMed]
53. Donati, M.; Ekestubbe, A.; Lindhe, J.; Wennstrom, J.L. Marginal bone loss at implants with different surface characteristics—A 20-year follow-up of a randomized controlled clinical trial. *Clin. Oral Implant. Res.* **2018**, *29*, 480–487. [CrossRef]
54. Raes, M.; D'Hondt, R.; Teughels, W.; Coucke, W.; Quirynen, M. A 5-year randomized clinical trial comparing minimally with moderately rough implants in patients with severe periodontitis. *J. Clin. Periodontol.* **2018**, *45*, 711–720. [CrossRef] [PubMed]
55. De Waal, Y.C.; van Winkelhoff, A.J.; Meijer, H.J.; Raghoebar, G.M.; Winkel, E.G. Differences in peri-implant conditions between fully and partially edentulous subjects: A systematic review. *J. Clin. Periodontol.* **2013**, *40*, 266–286. [CrossRef] [PubMed]
56. De Waal, Y.C.; Winkel, E.G.; Meijer, H.J.; Raghoebar, G.M.; van Winkelhoff, A.J. Differences in peri-implant microflora between fully and partially edentulous patients: A systematic review. *J. Clin. Periodontol.* **2014**, *85*, 68–82. [CrossRef] [PubMed]

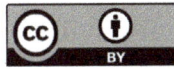

© 2019 by the authors. Licensee MDPI, Basel, Switzerland. This article is an open access article distributed under the terms and conditions of the Creative Commons Attribution (CC BY) license (http://creativecommons.org/licenses/by/4.0/).

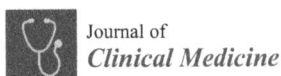

Article

Treatment of Peri-Implantitis—Electrolytic Cleaning Versus Mechanical and Electrolytic Cleaning—A Randomized Controlled Clinical Trial—Six-Month Results

Markus Schlee [1], Florian Rathe [2], Urs Brodbeck [3], Christoph Ratka [4], Paul Weigl [4] and Holger Zipprich [4],*

1. Private Practice and Department of Maxillofacial Surgery, Goethe University, 60590 Frankfurt am Main, Germany; markus.schlee@32schoenezaehne.de
2. Private Practice and Department of Prosthodontics, Danube University, 3500 Krems, Austria; florian.rathe@32schoenezaehne.de
3. Private Practice, 8051 Zürich, Switzerland; ursbrodbeck@bluewin.ch
4. Department of Prosthodontics, Goethe University, 60590 Frankfurt am Main, Germany; ratka@med.uni-frankfurt.de (C.R.); weigl@em.uni-frankfurt.de (P.W.)
* Correspondence: zipprich@em.uni-frankfurt.de; Tel.: +49-69-6301-4714; Fax: +49-69-6301-3711

Received: 29 October 2019; Accepted: 4 November 2019; Published: 7 November 2019

Abstract: Objectives: The present randomized clinical trial assesses the six-month outcomes following surgical regenerative therapy of periimplantitis lesions using either an electrolytic method (EC) to remove biofilms or a combination of powder spray and electrolytic method (PEC). Materials and Methods: 24 patients with 24 implants suffering from peri-implantitis with any type of bone defect were randomly treated by EC or PEC. Bone defects were augmented with a mixture of natural bone mineral and autogenous bone and left for submerged healing. The distance from implant shoulder to bone was assessed at six defined points at baseline (T0) and after six months at uncovering surgery (T1) by periodontal probe and standardized x-rays. Results: One implant had to be removed at T1 because of reinfection and other obstacles. None of the other implants showed signs of inflammation. Bone gain was 2.71 ± 1.70 mm for EC and 2.81 ± 2.15 mm for PEC. No statistically significant difference between EC and PEC was detected. Significant clinical bone fill was observed for all 24 implants. Complete regeneration of bone was achieved in 12 implants. Defect morphology impacted the amount of regeneration. Conclusion: EC needs no further mechanical cleaning by powder spray. Complete re-osseointegration in peri-implantitis cases is possible.

Keywords: periimplantitis; electrolytic cleaning; augmentation; air flow; re-osseointegration; classification of bone defects

1. Introduction

Increasing numbers of inserted dental implants cause an increasing number of infected implants [1]. Mucositis is a reversible inflammatory process limited to peri-implant soft tissue. Peri-implantitis (PI) is defined as an inflammatory process affecting peri-implant hard as well as soft tissue. Typical cup-shaped progressive bone defects, pus, and bleeding on probing (BoP) are clinical parameters which have to be verified simultaneously to justify the diagnosis of PI [2,3]. Mucositis and PI are correlated with bacterial biofilms colonizing the surfaces of implants or abutments [4]. In view of the difficulty in differentiating pathologic bleeding from bleeding caused by improper probing, as well as the discordance in the dental community about the acceptable threshold of bone loss, there is no consensus about when pathology starts and how PI can be diagnosed precisely. Hence, prevalence data vary from author to author [5,6]. Based on these data, up to 100 million dental implants may be infected worldwide. As implant surfaces, which are exposed to the oral cavity, are immediately colonized by the individual microbiome, the surfaces need to be re-osseointegrated for positive long-term results [7]. Treatment and replacement of implants cause immense costs and discomfort. Therefore, it is necessary to find more effective approaches to decontaminating infected implants.

Several methods, all of which are ablative for removing biofilms have been discussed. For example, mechanical debridement by hand or ultrasound-driven curettes, brushes, lasers, pellets, cold plasma, or air-powder sprays in conjunction with or without disinfection or antibiotic agents. Re-osseointegration of between 39% and 46% of treated implant surfaces was reported in a review [8]. Re-osseointegration in humans has not yet been proven. A review of the literature demonstrated that none of the assessed methods was superior to any other in removing the biofilm and no method was able to achieve a stable result over time [9]. Up to 100% relapse of the disease for some methods was demonstrated after one year, and evidence for the superiority of any treatment modality is lacking [10]. Powder spray systems (PSS) are commonly used to treat PI. Small particles (erythritol or glycine) are accelerated by air pressure and remove the biofilm when impacting the implant surface. Several animal studies investigating re-osseointegration after cleaning by PSS proved incomplete re-osseointegration [8]. Clinical parameters like BoP, pocket depth (PD), and pus improved. Furthermore, PSS failed to prove superiority to any other treatment modality [11–13]. Possible reasons for this limited efficacy might be craterlike bone defects with compromised access, thus improper working angle and distance of the device, macro- and micro-design of the implant surface, and particles too large for much smaller bacteria hidden in the microstructure of textured implants.

In an in vitro test, two bacterially contaminated implants were embedded in an electro-conductive gelatin block and were loaded with a continuous current of 0-10 mA – one acting as a cathode, the other as an anode. A reduction of bacteria was proved. This approach dramatically changed the pH at both implants [14]. Zipprich et al. covered implants with a mature biofilm, loaded them as cathode, and flooded the implants with a buffered potassium iodine solution which had passed an anode. Complete removal of the biofilm was demonstrated by SEM analysis [15]. The mode of action was investigated by a collaborative working group [16]. In an in vitro test, Ratka et al. used EC versus PSS to treat implants with different surfaces and alloys covered with a mature biofilm. In contrast to PSS, no bacteria could be cultivated in the EC groups. The difference was extremely significant [17]. Based on these findings, an electrolytic device was developed by the authors to remove the biofilm in a clinical setting.

The aim and endpoint of this controlled clinical trial was to compare the effectiveness of two processes of decontamination in terms of bone level changes.

2. Materials and Methods

2.1. Legal

The study was registered (BfArM DA/CA99, DIMDI 00010977) and approved by the "Ethik-Kommission der Bayerischen Landesärztekammer" (BASEC_No. DE/EKBY10) with the registration code 17075.

2.2. Sample Size Calculation

The data presented in this study were collected for a proof of principle study assessing the bacterial load before and after the treatment. This article describes the six-month results of the proof of principle study. Based on previous in vitro tests using a paired t-test with a power of 90% and a level of significance of 5%, a sample size of 12 per group was calculated. The sample size calculation was done using G*Power 3.1 (Heinrich Heine University of Düsseldorf).

2.3. Devices and Mode of Action

For the electrolytic approach (EL) the implant has to be loaded negatively with a voltage and a maximum current of 600 mA. This is achieved by a device (GS1000, GalvoSurge Dental AG, Widnau, Switzerland) providing the voltage and pumping a sodium formiate solution through a spray-head, which has to be pressed into the implant by finger pressure to achieve an electrical contact (Figure 1). Driven by a peristaltic pump, a sodium formiate solution passes an anode inside the spray-head and then covers the implant with a "film" of liquid (Figure 2). The current splits the water into hydrogen anions and cations. The cations penetrate the biofilm and take an electron from the implant. Hydrogen bubbles lift the biofilm off the implant surface.

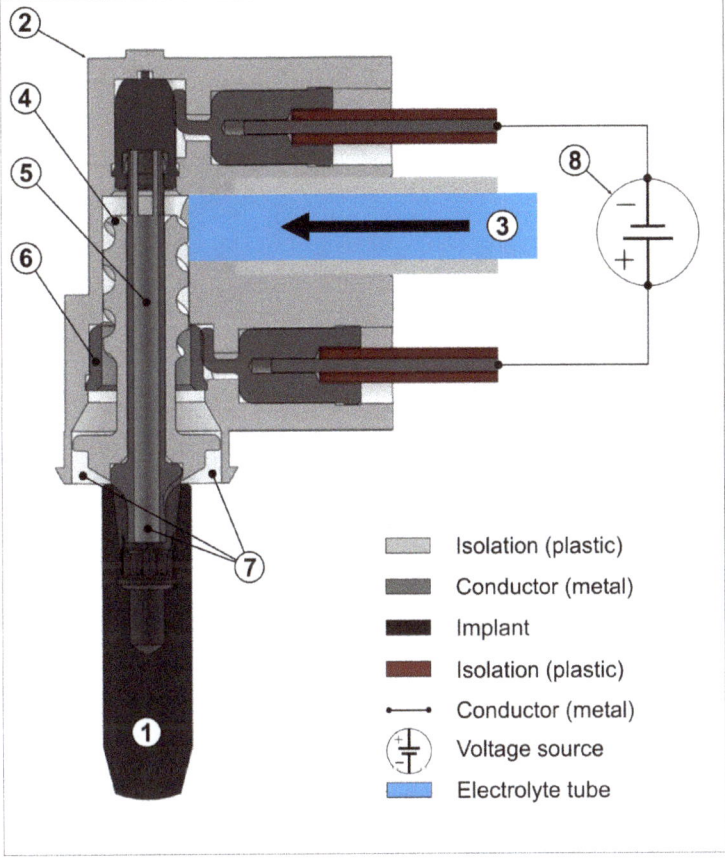

Figure 1. Composition of the spray-head. (1) Implant (loaded as a cathode); (2) spray head; (3) tube for electrolyte; (4) spiral-like threaded isolator; (5) connector (loaded as a cathode); (6) anode; (7) shower head (exit of electrolyte); (8) control unit and voltage source. Application of Figure 1: The spray-head (2) has to be pressed on containment of the implant (1) manually. The electrolyte will be pumped through the tube (3) and passes the spiral of the treaded isolator (4), reaches the anode (6), and will be sprayed by the shower head (7) onto the exposed implant surface. A second pathway branching off from the threaded isolator to the implant connector (5) pumps electrolyte in the implant containment (1). The positive current path derives from the voltage source (8), passes metallic conductors to the anode. The negative current path derives from the voltage source (8), passes metallic conductors to the connector (5), to the implant (1), which acts in the electrolytic process as the cathode.

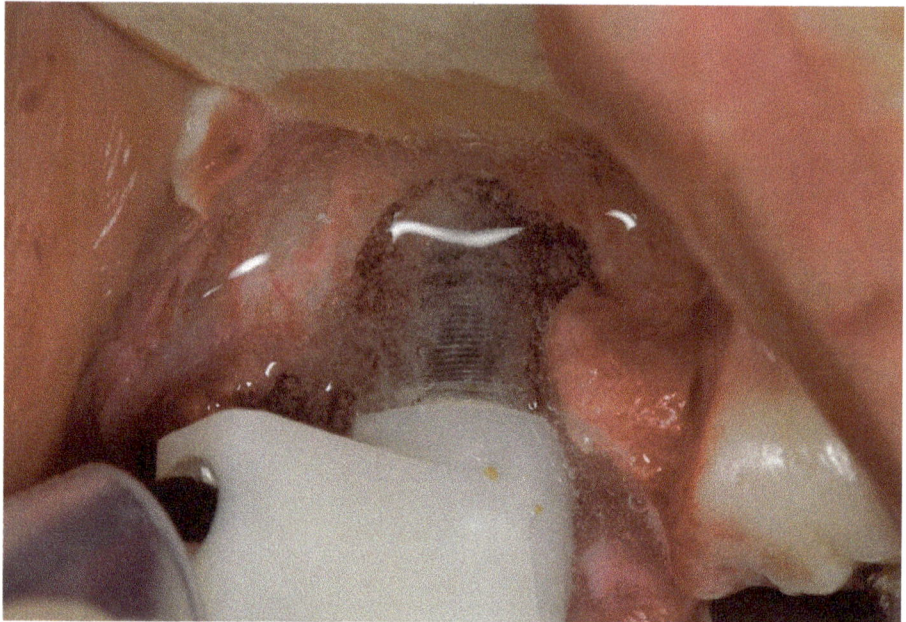

Figure 2. Spray-head during cleaning process.

2.4. Patient and Sample Selection, Randomization

24 patients with at least one titanium implant and diagnosed with periimplantitis (definition according to Berglund et al.) [3] were included in the study. If more than one implant was affected, one implant was chosen randomly. The patients were allocated to test group (EC) or control group (PEC) after randomization by using sealed envelopes immediately before surgery.

2.5. Inclusion Criteria

Patients older than 18 years, capable of understanding and signing an informed consent, smoking fewer than 10 cigarettes per day, without uncontrolled periodontitis, BoP < 20%, Plaque Index < 20%, no allergy to the drugs or materials used, and not pregnant or nursing were suitable to be enrolled in the study.

In contrast to most of the literature, the bone defects were not limited to intraosseous defects. All implants were included independently of their bone defect morphology, three-dimensional implant position, e.g. implant axis, inter-implant distance, etc.

2.6. Procedures and Measurements

Selected patients were instructed and motivated regarding proper oral hygiene and, if necessary, underwent periodontal treatment. Standardized photos were taken (occlusal, buccal, lingual view) and repeated in all appointments listed below. Suprastructures were removed 14 days before surgery. The implants were cleaned by powder spray (Nozzle, EMS, Nyon, Switzerland) and rinsed with chlorhexidine (Chlorhexamed forte, GlaxoSmithKline, Munich, Germany) to reduce soft tissue inflammation in line with standard procedures in periodontal therapy. A cover screw was placed. As a result of this pretreatment, in most cases the soft tissue grew over the implant, leaving a crestal fistula. PD and BoP were assessed at six defined points (m, mb, b, db, d, dl) (Figure 3) using a periodontal probe with a 1 mm scale (PCPUNC 15, HuFridy, Chicago, IL, USA). A crestal incision with releasing incisions was performed to enable a flap to be reflected so that access to the implant could be gained. Buccal and, in the mandible, additional lingual periosteal incisions were made so that the tissues could be mobilized over the implant. The granulation tissues were removed and, if applicable, tartar or cement remnants were removed mechanically by the use of curettes (DSC13/14, HuFridy, Chicago, IL, USA) and/or ultrasonic devices (Dentsply Sirona, Bensheim, Germany). This is necessary because the EC process can only work if the electrolyte is in direct contact with the conductive implant. The distance from implant platform to the most apical position of bone (P-B) was assessed as described in (Figure 3) at the same six points as PD and BoP were measured using the described periodontal probe. In the EC group, the spray-head was pressed into the implant and the GS1000 control unit started. The current was applied 5 s after the peristaltic pump was started and the electrolytic spray was initiated. The cleaning process took 120 s. In the PEC group, the implants were treated according to the manufacturer's manual by a powder spray (Airflow Plus powder, Airflow, EMS, Nyon, Switzerland) for 60 s followed by the treatment described for the EC group. After cleaning, the implants were rinsed with sterile saline and augmented with a mixture of autogenous bone harvested from the ramus area (Micross Safescraper, Zantomed, Duisburg, Germany) and Bio-Oss (Geistlich, Wohlhusen, Switzerland) in a 50:50 ratio. In cases with non-supporting infrabony defects, tenting screws were used for space maintaining (Umbrella-Screw, Ustomed, Tuttlingen, Germany). After placement of a collagen membrane (Bio-Gide, Geistlich, Wohlhusen, Switzerland) the flap was coronally advanced to cover the site passively. The 6-0 propylene monofilaments (Medipac, Kilis, Greece) were removed after two weeks, and wound healing was documented. A VAS (pain, acceptance) assessment was also done by the patients. When no exposure was present at the time of suture removal the patients were checked again four weeks later, then scheduled six months after surgery for second-stage surgery. In the case of exposure, the patients were instructed to brush the area carefully and rinse the site with chlorhexidine. These sites were checked monthly.

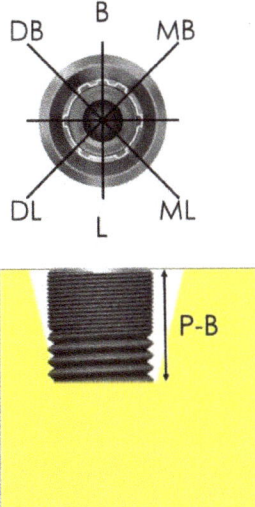

Figure 3. Bone defects were assessed at six defined points from implant shoulder to the most coronal position of the bone.

During the period of healing (six months) the patients were supervised, and exposures or infections were documented. After six months, second-stage surgery was performed. The implants and the surrounding bone were exposed and P-B was assessed under direct vision at the previous points. In cases with exposures, no second-stage surgery was necessary and P-B was assessed by bone sounding under local anesthesia using the described periodontal probe with sufficient pressure. Furthermore infections, BoP, and recessions were documented. For all implants, suprastructures were replaced, photographs were taken, and a standardized x-ray in the right-angle position was performed. Sutures were removed after 14 days, if applicable. Bone levels at baseline and after six months were assessed by two examiners using software (DBS Win, Dürr, Bietigheim-Bissingen, Germany). The examiners, not knowing the aim of the study, were calibrated until their results correlated adequately as measured by Cohen's Kappa ($\kappa \geq 0.6$). In addition, the measurements had to reach 90% agreement for ±0.5 mm as well as exact agreement in 75% of the radiologic measurements before assessment of the x-rays in this study.

Schwarz et al. [18] introduced a classification describing typical peri-implant bone defect anatomy. For clinical purposes, however, a classification providing information about the healing potential of a defect would be more helpful for the practitioner. Therefore, we hereby introduce the RP Classification differentiating the regenerative potential (RP) of a bone defect based on the risk-chance ratio of treatment. We assessed intrabony defects (RP1), intrabony defects with dehiscence defects (RP2) and horizontal bone defects (RP3) (Figure 4) and correlated them to total and median bone fill. Complete regain of bone is dependent on the type of implant. In most of the implants 1 mm remodeling occurs within the first year. It cannot be expected that these implants will re-osseointegrate up to the platform. Implants with a polished neck osseointegrate to the border rough-polished. They are placed at this level very often. More coronal re-osseointegration cannot be expected [19,20].

Therefore, we define bone-to-implant contact with a P-B < 1 mm as complete bone fill. Implants with polished necks are counted as complete bone fill, if the bone fill reaches the border rough-polished being visible at T2 after flap removal.

All the surgical procedures and clinical assessments such as PPD, recessions and BoP were performed by the first-named author.

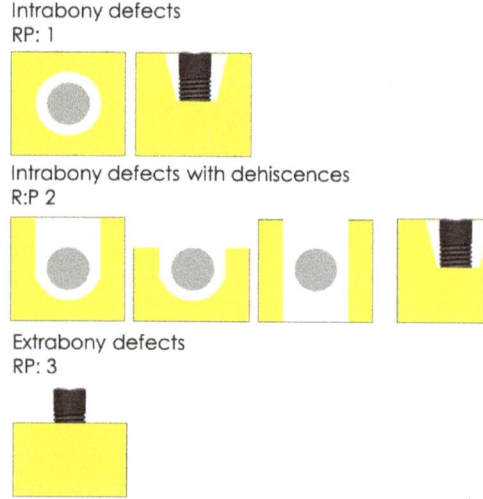

Figure 4. RP Classification of peri-implant bone defects based on risk-chance ratio of treatment.

2.7. Statistics

Quantitative values are presented as mean and standard deviation, and minimum and maximum, as well as quartiles. Gaussian distribution of data was assessed using the Saphiro-Wilk test. Comparisons were performed with the Mann-Whitney U test or *t*-test, as appropriate. The homogeneity of variance was verified by Levene's test before the *t*-tests. The level of significance was set at $\alpha = 0.05$ and all tests were two-sided. The statistical analysis was performed using R 3.6.1 with the package car 3.0-3. R. The package used is available from CRAN at http://CRAN.R-project.org/.

3. Results

The distribution of gender and age was homogeneous (12f/12m; mean age 57.13 y) and there were four smokers (3 EC, 1 PEC) < 10 cigarettes per day. All the sites were infected, BoP was positive, pus drained from pockets, and all sites probed deeper than 5 mm at baseline (Table 1). PD was 6.64 mm in the EC and 7.02 mm in the PEC group. No significant difference was assessable (Fisher's exact test, $p > 0.999$). Thus, the entity was considered to be homogeneous.

Table 1. Qualitative baseline data indicating homogenous data.

General Information	Specific Information	n/Mean Years	Percentage
gender	female	12	50.00%
	male	12	50.00%
age	female	59.2 y	
	male	51.4 y	
jaw	maxilla EL	4	16.67%
	maxilla PEL	8	33.33%
	mandible EL	8	33.33%
	mandible PEL	4	16.67%
	maxilla total	12	50.00%
	mandible total	12	50.00%
smokers	EL	3	12.50%
	PEL	1	4.17%
BoP		24	100.00%
pus		24	100.00%

Nineteen sites were exposed at suture removal, 15 after six months. Nevertheless, no implant was lost during the healing phase. One implant from the PEC group had to be removed after six months because of infection, incomplete bone regeneration, and the presence of infection. Compliance of this female patient was poor, and the implant was placed far too lingually in a compromised axis. The addition of these factors led to the recommendation to remove this implant.

The quality of regained bone was assessed by visual inspection with a microscope (24x magnification), bone sounding with high pressure, and interpretation of x-rays. Complete and solid bone in direct contact with the implant was confirmed.

Bone gain was assessed at six months as a difference between P-B$_{baseline}$ and P-B$_{6\,months}$ (ΔP-B) at the six defined points. There was no statistical significant difference either between the specific points or the median. Bone gain and differences between the EC and PEC groups are visualized in Table 2. Bone gain was 2.71 ± 1.70 mm in the EC group and 2.81 ± 2.15 for PEC. The difference (Δ PEC-EC) was not statistically significant (0.10 mm, p-value 0.87). The related boxplots are displayed in Figures 5 and 6.

The implants in the study population consisted of different implant brands and designs. Their distribution is displayed in Table 3. According to our definition, complete bone fill was achieved if ΔP-B was less than 1 mm. This was observed in nine implants (37.5%). In two cases with a polished implant shoulder (Camlog, Altatec, Wimsheim, Germany), the bone fill reached the border rough-polished (ΔP-B < 2). If those cases are accepted as complete bone fill, a total of 12 implants (50%) accomplished complete bone fill. The distribution of the different defect morphologies and regenerative potential was four implants RP1, 11 implants RP2, and nine implants RP3. Complete regain of visible and probable bone up to the implant shoulder was achieved in all the RP1 implants. Six implants in RP2 cases and only two implants in RP3 achieved complete bone fill. Median bone gain related to defect morphology was 4.02 ± 0.96 mm in RP1 cases, 2.64 ± 1.58 mm in RP2 and 2.34 ± 1.58 mm in RP3 (Table 4).

Table 2. Bone gain and differences between EC and AFL group.

Location	EC Group [mm]	PEC Group [mm]	Differences	
			AEL-EL	p-Value
db	3.00 ± 1.67	2.50 ± 2.10	−0.50	0.52
b	3.25 ± 1.63	2.83 ± 2.94	−0.42	0.71
mb	3.17 ± 1.61	3.00 ± 2.12	−0.17	0.83
ml	2.58 ± 1.84	3.13 ± 2.25	0.55	0.53
l	2.29 ± 1.79	2.96 ± 1.86	0.67	0.38
dl	1.96 ± 1.57	2.46 ± 1.83	0.50	0.48
Median	2.71 ± 1.70	2.81 ± 2.15	0.10	0.87

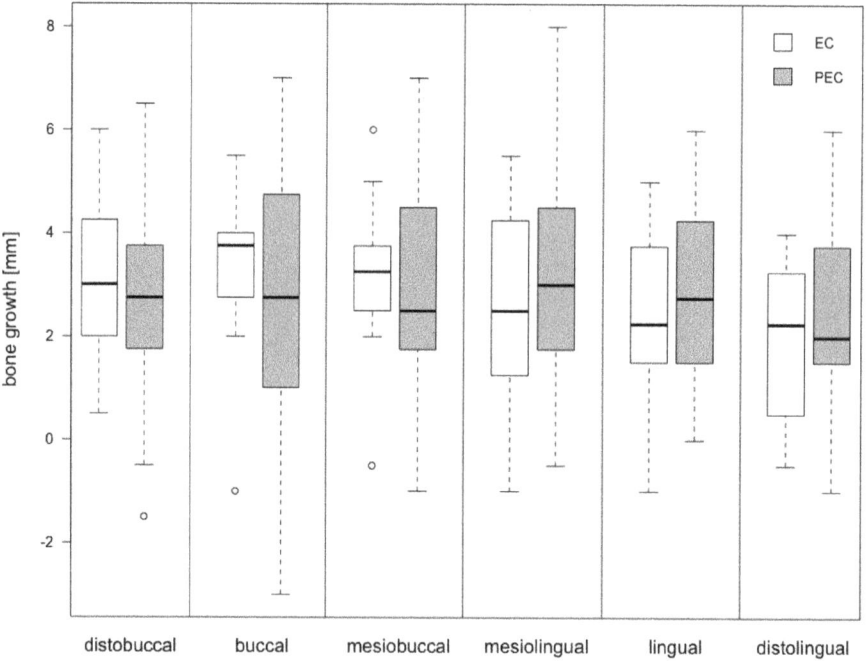

Figure 5. Boxplot indicating the distribution of the assessment points in EC and PEC.

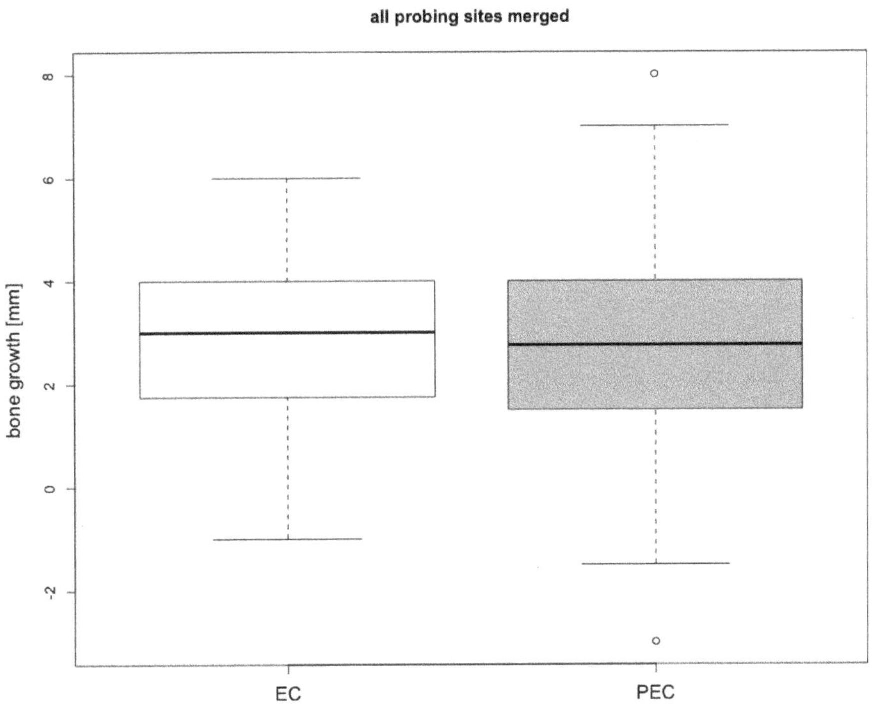

Figure 6. Boxplot indicating the merged distribution of the assessment points in EC and PEC.

Table 3. Allocation of different implant types.

Type of Implant	Number
Astra TX	5
Astra EV	2
Straumann tissue level	2
Straumann bone level	1
Conelog	2
Camlog	2
Ankylos	2
Sky	1
Branemark	2
Xive	1
Steri Oss	1
Zimmer	2
Nobel Active	1

Table 4. Bone gain in relation to RP class.

RP Class	Bone Gain
RP1	4.02 ± 0.96
RP2	2.64 ± 1.58
RP3	2.34 ± 1.58

In one case 1.5 mm bone grew over the top of the implant and 1.5 mm clinically hard and mature bone had to be removed to get access to the implant (Figures 7 and 8) [21]. In two cases, (both RP3) the implants were covered by tartar. In one case, complete bone fill was gained. In the other case, P-B improved slightly.

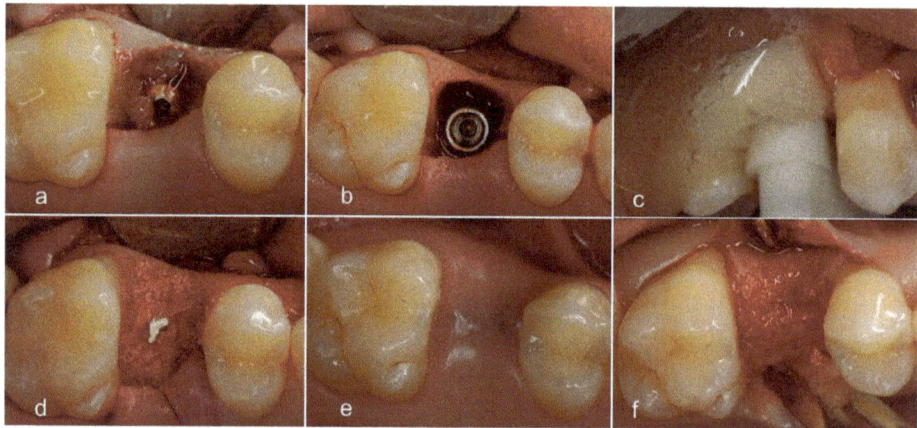

Figure 7. (**a**). A raised flap displays granulation tissue. (**b**). Deep peri-implant RP1 bone defect. (**c**). The spray-head is in place. The film of electrolyte is guided by a sponge. Hydrogen bubbles appear as a result of the process. (**d**). Defect augmented by a mixture of autogenous and natural bone mineral. (**e**). Healed defect after six months. (**f**). Solid bone overgrew the implant.

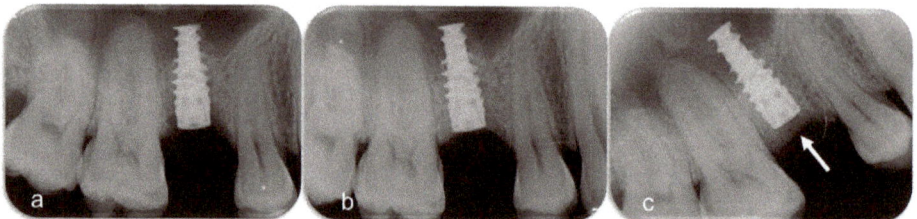

Figure 8. (**a**). The defect at baseline looks much less severe than in clinical reality. (**b**). Augmented defect. (**c**). Six months of healing.

4. Discussion

4.1. Design of Study

The study was designed as a randomized and controlled trial. As none of the current treatment modalities was superior to any other and all of them failed to prove long-term stability and re-osseointegration in a clinical setting [10], they were unsuitable to serve as a control method. None of these methods was considered ethical to use. After lengthy discussion with the ethics committee, we decided to investigate whether additional ablative methods are beneficial to the outcome of the electrolytic approach. For this purpose, we cannot compare the results of this study directly with current treatment modalities. Furthermore, this RCT investigated changes in bone level clinically while most of the published articles focus on the change in clinical parameters. In view of the different endpoints, the data presented in this article cannot be compared directly with existing literature. After six months of healing after second-stage surgery, we will have the chance to assess clinical data (PPD, BoP, secretion) and compare them to existing literature.

The definition of success in the therapy of periimplantitis is a matter of debate. Carcuac et al. approached this question by assessing three outcomes: 1. further marginal bone loss ≤ 0.5 mm, 2. outcome 1 + PD ≤ 5 mm, and 3. outcome 2 + BoP and/or suppuration on probing (SoP) = negative. According to this definition they were able to achieve 69.4%, 55.4% and 33.1% success in an RCT investigating resective surgery [22]. Assuming that elimination of a pocket should resolve the problems, these results are disheartening. In an RCT, after cleaning of the implant surface with plastic curettes and chlorhexidine gel in cases with intrabony defects, Schwarz et al. showed PD changes after four years from 7.1 mm to 4.6 mm when using Bio-Oss and a collagen membrane [23]. BoP reduced from 79 to 28%. Defect configuration seems to have a major effect on PD reduction. Schwarz et al. proved that circumferential intrabony defects exhibit a significantly higher reduction of PD compared to intrabony fenestration defects [24]. Roccuzzo et al. followed 24 patients (two dropouts) with intrabony defects in a case series for seven years. Implants were treated by mechanical debridement and application of EDTA and chlorhexidine gel followed by augmentation with Bio-Oss Collagen. The survival rate was 83.3% for SLA implants and 71.4% for TPS. PD was reduced from 6.6 ± 1.3 to 3.2 ± 0.7 mm in SLA, and 7.2 ± 1.5 to 3.4 ± 0.6 mm in TPS. BoP changed from 75.0 ± 31.2% to 7.5 ± 12.1% (SLA), and from 90.0 ± 12.9% to 30.0 ± 19.7% (TPS). The authors described successful therapy as PD ≤ 5 mm, negative BoP and no further bone loss. Success was achieved in two of 14 (14.3%) of the TPS and in seven of 12 (58.3%) of the SLA implants [25]. These results are difficult to understand as BoP, according to the definition of peri-implantitis, should have been 100% at baseline. It is not known whether non-infected implants with bone loss were enrolled in the study. This demonstrates the difficulty of using the parameter of BoP as a tool for diagnosing peri-implantitis, as discussed by Coli et al. [26].

4.2. Our Results

The potential of the electrolytic approach has previously been demonstrated in various in vitro tests [15–17,27]. We did not focus on intrabony defects, like the cited studies, but accepted all kinds of defects in our data. Therefore, because of the use of different endpoints, it is not possible to compare our data directly with the studies cited above. Achievement of re-osseointegration can be proved only histologically. In an animal study [27], we proved that complete re-osseointegration could be achieved after the use of EC, whereas with conventional cleaning, the bone filled the defect partially, but was never in direct contact with the implant. Clinically, bone fill cannot be equated with re-osseointegration, although this can happen with high probability after EC. The quality of the gained bone was evaluated by visual inspection, assessment of x-rays, and/or mechanical bone sounding of the most crestal position of the bone at the six predetermined points. Mature and solid bone in direct contact with the implant was detected. This still does not prove re-osseointegration. It may be stated, however, that we achieved complete bone fill (according to this definition) in all intrabony defects (RP1 cases). Complete bone fill was achieved in 50% of all cases – a number which, to the best knowledge of the authors, has not yet been quoted in the literature. In cases with exposure, no flap was raised after six months. The P-B distance could not be assessed under direct visual control. The potential bias seems to be negligible. Former studies demonstrated that even probing with 0.5 N completely lateralizes the peri-implant tissues [28]. In the study bone sounding was performed with high pressure under local anesthesia.

Published clinical studies focus on the change in radio-opalescence in x-rays. We will compare radiologic data in a further follow-up as well as PD and BoP assessments and answer the question of the long-term stability of the EC approach.

The exposure rates (15 sites at suture removal) were much higher than is usual in the hands of the author compared to simultaneous implant placement and augmentation. This happened even though a strict initial phase was applied in order to reduce infection and inflammation. It will be necessary to investigate this issue more closely in future and possibly adapt surgical techniques. Whether the soft tissues could be compromised by the former peri-implant infection is merely a matter of speculation.

Our in vitro data clearly prove the potential of EC for removing bacterial [17]. No data are available regarding whether periimplantitis impacts the healing potential of surrounding soft tissue. The number of exposures exceeds the number of exposures in cases of simultaneous implantation and augmentation according to the author's experience. This requires further studies.

Powder spray has to impact at an angle of 30–60° and a working distance of 3–5 mm according to the manufacturer's manual. Owing to micro- and macrostructure as well as defect anatomy, this prerequisite may not always be met. In our study, we compared EC with a combination of EC and powder spray in order to assess whether additional mechanical debridement enhances outcomes. Our data support previous in vitro results, namely that EC alone is able to clean the implant surface and regain a surface onto which bone grows [17].

Tartar had to be removed in two cases before EC cleaning. It was clearly visible that the surfaces of the implants were damaged by the curettes and the ultrasonic device. Our data prove that regain of bone above the former bone level and clinical reattachment of bone are nevertheless possible.

One implant had to be removed because of various factors (reinfection, malpositioning of the implant, and compliance of the patient). Which of these obstacles was causative for the decision is unclear. This raises the question of which implants should be treated or removed and leads to discussion about the etiology of the individual disease and the regenerative potential of this special defect. It is still a matter of discussion whether the bacterial biofilm is the only causal factor or whether bone loss caused by surgical, mechanical, or patient-related reasons, and bacterial colonization happens secondarily on the exposed surfaces [29]. This debate about etiology is not only an academic question. The success rate of possible treatments correlates with specimen susceptibility and uncorrectable surgical or mechanical obstacles. The number of implants included in the present study was too small to draw statistically significant conclusions about correlations between defect morphology and outcome. Conspicuously, all implants with completely preserved bone walls but intrabony defects (RP1) healed with complete bone fill of the defect. Only two out of nine cases with a vertical component (circumferential bone loss; RP3) achieved complete bone fill. Our data support the results of Schwarz et al. who stated that defect morphology has a major impact on healing [24]. We clearly state that the data from this study are too weak because of the sample size to justify the validity of the suggested RP classification. Initially, we did not plan to discuss the data in this way, but the results showed clear differences without reaching significance. Further studies are necessary to validate the RP classification. We treated all implants with the diagnosis of peri-implantitis. Implants placed with a bad axis, insufficient buccolingual inclination, and inter-implant distance < 3 mm were not excluded. Bone gain was smaller compared to perfectly placed implants according to the clinical impression of the authors. Statistical analysis was not performed because of small sample sizes. Further studies are recommended to clarify this issue. For treatment, planning a classification of bone defects to forecast treatment results would be helpful. Therefore, we herewith introduce a new classification focusing on risk-chance ratio: The Regenerative Potential (RP) Classification. Cup-shaped defects with complete bone walls surrounding the defect have the highest healing potential [24]. If more walls are missing and/or additional risk factors are present, removal of the infected implant may be considered. Further studies are necessary to develop a clear decision tree for determining which implants should be treated or removed and when electrolytic cleaning is helpful for long-term success.

5. Conclusions

Electrolytic cleaning of contaminated implants achieves an implant surface where complete re-osseointegration is possible. This was attained in 50% of the cases. Additional mechanical cleaning by the use of powder spray devices does not improve the results further. The amount of regeneration depends on the regenerative potential of the bone (multiwall craterlike defects perform better than horizontal bone loss). Further confounding factors could not be identified owing to the limited sample size of 24 patients.

Author Contributions: Conceptualization, M.S. and H.Z.; Data curation, M.S. and F.R.; Formal analysis, M.S., F.R., C.R. and H.Z.; Investigation, M.S. and F.R.; Methodology, M.S., U.B. and H.Z.; Project administration, M.S.; Resources, M.S.; Software, C.R.; Supervision, M.S.; Validation, M.S., F.R., C.R., P.W. and H.Z.; Visualization, M.S. and H.Z.; Writing—original draft, M.S. and H.Z.; Writing—review & editing, M.S., F.R., U.B., C.R., P.W. and H.Z.

Acknowledgments: The study was sponsored by GalvoSurge Dental AG; We appreciate Ümniye Balaban, Institute for Biostatistics and Mathematical Modeling Center of Health Sciences, Hospital and Department of Medicine of the Goethe University for her support with the statistics.

Conflicts of Interest: The authors Schlee, Zipprich and Brodbeck declare that they own shares in GalvoSurge Dental AG.

References

1. Sendyk, D.I.; Chrcanovic, B.R.; Albrektsson, T.; Wennerberg, A.; Deboni, Z.; Cristina, M. Does Surgical Experience Influence Implant Survival Rate? A Systematic Review and Meta-Analysis. *Int. J. Prosthodont.* **2017**, *30*, 341–347. [CrossRef]
2. Lang, N.P.; Berglundh, T. Periimplant diseases: Where are we now?—Consensus of the Seventh European Workshop on Periodontology. *J. Clin. Periodontol.* **2011**, *38*, 178–181. [CrossRef]
3. Berglundh, T.; Armitage, G.; Araujo, M.G.; Avila-Ortiz, G.; Blanco, J.; Camargo, P.M.; Chen, S.; Cochran, D.; Derks, J.; Figuero, E.; et al. Peri-implant diseases and conditions: Consensus report of workgroup 4 of the 2017 World Workshop on the Classification of Periodontal and Peri-Implant Diseases and Conditions. *J. Periodontol.* **2018**, *89*, S313–S318. [CrossRef]
4. Mombelli, A.; Décaillet, F. The characteristics of biofilms in peri-implant disease. *J. Clin. Periodontol.* **2011**, *38*, 203–213. [CrossRef]
5. Mombelli, A.; Müller, N.; Cionca, N. The epidemiology of peri-implantitis. *Clin. Oral Implant. Res.* **2012**, *23*, 67–76. [CrossRef]
6. Derks, J.; Tomasi, C. Peri-implant health and disease. A systematic review of current epidemiology. *J. Clin. Periodontol.* **2015**, *42*, S158–S171. [CrossRef]
7. Fürst, M.M.; Salvi, G.E.; Lang, N.P.; Persson, G.R. Bacterial colonization immediately after installation on oral titanium implants. *Clin. Oral Implant. Res.* **2007**, *18*, 501–508. [CrossRef]
8. Tastepe, C.S.; van Waas, R.; Liu, Y.; Wismeijer, D. Air powder abrasive treatment as an implant surface cleaning method: A literature review. *Int. J. Oral Maxillofac. Implant.* **2012**, *27*, 1461–1473.
9. Claffey, N.; Clarke, E.; Polyzois, I.; Renvert, S. Surgical treatment of peri-implantitis. *J. Clin. Periodontol.* **2008**, *35*, 316–332. [CrossRef]
10. Esposito, M.; Grusovin, M.G.; Worthington, H.V. Treatment of peri-implantitis: What interventions are effective? A Cochrane systematic review. *Eur. J. Oral Implantol.* **2012**, *5*, S21–S41.
11. de Almeida, J.M.; Matheus, H.R.; Rodrigues Gusman, D.J.; Faleiros, P.L.; Januário de Araújo, N.; Noronha Novaes, V.C. Effectiveness of Mechanical Debridement Combined With Adjunctive Therapies for Nonsurgical Treatment of Periimplantitis: A Systematic Review. *Implant Dent.* **2017**, *26*, 137–144. [CrossRef]
12. del Pozo, J.L.; Rouse, M.S.; Mandrekar, J.N.; Steckelberg, J.M.; Patel, R. The electricidal effect: Reduction of Staphylococcus and pseudomonas biofilms by prolonged exposure to low-intensity electrical current. *Antimicrob. Agents Chemother.* **2009**, *53*, 41–45. [CrossRef]
13. Schwarz, F.; Becker, K.; Sager, M. Efficacy of professionally administered plaque removal with or without adjunctive measures for the treatment of peri-implant mucositis. A systematic review and meta-analysis. *J. Clin. Periodontol.* **2015**, *42*, S202–S213. [CrossRef]

14. Mohn, D.; Zehnder, M.; Stark, W.J.; Imfeld, T. Electrochemical disinfection of dental implants—A proof of concept. *PLoS ONE* **2011**, *6*, e16157. [CrossRef]
15. Zipprich, H.; Ratka, C.; Schlee, M.; Brodbeck, U.; Lauer, H.C.; Seitz, O. Periimplantitistherapie: Durchbruch mit neuer Reinigungsmethode. *Dentalmagazin* **2013**, *31*, 14–17.
16. Schneider, S.; Rudolph, M.; Bause, V.; Terfort, A. Electrochemical removal of biofilms from titanium dental implant surfaces. *Bioelectrochemistry* **2018**, *121*, 84–94. [CrossRef]
17. Ratka, C.; Weigl, P.; Henrich, D.; Koch, F.; Schlee, M.; Zipprich, H. The Effect of In Vitro Electrolytic Cleaning on Biofilm-Contaminated Implant Surfaces. *J. Clin. Med.* **2019**, *8*, 1397. [CrossRef]
18. Schwarz, F.; Herten, M.; Sager, M.; Bieling, K.; Sculean, A.; Becker, J. Comparison of naturally occurring and ligature-induced peri-implantitis bone defects in humans and dogs. *Clin. Oral Implant. Res.* **2007**, *18*, 161–170. [CrossRef]
19. Alomrani, A.N.; Hermann, J.S.; Jones, A.A.; Buser, D.; Schoolfield, J.; Cochran, D.L. The effect of a machined collar on coronal hard tissue around titanium implants: A radiographic study in the canine mandible. *Int. J. Oral Maxillofac. Implant.* **2005**, *20*, 677–686.
20. Laurell, L.; Lundgren, D. Marginal bone level changes at dental implants after 5 years in function: A meta-analysis. *Clin. Implant Dent. Relat. Res.* **2011**, *13*, 19–28. [CrossRef]
21. Albrektsson, T.; Canullo, L.; Cochran, D.; de Bruyn, H. "Peri-Implantitis": A Complication of a Foreign Body or a Man-Made "Disease". Facts and Fiction. *Clin. Implant Dent. Relat. Res.* **2016**, *18*, 840–849. [CrossRef]
22. Carcuac, O.; Derks, J.; Abrahamsson, I.; Wennström, J.L.; Petzold, M.; Berglundh, T. Surgical treatment of peri-implantitis: 3-year results from a randomized controlled clinical trial. *J. Clin. Periodontol.* **2017**, *44*, 1294–1303. [CrossRef]
23. Schwarz, F.; Sahm, N.; Bieling, K.; Becker, J. Surgical regenerative treatment of peri-implantitis lesions using a nanocrystalline hydroxyapatite or a natural bone mineral in combination with a collagen membrane: A four-year clinical follow-up report. *J. Clin. Periodontol.* **2009**, *36*, 807–814. [CrossRef]
24. Schwarz, F.; Sahm, N.; Schwarz, K.; Becker, J. Impact of defect configuration on the clinical outcome following surgical regenerative therapy of peri-implantitis. *J. Clin. Periodontol.* **2010**, *37*, 449–455. [CrossRef]
25. Roccuzzo, M.; Pittoni, D.; Roccuzzo, A.; Charrier, L.; Dalmasso, P. Surgical treatment of peri-implantitis intrabony lesions by means of deproteinized bovine bone mineral with 10% collagen: 7-year-results. *Clin. Oral Implant. Res.* **2017**, *28*, 1577–1583. [CrossRef]
26. Coli, P.; Christiaens, V.; Sennerby, L.; de Bruyn, H. Reliability of periodontal diagnostic tools for monitoring peri-implant health and disease. *Periodontol. 2000* **2017**, *73*, 203–217. [CrossRef]
27. Schlee, M.; Naili, L.; Rathe, F.; Brodbeck, U.; Zipprich, H. Is complete re-osseointegration of an infected dental implant possible—Histological results of a dog study. A short communication. *J. Clin. Med.* **2019**, Submitted.
28. Ericsson, I.; Lindhe, J. Probing depth at implants and teeth. An experimental study in the dog. *J. Clin. Periodontol.* **1993**, *20*, 623–627. [CrossRef]
29. Canullo, L.; Schlee, M.; Wagner, W.; Covani, U. International Brainstorming Meeting on Etiologic and Risk Factors of Peri-implantitis, Montegrotto (Padua, Italy), August 2014. *Int. J. Oral Maxillofac. Implant.* **2015**, *30*, 1093–1104. [CrossRef]

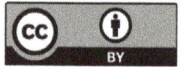

© 2019 by the authors. Licensee MDPI, Basel, Switzerland. This article is an open access article distributed under the terms and conditions of the Creative Commons Attribution (CC BY) license (http://creativecommons.org/licenses/by/4.0/).

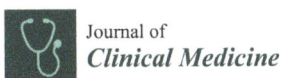

Review

Understanding Peri-Implantitis as a Plaque-Associated and Site-Specific Entity: On the Local Predisposing Factors

Alberto Monje [1,2,*], Angel Insua [2] and Hom-Lay Wang [3]

1. Department of Periodontology, Universitat Internacional de Catalunya, 08195 Barcelona, Spain
2. Division of Periodontics, CICOM Periodoncia, 06011 Badajoz, Badajoz, Spain Santiago de Compostela, Spain; ainsua@umich.edu
3. Department of Periodontics and Oral Medicine, University of Michigan School of Dentistry, Ann Arbor, MI 48109, USA; homlay@umich.edu
* Correspondence: amonjec@umich.edu; Tel.: +34-924-20-30-45

Received: 31 January 2019; Accepted: 21 February 2019; Published: 25 February 2019

Abstract: The prevalence of implant biological complications has grown enormously over the last decade, in concordance with the impact of biofilm and its byproducts upon disease development. Deleterious habits and systemic conditions have been regarded as risk factors for peri-implantitis. However, little is known about the influence of local confounders upon the onset and progression of the disease. The present narrative review therefore describes the emerging local predisposing factors that place dental implants/patients at risk of developing peri-implantitis. A review is also made of the triggering factors capable of inducing peri-implantitis and of the accelerating factors capable of interfering with the progression of the disease.

Keywords: peri-implantitis; peri-implant endosseous healing; dental implantation; dental implant; alveolar bone loss

1. Introduction

Implant dentistry, as a scientific discipline, has grown rapidly over the last four decades with the aim of facilitating early and effective osseointegration affording successful long-term outcomes. Over these years, the onset of complications has been neglected as representing only isolated events. Nowadays, however, due to the increase in prevalence of such problems, one of the major endeavors in this field is the prevention and efficient management of biological complications referred to as peri-implant diseases [1,2].

According to the bacterial theory, peri-implantitis by definition is a chronic inflammatory condition associated with a microbial challenge [3]. Nevertheless, in some cases there may be immunological reasons behind marginal bone loss [4–6] not primarily related to biofilm-mediated infectious processes [7]. Accordingly, a change from a stable immune system, seen during maintained osseointegration, to an active system may lead to the rejection of foreign bodies [7]. In this regard, implant surfaces types, surface wear, or contaminated particles may enhance these immunological reactions [8].

The conversion process from peri-implant mucositis mirrors the progression from gingivitis to periodontitis, with the constant formation of plaque features in the peri-implant tissues, characterized by erythema, bleeding, exudation, and tumefaction. At histological level, the establishment of B- and T-cell-dominated inflammatory cell infiltrates has been evidenced [9]. However, the clinical and histopathological characteristics during the conversion process are still not fully clear. Following conversion, peri-implantitis progresses in a nonlinear and accelerated manner [10].

The epidemiology of peri-implantitis varies widely depending on the given case definition. There has been important controversy regarding the threshold defining physiological peri-implant bone loss. As such, unspecific ranges have been observed in meta-analyses with heterogeneous case definitions. In 2012, the VIII European Workshop of Periodontology underscored that the diagnosis of peri-implantitis should be given on a longitudinal basis of overt progressive bone loss with clinical signs of inflammation [11]. In this regard, a threshold of ≥ 2 mm of peri-implant bone loss could be accepted for the diagnosis of peri-implantitis. More recently, the American Academy of Periodontology and the European Federation of Periodontology have jointly proposed a case definition based on a threshold of ≥ 3 mm [12]. Recent meta-analytical data have suggested the prevalence of peri-implantitis to be 18.5% at patient level and 12.8% at implant level [13], though the prevalence at patient level ranges widely between 1 and 47% [14]. Regardless of the diagnostic criteria proposed, peri-implantitis has been shown to be a site-specific condition. In contrast to periodontitis, which manifests with generalized loss of support, peri-implantitis commonly progresses conditioned by factors predisposing to biofilm accumulation which, under susceptible conditions, triggers a complex inflammatory response.

Strong evidence suggesting an increased risk of peri-implantitis has been obtained in subjects with poor personal- and professional-administered oral hygiene measures, and in individuals with a history of periodontitis [15,16]. Even though other factors and deleterious habits such as smoking [17] or hyperglycemia [18] have been identified as potential risk factors, there is a need for further and stronger evidence to validate their influence upon the development of peri-implantitis [3].

Moreover, in a site-specific condition, attention should focus on those factors which locally might be predisposing for the onset and progression of the disease [19]. Accordingly, the 2017 World Workshop identified evidence linking peri-implantitis to factors that complicate access to adequate oral hygiene, that is, those local conditions that predispose certain implants to develop disease [12].

2. Significance of Terminology for Reaching Consensus

As mentioned above, peri-implantitis and periodontitis occur more frequently under certain systemic conditions and in the presence of deleterious habits. For instance, it is known that major periodontal disease risk factors such as smoking and diabetes alter the epigenetics by downregulating the genic expression of bone matrix proteins that could influence the pathway from peri-implant mucositis to peri-implantitis by suppressing specific transcription factors for osteogenesis, or by activating certain transcription factors for osteoclastogenesis [20,21]. Hence, these systemic conditions may increase the risk of suffering peri-implant diseases.

On the other hand, emerging data point to the influence which certain local factors might have upon the onset and development of disease, since they induce plaque accumulation. These are the so-called predisposing factors. Terminologically, a predisposing factor is a condition that places the given element (dental implant)/individual (patient) at risk of developing a problem (peri-implantitis). In this regard, it is also of interest to underscore that a triggering factor, if not controlled after diagnosing and arresting (or not arresting) the problem (peri-implantitis), represents a perpetuating element that maintains the problem after it has become established [22]. Accelerating factors are therefore defined as those conditions that do not play a role in the onset of a problem (peri-implantitis) but can influence its progression.

3. Are Dental Implants Predisposed to Develop Biological Complications?

The evolution of dental implants and their incorporation to routine practice to restore function and aesthetics of lost or failing dentition have been described as one of the most revolutionary and innovative developments of the twentieth century. In fact, early dental implants were developed with a minimally rough surface microdesign. At that stage in modern implant dentistry, the osseointegration process proved slower and less effective. Long-term findings reported that these implants moreover tended to fail more frequently in the maxilla compared with the mandible. In addition, mean marginal bone loss using primitive implant–abutment connections was shown to be 1.5 mm, with an annual progressive bone loss of 0.1 mm [23,24].

With the development of new technology, the vast majority of commercial implants now have modified (moderately rough) surfaces with the primary aim of securing earlier osseointegration [25]. The incorporation of more biologically acceptable connections may be able to restrict inflammatory infiltration and thus minimize physiological bone loss. Indeed, a clinical study showed that 96% of the implants with a marginal bone loss of >2 mm at 18 months had lost 0.44 mm or more at 6 months postloading [26]. Thus, early healing dictates the long-term life of dental implants and the occurrence of biological complications, as it can be assumed that the establishment of a more anaerobic environment results in greater susceptibility to progressive bone loss.

Advances in the knowledge of bone biology and translational medicine summed to the development of novel armamentaria allow the clinician to minimize physiological bone remodeling. In this regard, excessive physiological bone remodeling (loss) may create a niche for the harboring of periopathogenic microorganisms that can lead to the development of implant biological complications.

4. Peri-Implant Monitoring: Diagnostic Accuracy of Clinical Peri-Implant Parameters

The prompt diagnosis of peri-implant disease is crucial to achieve favorable therapeutic outcomes. While the nonsurgical treatment of peri-implant mucositis is effective, the management of peri-implantitis proves more challenging [27]. Along these lines, it is worth mentioning that the severity and extensiveness of the lesion are crucial factors for successful and maintainable outcomes.

Peri-implantitis develops with progressive bone loss and signs of inflammation. As such, in order to secure an accurate diagnosis, the classical signs of inflammation (i.e., warmth, reddening, tumefaction) and an increased probing depth compared to baseline (assuming a measurement error) must be present [12] (Figure 1; Figure 2), as evidenced by clinical (Table 1) and preclinical studies. Interestingly, during the progression of ligature-induced experimental peri-implantitis, all the clinical parameters are worse due to the degree of inflammation present [28–31].

In this sense, it should be mentioned that disagreement persists concerning the sensitivity of bleeding on probing (BOP) and suppuration as diagnostic criteria. For instance, a human study showed the probability of positive BOP at a peri-implant site with a probing depth of 4 mm to be 27% [32]. The odds for positive BOP was seen to increase 1.6-fold per 1 mm of further probing depth. It has been further evidenced that BOP might be influenced by patient-related factors such as smoking [32]. In fact, understanding of the morphological differences of the periodontal apparatus compared with the peri-implant tissues supports the possibility that the former responds differently to mechanical stimulation. This might explain the poorer sensitivity in the detection of peri-implant diseases compared with periodontal diseases. Likewise, suppuration has been reported in about 10–20% of all peri-implant sites [28,33–36]. Hence, suppuration does not seem to exhibit high sensitivity in the diagnosis of peri-implantitis.

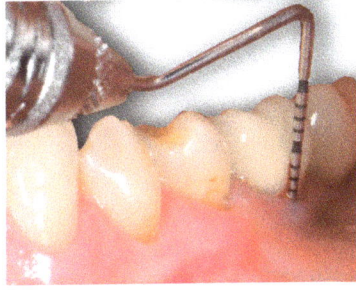 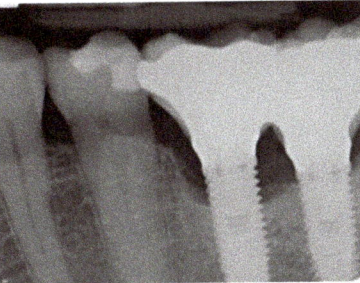

Figure 1. Bleeding on probing and increased probing pocket depth are clinical signs of peri-implantitis. The final diagnosis should be based on the correlation of the clinical data to the radiographic findings.

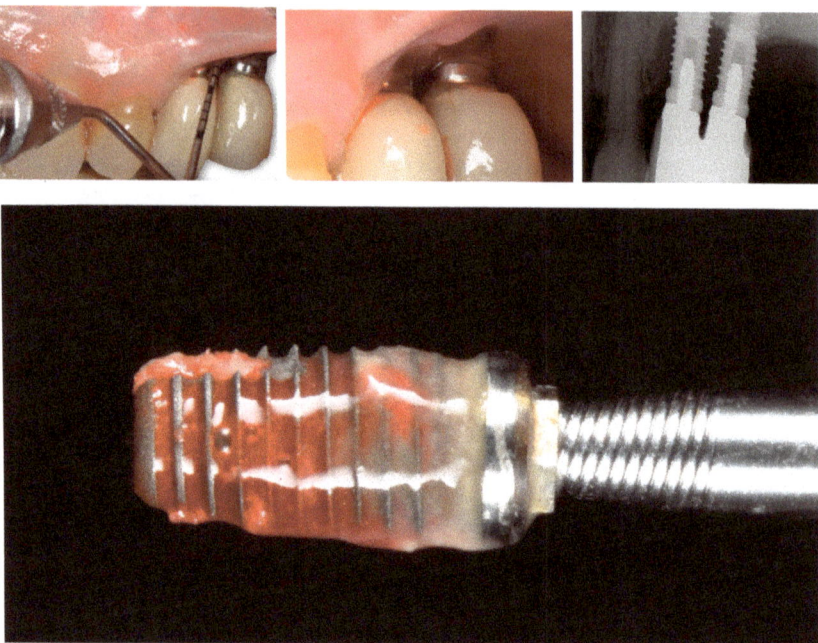

Figure 2. Bleeding on probing and increased probing pocket depth are clinical signs of peri-implantitis. The final diagnosis should be based on the correlation of the clinical data to the radiographic findings. When bone loss is advanced, implant removal is often the most predictable option for dealing with peri-implantitis.

In sum, clinical monitoring of peri-implantitis using a periodontal probe is indicated at each maintenance visit, with the purpose of preventing major biological complications. Nevertheless, the definite diagnosis should be based on the radiographic findings compared to baseline.

Table 1. Clinical characteristics of progressive peri-implant bone loss (peri-implantitis) based on the clinical findings.

Study	Study Design	Follow-Up (Mean)	Methods	Clinical Characteristics of Peri-Implantitis
Fransson et al. 2005, 2008 [37,38]	Cross-sectional	9.4 years	82 patients (197 implants with progressive bone loss/285 implants with stable bone)	• BOP, SUP, recession, and PPD ≥ 6 mm were greater at implants with than without 'progressive' bone loss • The proportion of affected implants that exhibited pus and PPD ≥ 6 mm was higher in smokers than in nonsmokers • SUP, recession, and PPD ≥ 6 mm at an implant in a smoking subject had a 69% accuracy in identifying progressive bone loss
Schwarz et al. 2017 [39]	Cross-sectional	-	60 patients (36 healthy implants/26 with mucositis/167 with peri-implantitis)	• Median PPD was 3 mm at healthy implant sites • Median PPD was 4 mm at peri-implant mucositis sites • Median PPD was 5 mm at peri-implantitis sites • PPD (i.e., by tactile sensation) revealed that 135 of 167 implant sites were associated with a missing buccal bone plate
Schwarz et al. 2017 [40]	Cross-sectional	2.2 years	238 patients (216 implants with mucositis/46 implants diagnosed with peri-implantitis)	• At mucositis sites, the BOP scores ranged between 33% and 50%, while the peak at peri-implantitis sites was 67% • Diseased implant sites were associated with higher frequencies of 4–6 mm PPD versus healthy sites • PPD values of ≥7 mm were only observed in one implant diagnosed with peri-implantitis
Monje et al. 2018 [35]	Case-control	3.17 years	141 patients (90 healthy implants/76 mucositis implants/96 peri-implantitis implants)	• Sites with peri-implant mucositis showed significant levels of BOP (OR = 3.56), redness (OR = 7.66), and PPD (OR = 1.48) compared to healthy sites • Sites exhibiting peri-implantitis showed significant levels of BOP (OR = 2.32), redness (OR = 7.21), PD (OR = 2.43), and SUP (OR = 6.81) compared to healthy sites • PPD was the only diagnostic marker displaying significance comparing peri-implant mucositis and peri-implantitis sites (OR = 1.76) • Tissue-level compared to bone-level implants were less associated with positive SUP (OR = 0.20) and PI (OR = 0.36)
Ramanauskaite et al. 2018 [36]	Cross-sectional	-	269 implants (77 healthy/77 mucositis/115 peri-implantitis)	• In patients diagnosed with peri-implant mucositis, the mean BOP values amounted to 20.83% (43% at implant level) • In patients diagnosed with peri-implantitis, the mean BOP values amounted to 71.33% (86% at implant level) • In patients diagnosed with peri-implantitis, the mean SUP values amounted to 30.16% (17.39% at implant level) • The mean PPD values at implant level were found to be 2.95 mm at healthy implant sites • The mean PPD values at implant level were found to be 3.10 mm at peri-implant mucositis • The mean PPD values at implant level were found to be 4.91 mm at peri-implantitis sites

BOP: bleeding on probing; SUP: suppuration; PPD: probing pocket depth; OR: odds ratio

5. Local Predisposing Factors

5.1. Significance of Soft Tissue Characteristics

The characteristics of the periodontal soft tissues and their association to periodontal conditions have been the subject of debate [41–45]. Based on the existing literature, it seems that attached keratinized gingiva is beneficial in patients with deficient oral hygiene. In contrast, patients with adequate personal- and professional-administered oral hygiene measures do not benefit from attached keratinized gingiva. In fact, movable mucosa facilitates the penetration of biofilm into the crevice, which would trigger the activation of neutrophils and lymphocytes [43]. Hence, in patients not adhering to adequate hygiene, the presence of keratinized attached gingiva might play a pivotal role in the prevention of the disease, in particular in the presence of subgingival restorations.

The influence of keratinized mucosa around dental implants has not been without controversy (Table 2). Early findings indicated that a lack of keratinized mucosa was not associated with less favorable peri-implant conditions [46]. More recent data have shown a wide band of keratinized mucosa to favor improved scores referred to as plaque index, modified gingival index, mucosal recession, and attachment loss [47]. Likewise, it has been demonstrated that the presence of keratinized mucosa around dental implants has a positive impact upon the immunological features, with a negative correlation to prostaglandin E2 levels [48]. This is due in part to a reduced inflammatory condition as a consequence of less discomfort during personal-administered oral hygiene. In fact, two recent clinical studies have shown the presence of ≥2 mm of keratinized mucosa to be crucial for the prevention of peri-implant diseases in erratic maintenance compliers [49] (Figure 3; Figure 4).

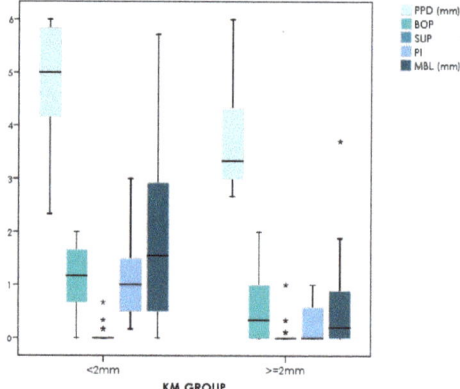

Figure 3. Comparative plot showing the clinical and radiographic differences between <2 mm versus ≥2 mm of peri-implant keratinized mucosa in erratic maintenance compliers [49]. Note: * stand for the outliers

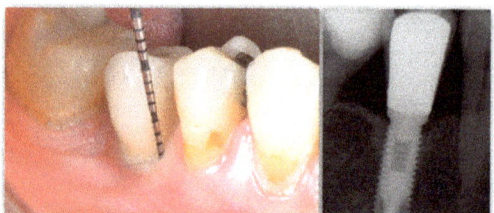

Figure 4. Representative case of an erratic maintenance complier with inadequate personal-administered oral hygiene presenting with healthy clinical and radiographic peri-implant conditions in the presence of 2 mm of keratinized and attached mucosa.

Table 2. Conflicting findings concerning the significance of the presence or lack of keratinized mucosa around dental implants.

Study	Study Design	Implant Function Time (Mean)	Methods	Clinical, Radiographic, and Patient-Reported Outcomes
Wennstrom et al. 1994 [46]	Prospective	5–10 years	39 patients (171 Branemark pure titanium implants)	• 24% of the implants presented with no KM • 13% of the implants presented with <2 mm of KM • 39% of the implants had attached mucosa • Neither attached nor keratinized mucosa were associated to peri-implant conditions
Romanos et al. 2015 [50]	Cross-sectional	9.4 years	118 patients (320 implants) Platform switched dental implants	• A wide band of ≥2 mm of KM was associated with a significantly lower mBI (0.12 ± 0.37; $p < 0.0001$), plaque index (0.45 ± 0.56; $p = 0.001$), and less mucosal recession (0.06 ± 0.23; $p < 0.0001$) than a narrow band of KM (<2 mm) • Considering regular and irregular implant maintenance therapy, a statistically significant difference was found between wide and narrow width of KM • In irregular compliers, the presence of KM is a protective mechanism for better peri-implant conditions
Roccuzzo et al. 2016 [51]	Prospective	10 years	98 patients	• The absence of KM was associated with greater plaque accumulation, greater soft-tissue recession, and a larger number of sites requiring additional surgical and/or antibiotic treatment • Patient-reported outcomes regarding maintenance procedures showed major differences between the groups, favoring the presence of KM
Bonino et al. 2018 [52]	Prospective	6 months	238 patients (216 implants with mucositis/46 implants diagnosed with peri-implantitis)	• Patients without peri-implant KM were less satisfied with the esthetics of the soft tissues around their implants ($p < 0.01$) • Lack of KM was not associated with discomfort during brushing • There was greater recession around implants without KM after 3 months ($p < 0.01$), but not after 6 months
Perussolo et al. 2018 [53]	Prospective	4 years	54 patients (202 implants)	• The values of the clinical parameters were greater in the <2 mm KM band: mean mPI (0.91 ± 0.60), BOP (0.67 ± 0.21), and BD (12.28 ± 17.59) • Marginal bone loss was greater in the KM < 2 mm group (0.26 ± 0.71) than in the KM ≥ 2 mm group (0.06 ± 0.48) • KM width and time in function had a statistically significant effect on marginal bone loss • In the <2 mm KM group, 51.4% presented with discomfort during brushing
Monje et al. 2018 [49]	Cross-sectional	5.73 years	37 patients (66 implants: 26 implants <2 mm/40 implants ≥2 mm) Erratic maintenance compliers (<2×/year)	• On comparing a KM band of <2 mm versus ≥2 mm, and with the exception of suppuration ($p = 0.6$), all the clinical and radiographic parameters were significantly increased when the KM band was <2 mm ($p < 0.001$) • A significant correlation was observed between KM and KT ($r = 0.55$) • A lack of KM did not condition a lack of KT • In the presence of peri-implantitis, only bleeding on probing at the adjacent dentate sites was seen to be increased • Patients had no brushing discomfort with a mean band of KM ≥ 2.5 mm

KM: keratinized mucosa; KT: keratinized gingival tissue; mBI: modified bleeding index; BOP: bleeding on probing; mPI: modified plaque index; BD: brushing discomfort.

Thus, a lack of keratinized mucosa in patients with inadequate oral hygiene could be regarded as a predisposing factor for peri-implant diseases, since it is associated with more recession, less vestibular depth, and more plaque accumulation, which, in turn, may be predisposing to inflammation (i.e., peri-implantitis).

5.2. Surgical Predisposing Factors

5.2.1. Significance of Implant Malpositioning as an Iatrogenic Factor: Critical Bone Dimensions

In the 2017 World Workshop on the classification of Periodontal and Peri-Implant Diseases and Conditions, implant malpositioning was suggested to be a predisposing factor for peri-implantitis due to the limited access for adequate oral hygiene often associated with these implant-supported restorations. If fact, a retrospective study associated implant malpositioning (OR = 48), occlusal overload (OR = 18.7), prosthetic problems (OR = 3.7), and bone grafting procedures (OR = 2.4) with peri-implantitis [54]. An early survey of cases reported in the literature as corresponding to peri-implantitis, following evaluation by a group of independent experts in the field, agreed that >40% of the implants diagnosed with peri-implantitis presented with a too-buccal position, with perfect interexaminer agreement (k = 0.81) [55]. This is in contrast to a four-year clinical study which found implants with residual buccal dehiscence defects to be more prone to develop peri-implantitis [56].

A comprehensive understanding of bone biology is crucial to conceive implant positioning, in particular, too-buccal positioning, as a predisposing factor for peri-implantitis. In a healed ridge, the alveolar process is composed of cortical bone at the outer side, while cancellous bone is featured in the inner structure. The cortical bone receives a blood supply branched from the outside through blood vessels of the periosteal surface, and from the inside from the endosteum [57]. When an implant is inserted with an open-flap procedure, elevation of the periosteum eliminates the periosteal blood supply from the outside. The same process occurs from the inside, since insertion of the implant interrupts the endosteal blood supply. This phenomenon of avascular necrosis is well known in bone biology [58] (Figure 5). A recent study has demonstrated that the critical buccal bone thickness for preventing marked physiological buccal–lingual bone resorption is 1.5 mm. In the absence of this thickness, more pronounced peri-implantitis may occur as a consequence of the microrough surface exposed to the oral cavity-facilitating surface contamination and the chronification of peri-implant infection [59] (Figure 6).

Likewise, apico-coronal implant positioning might dictate the long-term stability of the peri-implant tissues (Figure 7). Based on the hypothesis that too-apical implant positioning may favor the establishment of a microbial anaerobic environment, it is advised that implants be placed within the apico-coronal safety threshold. A recent retrospective analysis has validated this idea. Kumar et al., in nonsplinted single implants in function for at least five years, demonstrated that implant placement at a depth of ≥ 6 mm from the cementoenamel junction of the adjacent teeth is more commonly associated with peri-implantitis (OR = 8.5) [60]. Similarly, it should be noted that other factors could increase bone loss in these scenarios such as the type of implant–abutment connection (external vs internal vs conical) [61], number of abutment connection/disconnection [62], or the increased difficulty in removing cement remnants in case of cemented restorations [63].

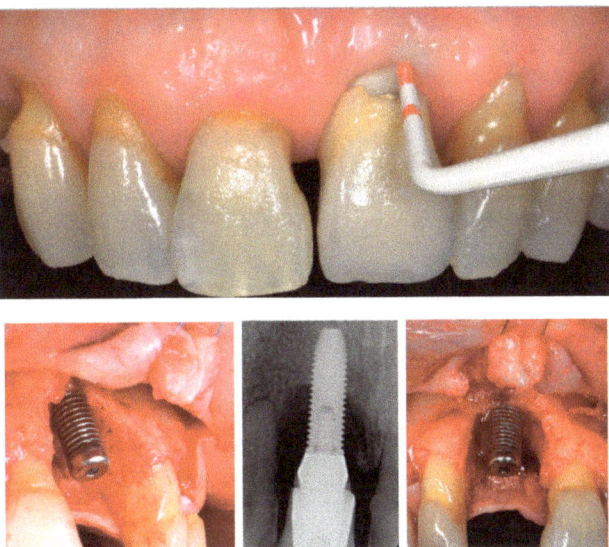

Figure 5. A critical buccal bone thickness of 1.5 mm is essential for preventing excessive physiological and pathological bone loss as a consequence of early avascular necrosis leading to peri-implant bone loss and thus to an increased risk of surface contamination.

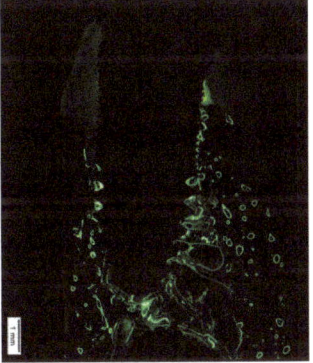

Figure 6. Histological analysis with fluorescent dyes illustrating excessive bone loss as a consequence of ligature-induced peri-implantitis. Note that the lack of fluorescence on the buccal side demonstrates the severe vertical bone resorption that occurs after physiological bone remodeling due to the insufficient critical buccal bone thickness (<1.5 mm).

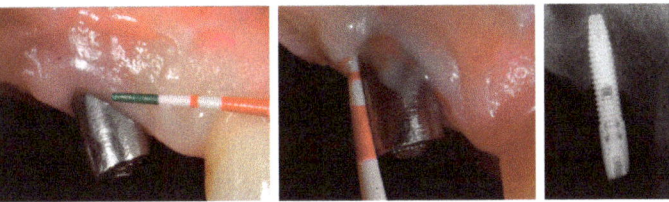

Figure 7. Inadequate apico-coronal implant positioning may favor the establishment of a microbial anaerobic environment that can be predisposing to progressive pathological peri-implant bone loss.

The mesiodistal implant position could be regarded as a predisposing factor for peri-implant bone loss, leading to peri-implantitis due to two main factors: (1) inadequate access for performing correct oral hygiene; and (2) excessive physiological bone remodeling if no safety distance is ensured between two adjacent dental implants or one implant with the adjoining dentition (Figure 8). Classically, the recommendation was to leave 3 mm between dental implants [64]. Even though this is no longer applicable to current implant dentistry due to advances in implant–abutment designs, a safety distance must be observed in order to avoid avascular necrosis of the interimplant cortical bone, with sufficient space to favor adequate personal oral hygiene.

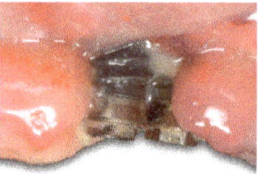
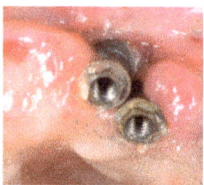
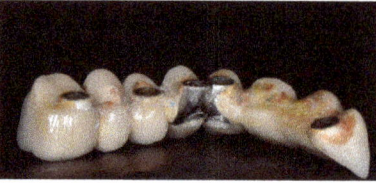

Figure 8. Incorrect implant positioning predisposes dental implants to peri-implant diseases due to the inability to perform correct oral hygiene.

5.2.2. Implant Insertion Torque and Its Interplay with the Hard Tissue Substratum

Implant placement in low-density bone can prove challenging. Thus, in order to ensure adequate primary stability and reduce early osseointegration implant failures, adaptation of the drilling protocol to the bone features has been recommended [65]. In fact, modifications in implant macrodesign, the use of osteotome condenser drills, and underpreparation of the implant socket may increase primary stability and osseointegration [65]. It is important to note that the connections between the trabecular mesh give cancellous bone the capacity to bear loads [66]; atraumatic surgical procedures therefore minimize the risk of bone loss. Thus, the use of drills to condense and densify trabecular bone might disrupt the connectivity of the trabecular network, reduce the capacity of bone to transmit occlusal forces, and result in weak bone that might not guarantee secondary stability due to higher bone turnover [66]. In fact, excessive compression of peri-implant bone by using osteotomes or increased torque may lead to 22–50% more crestal bone loss than conventional implantation [67,68] and also to a 41% reduction in the amount of bone-to-implant contact [69]. Such mechanical devices may damage the canalicular network of the trabecular bone, leading to a change in fluid flow mechanisms, impairment of mechanical stimulation, and delayed new bone formation [69]. Similar undesirable effects may be caused by excessive torque [70], leading to bone compression and delaying bone healing [71] (Figure 9). Areas with minimal bone-to-implant contact and therefore low strain seem to promote faster osteoblast differentiation [66,71,72]. During the first weeks, bone in contact areas around the implant threading is reabsorbed, and bone formation occurs earlier in contact-free areas [73].

The assessment of bone architecture is also relevant for implant drilling [74]. Larger osteocyte necrosis areas were found in trabecular bone versus cortical bone (550 versus 1400 μm, respectively) [65]. A similar increase in osteocyte damaged area was found when drilling speed was raised from 500 to 1500 rpm (600 versus 1400 μm, respectively) [65]. When using a 1.6 mm drill, a distance of 1050 μm of bone damage from the osteotomy center is expected, whereas the distance is about 1400 μm if a 5 mm drill is used [74]. The larger the drill diameter, the greater the tangential speed and centrifugal force, and therefore also the drilling power and energy transmitted to the bone. Lower values of early bone area formation around 5 mm implants versus 3.75 mm implants were found, and the use of large-diameter drills may be one of the underlying reasons [75]. Recently, simplified protocols have been proposed to reduce drilling time. Some authors reported no detrimental effects upon bone formation [75], but less bone formation was found in early stages in other studies [76]. It is important to note that simplified protocols might increase bone compression [76]. Moreover, the drill torque energy applied to the bone increases as the diameters of two consecutive drills increase. This fact might elevate the bone temperature and consequently the area of bone damage [65]. Further, other approaches, such as ultrasonic site preparation, have evidenced better preservation of the bone microarchitecture, resulting in a faster healing response [77].

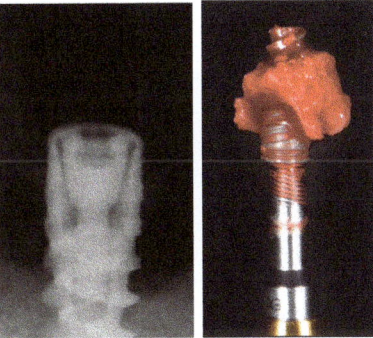

Figure 9. Implant removed four months after placement in the mandible. Note that the implant macrodesign, together with a highly corticalized bone structure, have induced excessive bone loss extending on the coronal portion of the implant and creating bone necrosis on the apical part. The severe bone resorption in the coronal area might have been predisposing to peri-implantitis as a biological complication if the implant had not been removed.

5.3. Significance of Prosthetic Design

Assuming the role of biofilm and its bacterial byproducts in the onset and progression of peri-implantitis, it is conceivable that retentive prosthetic components may promote inflammation (Figure 10). In this regard, Serino and Strom demonstrated that regardless of adequate oral hygiene of the natural dentition in partially edentulous patients, prosthetic design plays a major role in plaque accumulation around implant-supported prostheses. The authors found that adequate oral hygiene could not be performed in 53 out of 58 implants, and that peri-implantitis therefore could be attributed to deficient access for personal oral hygiene [78]. This is a typical scenario in hybrid prostheses, where esthetic requirements are satisfied but long-term implant maintenance is jeopardized owing to poor access for oral hygiene. Similarly, bone-level, implant-supported single crowns with an emergence angle of over 30 degrees and a convex profile have been shown to be factors strongly associated with peri-implantitis. This was not consistent with the findings in tissue-level implants [79]. Hence, convexities and marked emergence profiles should be avoided in the design of single crowns. In any case, patients should be comprehensively instructed to use interproximal brushes to remove food debris or plaque within the implant surroundings [2].

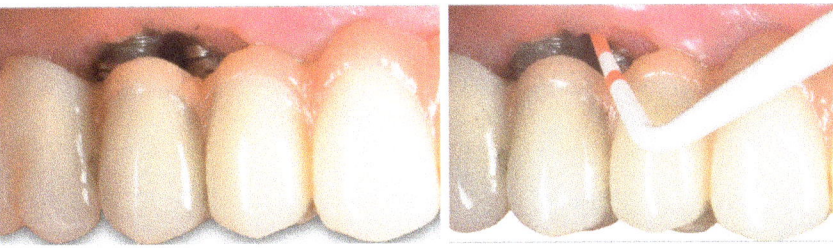

Figure 10. A hybrid prosthesis does not facilitate adequate oral hygiene and favors plaque retention, thereby triggering peri-implantitis.

Into the bargain, conceiving that excessive early bone resorption is often associated with greater late bone loss [26], prosthetic factors associated with minimal physiological bone loss should be noted. In this sense, longer transmucosal abutments (>2 mm) [80] and internal connection (including platform-switching [81] and Morse cone connections [82]) have demonstrated efficient preservation of the peri-implant hard tissue levels.

6. Local Precipitant Factors

The literature describes a few factors (so-called precipitant factors) associated with the triggering of inflammation within the peri-implant sulcus.

6.1. Residual Submucosal Cement

While screw-retained restorations do not necessarily outperform cement-retained prostheses, the presence of residual cement has been shown to have a deleterious effect upon the peri-implant tissues. Wilson et al. demonstrated the triggering role of residual cement, since 81% of the cases developed peri-implantitis, with spontaneous resolution in 74% following mechanical removal of the excess cement [63]. Likewise, Linkevicius et al. demonstrated the effect of residual cement upon peri-implant tissue response. In this scenario, 85% of the cases developed peri-implant disease [83]. Similar findings were obtained by Korsch et al. in a later study affording further insight into the effect of cement type upon the development of pathological complications. It was seen that while methacrylate cement was present in 62% of the suprastructures, zinc oxide eugenol cement could not be detected [84]. As a matter of fact, it was seen that the clinical and radiographic peri-implant conditions were generally unfavorable for implant-retained suprastructures using methacrylate cement, irrespective of cement excess [84]. In view of the significance of the presence of residual cement upon peri-implant tissue stability, it is advisable to use radiopaque cement if needed, with the aim of promptly detecting and removing it.

6.2. Residual Dental Floss

The remnants of floss in the peri-implant sulcus have also been regarded as a triggering factor for peri-implantitis. Van Velzen et al. reported 10 cases with progressive peri-implantitis related to floss remnants. Interestingly, in 90% of the cases, the inflammation resolved spontaneously after mechanical removal of the remnants [85]. Thus, caution is required when providing personal oral hygiene instructions involving the use of floss, and patients should be further encouraged to employ interproximal brushes.

7. Local Accelerating Factors: Influence of Surface Topography upon Progressive Bone Loss

In the course of the evolution of implant dentistry, advances in the form of implant surface modifications have led to stronger bone responses and higher implant survival rates [86]. Associations have been reported between significantly greater crestal bone loss and different implant surfaces and topographic features [86]. Furthermore, it has been suggested that surface roughness might have some role in the incidence of peri-implantitis [87] (Figure 11). In contrast, other authors consider that there are no available data confirming an association between implant surface features and the initiation of peri-implantitis or the progression of established peri-implantitis [88]. Ligature animal models have shown an increased risk of peri-implantitis with SLA implants in comparison to machined implants [89], and with TiUnite implants in comparison to machined, SLA, and TiOblast implants [31,90,91]. Similarly, another preclinical study noted significantly greater intrasurgical defect depths, defect widths, probing depths, and radiographic bone loss with TiUnite implants than with Straumann SLA or Biomet T3 implants [92]. Other factors apart from surface features might be relevant in the initial phase; for example, the invaginating grooves and pits on the TiUnite surface might favor bacterial adhesion and protect bacteria from shear forces [92]. Interestingly, a recent systematic review failed to find a long-term association between different surface modifications. Hence, these data in humans suggest that it is possible to achieve very good long-term results with all types of moderately rough implant surfaces [93].

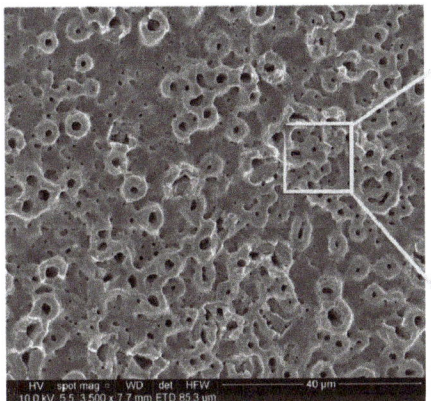 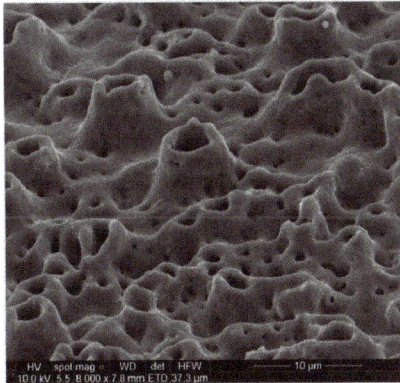

Figure 11. Moderately rough topographic characteristics (RA~1.3 µm) may induce chronification of the inflammatory condition by harboring pathogenic bacteria. This, in turn, may influence the therapeutic outcome. Note the scanning electron microscopic features of the implant surface under high magnification.

Furthermore, the management of established peri-implantitis is possible after surgical treatment, but the therapeutic outcome is also influenced by the implant surface characteristics [90]. In a randomized clinical trial on the effect of adjunctive systemic and local antimicrobial therapy in patients with peri-implantitis, treatment success was reported in 79% of the implants with nonmodified surface features, but in only 34% of the implants with modified surfaces [94]. Similarly, a three-year randomized controlled trial found the surgical treatment of peri-implantitis to be effective, with stable peri-implant marginal bone levels, but here again the nonmodified surfaces yielded significantly better results [95].

Depending on the surface modification methods used, some remnants may persist on the surface and have deleterious effects upon the clinical performance of the implant [87]. These particles and others released from the surface as a result of corrosion and mechanical wear may have cytotoxic effects and stimulate inflammatory reactions [8], leading to osteoclast activation and further peri-implant bone loss. Likewise, it has been recently evidenced that titanium particles derived from implants containing phosphate-enriched titanium oxide, fluoride-modified, and grit-blasted (GB) surface treatments are able to activate CHK2 and trigger the recruitment of BRCA1 in oral epithelial cells. These are markers for detecting activation of the DNA damage response. Accordingly, it can be inferred that titanium particles released into a surgical wound may contribute to the disruption of epithelial homeostasis, and potentially compromise the oral epithelial barrier [96].

8. Other Perspectives to Conceive Peri-Implantitis

Different perspectives to understand peri-implantitis have been further proposed. As such, it has been advocated that peri-implant marginal bone loss might be related to a change in the foreign body equilibrium between the host immune system and the implant device [97]. The biological behavior of the bone cells is mediated by the interaction among immune cells (neutrophils, macrophages, and lymphocytes) and the dental implant (or any kind of foreign body). Briefly, one of the very first interplays around the foreign body is carried out by neutrophils for 24–48 h [98]. The insertion of a dental implant induces a status of hypoxia in the surrounding bone that leads to neutrophil accumulation in order to promote angiogenesis. Also, neutrophil cells may discharge proteolytic enzymes and reactive oxygen species during their function that can erode the implant surface and release metal particles to the tissues [99]. After 48 h, the population of macrophages is higher around the foreign body and these cells may lead the evolution of the immune response. In fact, these cells promote osteoclastogenesis, matrix deposition, and bone anabolism [100], whereas macrophages' absence might impair osteoblast viability and bone formation [101,102]. Neutrophil apoptosis is mediated by macrophages during the shift between inflammatory phase to the healing phase. Also, the polarization between macrophages M1 to M2 and the length of each phase may have clinical effects, thereby an extended M1 phase may lead to a fibrous encapsulation of the fixture and implant failure [103]. On the contrary, higher presence of M2 macrophages has been reported on commercial pure implants [99,104], leading to bone deposition on the surface to isolate the fixture from the surrounding bone.

In addition, macrophages can differentiate into osteoclasts during bone remodeling and have phagocytosis capabilities until 5 μm of particle size [98]. Under presence of larger particles, macrophages tend to fuse to become foreign body giant cells (FBGCs). FBGCs are more frequent around the implant interface [105] than around healthy tissues and this fact might indicate the presence of a foreign body reaction around the dental fixture or the allogenic material.

Hence, under this concept of foreign body reaction, osseointegration is a mild chronic inflammatory and immunologically driven response where the bone–implant interface remains in a state of equilibrium but susceptible to changes in the environment [7,106]. Macrophages, FBGCs, and others approach this new bone barrier and if any disturbing factor occurs, a reactivation of the immuno-inflammatory cells against the foreign body material takes place. The loss of the foreign body equilibrium may thus stand as one of the reasons for this peri-implant bone loss [98].

9. Conclusions

Site-specific diseases are often attributable to local predisposing factors. In the case of plaque-associated peri-implantitis, local contributors, including surgical and prosthetic factors, as well as soft and hard tissue characteristics, may be predisposing factors to biofilm adherence around dental implants, thus leading to inflammation. Moreover, two major precipitant or triggering factors can be identified: residual cement and residual floss. In addition, current evidence seems to suggest that certain surface topographies can further accelerate the process of peri-implantitis.

Funding: The present review was partially founded by FEDICOM Foundation (Badajoz, Spain).

Conflicts of Interest: The authors declare no direct and potential conflict of interest with respect to the authorship or concepts presented in this article.

References

1. Tonetti, M.S.; Chapple, I.L.; Jepsen, S.; Sanz, M. Primary and secondary prevention of periodontal and peri-implant diseases: Introduction to, and objectives of the 11th European Workshop on Periodontology consensus conference. *J. Clin. Periodontol.* **2015**, *42* (Suppl. 16), S1–S4. [CrossRef]
2. Jepsen, S.; Berglundh, T.; Zitzmann, N.U.; Genco, R.; Aass, A.M.; Demirel, K.; Derks, J.; Figuero, E.; Giovannoli, J.L.; Goldstein, M.; et al. Primary prevention of peri-implantitis: Managing peri-implant mucositis. *J. Clin. Periodontol.* **2015**, *42* (Suppl. 16), S152–S157. [CrossRef]
3. Schwarz, F.; Derks, J.; Monje, A.; Wang, H.L. Peri-implantitis. *J. Periodontol.* **2018**, *89* (Suppl. 1), S267–S290. [CrossRef]
4. Albrektsson, T.; Jemt, T.; Mölne, J.; Tengvall, P.; Wennerberg, A. On inflammation-immunological balance theory-A critical apprehension of disease concepts around implants: Mucositis and marginal bone loss may represent normal conditions and not necessarily a state of disease. *Clin. Implant Dent. Relat. Res.* **2019**, *21*, 183–189. [CrossRef] [PubMed]
5. Albrektsson, T.; Chrcanovic, B.; Mölne, J.; Wennerberg, A. Foreign body reactions, marginal bone loss and allergies in relation to titanium implants. *Eur. J. Oral Implantol.* **2018**, *11* (Suppl. 1), S37–S46.

6. Tomas, A.; Luigi, C.; David, C.; Hugo, D.B. "Peri-Implantitis": A Complication of a Foreign Body or a Man-Made "Disease". Facts and Fiction. *Clin. Implant Dent. Relat. Res.* **2016**, *18*, 840–849.
7. Dahlin, C.; Sennerby, L.; Turri, A.; Albrektsson, T.; Jemt, T.; Wennerberg, A. Is Marginal Bone Loss around Oral Implants the Result of a Provoked Foreign Body Reaction? *Clin. Implant Dent. Relat. Res.* **2014**, *16*, 155–165.
8. Apaza-Bedoya, K.; Tarce, M.; Benfatti, C.A.M.; Henriques, B.; Mathew, M.T.; Teughels, W.; De Souza, J.C.M.; Apaza-Bedoya, K. Synergistic interactions between corrosion and wear at titanium-based dental implant connections: A scoping review. *J. Periodontal. Res.* **2017**, *52*, 946–954. [CrossRef] [PubMed]
9. Berglundh, T.; Zitzmann, N.U.; Donati, M. Are peri-implantitis lesions different from periodontitis lesions? *J. Clin. Periodontol.* **2011**, *38* (Suppl. 11), 188–202. [CrossRef]
10. Derks, J.; Schaller, D.; Håkansson, J.; Wennström, J.L.; Tomasi, C.; Berglundh, T. Peri-implantitis—Onset and pattern of progression. *J. Clin. Periodontol.* **2016**, *43*, 383–388. [CrossRef] [PubMed]
11. Sanz, M.; Chapple, I.L.; Working Group 4 of the VIII European Workshop on Periodontology. Clinical research on peri-implant diseases: Consensus report of Working Group 4. *J. Clin. Periodontol.* **2012**, *39* (Suppl. 12), 202–206. [CrossRef] [PubMed]
12. Berglundh, T.; Armitage, G.; Araújo, M.G.; Avila-Ortiz, G.; Blanco, J.; Camargo, P.M.; Chen, S.; Cochran, D.; Derks, J.; Figuero, E.; et al. Peri-implant diseases and conditions: Consensus report of workgroup 4 of the 2017 World Workshop on the Classification of Periodontal and Peri-Implant Diseases and Conditions. *J. Periodontol.* **2018**, *89* (Suppl. 1), S313–S318. [CrossRef]
13. Rakic, M.; Galindo-Moreno, P.; Monje, A.; Radovanovic, S.; Wang, H.-L.; Cochran, D.; Sculean, A.; Canullo, L. How frequent does peri-implantitis occur? A systematic review and meta-analysis. *Clin. Oral Investig.* **2018**, *22*, 1805–1816. [CrossRef] [PubMed]
14. Derks, J.; Tomasi, C. Peri-implant health and disease. A systematic review of current epidemiology. *J. Clin. Periodontol.* **2015**, *42* (Suppl. 16), 158–171. [CrossRef]
15. Aranda, L.; Diaz, K.; Alarcón, M.; Bagramian, R.; Catena, A.; Wang, H.; Monje, A. Impact of Maintenance Therapy for the Prevention of Peri-implant Diseases. A Systematic Review and Meta-analysis. *J. Dent. Res.* **2015**, *95*, 372–379.
16. Renvert, S.; Persson, G.R. Periodontitis as a potential risk factor for peri-implantitis. *J. Clin. Periodontol.* **2009**, *36* (Suppl. 10), 9–14. [CrossRef]
17. Sgolastra, F.; Petrucci, A.; Severino, M.; Gatto, R.; Monaco, A. Smoking and the risk of peri-implantitis. A systematic review and meta-analysis. *Clin. Oral Implant Res.* **2015**, *26*, e62–e67. [CrossRef] [PubMed]
18. Monje, A.; Catena, A.; Borgnakke, W.S. Association between diabetes mellitus/hyperglycaemia and peri-implant diseases: Systematic review and meta-analysis. *J. Clin. Periodontol.* **2017**, *44*, 636–648. [CrossRef] [PubMed]
19. Monje, A.; Galindo-Moreno, P.; Canullo, L.; Greenwell, H.; Wang, H.-L. Editorial: From Early Physiological Marginal Bone Loss to Peri-Implant Disease: On the Unknown Local Contributing Factors. *Int. J. Periodontics Restor. Dent.* **2016**, *35*, 764–765.
20. Monje, A.; Asa'Ad, F.; Larsson, L.; Giannobile, W.; Wang, H.-L. Editorial Epigenetics: A Missing Link Between Periodontitis and Peri-implantitis? *Int. J. Periodontics Restor. Dent.* **2018**, *38*, 476–477. [CrossRef] [PubMed]
21. Larsson, L.; Castilho, R.M.; Giannobile, W.V. Epigenetics and Its Role in Periodontal Diseases: A State-of-the-Art Review. *J. Periodontol.* **2015**, *86*, 556–568. [CrossRef] [PubMed]
22. Racine, N.M.; Riddell, R.R.P.; Khan, M.; Calic, M.; Taddio, A.; Tablon, P. Systematic Review: Predisposing, Precipitating, Perpetuating, and Present Factors Predicting Anticipatory Distress to Painful Medical Procedures in Children. *J. Pediatr. Psychol.* **2016**, *41*, 159–181. [CrossRef] [PubMed]
23. Brånemark, P.-I.; Adell, R.; Albrektsson, T.; Lekholm, U.; Lundkvist, S.; Rockler, B. Osseointegrated titanium fixtures in the treatment of edentulousness. *Biomaterials* **1983**, *4*, 17–20. [CrossRef]
24. Adell, R.; Lekholm, U.; Rockler, B.; Brånemark, P.-I. A 15-year study of osseointegrated implants in the treatment of the edentulous jaw. *Int. J. Oral Surg.* **1981**, *10*, 387–416. [CrossRef]
25. Teughels, W.; Van Assche, N.; Sliepen, I.; Quirynen, M. Effect of material characteristics and/or surface topography on biofilm development. *Clin. Oral Implants Res.* **2006**, *17* (Suppl. 2), 68–81. [CrossRef]

26. Galindo-Moreno, P.; León-Cano, A.; Ortega-Oller, I.; Monje, A.; O'valle, F.; Catena, A.; Galindo-Moreno, P.; León-Cano, A.; Ortega-Oller, I. Marginal bone loss as success criterion in implant dentistry: Beyond 2 mm. *Clin. Oral Implants Res.* **2015**, *26*, e28–e34. [CrossRef] [PubMed]
27. Figuero, E.; Graziani, F.; Sanz, I.; Herrera, D.; Sanz, M. Management of peri-implant mucositis and peri-implantitis. *Periodontol. 2000* **2014**, *66*, 255–273. [CrossRef] [PubMed]
28. Monje, A.; Insua, A.; Rakic, M.; Nart, J.; Moyano-Cuevas, J.L.; Wang, H.-L. Estimation of the diagnostic accuracy of clinical parameters for monitoring peri-implantitis progression: An experimental canine study. *J. Periodontol.* **2018**, *89*, 1442–1451. [CrossRef] [PubMed]
29. Carcuac, O.; Albouy, J.-P.; Linder, E.; Larsson, L.; Abrahamsson, I.; Albouy, J.; Berglundh, T. Experimental periodontitis and peri-implantitis in dogs. *Clin. Oral Implants Res.* **2013**, *24*, 363–371. [CrossRef] [PubMed]
30. Albouy, J.-P.; Abrahamsson, I.; Berglundh, T. Spontaneous progression of experimental peri-implantitis at implants with different surface characteristics: An experimental study in dogs. *J. Clin. Periodontol.* **2012**, *39*, 182–187. [CrossRef] [PubMed]
31. Albouy, J.-P.; Abrahamsson, I.; Persson, L.G.; Berglundh, T. Spontaneous progression of peri-implantitis at different types of implants. An experimental study in dogs. I: Clinical and radiographic observations. *Clin. Oral Implants Res.* **2008**, *19*, 997–1002. [CrossRef] [PubMed]
32. Farina, R.; Filippi, M.; Brazzioli, J.; Tomasi, C.; Trombelli, L. Bleeding on probing around dental implants: A retrospective study of associated factors. *J. Clin. Periodontol.* **2016**, *44*, 115–122. [CrossRef] [PubMed]
33. Fransson, C.; Tomasi, C.; Pikner, S.S.; Gröndahl, K.; Wennström, J.L.; Leyland, A.H.; Berglundh, T. Severity and pattern of peri-implantitis-associated bone loss. *J. Clin. Periodontol.* **2010**, *37*, 442–448. [CrossRef] [PubMed]
34. Fransson, C.; Wennström, J.; Tomasi, C.; Berglundh, T. Extent of peri-implantitis-associated bone loss. *J. Clin. Periodontol.* **2009**, *36*, 357–363. [CrossRef] [PubMed]
35. Monje, A.; Caballe-Serrano, J.; Nart, J.; Penarrocha, D.; Wang, H.-L.; Rakić, M. Diagnostic accuracy of clinical parameters to monitor peri-implant conditions: A matched case-control study. *J. Periodontol.* **2018**, *89*, 407–417. [CrossRef] [PubMed]
36. Ramanauskaite, A.; Becker, K.; Schwarz, F. Clinical characteristics of peri-implant mucositis and peri-implantitis. *Clin. Oral Implants Res.* **2018**, *29*, 551–556. [CrossRef] [PubMed]
37. Fransson, C.; Wennström, J.; Berglundh, T. Clinical characteristics at implants with a history of progressive bone loss. *Clin. Oral Implants Res.* **2008**, *19*, 142–147. [CrossRef] [PubMed]
38. Fransson, C.; Lekholm, U.; Jemt, T.; Berglundh, T. Prevalence of subjects with progressive bone loss at implants. *Clin. Oral Implants Res.* **2005**, *16*, 440–446. [CrossRef] [PubMed]
39. Schwarz, F.; Claus, C.; Becker, K. Correlation between horizontal mucosal thickness and probing depths at healthy and diseased implant sites. *Clin. Oral Implants Res.* **2017**, *28*, 1158–1163. [CrossRef] [PubMed]
40. Schwarz, F.; Becker, K.; Sahm, N.; Horstkemper, T.; Rousi, K.; Becker, J. The prevalence of peri-implant diseases for two-piece implants with an internal tube-in-tube connection: A cross-sectional analysis of 512 implants. *Clin. Oral Implants Res.* **2017**, *28*, 24–28. [CrossRef] [PubMed]
41. Wennström, J.L. Lack of association between width of attached gingiva and development of soft tissue recession. A 5-year longitudinal study. *J. Clin. Periodontol.* **1987**, *14*, 181–184. [CrossRef] [PubMed]
42. Wennström, J.; Lindhe, J. Plaque-induced gingival inflammation in the absence of attached gingiva in dogs. *J. Clin. Periodontol.* **1983**, *10*, 266–276. [CrossRef] [PubMed]
43. Lang, N.P.; Löe, H. The Relationship Between the Width of Keratinized Gingiva and Gingival Health. *J. Periodontol.* **1972**, *43*, 623–627. [CrossRef] [PubMed]
44. Stetler, K.J.; Bissada, N.F. Significance of the Width of Keratinized Gingiva on the Periodontal Status of Teeth with Submarginal Restorations. *J. Periodontol.* **1987**, *58*, 696–700. [CrossRef] [PubMed]
45. Coatoam, G.W.; Behrents, R.G.; Bissada, N.F. The Width of Keratinized Gingiva During Orthodontic Treatment: Its Significance and Impact on Periodontal Status. *J. Periodontol.* **1981**, *52*, 307–313. [CrossRef] [PubMed]
46. Wennström, J.L.; Bengazi, F.; Lekholm, U. The influence of the masticatory mucosa on the peri-implant soft tissue condition. *Implant Dent.* **1994**, *3*, 266. [CrossRef]
47. Lin, G.-H.; Chan, H.-L.; Wang, H.-L. The Significance of Keratinized Mucosa on Implant Health: A Systematic Review. *J. Periodontol.* **2013**, *84*, 1755–1767. [CrossRef] [PubMed]

48. Zigdon, H.; Machtei, E.E. The dimensions of keratinized mucosa around implants affect clinical and immunological parameters. *Clin. Oral Implants Res.* **2008**, *19*, 387–392. [CrossRef] [PubMed]
49. Monje, A.; Blasi, G. Significance of keratinized mucosa/gingiva on peri-implant and adjacent periodontal conditions in erratic maintenance compliers. *J. Periodontol.* **2018**. [CrossRef] [PubMed]
50. Romanos, G.; Grizas, E.; Nentwig, G.H. Association of Keratinized Mucosa and Periimplant Soft Tissue Stability Around Implants with Platform Switching. *Implant Dent.* **2015**, *24*, 422–426. [PubMed]
51. Roccuzzo, M.; Grasso, G.; Dalmasso, P. Keratinized mucosa around implants in partially edentulous posterior mandible: 10-year results of a prospective comparative study. *Clin. Oral Implants Res.* **2016**, *27*, 491–496. [CrossRef] [PubMed]
52. Bonino, F.; Steffensen, B.; Natto, Z.; Hur, Y.; Holtzman, L.P.; Weber, H.-P. Prospective study of the impact of peri-implant soft tissue properties on patient-reported and clinically assessed outcomes. *J. Periodontol.* **2018**, *89*, 1025–1032. [CrossRef] [PubMed]
53. Perussolo, J.; Souza, A.B.; Matarazzo, F.; Oliveira, R.P.; Araújo, M.G. Influence of the keratinized mucosa on the stability of peri-implant tissues and brushing discomfort: A 4-year follow-up study. *Clin. Oral Implants Res.* **2018**, *29*, 1177–1185. [CrossRef] [PubMed]
54. Canullo, L.; Peñarrocha-Oltra, D.; Covani, U.; Botticelli, D.; Serino, G.; Peñarrocha, M.; Peñarrocha-Oltra, D. Clinical and microbiological findings in patients with peri-implantitis: A cross-sectional study. *Clin. Oral Implants Res.* **2016**, *27*, 376–382. [CrossRef] [PubMed]
55. Monje, A.; Galindo-Moreno, P.; Tözüm, T.; Del Amo, F.S.-L.; Wang, H.-L. Into the Paradigm of Local Factors as Contributors for Peri-implant Disease: Short Communication. *Int. J. Oral Maxillofac. Implants* **2016**, *31*, 288–292. [CrossRef] [PubMed]
56. Sahm, N.; Schwarz, F.; Becker, J. Impact of the outcome of guided bone regeneration in dehiscence-type defects on the long-term stability of peri-implant health: Clinical observations at 4 years. *Clin. Oral Implants Res.* **2011**, *23*, 191–196.
57. Roush, J.K.; E Howard, P.; Wilson, J.W. Normal blood supply to the canine mandible and mandibular teeth. *Am. J. Vet. Res.* **1989**, *50*, 904–907. [PubMed]
58. Roux, S.; Orcel, P. Bone loss. Factors that regulate osteoclast differentiation: An update. *Arthritis Res.* **2000**, *2*, 451. [CrossRef] [PubMed]
59. Monje, A.; Insua, A.; Monje, F.; Muñoz, F.; Salvi, G.E.; Buser, D.; Chappuis, V. Diagnostic accuracy of the implant stability quotient in monitoring progressive peri-implant bone loss: An experimental study in dogs. *Clin. Oral Implants Res.* **2018**, *29*, 1016–1024. [CrossRef] [PubMed]
60. Hegde, R.; Ranganathan, N.; Mariotti, A.; Kumar, P.S.; Dabdoub, S.M. Site-level risk predictors of peri-implantitis: A retrospective analysis. *J. Clin. Periodontol.* **2018**, *45*, 597–604.
61. Galindo-Moreno, P.; Fernández-Jiménez, A.; O'Valle, F.; Monje, A.; Silvestre, F.J.; Juodzbalys, G.; Sánchez-Fernández, E.; Catena, A. Influence of the Crown-Implant Connection on the Preservation of Peri-Implant Bone: A Retrospective Multifactorial Analysis. *Int. J. Oral Maxillofac. Implants* **2015**, *30*, 384–390. [CrossRef] [PubMed]
62. Abrahamsson, I.; Berglundh, T.; Lindhe, J. The mucosal barrier following abutment dis/reconnection. An experimental study in dogs. *J. Clin. Periodontol.* **1997**, *24*, 568–572. [CrossRef] [PubMed]
63. Wilson, T.G., Jr. The Positive Relationship Between Excess Cement and Peri-Implant Disease: A Prospective Clinical Endoscopic Study. *J. Periodontol.* **2009**, *80*, 1388–1392. [CrossRef] [PubMed]
64. Tarnow, D.P.; Magner, A.W.; Fletcher, P. The Effect of the Distance from the Contact Point to the Crest of Bone on the Presence or Absence of the Interproximal Dental Papilla. *J. Periodontol.* **1992**, *63*, 995–996. [CrossRef] [PubMed]
65. Aghvami, M.; Brunski, J.B.; Tulu, U.S.; Chen, C.-H.; Helms, J.A. A Thermal and Biological Analysis of Bone Drilling. *J. Biomech. Eng.* **2018**, *140*, 101010. [CrossRef] [PubMed]
66. Wang, L.; Wu, Y.; Perez, K.; Hyman, S.; Brunski, J.; Tulu, U.; Bao, C.; Salmon, B.; Helms, J. Effects of Condensation on Peri-implant Bone Density and Remodeling. *J. Dent. Res.* **2017**, *96*, 413–420. [CrossRef] [PubMed]
67. Buhite, R. Implants in the Posterior Maxilla: A Comparative Clinical and Radiologic Study. *Int. J. Oral Maxillofac. Implants* **2005**, *20*, 231–237. [CrossRef]
68. Anitua, E.; Murias-Freijo, A.; Alkhraisat, M.H. Implant Site Under-Preparation to Compensate the Remodeling of an Autologous Bone Block Graft. *J. Craniofac. Surg.* **2015**, *26*, 374–377. [CrossRef] [PubMed]

69. Büchter, A.; Kleinheinz, J.; Wiesmann, H.P.; Jayaranan, M.; Joos, U.; Meyer, U. Interface reaction at dental implants inserted in condensed bone. *Clin. Oral Implants Res.* **2005**, *16*, 509–517. [CrossRef] [PubMed]
70. Insua, A.; Monje, A.; Wang, H.-L.; Miron, R.J.; Wang, H. Basis of bone metabolism around dental implants during osseointegration and peri-implant bone loss. *J. Biomed. Mater. Res.* **2017**, *105*, 2075–2089. [CrossRef] [PubMed]
71. Yin, X.; Mouraret, S.; Cha, J.Y.; Pereira, M.; Smith, A.; Houschyar, K.; Brunski, J.; Helms, J. Multiscale analyses of the bone-implant interface. *J. Dent. Res.* **2015**, *94*, 482–490.
72. Wang, L.; Aghvami, M.; Brunski, J.; Helms, J. Biophysical regulation of osteotomy healing: An animal study. *Clin. Implant Dent. Relat. Res.* **2017**, *19*, 590–599. [CrossRef] [PubMed]
73. Berglundh, T.; Abrahamsson, I.; Lang, N.P.; Lindhe, J. De novo alveolar bone formation adjacent to endosseous implants. *Clin. Oral Implants Res.* **2003**, *14*, 251–262. [CrossRef] [PubMed]
74. Monje, A.; Chan, H.-L.; Galindo-Moreno, P.; Elnayef, B.; Del Amo, F.S.-L.; Wang, F.; Wang, H.-L. Alveolar Bone Architecture: A Systematic Review and Meta-Analysis. *J. Periodontol.* **2015**, *86*, 1231–1248. [CrossRef] [PubMed]
75. Jimbo, R.; Janal, M.N.; Marin, C.; Giro, G.; Tovar, N.; Coelho, P.G. The effect of implant diameter on osseointegration utilizing simplified drilling protocols. *Clin. Oral Implants Res.* **2014**, *25*, 1295–1300. [CrossRef] [PubMed]
76. Gil, L.; Sarendranath, A.; Neiva, R.; Marão, H.; Tovar, N.; Bonfante, E.; Janal, M.; Castellano, A.; Coelho, P. Bone Healing Around Dental Implants: Simplified vs Conventional Drilling Protocols at Speed of 400 rpm. *Int. J. Oral Maxillofac. Implants* **2017**, *32*, 329–336. [CrossRef] [PubMed]
77. Rashad, A.; Sadr-Eshkevari, P.; Weuster, M.; Schmitz, I.; Prochnow, N.; Maurer, P.; Sadr-Eshkevari, P. Material attrition and bone micromorphology after conventional and ultrasonic implant site preparation. *Clin. Oral Implants Res.* **2013**, *24* (Suppl. A100), 110–114. [CrossRef]
78. Serino, G.; Strom, C. Peri-implantitis in partially edentulous patients: Association with inadequate plaque control. *Clin. Oral Implants Res.* **2009**, *20*, 169–174. [CrossRef] [PubMed]
79. Katafuchi, M.; Weinstein, B.F.; Leroux, B.G.; Daubert, D.M.; Chen, Y.-W.; Chen, Y. Restoration contour is a risk indicator for peri-implantitis: A cross-sectional radiographic analysis. *J. Clin. Periodontol.* **2018**, *45*, 225–232. [CrossRef] [PubMed]
80. Ortega-Oller, I.; Monje, A.; Spinato, S.; Catena, A.; León-Cano, A.; Galindo-Moreno, P.; Suárez, F.; Óvalle, F. Prosthetic Abutment Height is a Key Factor in Peri-implant Marginal Bone Loss. *J. Dent. Res.* **2014**, *93* (Suppl. 7), 80–85.
81. Galindo-Moreno, P.; León-Cano, A.; Monje, A.; Ortega-Oller, I.; O′valle, F.; Catena, A.; Galindo-Moreno, P.; León-Cano, A.; Ortega-Oller, I. Abutment height influences the effect of platform switching on peri-implant marginal bone loss. *Clin. Oral Implants Res.* **2015**, *27*, 167–173. [CrossRef] [PubMed]
82. Degidi, M.; Daprile, G.; Piattelli, A. Marginal bone loss around implants with platform-switched Morse-cone connection: A radiographic cross-sectional study. *Clin. Oral Implants Res.* **2017**, *28*, 1108–1112. [CrossRef] [PubMed]
83. Linkevicius, T.; Puisys, A.; Vindasiute, E.; Linkeviciene, L.; Apse, P. Does residual cement around implant-supported restorations cause peri-implant disease? A retrospective case analysis. *Clin. Oral Implants Res.* **2013**, *24*, 1179–1184. [CrossRef] [PubMed]
84. Korsch, M.; Walther, W. Peri-Implantitis Associated with Type of Cement: A Retrospective Analysis of Different Types of Cement and Their Clinical Correlation to the Peri-Implant Tissue. *Clin. Implant Dent. Relat. Res.* **2015**, *17* (Suppl. 2), 434–443. [CrossRef]
85. Van Velzen, F.J.J.; Lang, N.P.; Schulten, E.A.J.M.; Bruggenkate, C.M.T. Dental floss as a possible risk for the development of peri-implant disease: An observational study of 10 cases. *Clin. Oral Implants Res.* **2016**, *27*, 618–621. [CrossRef] [PubMed]
86. Jimbo, R.; Albrektsson, T. Long-term clinical success of minimally and moderately rough oral implants: A review of 71 studies with 5 years or more of follow-up. *Implant Dent.* **2015**, *24*, 62–69. [CrossRef] [PubMed]
87. De Bruyn, H.; Christiaens, V.; Doornewaard, R.; Jacobsson, M.; Cosyn, J.; Jacquet, W.; Vervaeke, S. Implant surface roughness and patient factors on long-term peri-implant bone loss. *Periodontology 2000* **2017**, *73*, 218–227. [CrossRef] [PubMed]
88. Renvert, S.; Polyzois, I.; Claffey, N. How do implant surface characteristics influence peri-implant disease? *J. Clin. Periodontol.* **2011**, *38* (Suppl. 11), 214–222. [CrossRef]

89. Berglundh, T.; Abrahamsson, I.; Welander, M.; Lang, N.P.; Lindhe, J. Morphogenesis of the peri-implant mucosa: An experimental study in dogs. *Clin. Oral Implants Res.* **2007**, *18*, 1–8. [CrossRef] [PubMed]
90. Albouy, J.-P.; Abrahamsson, I.; Persson, L.G.; Berglundh, T. Implant surface characteristics influence the outcome of treatment of peri-implantitis: An experimental study in dogs. *J. Clin. Periodontol.* **2010**, *38*, 58–64. [CrossRef] [PubMed]
91. Albouy, J.-P.; Abrahamsson, I.; Persson, L.G.; Berglundh, T. Spontaneous progression of ligatured induced peri-implantitis at implants with different surface characteristics. An experimental study in dogs II: Histological observations. *Clin. Oral Implants Res.* **2009**, *20*, 366–371. [CrossRef] [PubMed]
92. Fickl, S.; Kebschull, M.; Calvo-Guirado, J.L.; Hürzeler, M.; Zuhr, O.; Calvo-Guirado, J.L. Experimental Peri-Implantitis around Different Types of Implants—A Clinical and Radiographic Study in Dogs. *Clin. Implant Dent. Relat. Res.* **2015**, *17* (Suppl. 2), 661–669. [CrossRef]
93. Wennerberg, A.; Albrektsson, T.; Chrcanovic, B. Long-term clinical outcome of implants with different surface modifications. *Eur. J. Oral Implantol.* **2018**, *11* (Suppl. 1), S123–S136. [PubMed]
94. Carcuac, O.; Derks, J.; Charalampakis, G.; Abrahamsson, I.; Berglundh, T.; Wennström, J. Adjunctive Systemic and Local Antimicrobial Therapy in the Surgical Treatment of Peri-implantitis. *J. Dent. Res.* **2016**, *95*, 50–57. [CrossRef] [PubMed]
95. Carcuac, O.; Derks, J.; Abrahamsson, I.; Wennström, J.L.; Petzold, M.; Berglundh, T. Surgical treatment of peri-implantitis: 3-year results from a randomized controlled clinical trial. *J. Clin. Periodontol.* **2017**, *44*, 1294–1303. [CrossRef] [PubMed]
96. Del Amo, F.S.-L.; Rudek, I.; Wagner, V.; Martins, M.; O'Valle, F.; Galindo-Moreno, P.; Giannobile, W.; Wang, H.-L.; Castilho, R. Titanium Activates the DNA Damage Response Pathway in Oral Epithelial Cells: A Pilot Study. *Int. J. Oral Maxillofac. Implants* **2017**, *32*, 1413–1420. [CrossRef] [PubMed]
97. Albrektsson, T.; Buser, D.; Sennerby, L. Crestal Bone Loss and Oral implants. *Clin. Implant Dent. Relat. Res.* **2012**, *14*, 783–791. [CrossRef] [PubMed]
98. Amengual-Peñafiel, L.; Brañes-Aroca, M.; Marchesani-Carrasco, F.; Jara-Sepúlveda, M.C.; Parada-Pozas, L.; Cartes-Velásquez, R. Coupling between Osseointegration and Mechanotransduction to Maintain Foreign Body Equilibrium in the Long-Term: A Comprehensive Overview. *JCM* **2019**, *8*, 139. [CrossRef] [PubMed]
99. Trindade, R.; Albrektsson, T.; Galli, S.; Prgomet, Z.; Tengvall, P.; Wennerberg, A. Osseointegration and foreign body reaction: Titanium implants activate the immune system and suppress bone resorption during the first 4 weeks after implantation. *Clin. Implant Dent. Relat. Res.* **2018**, *20*, 82–91. [CrossRef] [PubMed]
100. Batoon, L.; Millard, S.M.; Raggatt, L.J.; Pettit, A. R Osteomacs and Bone Regeneration. *Curr. Osteoporos. Rep.* **2017**, *15*, 385–395. [CrossRef] [PubMed]
101. Pettit, A.R.; Chang, M.K.; Hume, D.A.; Raggatt, L.-J. Osteal macrophages: A new twist on coupling during bone dynamics. *Bone* **2008**, *43*, 976–982. [CrossRef] [PubMed]
102. Chang, M.K.; Raggatt, L.-J.; Alexander, K.A.; Kuliwaba, J.S.; Fazzalari, N.L.; Schröder, K.; Maylin, E.R.; Ripoll, V.M.; Hume, D.A.; Pettit, A.R.; et al. Osteal Tissue Macrophages Are Intercalated throughout Human and Mouse Bone Lining Tissues and Regulate Osteoblast Function In Vitro and In Vivo. *J. Immunol.* **2008**, *181*, 1232–1244. [CrossRef] [PubMed]
103. Li, B.; Gao, P.; Zhang, H.; Guo, Z.; Zheng, Y.; Han, Y. Osteoimmunomodulation, osseointegration, and in vivo mechanical integrity of pure Mg coated with HA nanorod/pore-sealed MgO bilayer. *Biomater. Sci.* **2018**, *6*, 3202–3218. [CrossRef] [PubMed]
104. Trindade, R.; Albrektsson, T.; Galli, S.; Prgomet, Z.; Tengvall, P.; Wennerberg, A. Bone Immune Response to Materials, Part I: Titanium, PEEK and Copper in Comparison to Sham at 10 Days in Rabbit Tibia. *JCM* **2018**, *7*, 526. [CrossRef] [PubMed]
105. Anderson, J.M.; Rodriguez, A.; Chang, D.T. Foreign body reaction to biomaterials. *Semin. Immunol.* **2008**, *20*, 86–100. [CrossRef] [PubMed]
106. Trindade, R.; Albrektsson, T.; Tengvall, P.; Wennerberg, A. Foreign Body Reaction to Biomaterials: On Mechanisms for Buildup and Breakdown of Osseointegration. *Clin. Implant Dent Relat. Res.* **2016**, *18*, 192–203. [CrossRef] [PubMed]

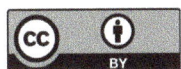

© 2019 by the authors. Licensee MDPI, Basel, Switzerland. This article is an open access article distributed under the terms and conditions of the Creative Commons Attribution (CC BY) license (http://creativecommons.org/licenses/by/4.0/).

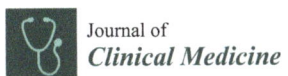

Editorial

Are Oral Implants the Same As Teeth?

Tomas Albrektsson

Department of Biomaterials, University of Gothenburg, 40530 Gothenburg, Sweden; tomas.albrektsson@biomaterials.gu.se; Tel.: +46-705916607

Received: 9 September 2019; Accepted: 10 September 2019; Published: 19 September 2019

Osseointegration of oral implants was initially discovered by Brånemark. The time for his discovery has incorrectly been said to have been during the 1950s [1,2], but in reality, the year was 1962 [3]. Brånemark operated the first patient with oral implants in 1965, only three years after his discovery. Osseointegration has meant a breakthrough for clinical results in oral and craniofacial implants [4,5] and has been applied, if in relatively small numbers, for anchorage of orthopedic implants in amputees [6]. The original definition of the term implied a direct contact, at the light microscopic level of resolution, between bone tissue and load-bearing implants [7,8]. Hip and knee arthroplasties do not present a direct bone anchorage, but instead display distance osteogenesis [9], probably due to the substantial clinical trauma at insertion. Nevertheless, clinical results of orthopedic implants have remained quite good, with 88% of operated hip replacements still in situ 25 years after surgery [10].

In 1985, I started seeing a researcher who later became a good friend. "Tomas" said this man to me in German, you must realize that osseointegration is but a "fremderkörperreaktion"—a foreign body reaction. It took me too many years to realize that this researcher, the now late Karl Donath of Hamburg University, was right [11,12]. Karl Donath was a pioneer. As happens to many pioneers his work was forgotten when later American colleagues started discussing implants as foreign bodies well into our new millennium and Donaths' papers published 15–20 years earlier were not even quoted.

What is then an oral implant? Some colleagues of ours saw the implant as being the same as the tooth it was replacing, exemplified in this volume in the paper by Monje and co-workers [13]. In fact, such a coupling between the tooth and the implant once lead to the assumption that since teeth display a disease entitled periodontitis, then implants will display a similar disease that was named peri-implantitis. The original reason for the alleged disease was bacterial attack, even if, at least in the case of tooth disease, hereditary factors were also acknowledged. This is the background to seeing marginal bone loss around oral implants as solely a disease phenomenon. This outlook stands in clear contrast to orthopedic implants. In orthopedics marginal bone loss may be seen in a pattern similar to an oral implant. However, the reason for marginal bone loss in a hip arthroplasty is assumed to depend on a condition named aseptic loosening, i.e., something quite in contrast to what is believed with respect to oral implants. Aseptic loosening has in recent studies, one of them included in this volume [14], been shown to depend on immunological reactions. As summarized by Harris [15], massive immune reactions triggering osteoclasts may lead to bone resorption around hip arthroplasties.

It would in fact seem very easy to conclude that the pathology of an oral implant is as little related to a tooth as is pathology of a hip arthroplasty to a normally functioning, pristine hip joint [16]. What then is behind the different opinion displayed by some dental colleagues? To my dismay, I must profess to clear guilt of the pioneering team of osseointegration of which I once was a member. When we worked to find out why we had seen oral implant success in clear contrast to all others who at the time had tried placing foreign devices in the oral cavity, we had several explanations. Among those were using minimal surgical trauma and commercially pure titanium implants that we at the time saw as being quite inert biologically, and presenting a simple wound healing phenomenon when placed in bone tissue [8,17]. Today we are aware of our misinterpretations. Trindade et al. [18,19] published two papers in this volume with evidence that titanium is not at all inert; the material causes clearly observable immune reactions in the tissue. Other biomaterials such as Poly-ether-ether-ketone, covered by Han et al. [20] in this volume, displayed significantly greater immune reactions than did titanium [19].

Another set of studies believed to prove that the presence of bacteria was the primary cause of problems with bone loss around implants relate to ligatures placed around experimental implants. One paper in this volume [21], summarized 133 such papers that generally reported a primary bacterial response to be behind the observed bone loss around the implants. However, in a ligature study conducted in a site where bacteria are usually absent, the tibia of research animals, Reinedahl and co-workers [22] reported of strong immunological reactions to the ligatures and subsequent marginal bone loss. Again, it seemed that the primary adverse reaction was immunological in nature and that bacteria were not needed for marginal bone loss which does not exclude a secondary bacterial action once the immune system has overreacted [23].

No, oral implants are not the same as a tooth. Neither does the primary bacterial theory explain why bone is lost around oral implants. We need a lot more research, such as several papers published in this volume of *Journal of Clinical Medicine*, to learn more about the true background of threats to osseointegration [24–26]. We must recognize that marginal bone loss commonly represents a complication to treatment; i.e., a condition, and not a disease. In addition, we can rejoice by the fact that moderately rough oral implant failure rates at 10 years of follow up are in the range of only 1–3% [27], that we see quite good clinical outcomes over 30 years of follow up [28] and that oral implants in case studies have been successfully followed up in excess of 50 years of clinical function [23].

Osseointegration is but an immunologically based reaction [29], representing demarcation of the foreign object [12], but if the immune system runs berserk the oral implant may be rejected from the body as a secondary response [12]. When the immune system in this manner overreacts and decides to reject the implant, at the same time the bacterial defense will go down, which explains the secondary presence of bacteria in failing implants [30].

Conflicts of Interest: The author declares no conflict of interest.

References

1. Osseointegration. Available online: https://en.wikipedia.org/wiki/Osseointegration (accessed on 9 September 2019).
2. Davies, J.E. Is osseointegration a foreign body reaction? *Int. J. Pros.* **2019**, *32*, 133–136.
3. Albrektsson, T. Per-Ingvar Brånemark´s Early Research on Osseointegration and Its Meaning on the Histological and Ultrastructural Levels. In Proceedings of the PI Brånemark Memorial Symposium, Stockholm, Sweden, 24 September 2015; van Steenberghe, D., Ed.; QUINTESSENCE Co.: Berlin, Germany, 2015; pp. 29–32.
4. Albrektsson, T.; Zarb, G.; Worthington, P.; Eriksson, R.A. The long-term efficacy of currently used dental implants: A review and proposed criteria of success. *Int. J. Oral Maxillofac. Implant.* **1986**, *1*, 11–25.
5. Albrektsson, T.; Tjellström, A. Bone healing concepts in craniofacial reconstructive and corrective bone surgery. In *Craniofacial Reconstructive and Corrective Bone Surgery*, 2nd ed.; Greenberg, A.M., Schmelzeisen, R., Eds.; Springer: New York, NY, USA, 2019; pp. 129–142.
6. Zaborowska, M.; Welch, K.; Brånemark, R.; Khalilpour, P.; Engqvist, H.; Thomsen, P.; Trobos, M. Bacteria-material surface intereactions: Methodological development for the assessment of implant surface induced antibacterial effects. *J. Biomed. Mater. Res. B Appl. Biomater.* **2014**, *1038*, 179–187.
7. Brånemark, P.I.; Adell, R.; Breine, U.; Lindström, J.; Hallén, O. Öhman, A. Osseointegrated implants in the treatment of the edentulous jaw. *Scand. J. Plast. Reconstr. Surg.* **1977**, *11*, 1–132.
8. Albrektsson, T.; Brånemark, P.I.; Hansson, H.A.; Lindström, J. Osseointegrated titanium implants. Requirements for ensuring a long-lasting, direct bone anchorage in man. *Acta. Orthop. Scand.* **1981**, *52*, 155–170. [CrossRef] [PubMed]

9. Shah, F.; Thomsen, P.; Palmquist, A. Osseointegration and current interpretations of the bone-implant interface. *Acta Biomater.* **2018**, *84*, 1–15. [CrossRef] [PubMed]
10. Buckwalter, A.; Callaghan, J.; Liu, S.; Douglas, P.R.; Goetz, D.; Sullivan, P.M.; Leinen, J.A.; Johnston, R. Results of Charnley total hip arthroplasty with use of improved femoral cementing techniques: A concise follow-up at a minimum of twenty-five years of a previous report. *J. Bone Jt. Surg.* **2006**, *88*, 1481–1485. [CrossRef] [PubMed]
11. Donath, K. Klinische und histopatologische Befunde im Implantgewebe bei Titan-implantaten. *ZWR Zahnaertzl Rundsch. Zahnaerztl Reform Stoma* **1987**, *96*, 14–21.
12. Donath, K.; Laass, M.; Günzl, H. The histopathology of different foreign body reactions in oral soft tissue and bone tissue. *Virchows Arch. A Pathol. Anat. Hist. Opathol.* **1992**, *420*, 131–137. [CrossRef] [PubMed]
13. Monje, A.; Insua, A.; Wang, H.L. Understanding peri-implantitis as a plaque-associated and site specific entity: On the local predisposing factors. *J. Clin. Med.* **2019**, *8*, 279. [CrossRef]
14. Christiansen, R.; Münch, H.; Bonefeld, M.; Thyssen, J.; Sloth, J.; Geisler, C.; Söballe, K.; Jellesen, M.; Jakobsen, S. Cytokine profile in patients with aseptic loosening of total hip replacements and its relation to metal release and metal allergy. *J. Clin. Med.* **2019**, *8*, 1259. [CrossRef] [PubMed]
15. Harris, W. *Vanishing Bone–Conquering A Stealth Disease Caused by Total Hip Replacements*; Oxford Press: Oxford, UK, 2018.
16. Albrektsson, T.; Becker, W.; Coli, P.; Jemt, T.; Mölne, J.; Sennerby, L. Bone loss around oral and orthopedic implants: An immunologically based condition. *Clin. Implant. Dent. Relat. Res.* **2019**, *21*, 786–795. [CrossRef] [PubMed]
17. Albrektsson, T.; Brånemark, P.I.; Hansson, H.A.; Kasemo, B.; Larsson, K.; Lundström, I.; McQueen, D.; Skalak, R. The interface zone of inorganic implants in vivo: Titanium implants in bone. *Ann. Biomed. Eng.* **1983**, *11*, 1–27. [CrossRef]
18. Trindade, R.; Albrektsson, T.; Galli, S.; Prgomet, Z.; Tengvall, P.; Wennerberg, A. Bone immune response to materials, Part I: Titanium, PEEKS and copper in comparison to sham at 10 days in rabbit tibia. *J. Clin. Med.* **2018**, *7*, 526. [CrossRef] [PubMed]
19. Trindade, R.; Albrektsson, T.; Galli, S.; Prgomet, Z.; Tengvall, P.; Wennerberg, A. Bone immune response to materials, Part II: Copper and polyetheretherketone (PEEK) compared to titanium at 10 and 28 days in rabbit tibia. *J. Clin. Med.* **2019**, *8*, 814. [CrossRef] [PubMed]
20. Han, X.; Yang, D.; Yang, C.; Spintzyk, S.; Scheideler, L.; Li, D.; Li, P.; Geis-Gerstorfer, D.; Rupp, J. Carbon fiber reinforced PEEK composites based on 3D-printing technology for orthopedic and dental applications. *J. Clin. Med.* **2019**, *8*, 240. [CrossRef] [PubMed]
21. Reinedahl, D.; Chrcanovic, B.; Albrektsson, T.; Tengvall, P.; Wennerberg, A. Ligature-induced peri-implantitis—A systematic review. *J. Clin. Med.* **2018**, *7*, 492. [CrossRef] [PubMed]
22. Reinedahl, D.; Galli, S.; Albrektsson, T.; Tengvall, P.; Johansson, C.; Hammarström, P.; Wennerberg, A. Aseptic ligatures induce marginal peri-implant bone loss—An 8-week trial in rabbits. *J. Clin. Med.* **2019**, *8*, 1248. [CrossRef] [PubMed]
23. Albrektsson, T.; Jemt, T.; Mölne, J.; Tengvall, P.; Wennerberg, A. On inflammation-immunological (I-I) balance theory. In a critical apprehension of disease concepts around implants: Mucositis and marginal bone loss may represent normal conditions and not necessarily a state of disease. *Clin. Implant. Dent. Rel. Res.* **2019**, *21*, 183–189. [CrossRef] [PubMed]
24. Naveau, A.; Shinmyouzu, K.; Moore, C.; Avivi-Arber, L.; Jokerst, J.; Koka, S. Etiology and measurement of peri-implant crestal bone loss (CBL). *J. Clin. Med.* **2019**, *8*, 166. [CrossRef] [PubMed]
25. Mengual-penafiel, L.; Brañes-Aroca, M.; Marchesani-Carrasco, F.; Jara-Sepúlveda, M.; Leopoldo Parada-Pozas, L.; Cartes-Velásquez, R. Coupling between osseointegration and mechanotransduction to maintain foreign body equilibrium in the long-term: A comprehensive overview. *J. Clin. Med.* **2019**, *8*, 139. [CrossRef] [PubMed]
26. Menini, M.; Pesce, P.; Baldi, D.; Coronel, V.; Paolo, G.; Pera, P.; Izzotti, A. Prediction of titanium implant success by analysis of microRNA expression in peri-implant tissue. A 5-year follow-up study. *J. Clin. Med.* **2019**, *8*, 888. [CrossRef] [PubMed]
27. Wennerberg, A.; Albrektsson, T.; Chrcanovic, B. Long-term clinical outcome of implants with different surface modifications. *Eur. J. Oral Implant.* **2018**, *11*, 123–136.

28. Jemt, T. Implant survival in the edentulous jaw—30 years of experience. Part I: A retrospective multivariate regression analysis of overall implant failure in 4585 consecutively treated arches. *Int. J. Prosthodont* **2018**, *31*, 425–435. [CrossRef]
29. Albrektsson, T.; Chrcanovic, B.; Jacobsson, M.; Wennerberg, A. Osseointegration of implants—A biological and clinical overview. *JSM Dent. Surg.* **2017**, *2*, 1022–1028.
30. Albrektsson, T.; Canullo, L.; Cochran, D.; De Bruyn, H. "Peri-implantitis": A complication of a foreign body or a man—Made "disease", facts and fictions. *Clin. Implant. Dent. Relat. Res.* **2016**, *18*, 840–849. [CrossRef] [PubMed]

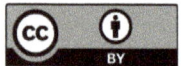

© 2019 by the author. Licensee MDPI, Basel, Switzerland. This article is an open access article distributed under the terms and conditions of the Creative Commons Attribution (CC BY) license (http://creativecommons.org/licenses/by/4.0/).

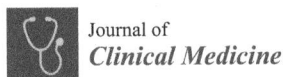

Article

Prediction of Titanium Implant Success by Analysis of microRNA Expression in Peri-Implant Tissue. A 5-Year Follow-Up Study

Maria Menini [1], Paolo Pesce [1,*], Domenico Baldi [1], Gabriela Coronel Vargas [2], Paolo Pera [1] and Alberto Izzotti [2,3]

1. Division of Implant Prosthodontics, Department of Surgical Sciences, University of Genoa, 16132 Genoa, Italy; maria.menini@unige.it (M.M.); baldi.domenico@unige.it (D.B.); paolopera@unige.it (P.P.)
2. Department of Health Sciences, University of Genoa, 16126 Genoa, Italy; gabrielafernanda.coronelvargas@edu.unige.it (G.C.V.); izzotti@unige.it (A.I.)
3. IRCCS Ospedale Policlinico San Martino, 16132 Genoa, Italy
* Correspondence: paolo.pesce@unige.it; Tel.: +39-0103-5374-21

Received: 12 June 2019; Accepted: 18 June 2019; Published: 21 June 2019

Abstract: The aim of the present study is to evaluate the expression of microRNA (miRNA) in peri-implant soft tissue and to correlate epigenetic information with the clinical outcomes of the implants up to the five-year follow-up. Seven patients have been rehabilitated with fixed screw-retained bridges each supported by implants. Peri-implant bone resorption and soft tissue health parameters have been recorded over time with a five-year follow-up. Mini-invasive samples of soft peri-implant tissue have been taken three months after implant insertion. miRNA have been extracted from cells of the soft tissue samples to evaluate gene-expression at the implant sites by microarray analysis. The epigenomic data obtained by microarray technology has been statistically analyzed by dedicated software and compared with measured clinical parameters. Specific miRNA expression profiles predictive of specific clinical outcomes were found. In particular, some specific miRNA signatures appeared to be "protective" from bone resorption despite the presence of plaque accumulation. miRNA may be predictors of dental implant clinical outcomes and may be used as biomarkers for diagnostic and prognostic purposes in the field of implant dentistry.

Keywords: dental implants; micro-RNA; microarray; predictive biomarker; epigenomics

1. Introduction

Currently dental implants are widely used for fixed rehabilitation of partially or completely edentulous patients and demonstrate predictable outcomes. However, the biological mechanisms of possible complications and implant failure are not clear and are debated in the dental scientific community.

In particular, the specific endogenous characteristic of the host (i.e., individual susceptibility) may strongly affect the success of the rehabilitation. Modern innovative technologies using molecular biomarkers may help in identifying individual susceptibility.

In a previous paper [1] we provided evidence that microRNA (miRNA) expression in peri-implant tissue reflects the pathological processes occurring in peri-implant tissues.

miRNAs are small noncoding RNAs (ncRNAs) of approximately 22 nucleotides responsible for specific regulation of gene expression in a post-transcriptional manner. They are the main regulator of gene transcription and bear relevance in predicting clinical outcomes. Indeed, only less than 5% of expressed genes producing messenger RNA is really translated into proteins while microRNAs are fully functionally active in cell cytoplasm [2]. They have an important role in several biological processes, such as development, cell proliferation, apoptosis and carcinogenesis [3,4].

A major problem is currently represented by the lack of a predictive marker to personalize risk after peri-implant surgery. Indeed, some authors have suggested peri-implant soft tissue biotype as a risk indicator of peri-implants tissue disease [5,6]. However, this biomarker is rough and does not reflect the multiple pathogenic mechanisms occurring in the peri-implant tissue hampering or favoring the outcome of implant surgery. Conversely the accurate classification of patients in high or low-risk categories is fundamental to set up follow-up procedures and therapies according to the real risk of each subject. This is a pivotal step in the era of personalized medicine.

Molecular biomarkers are already extensively used in medicine to accurately classify each patient according to their real risk of developing complications. This approach, referred to as personalized or "theranostic" medicine, has been already well developed in oncology but is still under development in dental science.

Molecular predictive biomarkers should reflect the pathogenic process modulating clinical outcome in the target tissue of the diseases. Furthermore, the molecular alteration investigated may occur years before the appearance of the related clinical consequence thus opening the possibility of preventing adverse clinical outcomes before their onset.

At this regard, miRNAs are currently identified as predictive biomarkers for degenerative diseases, because they do not undergo a post-transcriptional selection, being themselves the controllers of gene transcription. Consequently, compared to genomic or transcriptomic biomarkers, miRNA expression has by far a higher probability of being related with clinical variables representing a new tool for predictive medicine.

On the other side, several factors, including the implant surface [7], might affect dental implant success possibly through miRNA expression. Our research group demonstrated in vitro that osteoblasts change their gene expression profile according to the type of implant surface in contact with them [8].

The role of miRNA in implant dentistry has been established. In a clinical trial, we demonstrated that miRNA expressed by peri-implant tissues are related with the clinical outcome [2]. However, it remains to be established the long-term predictivity of miRNA analysis in a long-term follow-up study.

The aim of the present study is to examine the predictivity of miRNA profiling to categorize patients according to risk categories of developing more or less probably adverse consequences of oral implants on a long-term basis.

In particular, the expression of micro-RNA (miRNA) in peri-implant soft tissue will be correlated with the clinical outcomes of dental implants recorded up to the five-year follow-up.

2. Experimental Section

Between January 2013 and July 2014, 7 patients (4 women, 3 men; mean age: 64.6, range: 52–76) who were referred to the Division of Implant and Prosthetic Dentistry of the Surgical Sciences Department (DISC) of the University of Genoa (Genoa, Italy) and that required the insertion of two implants into an edentulous area were recruited if they met the following criteria: desire to be treated with fixed prostheses supported by dental implants and good general health without any contraindications for undergoing oral surgery and the related prosthodontic protocols.

Exclusion criteria included: an uncontrolled medical condition such as diabetes mellitus, immune suppression, intravenous bisphosphonate medication, oro-facial cancer, chemotherapy or head and neck radiotherapy, infarct during the preceding 6 months, heavy smokers (≥20 cigarettes/day).

Healing time since tooth extraction in the intended implant sites had to be longer than 1 year. Post-extractive implants and implant sites that required a bone graft were excluded.

The present report was conducted in accordance with the Helsinki Declaration and was approved by the local Scientific Ethical Committee of the University of Genoa.

Patients were instructed in detail on the planned clinical procedure and signed an informed consent before being scheduled in the experimental protocol.

Each patient of the sample received two adjacent implants: Osseotite implants (Biomet 3i, Palmbeach Gardens, FL) with a dual acid-etched (DAE) surface in the apical portion and a machined coronal part (hybrid implants), and Full Osseotite implants (Biomet 3i) completely DAE (DAE implants).

All the implants had identical macro- and micro-structure, external hexagon connection, a 4 mm diameter, a 10–13 mm length (depending on available bone).

Implants were placed with a single-stage delayed loading approach and were assigned specific codes for blinding.

The healing abutments remained in situ up to the 4-month follow-up appointment when impressions of the implants were taken to fabricate the fixed prostheses. No bone nor soft tissue grafting procedures were performed at the implant sites.

Patients were accurately instructed on the hygienic procedures to be followed and were prescribed adequate dietary guidelines in order to ensure optimal recovery.

Screw-retained prostheses, provided with a metal framework and composite resin veneering material, were delivered 5–6 months (mean 24 weeks) after surgery (Figure 1).

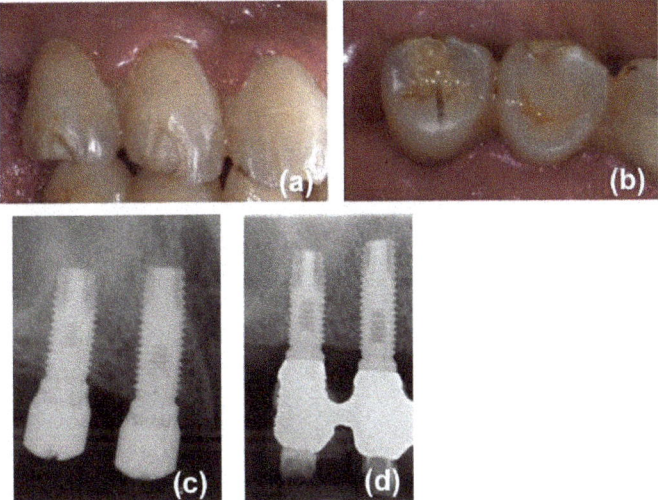

Figure 1. One of the patients included in the present research: (**a**) intraoral view of the bridge at the five-year follow-up appointment; (**b**) occlusal view of the bridge at the five-year follow-up appointment; (**c**) endoral radiograph three months after implant insertion; (**d**) endoral radiograph taken at the five-year follow-up appointment.

Spontaneous bleeding, probing depth (PD), bleeding on probing (BoP), plaque index (PI), and suppuration were recorded at 3 and 6 weeks and at 3-, 6- and 12-months post-surgery and then at the five-year follow-up appointment. At the five-year appointment the fixed prostheses were unscrewed in order to record the parodontal parameters. PD was recorded in four points for each implant (mesial, distal, buccal and lingual) using a non-metallic probe. BoP was simultaneously evaluated in four points for each implant (values from 0 to 4 for each implant). PI was measured at four points for each implant using an erythrosine gel (values from 0 to 4 for each implant).

Technical and biological complications were also recorded.

Intraoral radiographs were taken at the time of implant placement and at 3-, 6- and 12-months post-surgery and then at the five-year follow-up appointment. The implant–abutment interface was used as the reference point for interproximal bone level measurements over time. Bone resorption (BR) over the duration of the study was assessed from these reference points to the most coronal bone at the mesial and distal aspects of each implant.

The above-mentioned clinical parameters recorded at the five-year follow-up appointment were statistically analyzed and differences between DAE and hybrid implants were evaluated by Student's *t*-test.

After 3 months from surgery, a sample of soft tissue containing both epithelium and connective tissue was collected: a mini-invasive sample of soft tissue (diameter < 3 mm) surrounding each implant was taken using a surgical blade to be histologically analyzed by miRNA microarray at the Department of Health Sciences (DISSAL) of Genoa University.

MicroRNA microarray analysis is an innovative technology, which allows the evaluations of thousands of genes in a single experiment. MicroRNAs (miRNA) have been extracted from cells of the soft tissue samples to evaluate gene-expression at the implant sites by microarray analysis.

miRNA expression data was evaluated in the peri-implant tissue as previously reported [1]. The expression of 1928 human miRNA was determined by using a commercially available microarray (miRCURY LNATM, Exiqon, Vedbaek, Denmark).

The results of miRNA microarray have been compared with clinical parameters measured over time for five years since miRNA analysis. The previously published paper reported correlation between miRNA data and one-year outcomes (T0). The present paper reports the correlation between miRNA data and clinical outcomes recorded at the five-year follow-up appointment (T1).

All clinical continuous variables recorded at the five-year follow-up have been turned into categorical ones depending on the following criteria arbitrarily chosen by the authors:

- mean bone resorption (BR): normal/increased (normal ≤ 1 mm, increased > 1 mm)
- mean probing depth (PD): normal/increased (normal ≤ 3 mm, increased > 3 mm)
- mean plaque index (PI): low/high (low ≤ 1, high > 1)
- mean bleeding on probing (BOP): yes/no (yes ≥ 0.5, no < 0.5)

On the base of these parameters, several categories of implants (i.e., implants with normal BR vs. implants with increased BR) have been determined.

In addition, implants with the contemporary presence of BOP, altered PD and bone resorption were considered affected by peri-implantitis (PITI).

Implant sites were also divided in two categories according to the periodontal biotype: thin (TH) and thick (TK). To evaluate the biotype, a periodontal probe was placed into the facial aspect of the peri-implant mucosa. The peri-implant biotype was categorized as thin if the outline of the underlying periodontal probe could be seen through the gingiva and thick if the probe could not be seen [9].

Relationship between miRNA and clinical events were tested by Genespring software (Agilent technologies, Palo Alto, CA, USA).

3. Results

During the five-year follow-up, there were no dropouts and all the patients attended the five-year recall appointment. No implant failure occurred resulting in an implant cumulative survival rate (CSR) of 100%. No technical complications were detected, resulting in a prosthodontic CSR of 100%. All the patients anecdotally reported to be satisfied with their implant rehabilitation.

Five patients presented a thin periodontal biotype and two a thick periodontal biotype.

Mean bone resorption at the five-year follow-up appointment was 1.98 mm (min: 0.7, max: 4 mm): 1.8 mm and 2.2 mm for implants with a machined coronal portion and DAE implants respectively.

No patient presented spontaneous bleeding or suppuration.

No statistically significant differences were found between hybrid implants and DAE implants for the clinical variables recorded at the five-year follow-up.

Mean and median values of the other soft tissue health parameters are reported in Table 1.

Table 1. Bone level and peri-implant health parameters recorded at the five-year follow-up appointment.

	Interproximal Bone Resorption (mm)	Plaque Index	Bleeding on Probing	Probing Depth (mm)
Mean	1.98	2.9	2.1	3.7
Median	2	3	2	4
Min	0.7	0	0	1
Max	4	4	4	6.5
P for DAE vs. hybrid implants	0.1466	0.8641	0.5817	0.6215

An overall view of the miRNA alterations as related to clinical outcomes occurring in the five years after surgery was performed using scatter plot (Figure 2) and volcano plot analyses (Figure 3).

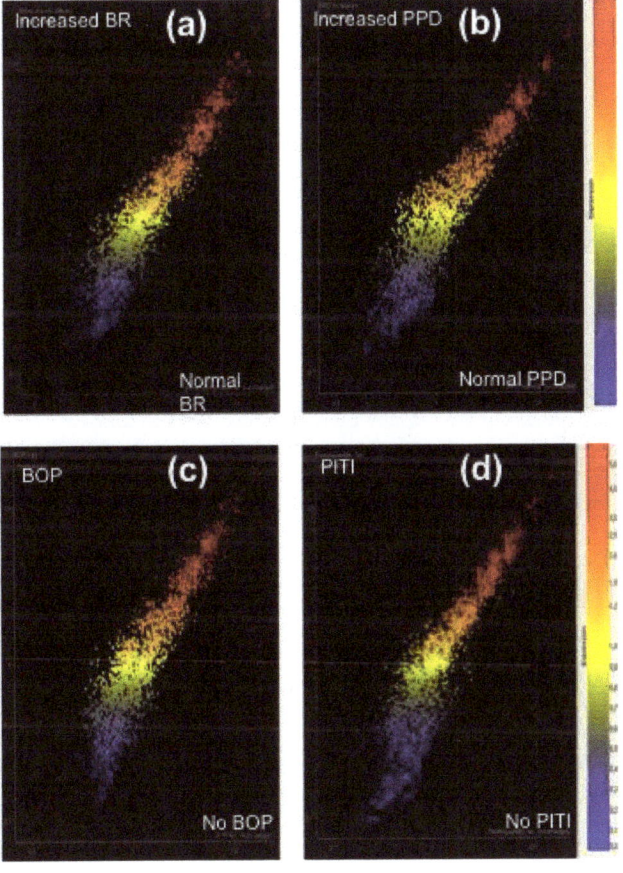

Figure 2. Scatter plot analyses reporting the alteration of microRNA (miRNA) profile as related to the outcome of the following clinical variables recorded at the five-year follow-up appointment: (**a**) bone resorption (BR), (**b**) peri-implant probing depth (PPD), (**c**) bleeding on probing (BOP), (**d**) peri-implantits (PITI).

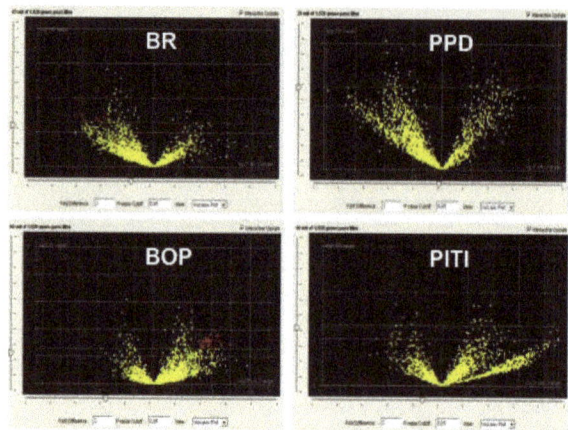

Figure 3. Volcano plot analyses reporting the number of significantly (<2-fold, $p < 0.05$) altered miRNAs as related to the outcome of the following clinical variables recorded at the five-year follow-up appointment: BR, PPD, BOP, PITI.

For each clinical variable, the predictor miRNAs were identified by volcano plot analysis (Table 2).

Table 2. Identity of miRNAs predictor of five-year clinical outcomes of dental implants.

Clinical Variable Predicted	miRNA
Bone Resorption (BR)	miR-33, miR-134, miR-200, miR-378
Bleeding on probing (BOP)	let-7f miR-425, miR-548
Peri-implant pocket depth (PPD)	miR-30, miR-197, miR-218, miR-548, miR-613
Perimplantitis (PITI)	miR-517, miR-525, miR-624, miR-3128, miR-3658, miR-3692, miR-3912, miR-3920, miR-4683, miR-4690

BR: 48 miRNA were significantly (Figure 3) dysregulated at T0 in patients with altered BR (altered) as compared to those with normal BR (normal) in the five years following implant surgery. Venn diagram analyses indicated that in these patients among the miRNAs altered at T0, four were predictors of BR in the following five years. These miRNAs are miR-33, miR-134, miR-200 and miR-378 (Table 2). They play a regulatory role in cell proliferation, stem cell recruitment and differentiation, osteogenesis and inflammation.

Hierarchical cluster analyses were used to classify patients according to their miRNA expression profile as related to BR in the five years following implant surgery. Implants with a normal miRNA expression level (yellow, red) are located in the left part of the cluster, while implants with a decreased miRNA expression (blue) are located in the right part of the cluster. A severe alteration of miRNA expression at three months occurs in patients with BR ≥ 2 mm at the five-year follow-up appointment (Figure 4a). These findings were confirmed by unsupervised principal component analysis of variance (PCA) of miRNA expression profile for each implant. Indeed, all implants that had a BR ≥ 2 mm in the five years after surgery were located in a different quadrant as compared to other implants (Figure 4b).

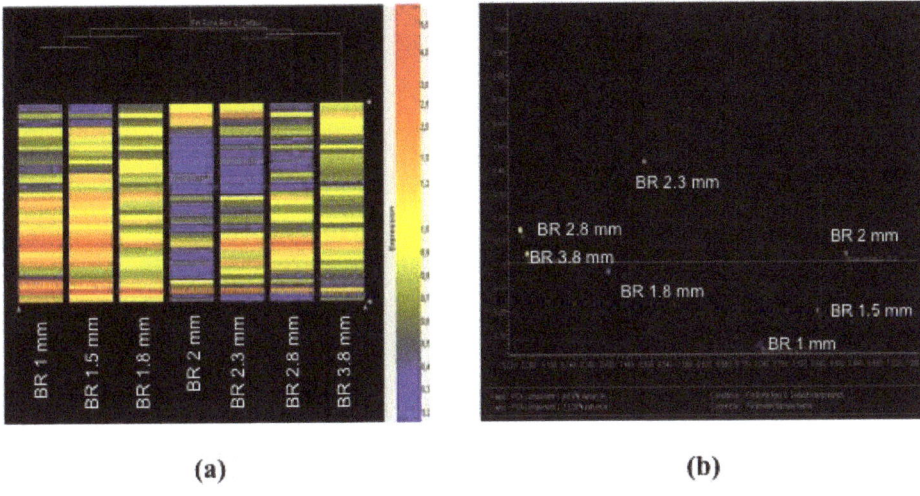

Figure 4. Hierarchical cluster (**a**) and principal component analysis of variance (**b**) analyses showing the occurrence of miRNA alteration in implants with BR > 2 mm.

PD: 29 miRNA were significantly (Figure 3, volcano plot) altered at T0 in patients with PD increase (increased) as compared to those having normal PD (normal) in the five years following implant surgery. Venn diagram analyses indicated that among the 10 miRNA altered in these implants at T0 (see data reported in Menini et al. [1] first year after surgery) five were predictors of PD increase in the following five years. These miRNAs are miR-30, miR-197, miR-218, miR-548 and miR-613 (Table 2). They play a regulatory role in the following biological functions: osteogenesis and cartilage homeostasis.

BOP: 66 miRNA were significantly (Figure 3, volcano plot) altered at T0 in patients with BOP (yes) as compared to those without BOP (no) at five years following implant surgery. Venn diagram analyses indicated that among the six miRNA altered in these patients at T0 (see data reported in Menini et al. [1] first year after surgery) three were predictors of BOP increase in the following five years. These miRNAs are let-7f, miR-425 and miR-548 (Table 2). They play a regulatory role in the following biological function: inflammation.

PITI: 10 miRNA were significantly (Figure 3, volcano plot) altered at T0 in patients having PITI (yes) as compared to those not having PITI (no) at five years following implant surgery. This condition was not evaluated at T0 (at the one-year follow-up appointment only two implants in one single patient presented PITI). These miRNAs are miR-517, miR-525, miR-624, miR-3128, miR-3658, miR-3692, miR-3912, miR-3920, miR-4683 and miR-4690 (Table 2). They play a regulatory role in the following biological functions: inflammation, cellular proliferation and cartilage homeostasis.

The number of altered miRNAs as related to BR, peri-implant probing depth (PD) and BOP recorded at the five-year follow-up was dramatically increased (T1) as compared to T0 (Table 3). These findings reflect the progressive recruitment of new pathogenic mechanisms during the progression of the diseases.

Table 3. Number of altered miRNAs as related to BR, PD and BOP recorded at the one-year (T0) and at the five-year follow-up (T1).

	BR	PD	BOP
T0	7	10	6
T1	48	29	66

The efficacy of miRNA as biomarkers predicting clinical outcome was compared with those of periodontal biotype classified for each patient as thick (low-risk) or thin (high-risk). The ability of periodontal biotype to predict the clinical outcome of dental implants in the following five years was tested by chi square analysis (Figure 5). Of the patients with a thick biotype 33% underwent PITI, while none of the patients with a thin biotype underwent PITI. These differences were not significantly different (chi square = 2.727; chi square p-value = 0.0986; Fischer's exact p-value = 0.2308). Conversely, miRNA expression as focused on the cluster of PITI miRNA predictors (see Table 2 and Figure 6) was able to predict PITI occurrence in all (100%) patients.

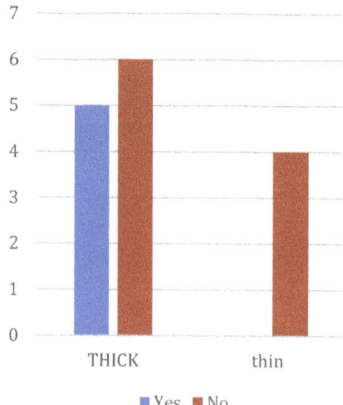

Summary table for PITI, Biotype	
Num. missing	0
DF	1
Chi Square	2.727
Chi Square p-Value	0.0986
G-Squared	*
G-Squared p-Value	*
Contingency Coef.	0.392
Phi	0.426
Cty. Cor. Chi Square	1.152
Cty. Cor. p-Value	0.2831
Fisher's exact p-Value	0.2308

Observed Frequencies for PITI, Biotype			
	THICK	Thin	Totals
PITI	5	0	5
No PITI	6	4	10
Totals	11	4	15

Figure 5. PITI occurrence as related to parodontal biotype.

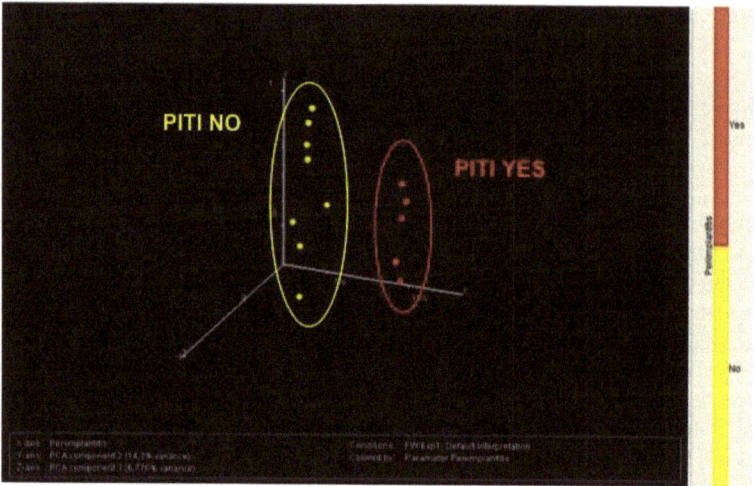

Figure 6. Principal component analysis of variance showing differences in miRNA expression in implants with or without PITI.

In fact, PCA of miRNA expression at T0 (Figure 6) distinguished between patients that would develop PITI in the following five years (red dots) from those who would not develop PITI (yellow dots) in a clear-cut manner, as highlighted by the lack of any overlap between the grouping circles. The ability of miRNA profiling in predicting PITI was also statistically evaluated by k-nearest neighbors and support vector machine algorithms. The sensitivity (percentage of patients with prediction) was 80%

and 93% respectively; the specificity (percentage of patients with true prediction) was 100% and 93% respectively. Accordingly, the accuracy of this test was >90% independently of the algorithm adopted.

The miRNA pattern was compared in patients undergoing plaque accumulation (high PI) between those with or without BR. The aim of this approach was to identify miRNA protecting peri-implant tissue from the adverse effect of plaque accumulation. Obtained results are reported in Figure 7.

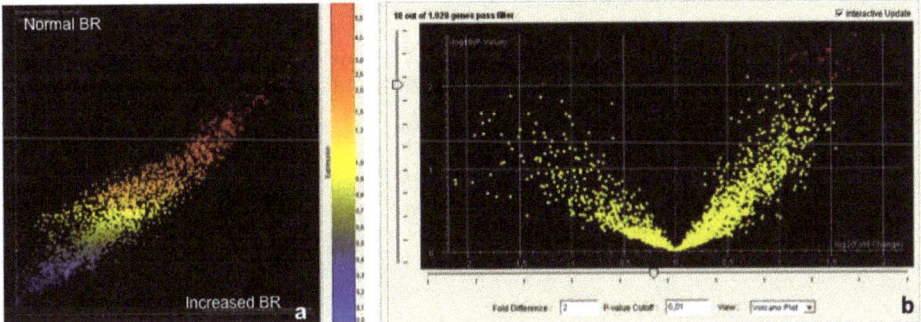

Figure 7. Scatter plot (**a**) and volcano plot (**b**) analyses reporting the alteration of miRNA profile as related to BR at the level of implants with high plaque index (PI).

Both scatter plot and volcano plot identified differences between these two groups of patients. The miRNAs that protected peri-implant tissue from BR despite the presence of plaque deposits are reported in Table 4.

Table 4. miRNA that were found to be "protective" from bone resorption despite the presence of plaque deposits (high PI) and their fold variation. The fold change indicates the ratio of miRNA expression intensity between the two categories of implants stratified according to differences in bone resorption (increased vs. normal) next to implants with high PI.

Gene Name	Fold Change
hsa-miR-4677-5p	3.328
hsa-miR-3914	3.189
hsa-miR-4679	2.948
hsa-miR-378b	2.929
hsa-miR-4434	2.858
hsa-miR-32-3p/mmu-miR-32-3p/rno-miR-32-3p	2.804
hsa-miR-1/mmu-miR-1a-3p	2.769
hsa-miR-4778-5p	2.681
hsa-miR-99b-3p/mmu-miR-99b-3p/rno-miR-99b-3p	2.615
hsa-miR-7-5p/mmu-miR-7a-5p/rno-miR-7a-5p	2.496
hsa-miR-3146	2.389
hsa-miR-4439	2.296
hsa-miR-539-3p	2.247
hsa-miR-222-3p/mmu-miR-222-3p/rno-miR-222-3p	2.225
hsa-miR-124-5p/mmu-miR-124-5p/rno-miR-124-5p	2.169
hsa-miR-4689	2.167

4. Discussion

miRNA are biomarkers of several diseases and in recent years, some studies have begun to focus on the regulatory role of miRNAs in the inflammatory response [10,11].

miRNA are fundamental in controlling cell function and also influence osteoinductive pathways and inflammation in several ways. On the other side, miRNA expression is influenced by many factors and some authors have suggested that different implant surfaces may condition miRNA expression [12,13].

However, studies investigating the role of miRNA in implant dentistry are still scarce. Some in vitro studies are present [12,14] and studies focused on the differences of miRNA profiles between periimplantitis and periodontitis [15].

A recent review [16] found only one clinical trial evaluating the role of miRNA expression in the osseointegration of dental implants. This study was the investigation conducted by the present team of authors [1] and the present paper reports follow-up data for the same patients' samples.

Our previous study suggested that miRNAs play an important role in conditioning clinical outcomes after implant insertion [1]. Specific miRNA profiles appeared to indicate lower susceptibility to peri-implant tissue inflammation and bone resorption. These findings highlighted the remarkable biological importance of miRNA expression in peri-implant tissue in determining the clinical outcome of dental implant rehabilitations.

The present study with a five-year follow-up confirmed the potential role of miRNA in patients' susceptibility to peri-implant disease and the potential role of miRNAs as predictors of clinical outcomes of dental implants. In fact, miRNA expression at three months of healing was predictive of the clinical variables recorded at five years of follow-up.

The miRNA mostly involved in the prediction of clinical outcomes was miR-548. Indeed, this miRNA predicted PD and BOP (Table 2). This miRNA is an established regulator of the balance between cell proliferation and apoptosis. This miRNA was found to be upregulated in patients undergoing these adverse events; indeed this upregulation results in cell proliferation arrest and apoptosis activation, two conditions fundamental in triggering degenerative diseases of the peri-implant tissue and to hamper wound healing.

The definition and etiology of peri-implant disease are controversial [17]. In particular, a clear link between plaque accumulation and bone loss has yet to be demonstrated [18,19]. The possible etiological effect of plaque accumulation on peri-implant disease may be decreased or enhanced by specific miRNAs.

Indeed, a specific miRNA expression profile was found in patients with normal BR at five years, despite the presence of plaque accumulation (6,7), and miRNA expression analysis was far more accurate than periodontal biotype in predicting PITI occurrence in the five years after implant surgery (5,6).

The present investigation shed light on possible biomarkers that may be predictable of dental implants clinical outcomes. The variables that can compromise implant therapy are numerous (systematic diseases, residual bone density and 3-D morphology, smoking, bruxism, regularity and effectiveness of the follow-up etc.) and the miRNA can be considered a useful tool for only evaluating the "predisposition" of the peri-implant tissues to a stable osseointegration process.

The integrated findings derived from clinical and laboratory analysis helped with understanding the biological mechanisms affecting peri-implant tissue healing and maintenance. This will help clinicians in the choice of a better treatment plan for a predictable success of dental implant rehabilitations. In fact, specific miRNA expression profiles are predictive of specific clinical outcomes in implant dentistry and may be used as diagnostic and prognostic tools, thus affecting therapeutic strategies. These findings can be tools for a more personalized medicine approach in the treatment of edentulous patients using dental implants.

Moreover, the possible identification of "protective" miRNA also discloses the possibility of using miRNAs in future studies as therapeutic agents in implant dentistry. miRNAs might be used as possible drugs or coatings for implant surfaces, in order to improve healing and maintenance of peri-implant tissues.

5. Conclusions

The results of the present clinical trial suggest that miRNA may be predictors of dental implants clinical outcomes and may be used as biomarkers for diagnostic and prognostic purposes in the field of implant dentistry.

Author Contributions: Conceptualization, M.M., P.P. (Paolo Pera)Paolo Pera, D.B. and A.I.; methodology, M.M., D.B. and A.I.; software, A.I. and G.C.V.; validation, M.M., P.P.(Paolo Pesce), D.B. and A.I.; formal analysis, M.M., P.P. (Paolo Pesce) and A.I.; investigation, M.M., P.P. (Paolo Pesce), D.B., G.C.V. and A.I.; resources, P.P.(Paolo Pera) and A.I.; data curation, P.P. (Paolo Pesce) and M.M.; writing—original draft preparation, M.M. and A.I.; writing—review and editing, M.M., A.I. and P.P. (Paolo Pesce); visualization, M.M., A.I. and P.P. (Paolo Pesce); supervision, P.P. (Paolo Pera); project administration, M.M.; funding acquisition, M.M. and P.P. (Paolo Pera).

Funding: This research was partly funded by an Atheneum Research Project—PRA 2012, University of Genoa, Genoa, Italy, and by Biomet 3i, Palmbeach Gardens, FL.

Conflicts of Interest: The authors declare no conflict of interest.

References

1. Menini, M.; Dellepiane, E.; Baldi, D.; Longobardi, M.G.; Pera, P.; Izzotti, A. Microarray expression in peri-implant tissue next to different titanium implant surfaces predicts clinical outcomes: A split-mouth study. *Clin. Oral. Implant. Res.* **2017**, *28*, e121–e134. [CrossRef] [PubMed]
2. Izzotti, A. Molecular medicine and development of cancer chemopreventive agents. *Ann. N. Y. Acad. Sci.* **2012**, *1259*, 26–32. [CrossRef] [PubMed]
3. Osada, H.; Takahashi, T. MicroRNAs in biological processes and carcinogenesis. *Carcinogenesis* **2007**, *28*, 2–12. [CrossRef] [PubMed]
4. Pasquinelli, A.E.; Reinhart, B.J.; Slack, F.; Martindale, M.Q.; Kuroda, M.I.; Maller, B.; Hayward, D.C.; Ball, E.E.; Degnan, B.; M€uller, P.; et al. Conservation of the sequence and temporal expression of let-7 heterochronic regulatory RNA. *Nature* **2000**, *408*, 86–89. [CrossRef] [PubMed]
5. Isler, S.C.; Uraz, A.; Kaymaz, O.; Cetiner, D. An Evaluation of the Relationship between Peri-implant Soft Tissue Biotype and the Severity of Peri-implantitis: A Cross-Sectional Study. *Int. J. Oral. Maxillofac. Implant* **2019**, *34*, 187–196. [CrossRef] [PubMed]
6. Mailoa, J.; Miron, R.J.; Wang, H.L. Risk Indicators and Prevention of Implant Soft-Tissue Complications: Interproximal Papillae Loss and Midfacial Implant Mucosal Recessions. *Compend. Contin. Educ. Dent.* **2017**, *38*, 436–443. [PubMed]
7. Menini, M.; Dellepiane, E.; Chvartszaid, D.; Baldi, D.; Schiavetti, I.; Pera, P. Influence of Different Surface Characteristics on Peri-implant Tissue Behavior: A Six-Year Prospective Report. *Int. J. Prosthodont.* **2015**, *28*, 389–395. [CrossRef] [PubMed]
8. Baldi, D.; Longobardi, M.G.; Cartiglia, C.; La Maestra, S.; Pulliero, A.; Bonica, P.; Micale, R.; Menini, M.; Pera, P.; Izzotti, A. Dental Implants Osteogenic Properties Evaluated by cDNA Microarrays. *Implant Dent.* **2011**, *20*, 299–304. [CrossRef] [PubMed]
9. Kan, J.Y.; Rungcharassaeng, K.; Umezu, K.; Kois, J.C. Dimensions of peri-implant mucosa: An evaluation of maxillary anterior single implants in humans. *J. Periodontol.* **2003**, *74*, 557–562. [CrossRef] [PubMed]
10. Lindsay, M.A. MicroRNAs and the immune response. *Trends Immunol.* **2008**, *29*, 343–351. [CrossRef] [PubMed]
11. O'Connell, R.M.; Taganov, K.D.; Boldin, M.P.; Cheng, G.; Baltimore, D. MicroRNA-155 is induced during the macrophage inflammatory response. *Proc. Natl. Acad. Sci. USA* **2007**, *104*, 1604–1609. [CrossRef] [PubMed]
12. Iaculli, F.; Di Filippo, E.S.; Piattelli, A.; Mancinelli, R.; Fulle, S. Dental pulp stem cells grown on dental implant titanium surfaces: An in vitro evaluation of differentiation and micro-RNAs expression. *J. Biomed. Mater. Res. Part B. Appl. Biomater.* **2017**, *105*, 953–965. [CrossRef] [PubMed]
13. Sartori, E.M.; Magro-Filho, O.; Silveira Mendonça, D.B.; Li, X.; Fu, J.; Mendonça, G. Modulation of Micro RNA Expression and Osteoblast Differentiation by Nanotopography. *Int. J. Oral. Maxillofac. Implant* **2018**, *33*, 269–280. [CrossRef] [PubMed]

14. Chakravorty, N.; Ivanovski, S.; Prasadam, I.; Crawford, R.; Oloyede, A.; Xiao, Y. The micro-RNA expression signature on modified titanium implant surfaces influences genetic mechanisms leading to osteogenic differentiation. *Acta. Biomater.* **2012**, *8*, 3516–3523. [CrossRef] [PubMed]
15. Xie, F.; Shu, R.; Jiang, S.; Liu, D.; Zhang, X. Comparison of microRNA profiles of human periodontal diseased and healthy gingival tissues. *Int. J. Oral. Sci.* **2011**, *3*, 125–134. [CrossRef] [PubMed]
16. Sartori, E.M.; das Neves, A.M.; Magro-Filho, O.; Mendonça, D.B.S.; Krebsbach, P.H.; Cooper, L.F.; Mendonça, G. The Role of MicroRNAs in the Osseointegration Process. *Int. J. Oral. Maxillofac. Implant.* **2019**, *34*, 397–410. [CrossRef] [PubMed]
17. Albrektsson, T.; Canullo, L.; Cochran, D.; De Bruyn, H. "Peri-Implantitis": A Complication of a Foreign Body or a Man-Made "Disease". Facts and Fiction. *Clin. Implant Dent. Relat. Res.* **2016**, *18*, 840–849. [CrossRef] [PubMed]
18. Pesce, P.; Menini, M.; Tealdo, T.; Bevilacqua, M.; Pera, F.; Pera, P. Peri-implantitis: A systematic review of recently published papers. *Int. J. Prosthodont.* **2014**, *27*, 15–25. [CrossRef] [PubMed]
19. Menini, M.; Setti, P.; Pera, P.; Pera, F.; Pesce, P. Peri-implant tissue health and bone resorption in immediately loaded, implant-supported full-arch prostheses. *Int. J. Prosthodont.* **2018**, *31*, 327–333. [CrossRef] [PubMed]

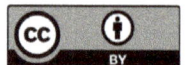

© 2019 by the authors. Licensee MDPI, Basel, Switzerland. This article is an open access article distributed under the terms and conditions of the Creative Commons Attribution (CC BY) license (http://creativecommons.org/licenses/by/4.0/).

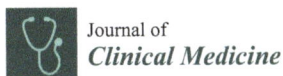

Review

Is Peri-Implant Probing Causing Over-Diagnosis and Over-Treatment of Dental Implants?

Pierluigi Coli [1] and Lars Sennerby [1,2,*]

[1] Edinburgh Dental Specialists, Edinburgh EH2 4BA, UK
[2] Department of Maxillofacial Surgery, University of Gothenburg, 413 90 Gothenburg, Sweden
* Correspondence: lars.sennerby@gu.se

Received: 16 June 2019; Accepted: 25 July 2019; Published: 29 July 2019

Abstract: Pocket probing depth (PPD) and bleeding on probing (BOP) measurements are useful indices for the assessment of periodontal conditions. The same periodontal indices are commonly recommended to evaluate the dental implant/tissue interface to identify sites with mucositis and peri-implantitis, which, if not treated, are anticipated to lead to implant failure. The aim of the present narrative review is to discuss the available literature on the effectiveness of probing at dental implants for identification of peri-implant pathology. There is substantial clinical evidence that PPD and BOP measurements are very poor indices of peri-implant tissue conditions and are questionable surrogate endpoints for implant failure. On the contrary, the literature suggests that frequent disturbance of the soft tissue barrier at implants may instead induce inflammation and bone resorption. Moreover, over-diagnosis and subsequent unnecessary treatment may lead to iatrogenic damage to the implant-tissue interface. Despite this, the recommendations from recent consensus meetings are still promoting the use of probing at dental implants. For evaluation of implants, for instance at annual check-ups, the present authors recommend a clinical examination that includes (i) a visual inspection of the peri-implant tissues for the assessment of oral hygiene and the detection of potential redness, swelling, (ii) palpation of the peri-implant tissues for assessment of the potential presence of swelling, bleeding, suppuration. In addition, (iii) radiography is recommended for the assessment of crestal bone level for comparison with previous radiographs to evaluate potential progressive bone loss even if there is a need for more scientific evidence of the true value of the first two clinical testing modes.

Keywords: dental implants; mucositis; peri-implantitis; diagnosis; over-treatment; iatrogenic damage

1. Introduction

The ultimate goals of the maintenance phase of implant treatment are to preserve the function and the aesthetics of the rehabilitation as well as the stability /health of the peri-implant tissues for as long as possible. From a research point of view, the goal is to monitor the treatment outcomes: implant survival and success/failure. One evident problem is that the definitions of survival, success/failure used in more recent publications do not necessarily reflect the patient/clinician perceived successful maintenance of the function and aesthetics of the treatment. In other words, the definitions of disease, which would motivate a clinical intervention to cure the disease, do not seem to reflect the clinical reality. Thus, the first questions to be answered are "what should be considered pathology at a dental implant?" and "what diagnostic tools are available?". With regards to the natural dentition, there has been a wide agreement within the scientific community in relation to disease definitions and available diagnostic tools [1]. Despite the recent World Consensus meeting in Chicago [1], a similar consensus with regards to definition of pathologies and available diagnostic tools does not seem to exist for peri-implant tissue conditions [2–5]. The controversy regarding the application of periodontal indices to dental implants is not a recent one [6]. The basis for the disagreement can be found in the difference in the viewing of the peri-implant tissues. Can similar disease definitions and diagnostic tools be used in natural dentition and in situations where the natural dentition has been replaced with implant-retained restorations? The question is logical since there are no doubts that the periodontium and the peri-implant tissues ought to be regarded as two very different entities [5,7,8].

Is it correct to assume that similar reactions to infection, occlusal trauma, trauma from probing can be expected for the periodontium and the peri-implant tissues? Is there a similar pattern of disease progression? And if these aspects differ between the two entities, is it correct to use similar diagnostic tools? There is evidence in the literature that the peri-implant tissues are more susceptible to inflammatory reactions, a phenomenon also confirmed immunohistochemically with increase of inflammatory infiltrate in comparison to teeth [9] that lesions around implants and teeth have critical histopathologic differences [10], and that there are differences in the onset and progression of the periodontal and peri-implant diseases [11]. Becker and co-workers examined the differences and similarities between peri-implantitis and periodontitis underlying disease mechanisms [12]. On the basis of quantitative transcriptome analysis, peri-implantitis and periodontitis exhibited significantly different mRNA signatures, supporting the hypothesis of peri-implantitis being a complex inflammatory disorder with a unique pathophysiology. While in peri-implantitis tissue, the regulation of transcripts related to innate immune responses and defense responses were dominating, in periodontitis tissues, bacterial response systems prevailed [12]. Several authors questioned the role of infection as a principal cause of peri-implant diseases. For instance, Koka and Zarb questioned whether peri-implantitis is a disease entity at all. The Authors refuted the bacterial implications and suggested terms such as osseoinsufficiency or osseoseparation to describe problematic implants [13]. Moreover, in a review article, Qian and co-workers failed to find evidence that primary infection causes marginal bone resorption around implants [14]. Osseointegration has been suggested to represent a foreign body reaction to biomaterials and its long-term clinical function depending on a foreign body equilibrium that, if disturbed, may lead to impaired clinical function of the implant [15]. Recently, dental implants have been suggested having more in common to orthopaedic implants in terms of foreign body reaction and failure pattern than to teeth [16]. Given these fundamental differences between the periodontal and peri-implant tissues, can periodontal indices be used as reliable diagnostic tools for peri-implant tissues?

2. The Risk of Using Surrogate Endpoints for Prediction of Fatal Events

In the most recent definition and diagnosis requirements for peri-mucositis and peri-implantitis, the use of probing around dental implants has been recommended for the detection of presence of bleeding on probing (BOP), of increases in pocket probing depth (PPD) or of presence of PPD equal or more than 6 mm [17]. Thus, periodontal indices are recommended as biologic measures to distinguish between health and disease conditions and as surrogate endpoints as substitutes for fatal events (implant failures) in clinical trial designs. The underlying assumption is that an improvement in the surrogates would benefit the patient and that it is equivalent to reducing the rate of implant losses [18]. Whenever surrogate endpoints (or biological markers) are used, the link between the surrogate and the true clinical event is critical since the use of non-validated endpoints may be more harmful than beneficial. A classic example in the field of medicine is the clinical investigation carried out on the assumption that arrhythmia is a risk factor for acute myocardial infarction and that, as a consequence, the suppression of arrhythmia would reduce the risk of death by infarction. The investigation had to be stopped when it became clear that the antiarrhythmic agents successfully reduced the number of arrhythmia episodes but increased the risk of dying by infarction. Clearly, the reduction of arrhythmia was not a good surrogate of treatment benefit to the patient [19]. One can question whether the high prevalence of periodontal diseases claimed in more recent years and the alarming possibility of peri-implantitis becoming a major future health problem [20] is correct or whether it is based on the wrong choice of surrogate endpoints (biologic markers), and therefore cause unnecessary alarmism and overtreatments which are of no benefit to the patients.

3. The Use of Periodontal Indices to Diagnose Peri-Implant Disease

A systematic review of peri-implantitis therapy published in 2010 showed that PPD, BOP and clinical attachment level (CAL) were the most frequently reported surrogate markers for important clinical events such as implant failure, despite the fact that these surrogate markers/endpoints had not yet been validated [18]. Has anything changed in the last nine years? Has the use of periodontal indices around dental implants been validated since then? Periodontal probing has been a common basic diagnostic tool around teeth since investigations in the 1970s demonstrated that PPD measurements around teeth provide information regarding the ability of the periodontium to withstand probe penetration as a measure of the inflammatory conditions of the tissues. In case of an inflamed periodontium, the tip of the probe penetrates the epithelium into the connective tissue, overestimating the depth of the histological pocket. In case of a healthy gingiva, the tip of the probe fails to reach the most apical cell of the epithelium due to the increased resistance of the periodontal tissues, thus underestimating the depth of the histological pocket [21–23]. Ericsson and Lindhe confirmed this finding in animals but also showed that in healthy soft tissues conditions, probe penetration was more advanced at implants than at teeth and concluded that the differences between the attachment structure of teeth versus peri-implant mucosa makes the conditions for PPD measurements at teeth and implants different [24]. In contrast, Lang and co-workers reported that in healthy and mucositis sites, the probe tip was located at the most apical cell of the junctional epithelium, whereas in the case of ligature-induced peri-implantitis sites, the probe tip penetrated into the connective tissue. They concluded that probing around implants represents a good technique for assessing the status of peri-implant mucosal health or disease. The difference in results between the two studies was attributed to the lower probing forces in the last study, which was 0.2 N versus 0.5 N [25].

More relevantly, on an evidence-based scale, investigations in humans failed to detect a positive correlation between the presence of periodontal signs of inflammation (PPD, BOP) and peri-implant bone loss. In a cross-sectional study by Lekholm and co-workers with a mean follow-up time of 7.6 years of 125 implants placed in 20 partially edentulous patients reported that 60% of the pockets measured more than 4 mm and that 80% of the sites were positive for BOP despite a limited mean bone loss of 0.07 mm annually. The microflora was periodontally non-pathogenic in nature in 94% of the samples and soft tissue biopsies showed a healthy mucosa in 95% of the cases. Thus, bleeding of the peri-implant tissues and deep pockets had no correlation to crestal bone loss or to the presence of a pathogenic microflora or to histological changes indicative for signs of periodontitis [26]. These findings were confirmed several years later by Dierens and co-workers, who reported of lack of correlations between PPD or BOP and crestal bone loss around single implants functional for 16–22 years. PPD and BOP were found to be of poor diagnostic value [27]. Recently also Winitsky and co-workers confirmed these observations, reporting of a lack of correlation between radiographically-detected crestal bone loss and periodontal indices such as PPD >6 mm and BOP in a 14–20 follow-up of 48 single anterior maxillary implants with a survival rate of 96%. The authors concluded by raising the question of whether PPD and BOP should be used as diagnostic measurements of implant health [28].

4. Evidences That Pocket Probing Depth Is a Poor Indicator of Ongoing Peri-Implant Pathology

The thickness of the healthy soft tissues surrounding implants has been reported to range between 1.85 and 5.75 mm in beagle dogs [29]. A clinical study showed values ranging from of 0.85 to 6.85 mm, but even papillae of 7–9 mm were observed [30]. Often, deeper PPDs are found at implant sites inserted in partially edentulous ridges compared to edentulous ridges [31]. Kan and co-workers reported the interproximal thickness of healthy peri-implant mucosa to be roughly 6 mm (SD 1.2) in maxillary anterior single implant with a mean functional time of 3 years [32]. Long-term clinical investigations have clearly shown that the probing depth of healthy peri-implant mucosa is often more than 4 mm (60% to 63%) [26,28,33] and up and over 6 mm (15% to 23%) [27,28] and that successful implants with over 18 years of function might have a history of PPD up to 9 mm [28,33]. From animal and human studies, it is evident that PPD depends on the thickness of the soft tissue at the time of implant placement and on the anatomical circumstances. For these reasons, there is no specific pocket depth that can indicate disease conditions. This fact is acknowledged in the new classification scheme for periodontal and peri-implant diseases and conditions, where in the peri-implant health definition it is stated that "it is not possible to define a range of probing depths compatible with peri-implant health" [1], and it is reflected in the fact that for the diagnosis of peri-implant health, it is mentioned that probing depths depend on the height of the soft tissue at the location of the implant [17]. Unfortunately, in the same paper, it is stated that in the absence of previous examination data, diagnosis of peri-implantitis requires the presence of bleeding and/or suppuration on gentle probing, probing depths ≥6 mm, and bone levels ≥3 mm apical of the most coronal portion of the intraosseous part of the implant.

Obviously, in light of what was discussed so far, the recommendation of using a 6-mm deep pocket (which appears to be an arbitrary choice) as one of the indicators of peri-implantitis appears to be highly questionable.

In the same paper, it is stated that for the diagnosis of peri-implantitis among other parameters, "an increased probing depth compared to previous examinations" is required.

The use of changes in PPD to establish a diagnosis of peri-implantitis has been questioned [5]. Schou and co-workers have shown in animal studies that PPD assessments could not distinguish between peri-implant sites with or without crestal bone loss and that the only correct indication of bone level stability was obtained by radiographs [34]. Furthermore, even mild inflammation was associated with deeper probe penetration around implants in comparison to teeth with no correlation to presence of bone loss [35]. In a more relevant 5-year clinical prospective investigation, Weber and co-workers assessed the ability of several clinical parameters (Suppuration, PI. BOP, PPD, PAL, mobility) to predict crestal bone loss as detected on radiographs in 112 ITI implants [36]. The authors reported no bone changes between years one and five in comparison to increasing PPD values during the five years. The cumulative predictive power of the six clinical parameters with regards to bone loss was reported to range from 2.8% to 14.3%. It was concluded that "the low levels of correlation between the individual and cumulative clinical parameters with radiographically measured bone loss, suggests that these measures are of limited clinical value in assessing and predicting future peri-implant bone loss". Healthy peri-implant soft tissues have been reported in sites with increased PPD values by Giannopoulou and co-workers in a 9-year follow-up of 61 maxillary anterior implants using clinical, microbiologic and biochemical parameters, thus showing a very poor correlation between PPD changes and the presence of pathology at the peri-implant tissues [37]. From the above discussed data, it appears that an increase in probing depth around implants does not necessarily mean that loss of bone or clinical attachment has occurred. Since the key parameter for establishing a diagnosis of peri-implantitis is bone loss and since the latter cannot be properly identified by a specific, pre-established PPD value or by changes in PPD, the use of probing for PPD assessments around implants does not appear to be a validated diagnostic tool.

5. Evidences That Bleeding on Probing Is a Poor Indicator of Ongoing Peri-Implant Pathology

For the detection of pathology and consequent treatment needs, BOP is a key parameter, according to the most recent recommendations, since BOP is used as a diagnostic parameter for the detection of both peri-mucositis and peri-implantitis [17]. This recommendation assumes that healthy peri-implant soft tissues do not test positive to BOP, whereas only diseased sites do (or, at least, that there is a statistically significant clinical difference between healthy and diseased sites when it comes to BOP positivity test). While Lang and co-workers' Beagle dog investigation detected constant increases in BOP from healthy peri-implant sites to ligature-induced peri-mucositis sites to ligature-induced peri-implantitis [25], Ericsson and Lindhe's Beagle dog investigation reported of the presence of

BOP for the majority of the healthy peri-implant sites [24]. One investigation comparing teeth and implants with respect to soft tissue healing revealed that peri-implant healing as determined by crevicular molecular composition differs from periodontal healing and suggested that peri-implant tissues represent a higher pro-inflammatory state [38]. Thus, the peri-implant soft tissues could be considered to be in a state of subclinical chronic inflammation. In fact, cross-sectional studies have shown that BOP can be detected at the majority of sites, showing stable peri-implant tissues.

With a definition of peri-implantitis as an association of BOP and any bone-level alterations at implant sites occurring between the 1-year and the 5-year (up to 23 years) follow-up examinations, Fransson and co-workers reported the presence of BOP in 93.9% of the 197 implants with "progressive" bone loss and in 90.9% of the 285 implants with stable bone level [39].

Roos-Jansåker et al reported that peri-implant mucositis, diagnosed by BOP, was detected in approximately 70% of functioning implants after 9 to 14 years. The prevalence of peri-implantitis, defined as bone loss of at least 1.8 mm following the first year of function, combined with BOP and/or pus, was 16% at patient level and 6.6% at implant level. Interestingly, 42.2% of the implants had stable bone levels and still showed BOP or suppuration, and 8.4% of the implants showed bone level gain even in the presence of BOP or suppuration [40]. A very poor correlation between presence of BOP and presence of peri-implant diseases has been reported in several long-term clinical studies. Lekholm at al reported the BOP of 80% around implants, showing an annual bone loss of 0.07 mm and a 95% healthy mucosa at biopsies [26]. Dierens and coworkers reported 81% BOP around implants, showing stable conditions for 16 to 22 years of function [27]. Winitsky and co-workers reported 71% BOP around implants, showing stable conditions for 14 to 20 years of function [28]. French and co-workers, in a large cohort study including 4591 Straumann implants from 2060 subjects evaluated up to ten-year follow-up, reported that BOP was a common finding, detected in more than 40% of the implants during the study. Despite the high prevalence of bleeding, less than 3% of implants exhibited more than 1 mm crestal bone. The presented data indicated that minimal bleeding did not correlate with bone loss, whereas profuse bleeding or suppuration did [41].

The type of implant, two-piece vs. one-piece, may affect the soft tissue bleeding response to probing. The presence of a chronic infiltrate at the implant-abutment interface of two-piece implants has been reported and has been attributed to the microgap between the implant and the abutment [42,43]. In contrast, the connective tissue surrounding one-piece implants has been reported to be inflammation-free, possibly due to the absence of a microgap [44]. This could partially explain the high BOP prevalence detected at stable peri-implant sites in investigations on two-piece implants [26–28,39,40] and the lower percentage of BOP (40%) detected at stable peri-implant sites around one-piece implants. In case of one-piece implants, the presence of profuse BOP had a higher correlation to crestal bone loss compared to the poor correlation of minimal BOP [41].

The type of abutment material has been demonstrated to have an effect on BOP values in a recent systematic review, where increased BOP values over time were demonstrated for Ti when compared to Zi abutments [45]. Implant position (anterior v posterior), gender and PPD have been shown to be factors affecting the probability of a peri-implant site to be positive to BOP. In 112 patients, data related to 1725 peri-implant sites showed that the probability to bleed on probing increases for implants placed in anterior compared to posterior areas of the dentition, for implants placed in female patients compared to male patients, and that for each mm increase in PPD, there is a corresponding 10% increase in the probability of detecting BOP at the site [46].

Thus, BOP seems to depend on the implant type (two-piece/one-piece), the type of abutment material, the implant position (anterior/posterior), the patient's gender and the PPD of the probed site without correlation to disease presence.

It has been shown that BOP can be detected in the majority of healthy peri-implant sites and cannot therefore be reasonably used to distinguish between peri-implant health and disease.

The investigations that attempted to establish the validity of the use of BOP as a predictor of future crestal bone loss around implants have failed to produce convincing result to justify the use of BOP as an appropriate diagnostic test. Jepsen and co-workers reported no difference in BOP between sites with progressive peri-implant PAL loss (rather than progressive bone loss) or stable sites. The authors pointed out that probing might provoke a nonspecific bleeding that is unrelated to the amount of inflammation. Thus, BOP as a diagnostic test for progressive PAL loss had a sensitivity of 70% and a specificity of 32%. In other words, BOP was of limited value in the implant-specific diagnosis when examined as positive predictors for peri-implant attachment loss. However, BOP demonstrated a higher negative predictive value and it was concluded that negative scores can serve as indicators of stable peri-implant conditions [47]. Monje and co-workers found that the diagnostic accuracy of BOP was not enough to distinguish healthy from peri-implantitis sites (defined as presence of inflammation and 2 mm crestal bone loss). A visual sign, such as mucosa redness, was reported having a much better diagnostic accuracy in monitoring the presence of pathology. For the clinical parameters investigated (PPD, BPO, mucosa redness, PI), it was found that, as diagnostic tests, their specificity surpasses their sensitivity in the detection of peri-implant diseases. The authors therefore concluded that the diagnosis of peri-implant diseases cannot rely on a single clinical parameter but rather requires a combination. More interestingly, it was pointed out that progressive radiographic bone loss must be cautiously examined to reach definitive diagnosis and avoid overtreatment [48]. Weber and co-workers reported that the cumulative predictive power of six clinical parameters (Suppuration, PI. BOP, PPD, PAL) with regards to bone loss ranges from 2.8% to 14.3% and concluded that "these measures are of limited clinical value in assessing and predicting future peri-implant bone loss" [36]. A recent systematic review and meta-analysis demonstrated that for BOP-positive implants, there was a 24.1% chance of being diagnosed with peri-implantitis, while for BOP-positive patients, there was a 33.8% probability of being diagnosed with peri-implantitis. It was concluded that clinicians should be aware of the considerable false-positive rate of BOP to diagnose peri-implantitis [49].

6. Mismatch between Known Clinical Facts and Recommendations from Consensus Meetings

It is interesting to note that review articles [5,49,50] and prospective studies [36,48] conclude that periodontal indices are unreliable tools for examining implants. Yet, the consensus meetings that often commission the reports keep recommending the use of periodontal indices around implants.

As discussed by Coli and co-workers, the efficacy of a diagnostic test is affected by the prevalence of the disease in the investigated population [5]. With increases in the disease prevalence, the probability that a person with a positive test result does in fact have the disease increases. Thus, two factors are of importance in order to properly establish an accurate disease diagnosis and avoid high figures of false positives. The first factor is the availability of a diagnostic test with high sensitivity and specificity. This has not yet been proven to be the case for any of the periodontal indices usually applied around dental implants. The second factor is the application of the diagnostic test to a population that has a high prevalence of the disease. Studies using the presence of BOP and a pre-established amount of crestal bone loss can result in high prevalence of peri-mucositis and peri-implantitis, however, if more stringent values of crestal bone loss are applied, much lower prevalence values are presented [50].

Long-term clinical investigations on machined implants are showing that despite the presence of several clinical parameters that would be considered indicative of pathology in the case of natural dentition (BOP, increases in PPD, suppuration), peri-implant tissue conditions were generally stable for over 18 years with only 2.5%–5% of implants showing progressive bone loss [27,28,33,51,52]. A review including ten different publications on three brands of moderately rough surfaces with ten- year or longer follow-up times reported a 2.7% peri-implantitis prevalence [7]. Jemt and co-workers reported that the incidence of surgery related to peri-implantitis problems carried out at the Branemark clinic was on an average 1.2% of followed-up patients per year (on an average, 1294 patients per year) during an 8-years period [53]. Thus, long-term clinical studies on machined as well as on modern micro-rough implant surfaces are indicative of a low 1.2%–5% prevalence of peri-implantitis and implant losses due to peri-implantitis. With such low peri-implantitis prevalence figures and with clinical parameters with poor accuracy as diagnostic tests, the probability of a dental implant being correctly diagnosed as suffering from peri-implant diseases appears to be very low and the risk of overtreatment very high.

Two investigations highlight the poor accuracy of periodontal indices causing overdiagnosis in several cases and failing to correctly identify implants that will suffer crestal bone loss in the future. In a follow-up study based on the population described by Fransson and co-workers [39,54], Jemt and co-workers showed that 9 years after the initial diagnosis of peri-implantitis, 31% of the patients presented with implants with bone loss >2mm/year or with implant failures, whereas 69% of them showed no problems with their implants [55]. A total of 91.4% of the implants in the peri-implantitis diagnosed patients showed no or smaller annual bone loss than <0.2mm during the 9 years from the diagnosis. The authors reported a low prevalence of obvious bone loss at implants (>0.2 mm/year) with a comparable distribution between "affected" and "not affected" implants. Hence, the definition of peri-implantitis used in the Fransson and co-workers study [39], bone loss associated with BOP, was shown to be a poor predictor of future bone loss and implant failure and, consequently, a poor indicator of treatment needs. In a follow-up study based on the population described by Roos-Jansåker and co-workers in 2006 [40], Renvert and co-workers reported that 12 years after the initial diagnosis of peri-implantitis and surgical treatment, 23% of the patients presented with implants with further bone loss ≥3 threads. In the remaining 77% of the subjects, bone gains (15%) or no further bone loss or bone loss <3 threads were detected [56]. Out of the subjects that at the first examination did not have peri-implantitis, 15% were diagnosed as having at least one implant with bone loss of ≥3 threads in the 21–26-year examination. For the 9–14 years examination, 58% of the individuals had been diagnosed with mucositis. Of those, 14% were found to have developed peri-implantitis at the 21–26-year examination. On the other hand, 22% of the patients without any sign of mucositis after 9–14 years had developed peri-implantitis at a later stage. Thus, a diagnosis of mucositis established after 9–14 years was not predictive for development of peri-implantitis after 21–26 years, nor was the diagnosis of peri-implantitis after 9–14 years predictive of further bone loss at 21–26 years. It seems evident that the use of a dichotomous diagnostic criterion (bleeding yes or no) for the definition of peri-mucositis and the arbitrary choice of a defined bone loss in association with BOP (surrogate endpoints) for the definition of peri-implantitis, does not capture the long-term true outcome (endpoint) in the form of implant failure and could result in massive overtreatment of implant patients. In fact, patients treated by oral hygienists and/or had experienced peri-implantitis surgery did not seem to show any more favourable progression of bone loss as compared with non-treated patients [55,56].

7. The Risk of Iatrogenic Damage by Probing of Dental Implants

One important aspect that has not been debated in the literature and that has not yet been properly tested is the fact that probing around implants could potentially result in trauma to the peri-implant soft tissues with consequent inflammation, apical proliferation of the epithelium and consequent bone loss. There is strong evidence in the literature that the mechanical disruption of the mucosal barrier around an implant should be considered as a connective tissue wound resulting in epithelial proliferation to cover the wound and in bone resorption to allow a connective tissue barrier of proper dimensions to reform in order to re-establish a "biological width". Repeated abutment dis/reconnections with a consequent disruption of the peri-implant soft tissue barrier have been shown to cause crestal bone resorption around dental implants in animal studies [57,58] and in short-term and long-term clinical investigations, as confirmed in several meta-analysis reports [59–61]. Although this limited crestal bone resorption does not seem to be clinically relevant, this established fact should at least raise the doubt that regular peri-implant tissue probing assessments might repeatedly disrupt the soft tissue barrier with consequent serious iatrogenic effects on the stability of the peri-implant tissues in the long term.

Another serious aspect to be considered is the overdiagnosis and overtreatment caused by the use of periodontal indices. In periodontology, it is well established that the presence of BOP is not an indicator of future periodontal tissue loss, but rather that the absence of BOP is a good predictor of periodontal stability [62]. For this reason, during the active and maintenance phases of periodontal treatment, 4-mm-deep or deeper sites showing BOP are treated by scaling and root planing. This zero-tolerance approach certainly results in overtreatment in several cases but does not result in damages to the periodontal tissues and is therefore accepted and recommended. The same approach in the case of dental implants seems to be unjustified and potentially dangerous. As discussed above, there is no evidence in the literature that the presence of BOP at an implant site is a sign of pathology (peri-mucositis or peri-implantitis) with a consequent treatment needed. The zero-tolerance approach to bleeding in the case of dental implants could not only result in overtreatment, but, in fact, in the triggering and the establishment of a difficult-to-manage inflammation in the soft tissues and excruciate into a foreign-body reaction.

Different techniques are used to achieve decontamination of the abutment/implant surfaces. Calculus is removed by manual debridement, such as conventional or ultrasonic scaling, resulting in the release of Ti particles in the surrounding tissues and in surface changes affecting the corrosion resistance of the material [63–67]. Orthopaedic studies have shown that the presence of titanium particles from wear of limb prosthesis could over-express pro-inflammatory cytokines, that are related to the osteolysis process, culminating in bone loss around the implant and prosthesis failure [68]. A recent review concluded that Ti particles and corrosion products from dental implants can have adverse effects on biological tissue [69]. Titanium particles released by ultrasonic scaling on dental implants have been shown to activate inflammatory responses in in vitro studies: activating the DNA damage response pathway in oral epithelial cells [70] or resulting in an increased secretion of IL-1β, IL-6, and TNF-α in cultured human macrophages [71–73], inducing bone resorption [71]. In vivo, titanium particles have been found in soft and hard tissue biopsies retrieved from sites with peri-implantitis [74,75]. Peri-implantitis tissues have been shown to contain high concentrations of Ti compared to controls from periodontitis tissues, leading to the conclusion that the high Ti content in peri-implant mucosa has the potential to aggravate inflammation [76]. Furthermore, greater levels of dissolved titanium have been detected in submucosal plaque around implants with peri-implantitis compared with healthy implants, indicating an association between titanium dissolution and peri-implantitis [77].

Since Ti particles can be released from surfaces of dental implants because of mechanical wear and because of contact to chemical agents and/or with substances produced by adherent biofilm and inflammatory cells, Mombelli and co-workers suggested that rather than being the trigger of disease, the observed higher concentration of Ti particles in inflamed peri-implant tissues could be the consequence of the presence of biofilms and inflammation [78]. However, in a recent animal model, it was shown that Ti particles induce an inflammatory response with consequent bone loss and that both inflammation and bone loss can be inhibited by the use of blockers targeting specific inflammatory cytokines. The specific role of inflammatory cytokines in the development of Ti particle-induced peri-implantitis was therefore clearly demonstrated [79]. Another investigation using a different animal model further confirms that Ti particles can induce inflammatory bone loss even in the absence of a bacteria infection and that the inflammatory response can be inhibited by blocking macrophage activity [80]. Thus, there is increasing evidence that dental implant degradation products released by corrosion and/or abrasion during mechanical debridement can act as foreign bodies, initiating the release of inflammatory mediators associated with bone resorption, as already described in the case of orthopaedic implants [81]. Hence, non-surgical implant debridement, incorrectly triggered by the detection of BOP at one otherwise healthy and stable implant site, could result in alterations of the implant surface, with the release of Ti particles (at the time of debridement and/or as a later consequence of the surface corrosion) and initiation of a foreign-body reaction.

8. Conclusions and Recommendations Regarding Evaluation of the Implant-Tissue Interface

Periodontal indices do not seem to be reliable indicators for appropriate diagnosis and treatment needs around dental implants. Apparently, they do not provide better information than visual inspection and detection of mucosa redness. Probing around dental implant is more uncomfortable for the patient compared to probing around teeth. Probing around implants could potentially create a trauma in the peri-implant scar tissue that could become difficult to manage. All the information gathered from probing (BOP, PPD, CAL) needs to be associated to the radiographic assessment of crestal bone levels to establish a definitive diagnosis and avoid overtreatment. Therefore, it appears to be more logical to avoid any risks of disturbing the peri-implant tissues with probing and instead proceeding with a clinical examination that includes (1) a visual inspection of the peri-implant tissues for the assessment of oral hygiene and the detection of potential redness, swelling, (2) palpation of the peri-implant tissues for assessment of the potential presence of swelling, bleeding, and suppuration, and (3) radiography for the assessment of crestal bone level for comparison with previous radiographs to evaluate potential progressive bone loss even if there is a need for more scientific evidence of the true value of the first two clinical testing modes.

Conflicts of Interest: The authors declare no conflict of interest.

References

1. Caton, J.G.; Armitage, G.; Berglundh, T.; Chapple, I.L.C.; Jepsen, S.; Kornman, K.S.; Mealey, B.L.; Papapanou, P.N.; Sanz, M.; Tonetti, M.S. A new classification scheme for periodontal and peri-implant diseases and conditions—Introduction and key changes from the 1999 classification. *J. Clin. Periodontol.* **2018**, *45* (Suppl. 20), S1–S8. [CrossRef] [PubMed]
2. Tomasi, C.; Derks, J. Clinical research of peri-implant diseases—Quality of reporting, case definitions and methods to study incidence, prevalence and risk factors of peri-implant diseases. *J. Clin. Periodontol.* **2012**, *39* (Suppl. 12), 207–223. [CrossRef]
3. Derks, J.; Tomasi, C. Peri-implant health and disease. A systematic review of current epidemiology. *J. Clin. Periodontol.* **2015**, *42* (Suppl. 16), S158–S171. [CrossRef] [PubMed]
4. Albrektsson, T.; Chrcanovic, B.; Ostman, P.O.; Sennerby, L. Initial and long-term crestal bone responses to modern dental implants. *Periodontology 2000* **2017**, *73*, 41–50. [CrossRef] [PubMed]
5. Coli, P.; Christiaens, V.; Sennerby, L.; Bruyn, H. Reliability of periodontal diagnostic tools for monitoring peri-implant health and disease. *Periodontology 2000* **2017**, *73*, 203–217. [CrossRef] [PubMed]
6. Brånemark, P.I.; Hansson, B.O.; Adell, R.; Breine, U.; Lindström, J.; Hallén, O.; Ohman, A. Osseointegrated implants in the treatment of the edentulous jaw. Experience from a 10-year period. *Scand. J. Plast. Reconstr. Surg. Suppl.* **1977**, *16*, 1–132. [PubMed]
7. Albrektsson, T.; Buser, D.; Sennerby, L. Crestal bone loss and oral implants. *Clin. Implant Dent. Relat. Res.* **2012**, *14*, 783–791. [CrossRef]
8. Albrektsson, T.; Dahlin, C.; Jemt, T.; Sennerby, L.; Turri, A.; Wennerberg, A. Is marginal bone loss around oral implants the result of a provoked foreign body reaction? *Clin. Implant Dent. Relat. Res.* **2014**, *16*, 155–165. [CrossRef]
9. Degidi, M.; Artese, L.; Piattelli, A.; Scarano, A.; Shibli, J.A.; Piccirilli, M.; Perrotti, V.; Iezzi, G. Histological and immunohistochemical evaluation of the peri-implant soft tissues around machined and acid-etched titanium healing abutments: A prospective randomised study. *Clin. Oral Investig.* **2012**, *16*, 857–866. [CrossRef]
10. Carcuac, O.; Berglundh, T. Composition of Human Peri-implantitis and Periodontitis Lesions. *J. Dent. Res.* **2014**, *93*, 1083–1088. [CrossRef]
11. Lang, N.P.; Berglundh, T. Periimplant diseases: Where are we now? Consensus of the Seventh European Workshop on periodontology. *J. Clin. Periodontol.* **2011**, *38*, 178–181. [CrossRef] [PubMed]
12. Becker, S.T.; Beck-Broichsitter, B.E.; Graetz, C.; Dörfer, C.E.; Wiltfang, J.; Häsler, R. Peri-implantitis versus periodontitis: Functional differences indicated by transcriptome profiling. *Clin. Implant Dent. Relat. Res.* **2014**, *16*, 401–411. [CrossRef] [PubMed]
13. Koka, S.; Zarb, G. On osseointegration: The healing adaptation principle in the context of osseosufficiency, osseoseparation, and dental implant failure. *Int. J. Prosthodont.* **2012**, *25*, 48–52. [PubMed]
14. Qian, J.; Wennerberg, A.; Albrektsson, T. Reasons for marginal bone loss around oral implants. *Clin. Implant Dent. Relat. Res.* **2012**, *14*, 792–807. [CrossRef] [PubMed]

15. Trindade, R.; Albrektsson, T.; Tengvall, P.; Wennerberg, A. Foreign Body Reaction to Biomaterials: On Mechanisms for Buildup and Breakdown of Osseointegration. *Clin. Implant Dent. Relat. Res.* **2016**, *18*, 192–203. [CrossRef] [PubMed]
16. Albrektsson, T.; Becker, W.; Coli, P.; Jemt, T.; Mölne, J.; Sennerby, L. Bone loss around oral and orthopedic implants: An immunologically based condition. *Clin. Implant Dent. Relat. Res.* **2019**. [CrossRef]
17. Berglundh, T.; Armitage, G.; Araujo, M.G.; Avila-Ortiz, G.; Blanco, J.; Camargo, P.M.; Chen, S.; Cochran, D.; Derks, J.; Figuero, E.; et al. Peri-implant diseases and conditions: Consensus report of workgroup 4 of the 2017 World Workshop on the Classification of Periodontal and Peri-Implant Diseases and Conditions. *J. Clin. Periodontol.* **2018**, *45* (Suppl. 20), S286–S291. [CrossRef]
18. Faggion, C.M., Jr.; Listl, S.; Tu, Y.K. Assessment of endpoints in studies on peri-implantitis treatment—A systematic review. *J. Dent.* **2010**, *38*, 443–450. [CrossRef]
19. Echt, D.S.; Liebson, P.R.; Mitchell, L.B.; Peters, R.W.; Obias-Manno, D.; Barker, A.H.; Arensberg, D.; Baker, A.; Friedman, L.; Greene, H.L.; et al. Mortality and Morbidity in Patients Receiving Encainide, Flecainide, or Placebo—The Cardiac Arrhythmia Suppression Trial. *N. Engl. J. Med.* **1991**, *324*, 781–788. [CrossRef]
20. Giannobile, W.V.; Lang, N.P. Are Dental Implants a Panacea or Should We Better Strive to Save Teeth? *J. Dent. Res.* **2016**, *95*, 5–6. [CrossRef]
21. Listgarten, M.A.; Mao, R.; Robinson, P.J. Periodontal probing and the relationship of the probe tip to periodontal tissues. *J. Periodontol.* **1976**, *47*, 511–513. [CrossRef]
22. Armitage, G.C.; Svanberg, G.K.; Loë, H. Microscopic evaluation of clinical measurements of connective tissue attachment levels. *J. Clin. Periodontol.* **1977**, *4*, 173–190. [CrossRef]
23. Spray, J.R.; Garnick, J.J.; Doles, L.R.; Klawitter, J.J. Microscopic demonstration of the position of periodontal probes. *J. Periodontol.* **1978**, *49*, 148–152. [CrossRef]
24. Ericsson, I.; Lindhe, J. Probing depth at implants and teeth. An experimental study in the dog. *J. Clin. Periodontol.* **1993**, *20*, 623–627. [CrossRef]
25. Lang, N.P.; Wetzel, A.C.; Stich, H.; Caffesse, R.G. Histologic probe penetration in healthy and inflamed peri-implant tissues. *Clin. Oral Implants Res.* **1994**, *5*, 191–201. [CrossRef]
26. Lekholm, U.; Adell, R.; Lindhe, J.; Brånemark, P.I.; Eriksson, B.; Rockler, B.; Lindvall, A.M.; Yoneyama, T. Marginal tissue reactions at osseointegrated titanium fixtures. (II) A cross-sectional retrospective study. *Int. J. Oral Maxillofac. Surg.* **1986**, *15*, 53–61. [CrossRef]
27. Dierens, M.; Vandeweghe, S.; Kisch, J.; Nilner, K.; De Bruyn, H. Long-term follow-up of turned single implants placed in periodontally healthy patients after 16–22 years: Radiographic and peri-implant outcome. *Clin. Oral Implants Res.* **2012**, *23*, 197–204. [CrossRef]
28. Winitsky, N.; Olgart, K.; Jemt, T.; Smedberg, J.I. A retro-prospective long-term follow-up of Brånemark single implants in the anterior maxilla in young adults. Part 1: Clinical and radiographic parameters. *Clin. Implant Dent. Relat. Res.* **2018**, *20*, 937–944. [CrossRef]
29. Berglundh, T.; Lindhe, J.; Ericsson, I.; Marinello, C.P.; Liljenberg, B.; Thomsen, P. The soft tissue barrier at implants and teeth. *Clin. Oral Implants Res.* **1991**, *2*, 81–90. [CrossRef]
30. Choquet, V.; Hermans, M.; Adriaenssens, P.; Daelemans, P.; Tarnow, D.P.; Malevez, C. Clinical and radiographic evaluation of the papilla level adjacent to single-tooth dental implants. A retrospective study in the maxillary anterior region. *J. Periodontol.* **2001**, *72*, 1364–1371. [CrossRef]
31. Serino, G.; Turri, A.; Lang, N.P. Probing at implants with peri-implantitis and its relation to clinical peri-implant bone loss. *Clin. Oral Implants Res.* **2013**, *24*, 91–95. [CrossRef]
32. Kan, J.Y.; Rungcharassaeng, K.; Umezu, K.; Kois, J.C. Dimensions of peri-implant mucosa: An evaluation of maxillary anterior single implants in humans. *J. Periodontol.* **2003**, *74*, 557–562. [CrossRef]
33. Bergenblock, S.; Andersson, B.; Fürst, B.; Jemt, T. Long-term follow-up of CeraOne single-implant restorations: An 18-year follow-up study based on a prospective patient cohort. *Clin. Implant Dent. Relat. Res.* **2012**, *14*, 471–479. [CrossRef]
34. Schou, S.; Holmstrup, P.; Stoltze, K.; Hjørting-Hansen, E.; Kornman, K.S. Ligature-induced marginal inflammation around osseointegrated implants and ankylosed teeth. *Clin. Oral Implants Res.* **1993**, *4*, 12–22. [CrossRef]
35. Schou, S.; Holmstrup, P.; Stoltze, K.; Hjørting-Hansen, E.; Fiehn NESkovgaard, L.T. Probing around implants and teeth with healthy or inflamed peri-implant mucosa/gingiva. A histologic comparison in cynomolgus monkeys (Macaca fascicularis). *Clin. Oral Implants Res.* **2002**, *13*, 113–126. [CrossRef]

36. Weber, H.P.; Crohin, C.C.; Fiorellini, J.P. A 5-year prospective clinical and radiographic study of non-submerged dental implants. *Clin. Oral Implants Res.* **2000**, *11*, 144–153. [CrossRef]
37. Giannopoulou, C.; Bernard, J.P.; Buser, D.; Carrel, A.; Belser, U.C. Effect of intracrevicular restoration margins on peri-implant health: Clinical, biochemical, and microbiologic findings around esthetic implants up to 9 years. *Int. J. Oral Maxillofac. Implants* **2003**, *18*, 173–181.
38. Emecen-Huja, P.; Eubank, T.D.; Shapiro, V.; Yildiz, V.; Tatakis, D.N.; Leblebicioglu, B. Peri-implant versus periodontal wound healing. *J. Clin. Periodontol.* **2013**, *40*, 816–824. [CrossRef]
39. Fransson, C.; Wennström, J.; Berglundh, T. Clinical characteristics and implant with a history of progressive bone loss. *Clin. Oral Implants Res.* **2008**, *19*, 142–147. [CrossRef]
40. Roos-Jansåker, A.M.; Lindahl, C.; Renvert, H.; Renvert, S. Nine to fourteen-year follow-up of implant treatment. Part II: Presence of peri-implant lesions. *J. Clin. Periodontol.* **2006**, *33*, 290–295. [CrossRef]
41. French, D.; Cochran, D.L.; Ofec, R. Retrospective cohort study of 4591 Straumann implants placed in 2060 patients in private practice with up to 10-year follow-up: The relationship between crestal bone level and soft tissue condition. *Int. J. Oral Maxillofac. Implants* **2016**, *31*, e168–e178. [CrossRef]
42. Broggini, N.; McManus, L.M.; Hermann, J.S.; Medina, R.U.; Oates, T.W.; Schenk, R.K.; Buser, D.; Mellonig, J.T.; Cochran, D.L. Persistent acute inflammation at the implant-abutment interface. *J. Dent. Res.* **2003**, *82*, 232–237. [CrossRef]
43. Broggini, N.; McManus, L.M.; Hermann, J.S.; Medina, R.; Schenk, R.K.; Buser, D.; Cochran, D.L. Peri-implant inflammation defined by the implant-abutment interface. *J. Dent. Res.* **2006**, *85*, 473–478. [CrossRef]
44. Buser, D.; Weber, H.P.; Donath, K.; Fiorellini, J.P.; Paquette, D.W.; Williams, R.C. Soft tissue reactions to non-submerged unloaded titanium implant in beagle dogs. *J. Periodontol.* **1992**, *63*, 225–235. [CrossRef]
45. Sanz-Martín, I.; Sanz-Sánchez, I.; Carrillo de Albornoz, A.; Figuero, E.; Sanz, M. Effects of modified abutment characteristics on peri-implant soft tissue health: A systematic review and meta-analysis. *Clin. Oral Implants Res.* **2018**, *29*, 118–129. [CrossRef]
46. Farina, R.; Filippi, M.; Brazzioli, J.; Tomasi, C.; Trombelli, L. Bleeding on probing around dental implants: A retrospective study of associated factors. *J. Clin. Periodontol.* **2017**, *44*, 115–122. [CrossRef]
47. Jepsen, S.; Rühling, A.; Jepsen, K.; Ohlenbusch, B.; Albers, H.K. Progressive peri-implantitis. Incidence and prediction of peri-implant attachment loss. *Clin. Oral Implants Res.* **1996**, *7*, 133–142. [CrossRef]
48. Monje, A.; Caballé-Serrano, J.; Nart, J.; Peñarrocha, D.; Wang, H.L.; Rakic, M. Diagnostic accuracy of clinical parameters to monitor peri-implant conditions: A matched case-control study. *J. Periodontol.* **2018**, *89*, 407–417. [CrossRef]
49. Hashim, D.; Cionca, N.; Combescure, C.; Mombelli, A. The diagnosis of peri-implantitis: A systematic review on the predictive value of bleeding on probing. *Clin. Oral Implants Res.* **2018**, *29* (Suppl. 16), 276–293. [CrossRef]
50. Doornewaard, R.; Jacquet, W.; Cosyn, J.; De Bruyn, H. How do peri-implant biologic parameters correspond with implant survival and peri-implantitis? A critical review. *Clin. Oral Implants Res.* **2018**, *29* (Suppl. 18), 100–123. [CrossRef]
51. Attard, N.J.; Zarb, G.A. Long-term treatment outcomes in edentulous patients with implant-fixed prostheses: The Toronto study. *Int. J. Prosthodont.* **2004**, *17*, 417–424. [CrossRef]
52. Astrand, P.; Ahlqvist, J.; Gunne, J.; Nilson, H. Implant treatment of patients with edentulous jaws: A 20-year follow-up. *Clin. Implant Dent. Relat. Res.* **2008**, *10*, 207–217. [CrossRef]
53. Jemt, T.; Gyzander, V.; Britse, A.Ö. Incidence of surgery related to problems with peri-implantitis: A retrospective study on patients followed up between 2003 and 2010 at one specialist clinic. *Clin. Implant Dent. Relat. Res.* **2015**, *17*, 209–220. [CrossRef]
54. Fransson, C.; Lekholm, U.; Jemt, T.; Berglundh, T. Prevalence of subjects with progressive bone loss at implants. *Clin. Oral Implants Res.* **2005**, *16*, 440–446. [CrossRef]
55. Jemt, T.; Sundén Pikner, S.; Gröndahl, K. Changes of marginal bone level in patients with progressive bone loss at Brånemark System®implants: A radiographic follow-up study over an average of 9 years. *Clin. Implant Dent. Relat. Res.* **2015**, *17*, 619–628. [CrossRef]
56. Renvert, S.; Lindahl, C.; Persson, G.R. Occurrence of cases with peri-implant mucositis or peri-implantitis in a 21-26 year follow up study. *J. Clin. Periodontol.* **2018**, *45*, 233–240. [CrossRef]
57. Abrahamsson, I.; Berglundh, T.; Lindhe, J. The mucosal barrier following abutment dis/reconnection. An experimental study in dogs. *J. Clin. Periodontol.* **1997**, *24*, 568–572. [CrossRef]

58. Rodríguez, X.; Vela, X.; Méndez, V.; Segalà, M.; Calvo-Guirado, J.L.; Tarnow, D.P. The effect of abutment dis/reconnections on peri-implant bone resorption: A radiologic study of platform-switched and non-platform-switched implants placed in animals. *Clin. Oral Implants Res.* **2013**, *24*, 305–311. [CrossRef]
59. Koutouzis, T.; Gholami, F.; Reynolds, J.; Lundgren, T.; Kotsakis, G.A. Abutment Disconnection/Reconnection Affects Peri-implant Marginal Bone Levels: A Meta-Analysis. *Int. J. Oral Maxillofac. Implants* **2017**, *32*, 575–581. [CrossRef]
60. Wang, Q.Q.; Dai, R.; Cao, C.Y.; Fang, H.; Han, M.; Li, Q.L. One-time versus repeated abutment connection for platform-switched implant: A systematic review and meta-analysis. *PLoS ONE* **2017**, *12*, e0186385. [CrossRef]
61. Tallarico, M.; Caneva, M.; Meloni, S.M.; Xhanari, E.; Covani, U.; Canullo, L. Definitive Abutments Placed at Implant Insertion and Never Removed: Is It an Effective Approach? A Systematic Review and Meta-Analysis of Randomized Controlled Trials. *J. Oral Maxillofac. Surg.* **2018**, *76*, 316–324. [CrossRef]
62. Lang, N.P.; Adler, R.; Joss, A.; Nyman, S. Absence of bleeding on probing. An indicator of periodontal stability. *J. Clin. Periodontol.* **1990**, *17*, 714–721. [CrossRef]
63. Louropoulou, A.; Slot, D.E.; van der Weijden, F.A. Titanium surface alterations following the use of different mechanical instruments: A systematic review. *Clin. Oral Implants Res.* **2012**, *23*, 643–658. [CrossRef]
64. Ruhling, A.; Kocher, T.; Kreusch, J.; Plagmann, H.C. Treatment of subgingival implant surfaces with TeflonR-coated sonic and ultrasonic scaler tips and various implant curettes. An in vitro study. *Clin. Oral Implant Res.* **1994**, *5*, 19–29. [CrossRef]
65. Hallmon, W.W.; Waldrop, T.C.; Meffert, R.M.; Wade, B.W. A comparative study of the effects of metallic, nonmetallic, and sonic instrumentation on titanium abutment surfaces. *Int. J. Oral Maxillofac. Implants* **1996**, *11*, 96–100. [CrossRef]
66. Homiak, A.W.; Cook, P.A.; DeBoer, J. Effect of hygiene instrumentation on titanium abutments: A scanning electron microscopy study. *J. Prosthet. Dent.* **1992**, *67*, 364–369. [CrossRef]
67. Cross-Poline, G.N.; Shaklee, R.L.; Stach, D.J. Effect of implant curettes on titanium implant surfaces. *Am. J. Dent.* **1997**, *10*, 41–45.
68. Souza, P.P.; Lerner, U.H. The role of cytokines in inflammatory bone loss. *Immunol. Investig.* **2013**, *42*, 555–622. [CrossRef]
69. Noronha Oliveira, M.; Schunemann, W.V.H.; Mathew, M.T.; Henriques, B.; Magini, R.S.; Teughels, W.; Souza, J.C.M. Can degradation products released from dental implants affect peri-implant tissues? *J. Periodontal Res.* **2018**, *53*, 1–11. [CrossRef]
70. Suarez-Lopez del Amo, F.; Rudek, I.E.; Wagner, V.P.; Martins, M.D.; O'Valle, F.; Galindo-Moreno, P.; Giannobile, W.V.; Wang, H.L.; Castilho, R.M. Titanium activates the DNA damage response pathway in oral epithelial cells: A pilot study. *Int. J. Oral Maxillofac. Implants* **2017**, *32*, 1413–1420. [CrossRef]
71. Eger, M.; Sterer, N.; Liron, T.; Kohavi, D.; Gabet, Y. Scaling of titanium implants entrains inflammation-induced osteolysis. *Sci. Rep.* **2017**, *7*, 39612. [CrossRef] [PubMed]
72. Pettersson, M.; Kelk, P.; Belibasakis, G.N.; Bylund, D.; Molin Thoren, M.; Johansson, A. Titanium ions form particles that activate and execute interleukin-1beta release from lipopolysaccharide-primed macrophages. *J. Periodontal Res.* **2017**, *52*, 21–32. [CrossRef] [PubMed]
73. Dodo, C.G.; Meirelles, L.; Aviles-Reyes, A.; Ruiz, K.G.S.; Abranches, J.; Cury, A.A.D.B. Pro-inflammatory Analysis of Macrophages in Contact with Titanium Particles and Porphyromonas gingivalis. *Braz. Dent. J.* **2017**, *28*, 428–434. [CrossRef] [PubMed]
74. Wilson, T.G., Jr.; Valderrama, P.; Burbano, M.; Blansett, J.; Levine, R.; Kessler, H.; Rodrigues, D.C. Foreign bodies associated with peri-implantitis human biopsies. *J. Periodontol.* **2015**, *86*, 9–15. [CrossRef] [PubMed]
75. Fretwurst, T.; Buzanich, G.; Nahles, S.; Woelber, J.P.; Riesemeier, H.; Nelson, K. Metal elements in tissue with dental peri-implantitis: A pilot study. *Clin. Oral Implants Res.* **2016**, *27*, 1178–1186. [CrossRef] [PubMed]
76. Pettersson, M.; Pettersson, J.; Johansson, A.; Molin Thorén, M. Titanium release in peri-implantitis. *J. Oral Rehabil.* **2019**, *46*, 179–188. [CrossRef] [PubMed]
77. Safioti, L.M.; Kotsakis, G.A.; Pozhitkov, A.E.; Chung, W.O.; Daubert, D.M. Increased Levels of Dissolved Titanium Are Associated with Peri-Implantitis. A Cross-Sectional Study. *J. Periodontol.* **2017**, *88*, 436–442. [CrossRef]
78. Mombelli, A.; Hashim, D.; Cionca, N. What is the impact of titanium particles and biocorrosion on implant survival and complications? A critical review. *Clin. Oral Implants Res.* **2018**, *29* (Suppl. 18), 37–53. [CrossRef]

79. Eger, M.; Hiram-Bab, S.; Liron, T.; Sterer, N.; Carmi, Y.; Kohavi, D.; Gabet, Y. Mechanism and Prevention of Titanium Particle-Induced Inflammation and Osteolysis. *Front. Immunol.* **2018**, *18*, 2963. [CrossRef]
80. Wang, X.; Li, Y.; Feng, Y.; Cheng, H.; Li, D. Macrophage polarization in aseptic bone resorption around dental implants induced by Ti particles in a murine model. *J. Periodontal Res.* **2019**, *54*, 329–338. [CrossRef]
81. Purdue, P.E.; Koulouvaris, P.; Potter, H.G.; Nestor, B.J.; Sculco, T.P. The cellular and molecular biology of periprosthetic osteolysis. *Clin. Orthop. Relat. Res.* **2007**, *454*, 251–261. [CrossRef] [PubMed]

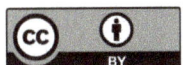

© 2019 by the authors. Licensee MDPI, Basel, Switzerland. This article is an open access article distributed under the terms and conditions of the Creative Commons Attribution (CC BY) license (http://creativecommons.org/licenses/by/4.0/).

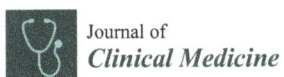

Review

Ligature-Induced Experimental Peri-Implantitis—A Systematic Review

David Reinedahl [1,*], Bruno Chrcanovic [2], Tomas Albrektsson [2,3], Pentti Tengvall [3] and Ann Wennerberg [1]

1   Department of Prosthodontics, Institute of Odontology, Sahlgrenska Academy, Gothenburg University, Gothenburg 405 30, Sweden; ann.wennerberg@odontologi.gu.se
2   Department of Prosthodontics, Faculty of Odontology, Malmö University, Malmö 205 06, Sweden; brunochrcanovic@hotmail.com (B.C.); tomas.albrektsson@biomaterials.gu.se (T.A.)
3   Department of Biomaterials, Institute of Clinical Sciences, Sahlgrenska Academy, Gothenburg University, Gothenburg 405 30, Sweden; pentti.tengvall@gu.se
*   Correspondence: d.reinedahl@gmail.com; Tel.: +46-73-390-57-26

Received: 4 November 2018; Accepted: 26 November 2018; Published: 28 November 2018

Abstract: This systematic review sought to analyze different experimental peri-implantitis models, their potential to induce marginal bone resorption (MBR) and the necessity of bacteria for bone loss to occur in these models. An electronic search in PubMed/Medline, Web of Science, and ScienceDirect was undertaken. A total of 133 studies were analyzed. Most studies induced peri-implantitis with ligatures that had formed a biofilm, sometimes in combination with inoculation of specific bacteria but never in a sterile environment. Most vertical MBR resulted from new ligatures periodically packed above old ones, followed by periodically exchanged ligatures and ligatures that were not exchanged. Cotton ligatures produced the most MBR, followed by steel, "dental floss" (not further specified in the studies) and silk. The amount of MBR varied significantly between different animal types and implant surfaces. None of the analyzed ligature studies aimed to validate that bacteria are necessary for the inducement of MBR. It cannot be excluded that bone loss can be achieved by other factors of the model, such as an immunological reaction to the ligature itself or trauma from repeated ligature insertions. Because all the included trials allowed plaque accumulation on the ligatures, bone resorbing capacity due to other factors could not be excluded or evaluated here.

Keywords: osseointegration; dental implant; peri-implantitis; ligature-induced peri-implantitis; aseptic loosening; systematic review

1. Introduction

Experiments that aimed to mimic peri-implantitis were first introduced in the early 1990s in response to reports on progressive peri-implant bone loss around dental implants [1,2]. These experiments have mainly been based on the infectious model of explanation where bacteria are the presumed cause of the phenomenon [2,3]. The view of peri-implantitis as a strictly infectious condition, as suggested in the studies these models were based on, is currently a matter of debate. Albrektsson and co-workers recently proposed that tissue responses to dental implants should be viewed similarly to other biomaterials; primarily as an immune mediated inflammatory and foreign body reaction (FBR), indicating that immunological reactions may be important also for MBR [4]. The initial, and most frequently used experimental peri-implantitis model was adopted from the ligature-induced periodontitis model. In short, ligatures made of silk, cotton, stainless-steel wire, or other materials, are placed around the neck of dental implants, usually in a sub-marginal position. The ligatures are then allowed to accumulate plaque for a few months, after which a certain amount of marginal bone resorption (MBR) can be expected. Previous authors have claimed that plaque accumulation is necessary for bone resorption to occur in response to ligation [2,5], but Baron et al. pointed out a lack of validation for this claim in their review from year 2000 and concluded that other factors, such as a foreign body reaction to the ligature may also trigger a peri-implant inflammatory response [6]. The aims of the present review were to categorize (1) the models that induce experimental peri-implantitis described in literature and (2) to verify whether the amount of vertical MBR varies between different ligature techniques (exchanged or non-exchanged ligature), material and size of ligatures, animals or implant surfaces used in these studies. With this information in mind, we then (3) critically analyzed the attempts to validate the presence of bacteria containing biofilms as a cause of MBR in ligature-induced peri-implantitis models.

2. Materials and Methods

The present study followed the PRISMA Statement for Transparent Reporting of Systematic Reviews and Meta-analyses [7].

2.1. Search Strategies

An electronic search without time restrictions for publications in English was undertaken in January 2018 in the following databases: PubMed/Medline, Web of Science, and ScienceDirect. The following terms were used in the search strategies:

(((dental implant) OR oral implant)) AND (experimentally induced periimplantitis) OR experimentally induced peri-implantitis) OR experimental periimplantitis) OR experimental peri-implantitis) OR ligature induced periimplantitis) OR ligature induced peri-implantitis) OR ligature) OR plaque induced periimplantitis) OR plaque induced peri-implantitis) OR plaque accumulation) OR mechanical overload) OR bacterial inoculation)

An additional manual search of related journals was conducted. The reference list of the identified studies and the relevant reviews on the subject were scanned for possible additional studies.

2.2. Inclusion and Exclusion Criteria

The inclusion criteria comprised in vivo studies performing experimentally induced peri-implantitis. All animal species used for the experiments and all methods to induce peri-implantitis were considered. Studies inducing periodontitis (around teeth) were not included, unless they were also investigating peri-implantitis around implants. Studies evaluating only mucositis around implants were excluded.

2.3. Study Selection

The titles and abstracts of all reports identified through the electronic searches were read independently by the authors. For studies appearing to meet the inclusion criteria, or for which there were insufficient data in the title and abstract to make a clear decision, the full report was obtained. Disagreements were resolved by discussion between the authors and the authors rapidly reached a consensus.

2.4. Data Extraction

Two review authors independently searched for trials aiming to validate the necessity of biofilm in order to induce MBR by means of ligatures. They then independently extracted data using specially designed data extraction forms. The data extraction forms were piloted on several papers, which were modified as required before use.

From the studies included in the final analysis, the following data was extracted (when available): Year of publication, animal species used in the experiments, number of animals, jaw receiving the implants, number of extracted teeth (to make room for the implants), implants' healing period, study design (split design, inter-quadrant, other), implant characteristics (shape, dimensions, material, surface, bone/tissue level), number of implants per animal, number of surgery stages, time between abutment connection and peri-implantitis induction, use or not of randomization, use or not of loading, pre- and post-operative care (antibiotic, and plaque control method, timing, and duration), method of induction of peri-implantitis (ligature, overload, bacterial inoculation, other), ligature (material, size, exchange regimen, duration, control side protocol), diagnostic markers (clinical measurements, mobility, microbiological sampling, radiographies, histometric measurements, histological evaluation, other), peri-implant bone defect (time of registration, vertical MBR, horizontal MBR, measurement method, development after ligature removal, number of lost implants). Contact with authors for possible missing data was performed.

2.5. Analyses

Descriptive statistics were utilized to report the data. In order to standardize and clarify ambiguous data, vertical MBR was reported for each publication. Vertical MBR was the continuous outcome evaluated, and the statistical unit was the implant (the implants used in the animals). The untransformed proportion (random-effects DerSimonian–Laird (1986) method) for vertical bone loss was calculated [8] with consideration for the different implant surfaces, the different animal species, the different methods to induce peri-implantitis and, when ligature was the method used, the different regimen applied, i.e., application of only one ligature, exchange of ligatures over time, and application of a new ligature on the top of an old one. Meta-regression was performed for the outcome of vertical MBR, using the time period of peri-implantitis induction as covariate. Statistical significance was set at $p < 0.05$. The data were analyzed using the software OpenMeta (Analyst) (MetaMorph Inc., Nashville, TN, USA) [9].

3. Results

3.1. Literature Search

The study selection process is summarized in Figure 1. The search strategy in the databases returned 3525 papers. A number of 745 articles were cited in more than one database (duplicates). The reviewers independently screened the abstracts for those articles related to the aim of the review. Of the resulting 2780 studies, 2642 were excluded for not being related to the topic or for not being induced peri-implantitis animal studies. Additional hand-searching of journals and of the reference lists of selected studies yielded 10 additional papers. The full-text reports of the remaining 148 articles led to the exclusion of 15 because they did not meet the inclusion criteria. Thus, a total of 133 publications were included in the review (see References S1).

3.2. Description of the Studies and Analyses

Regarding ligature-induced peri-implantitis; none of the included publications attempted to validate the presence of a bacterial biofilm in order to achieve MBR.

Detailed data of the 133 included studies are listed in Tables S1 and S2. Dogs were the most commonly used animal for the experiments (being the case of 94 studies) followed by monkeys (26 studies), mice (8 studies), micro-/mini-pigs (3 studies), and rats (2 studies).

Concerning the method of peri-implantitis induction, most of the studies ($n = 91$) induced peri-implantitis with the use of ligatures alone. Ligatures of cotton were used in 50 studies, silk in 31 studies, 3 metallic ligatures, one the resorbable suture Vicryl, one "dental floss", and 5 studies used a combination of ligatures of different materials. Thirteen studies applied a period of ligature and then a period of plaque accumulation (or vice-versa), 8 studies compared two or more groups concerning the method of peri-implantitis induction (ligature and/or overload and/or plaque accumulation), 5 studies used cotton ligatures followed by inoculation of *Porphyromonas gingivalis*. Seven studies provided a time of plaque accumulation alone, 4 studies exposed the implants to overload, 2 studies applied ligatures plus cyanoacrylate, 2 studies used bacterial inoculation alone, and 1 study immunized the animals followed by an injection of lipopolysaccharides.

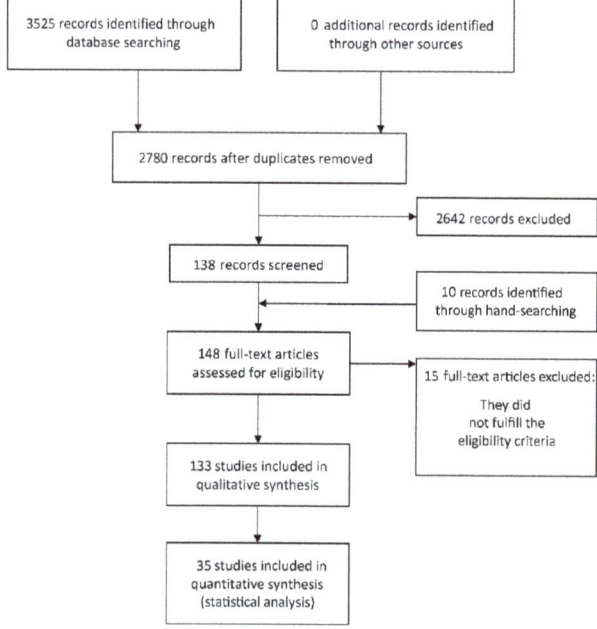

Figure 1. Study selection.

The implant healing period before the induction of experimental peri-implantitis was at average 96.0 ± 57.1 days (min–max, 0–365). Seventy-nine studies used bone-level implants, 46 tissue-level implants, 5 studies used both types of implants, 2 studies installed the implants at the sub-crestal level, and proper information was not provided in one study.

The ligature methods were of three different regimens: One ligature not replaced ($n = 53$), exchange of ligatures ($n = 43$), and periodical replacement of ligatures on top of old ones ($n = 11$). Information was not available in 4 studies. Only 30 studies provided information on ligature size, varying from suture size 7–0 to 2–0 United States Pharmacopeia (USP). Other examples included 0.010 inch, 0.254 mm, and 1.58 mm. The duration of ligature placement time varied between 7 and 660 days, and some studies intercalated the use of ligatures between periods of plaque accumulation or of plaque control.

Plaque control maintenance was performed in 111 studies, where the period varied between "only once" to 2 years. Information about plaque control was not available in 8 studies. The plaque control methods used varied considerably among studies and included one or a combination of two or more of the following activities: Daily brushing with toothpaste, interdental brushing, electric pencil brush, application of chlorhexidine, scrubbing with chlorhexidine, implant scaling with plastic scaler, gentle mechanical cleaning of pockets, manual irrigation with syringe, dental water jet, flossing, and curettage. The plaque control maintenance also varied considerably among studies concerning the duration period, the number of maintenance periods, and timing (for example; after teeth extraction, after implant installation, at abutment connection, and after ligature removal).

The studies usually made use of several diagnostic markers listed in Table S2, but the present review focused on the analysis of the vertical MBR. Table 1 shows the estimated vertical bone loss in relation to implant surface type, species, method of peri-implantitis induction, and ligature regimen, according to the untransformed proportion using the DerSimonian–Laird method (1986) analysis [6].

Only studies providing the number of implants used, mean value and standard deviation for bone loss were included here ($n = 35$ of the 133 reviewed studies) because these values are necessary for the analyses. Detailed data for these 35 studies are listed in Tables S3 and S4 and a reference list is available in References S2.

Table 1. Estimated vertical bone resorption in relation to implant surface type, species, method of peri-implantitis induction and ligature regimen.

Factor	MBR (in mm) (95% CI), p-Value, SE	Heterogeneity	Number of Measurements * Included for the Meta Regression (Number of Studies)
Surface			
Turned	2.265 (1.786, 2.745), $p < 0.001$, 0.245	$I^2 = 99.5\%$, $p < 0.001$	29 (21)
Acid-etched	2.864 (2.491, 3.237), $p < 0.001$, 0.190	$I^2 = 94.72\%$, $p < 0.001$	12 (6)
SB	2.509 (1.555, 3.463), $p < 0.001$, 0.487	$I^2 = 98.03\%$, $p < 0.001$	6 (5)
SB+F	1.697 (−0.640, 4.034), $p = 0.155$, 1.193	$I^2 = 98.94\%$, $p < 0.001$	3 (2)
SBAE	2.175 (1.658, 2.693), $p < 0.001$, 0.264	$I^2 = 98.44\%$, $p < 0.001$	21 (10)
SBAE/HA-coated	2.700 (2.174, 3.226), NA, 0.268	NA	1 (1)
HA-coated	2.349 (1.254, 3.444), $p < 0.001$, 0.559	$I^2 = 98.58\%$, $p < 0.001$	12 (7)
HA-plasma	1.650 (1.410, 1.890), $p < 0.001$, 0.122	$I^2 = 0\%$, $p = 0.683$	2 (1)
CaP-plasma sprayed	0.469 (−0.010, 0.949), $p = 0.055$, 0.245	$I^2 = 75.67\%$, $p < 0.043$	2 (1)
TPS	2.184 (1.523, 2.844), $p < 0.001$, 0.337	$I^2 = 98.16\%$, $p < 0.001$	13 (9)
Cancellous	1.932 (1.432, 2.431), $p < 0.001$, 0.255	$I^2 = 0\%$, $p = 0.990$	4 (1)
Anodized	3.462 (3.273, 3.651), $p < 0.001$, 0.097	$I^2 = 16.1\%$, $p = 0.311$	4 (2)
Overall	2.295 (2.042, 2.548), $p < 0.001$, 0.129	$I^2 = 99.18\%$, $p < 0.001$	109 (35 **)
Species			
Dog	2.389 (2.152, 2.626), $p < 0.001$, 0.121	$I^2 = 98.3\%$, $p < 0.001$	98 (30)
Monkey	1.649 (1.254, 2.044), $p < 0.001$, 0.202	$I^2 = 96.75\%$, $p < 0.001$	9 (4)
Rat	0.800 (0.393, 1.207), NA, 0.208	NA	1 (1)
Mouse	0.579 (0.549, 0.609), NA, 0.015	NA	1 (1)
Overall	2.295 (2.042, 2.548), $p < 0.001$, 0.129	$I^2 = 99.18\%$, $p < 0.001$	109 (35 **)
Method			
Plaque	0.689 (0.507, 0.871), $p < 0.001$, 0.093	$I^2 = 66.17\%$, $p = 0.007$	7 (2)
Inoculation	0.800 (0.393, 1.207), NA, 0.208	NA	1 (1)
Ligature			
Cotton	2.730 (2.478, 2.982), $p < 0.001$, 0.129	$I^2 = 97.88\%$, $p < 0.001$	66 (22)
Silk	1.683 (1.296, 2.070), $p < 0.001$, 0.197	$I^2 = 98.98\%$, $p < 0.001$	28 (8)
"Dental floss"	2.361 (1.675, 3.046), $p < 0.001$, 0.350	$I^2 = 86.05\%$, $p = 0.007$	2 (1)
Steel	2.607 (1.359, 3.856), $p < 0.001$, 0.637	$I^2 = 98.08\%$, $p < 0.001$	5 (2)
Overall	2.295 (2.042, 2.548), $p < 0.001$, 0.129	$I^2 = 99.18\%$, $p < 0.001$	109 (35 **)
Ligature regimen			
Only one	2.000 (1.647, 2.352), $p < 0.001$, 0.180	$I^2 = 98.91\%$, $p < 0.001$	37 (13)
Exchange	2.303 (2.030, 2.576), $p < 0.001$, 0.139	$I^2 = 97.89\%$, $p < 0.001$	48 (14)
New on top	3.123 (2.409, 3.838), $p < 0.001$, 0.365	$I^2 = 98.66\%$, $p < 0.001$	20 (6)
Overall	2.395 (2.098, 2.620), $p < 0.001$, 0.133	$I^2 = 99.2\%$, $p < 0.001$	105 (33) ***

CI—confidence interval, SE—standard error, MBL—marginal bone loss, SB—sandblasted, SB+F—sandblasted + fluoride modified, SBAE—Sandblasted/acid-etched, HA—hydroxyapatite, NA—not applicable (there is only one study for this category), TPS—Titanium plasma-sprayed. * Some studies performed measurements of MBL in different implant surfaces, and/or different time points, and/or different methods. ** The total number of studies is always 35 for the factors "surface", "species", and "method", even though the sum of the studies for all categories under the same factor is higher than 35. The reason for this is that some studies performed measurements of MBL in different conditions, as explained in the footnote "*" above. An exception is made for "ligature regimen" (see footnote "***" below). *** The ligature regimen was not clearly informed in four measurements performed in two studies.

4. Discussion

This systematic review presents a broad inclusion of experimental peri-implantitis studies that were all based on the infectious model except for a few studies that exposed the implants to overload. The infectious model of explanation for peri-implantitis stems from the traditional view that osseointegration results from ordinary bone healing adjacent to an inert implant and where all subsequent marginal bone loss is due to bacterial challenge [3,10]. Currently, it is becoming more and more clear that osseointegration is an FBR of demarcation type that is dependent on local and systemic factors [11–13]. Even though the demarcation type reaction serves a functional purpose by enabling dental implants to carry chewing forces, its immunological purpose is to shield off the material and limit its tissue damage. It has been well established that an FBR is initiated at the time of implantation of all biomaterials and that its expression may vary between encapsulation, dissolution, resorption or rejection, depending on the properties of the material or the trauma associated with its insertion. Its expression type may also vary over time in response to changing local or systemic factors [14,15].

Sub-marginal ligation remains the most commonly used means to induce experimental peri-implantitis and provides a relatively rapid and effective MBR. Plaque accumulation alone on the other hand, provides minimal or absent MBR as evident from the dog ($n = 5$) and monkey ($n = 2$) studies which used that technique in the present review [16–22]. Prior to its introduction in dental implant research in the early 1990s, the model had been used extensively in experimental periodontitis studies [23]. While it has been realized that ligature-induced peri-implantitis may not completely mimic the onset and progression of disease in humans [24], it is still generally regarded as a solely infectious model as evident from repeated claims that bone resorption results from exposition to biofilm, not the ligature per se [2,4,25]. The earliest studies on experimental peri-implantitis revealed that the infectious model of explanation was adopted from studies on native tissues (experimental periodontitis), rather than implanted material. For example, Lindhe et al. referred to a 1966 study on germ-free vs. conventional rats to support the theory [2]. In the provided reference, Rovin et al. described an increased inflammatory response in the gingival tissues of conventional rats compared to germ free rats after ligation with USP 3-0 braided silk sutures. However, none of the rats lost any bone and neither did the distance between the epithelial attachment and cemento-enamel junction vary between these groups at any time interval until the termination of the experiment after 6 months of ligation. Rovin et al. concluded that their specific rat type appeared unsusceptible to periodontitis [26]. We failed to identify any experimental peri-implantitis studies that attempted to validate that ligatures cannot induce MBR without the presence of a biofilm. As concluded in a previous review by Baron et al., it still "remains uncertain whether the peri-implant inflammatory response is really only the result of increased plaque accumulation or if the thread itself, as a foreign body, also acts as a stimulus" [5].

In the present review dogs displayed more bone loss in response to ligation than monkeys, which points to differences in their susceptibility to ligature-induced peri-implantitis. The time required to achieve a certain amount of bone loss also varied greatly within the groups of dogs or monkeys in single studies [27,28]. The difference in MBR between rodents and large animals in the present review may be due to the small implants and ligatures used in rodents compared to dogs and monkeys. One must also consider the small number of rodent studies ($n = 2$) included in the analysis. Recently, different mouse strains and knock out models have been used to better understand why the marginal bone resorption in response to ligation differs between animals [29,30].

The significant differences in the MBR that resulted from different ligature materials in the present meta-analysis, may be due to differences between the FBRs provoked by these materials. They could also be related to varying plaque carriage potentials for these materials, but this can hardly explain why smooth stainless-steel ligatures induced more bone loss than twined silk. Consider also the significant differences in MBR between different ligature regimens, with more bone loss generated from regularly exchanged ligatures and new ligatures packed on top of old ones, as compared to only one ligature. Studies that utilized the exchanged ligature technique in the present review typically carried out the exchange every 3 weeks by first removing the old ligature and then pushing a new one into the bottom of the existing peri-implant pocket. Assuming that an anaerobic flora exists in the apical part of a lesion prior to ligature exchange, it is likely that the removal procedure will disrupt the biofilm and also introduce air into the lesion (aeration is generally considered an important part of the surgical treatment of an anaerobic infection). It would also take some time for a new anaerobic biofilm to develop on the new, presumably clean ligature. This may indicate that a close proximity between ligature and bone, is more critical for continuous bone loss to occur than the type and composition of its bacterial flora. The general disregard of the ligature itself as a potential inducer of bone loss may perhaps explain why details about ligature size, material, structure, and sometimes composition, were left out in many studies. In fact, none of the included studies compared the effect of different ligature types or regimens.

The addition of ligature around a dental implant introduces a new foreign body on another foreign body. It is plausible to assume that the new foreign body will alter the biological response of adjacent tissues to a type more specific for the introduced ligature material. Because bacteria were always present on the ligatures of the included studies, their isolated effect could not be evaluated in the present review. However, the FBRs to some of the most common ligature materials have been described elsewhere in the literature. Silk, for example, is commonly used in in vivo applications and produced the least amount of marginal bone loss in the present review. Setzen et al. reported that twined silk sutures, identical with those commonly used in the trials of the present review, produced a relatively extensive foreign body reaction and the thickest fibrous capsule of 11 sterile suture materials that were placed subcutaneously in a rabbit model [31]. Cotton on the other hand, has been shown to induce intense FBRs and also produced the most vertical MBL in the present review. Even though cotton is generally avoided in vivo, it has sometimes been used as a negative control in studies that compared the FBR to different biomaterials [32]. From reports on iatrogenic injuries following surgery, it is known that retained sterile cotton sponges can cause large lesions of foreign body type in both hard and soft tissues, sometimes referred to as "cottonballomas". For example, Kalbermatten et al. reported a massive osteolytic process surrounded by a thin rim of bone next to a sterile cotton sponge that had been left 25 years earlier during the stabilization of a femoral fracture [33]. The case exemplifies the slow progression often seen in foreign body type lesions, as well as their potential to induce both bone resorption and bone remodelling. Even microscopic remnants of sterile lint retained from cotton sponges during routine surgery have been shown to cause considerable foreign body granulomas with ingested lint particles visible within macrophages and foreign body giant cells after 4 weeks in rats [34]. It is plausible that similar particles can disseminate from the cotton ligatures used to induce experimental peri-implantitis, but their presence or eventual role does not appear to have been investigated in experimental peri-implantitis models. Within the orthopedic field, macrophage activation after phagocytosis or cell-surface contact with wear particles is considered the key causal reason for aseptic implant loosening, which is the main cause for revision surgery over the mid- and long-term [35,36].

The addition of bacteria on ligatures, as was the case in all reviewed studies, will obviously alter the inflammatory reaction to the ligature and likely plays an important role in the initiation and progression of MBR, i.e. it is an offer to bacteria to invade new space. Bacteria may however not be the only cause, as indicated by the results of this meta-analysis and other cited literature. It therefore remains uncertain whether a ligature-induced lesion represents clinical peri-implantitis better than a man-made defect would, perhaps created at implant insertion and then allowed to accumulate biofilm for a short time. A man-made defect would probably decrease animal suffering significantly, considering that ligatures have sometimes been left in place for as long as 1 year to induce a few millimeters of bone loss [37–39]. A few experiments with man-made defects have been reported. For example, Takasaki et al. combined manually created bone defects with a shorter ligature period of 5 weeks [40].

It also remains uncertain as to what extent a ligature-induced lesion can represent clinical peri-implantitis and until further validation has been provided, clinical conclusions from ligature-induced peri-implantitis studies should be drawn with great care and the experimental and clinical conditions should be treated as separate entities at all times.

Supplementary Materials: The following are available online at http://www.mdpi.com/2077-0383/7/12/492/s1, Table S1: Main characteristics of the studies included in the qualitative synthesis; Table S2: Induction and outcome of experimentally induced peri-implant bone loss in studies included in the qualitative synthesis; Table S3: Main characteristics of the studies included in the quantitative synthesis; Table S4: Induction and outcome of experimentally induced peri-implant bone loss in studies included in the quantitative synthesis; References S1: List of 133 studies included in the qualitative synthesis and excluded full text studies; References S2: List of 35 studies included in the quantitative synthesis.

Author Contributions: Conceptualization, D.R., B.C., T.A., P.T., A.W.; Methodology, D.R., B.C., T.A., P.T., A.W.; Formal Analysis, B.C., D.R.; Investigation D.R., B.C.; Writing—Original Draft Preparation, D.R., B.C.; Writing—Review & Editing, all authors; Supervision, A.W., T.A., P.T.; Funding Acquisition, A.W.

Funding: This study was funded by the Swedish Research Council grant number 2015-02971.

Conflicts of Interest: The authors declare no conflicts of interest.

References

1. Hickey, J.S.; O'Neal, R.B.; Scheidt, M.J.; Strong, S.L.; Turgeon, D.; Van Dyke, T.E. Microbiologic characterization of ligature-induced peri-implantitis in the microswine model. *J. Periodontol.* **1991**, *62*, 548–553. [CrossRef] [PubMed]
2. Lindhe, J.; Berglundh, T.; Ericsson, I.; Liljenberg, B.; Marinello, C. Experimental breakdown of peri-implant and periodontal tissues. A study in the beagle dog. *Clin. Oral Implants Res.* **1992**, *3*, 9–16. [CrossRef] [PubMed]
3. Lindhe, J.; Meyle, J.; D.o.E.W.o.P. Group. Peri-implant diseases: Consensus Report of the Sixth European Workshop on Periodontology. *J. Clin. Periodontol.* **2008**, *35*, 282–285. [CrossRef] [PubMed]
4. Albrektsson, T.; Dahlin, C.; Jemt, T.; Sennerby, L.; Turri, A.; Wennerberg, A. Is marginal bone loss around oral implants the result of a provoked foreign body reaction? *Clin. Implant Dent. Relat. Res.* **2014**, *16*, 155–165. [CrossRef] [PubMed]
5. Carcuac, O.; Abrahamsson, I.; Albouy, J.P.; Linder, E.; Larsson, L.; Berglundh, T. Experimental periodontitis and peri-implantitis in dogs. *Clin. Oral Implants Res.* **2013**, *24*, 363–371. [CrossRef] [PubMed]
6. Baron, M.; Haas, R.; Dortbudak, O.; Watzek, G. Experimentally induced peri-implantitis: a review of different treatment methods described in the literature. *Int. J. Oral Maxillofac. Implants* **2000**, *15*, 533–544. [PubMed]
7. Moher, D.; Liberati, A.; Tetzlaff, J.; Altman, D.G.; Group, P. Preferred reporting items for systematic reviews and meta-analyses: the PRISMA statement. *Ann. Intern. Med.* **2009**, *151*, 264–269. [CrossRef] [PubMed]
8. DerSimonian, R.; Laird, N. Meta-analysis in clinical trials. *Control Clin. Trials.* **1986**, *7*, 177–188. [CrossRef]
9. Wallace, B.C.; Trikalinos, T.A.; Lau, J.; Trow, P.; Schmid, C.H. Closing the Gap between Methodologists and End-Users: R as a Computational Back-End. *J. Stat. Softw.* **2012**, *49*, 1–15. [CrossRef]
10. Zitzmann, N.U.; Berglundh, T. Definition and prevalence of peri-implant diseases. *J. Clin. Periodontol.* **2008**, *35*, 286–291. [CrossRef] [PubMed]
11. Albrektsson, T.; Chrcanovic, B.; Ostman, P.O.; Sennerby, L. Initial and long-term crestal bone responses to modern dental implants. *Periodontol 2000.* **2017**, *73*, 41–50. [CrossRef] [PubMed]
12. Trindade, R.; Albrektsson, T.; Tengvall, P.; Wennerberg, A. Foreign Body Reaction to Biomaterials: On Mechanisms for Buildup and Breakdown of Osseointegration. *Clin. Implant Dent. Relat. Res.* **2014**, *18*, 192–203. [CrossRef] [PubMed]
13. Trindade, R.; Albrektsson, T.; Galli, S.; Prgomet, Z.; Tengvall, P.; Wennerberg, A. Osseointegration and foreign body reaction: Titanium implants activate the immune system and suppress bone resorption during the first 4 weeks after implantation. *Clin. Implant Dent. Relat. Res.* **2018**, *20*, 82–91. [CrossRef] [PubMed]
14. Donath, K.; Laass, M.; Günzl, H.J. The histopathology of different foreign-body reactions in oral soft tissue and bone tissue. *Virchows Arch. A Pathol. Anat. Histopathol.* **1992**, *420*, 131–137. [CrossRef] [PubMed]
15. Anderson, J.M.; Rodriguez, A.; Chang, D.T. Foreign body reaction to biomaterials. *Semin. Immunol.* **2008**, *20*, 86–100. [CrossRef] [PubMed]
16. Abrahamsson, I.; Berglundh, T.; Lindhe, J. Soft tissue response to plaque formation at different implant systems. A comparative study in the dog. *Clin. Oral Implants Res.* **1998**, *9*, 73–79. [CrossRef] [PubMed]
17. Ericsson, I.; Berglundh, T.; Marinello, C.; Liljenberg, B.; Lindhe, J. Long-standing plaque and gingivitis at implants and teeth in the dog. *Clin. Oral Implants Res.* **1992**, *3*, 99–103. [CrossRef] [PubMed]
18. Ericsson, I.; Persson, L.G.; Berglundh, T.; Marinello, C.P.; Lindhe, J.; Klinge, B. Different types of inflammatory reactions in peri-implant soft tissues. *J. Clin. Periodontol.* **1995**, *22*, 255–261. [CrossRef] [PubMed]
19. Lang, N.P.; Brägger, U.; Walther, D.; Beamer, B.; Kornman, K.S. Ligature-induced peri-implant infection in cynomolgus monkeys. I. Clinical and radiographic findings. *Clin. Oral Implants Res.* **1993**, *4*, 2–11. [CrossRef] [PubMed]
20. Lang, N.P.; Wetzel, A.C.; Stich, H.; Caffesse, R.G. Histologic probe penetration in healthy and inflamed peri-implant tissues. *Clin. Oral Implants Res.* **1994**, *5*, 191–201. [CrossRef] [PubMed]
21. Watzak, G.; Zechner, W.; Tangl, S.; Vasak, C.; Donath, K.; Watzek, G. Soft tissue around three different implant types after 1.5 years of functional loading without oral hygiene: a preliminary study in baboons. *Clin. Oral Implants Res.* **2006**, *17*, 229–236. [CrossRef] [PubMed]
22. Saito, A.; Hosaka, Y.; Sekiguchi, K.; Kigure, T.; Isobe, S.; Shibukawa, Y.; Sumii, H.; Ito, T.; Nakagawa, T.; Yamada, S. Responses of peri-implant tissues to undisturbed plaque formation in dogs: clinical, radiographic, and microbiological findings. *Bull. Tokyo Dent. Coll.* **1997**, *38*, 13–20. [PubMed]

23. Oz, H.S.; Puleo, D.A. Animal models for periodontal disease. *J. Biomed. Biotechnol* **2011**, *2011*, 754857. [CrossRef] [PubMed]
24. Berglundh, T.; Stavropoulos, A. Preclinical in vivo research in implant dentistry. Consensus of the eighth European workshop on periodontology. *J. Clin. Periodontol.* **2012**, *39*, 1–5. [CrossRef] [PubMed]
25. Moest, T.; Wrede, J.; Schmitt, C.M.; Stamp, M.; Neukam, F.W.; Schlegel, K.A. The influence of different abutment materials on tissue regeneration after surgical treatment of peri-implantitis—A randomized controlled preclinical study. *J. Craniomaxillofac. Surg.* **2017**, *45*, 1190–1196. [CrossRef] [PubMed]
26. Rovin, S.; Costich, E.R.; Gordon, H.A. The influence of bacteria and irritation in the initiation of periodontal disease in germfree and conventional rats. *J. Period. Res.* **1966**, *1*, 193–204. [CrossRef] [PubMed]
27. You, T.M.; Choi, B.H.; Zhu, S.J.; Jung, J.H.; Lee, S.H.; Huh, J.Y.; Lee, H.J.; Li, J. Treatment of experimental peri-implantitis using autogenous bone grafts and platelet-enriched fibrin glue in dogs. *Oral Surg. Oral Med. Oral Pathol. Oral Radiol. Endod.* **2007**, *103*, 34–37. [CrossRef] [PubMed]
28. Schou, S.; Holmstrup, P.; Jørgensen, T.; Stoltze, K.; Hjørting-Hansen, E.; Wenzel, A. Autogenous bone graft and ePTFE membrane in the treatment of peri-implantitis. I. Clinical and radiographic observations in cynomolgus monkeys. *Clin. Oral Implants Res.* **2003**, *14*, 391–403. [CrossRef] [PubMed]
29. Hiyari, S.; Naghibi, A.; Wong, R.; Sadreshkevary, R.; Yi-Ling, L.; Tetradis, S.; Camargo, P.M.; Pirih, F.Q. Susceptibility of different mouse strains to peri-implantitis. *J. Period. Res.* **2018**, *53*, 107–116. [CrossRef] [PubMed]
30. Yu, X.; Hu, Y.; Freire, M.; Yu, P.; Kawai, T.; Han, X. Role of toll-like receptor 2 in inflammation and alveolar bone loss in experimental peri-implantitis versus periodontitis. *J. Period. Res.* **2018**, *53*, 98–106. [CrossRef] [PubMed]
31. Setzen, G.; Williams, E.F., 3rd. Tissue response to suture materials implanted subcutaneously in a rabbit model. *Plast. Reconstruct. Surg.* **1997**, *100*, 1788–1795. [CrossRef]
32. Ibrahim, M.; Bond, J.; Medina, M.A.; Chen, L.; Quiles, C.; Kokosis, G.; Bashirov, L.; Klitzman, B.; Levinson, H. Characterization of the Foreign Body Response to Common Surgical Biomaterials in a Murine Model. *Eur. J. Plast. Surg.* **2017**, *40*, 383–392. [CrossRef] [PubMed]
33. Kalbermatten, D.F.; Kalbermatten, N.T.; Hertel, R. Cotton-induced pseudotumor of the femur. *Skeletal Radiol.* **2001**, *30*, 415–417. [CrossRef] [PubMed]
34. Sari, A.; Basterzi, Y.; Karabacak, T.; Tasdelen, B.; Demirkan, F. The potential of microscopic sterile sponge particles to induce foreign body reaction. *Int. Wound J.* **2006**, *3*, 363–368. [CrossRef] [PubMed]
35. Landgraeber, S.; Jäger, M.; Jacobs, J.J.; Hallab, N.J. The pathology of orthopedic implant failure is mediated by innate immune system cytokines. *Mediat. Inflamm.* **2014**, *2014*, 185150. [CrossRef] [PubMed]
36. Jiang, Y.; Jia, T.; Wooley, P.H.; Yang, S.Y. Current research in the pathogenesis of aseptic implant loosening associated with particulate wear debris. *Acta Orthop. Belg.* **2013**, *79*, 1–9. [PubMed]
37. Akagawa, Y.; Matsumoto, T.; Hashimoto, M.; Tsuru, H. Clinical evaluation of the gingiva around single crystal sapphire endosseous implant after experimental ligature-induced plaque accumulation in monkeys. *J. Prosthet. Dent.* **1992**, *68*, 111–115. [CrossRef]
38. Akagawa, Y.; Matsumoto, T.; Kawamura, M.; Tsuru, H. Changes of subgingival microflora around single crystal sapphire endosseous implants after experimental ligature-induced plaque accumulation in monkeys. *J. Prosthet. Dent.* **1993**, *69*, 594–598. [CrossRef]
39. Kozlovsky, A.; Tal, H.; Laufer, B.Z.; Leshem, R.; Rohrer, M.D.; Weinreb, M.; Artzi, Z. Impact of implant overloading on the peri-implant bone in inflamed and non-inflamed peri-implant mucosa. *Clin. Oral Implants Res.* **2007**, *18*, 601–610. [CrossRef] [PubMed]
40. Takasaki, A.A.; Aoki, A.; Mizutani, K.; Kikuchi, S.; Oda, S.; Ishikawa, I. Er:YAG laser therapy for peri-implant infection: A histological study. *Lasers Med. Sci.* **2007**, *22*, 143–157. [CrossRef] [PubMed]

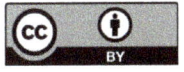

© 2018 by the authors. Licensee MDPI, Basel, Switzerland. This article is an open access article distributed under the terms and conditions of the Creative Commons Attribution (CC BY) license (http://creativecommons.org/licenses/by/4.0/).

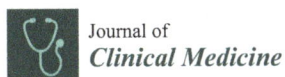

Article

Aseptic Ligatures Induce Marginal Peri-Implant Loss—An 8-Week Trial in Rabbits

David Reinedahl [1,*], Silvia Galli [2], Tomas Albrektsson [2,3], Pentti Tengvall [3], Carina B. Johansson [1], Petra Hammarström Johansson [1] and Ann Wennerberg [1]

1. Department of Prosthodontics, Institute of Odontology, Sahlgrenska Academy, University of Gothenburg, Gothenburg 405 30, Sweden
2. Department of Prosthodontics, Faculty of Odontology, Malmö University, Malmö 205 06, Sweden
3. Department of Biomaterials, Institute of Clinical Sciences, Sahlgrenska Academy, University of Gothenburg, Gothenburg 405 30, Sweden
* Correspondence: d.reinedahl@gmail.com

Received: 16 July 2019; Accepted: 16 August 2019; Published: 18 August 2019

Abstract: The clinical value of ligature-induced experimental peri-implantitis studies has been questioned due to the artificial nature of the model. Despite repeated claims that ligatures of silk, cotton and other materials may not induce bone resorption by themselves; a recent review showed that the tissue reaction toward them has not been investigated. Hence, the current study aimed to explore the hard and soft tissue reactions toward commonly used ligature materials. A total of 60 dental implants were inserted into the femur ($n = 20$) and tibia ($n = 40$) of 10 rabbits. The femoral implants were ligated with sterile 3-0 braided silk in one leg and sterile cotton retraction chord in the other leg. The tibial implants were ligated with silk or left as non-ligated controls. All wounds were closed in layers. After a healing time of 8 weeks, femoral (silk versus cotton) and proximal tibial (silk versus non-ligated control) implants were investigated histologically. Distal tibial (silk versus non-ligated control) implants were investigated with real time polymerase chain reaction (qPCR). The distance from the implant-top to first bone contact point was longer for silk ligated implants compared to non-ligated controls ($p = 0.007$), but did not vary between cotton and silk. The ligatures triggered an immunological reaction with cell infiltrates in close contact with the ligature materials, adjacent soft tissue encapsulation and bone resorption. qPCR further demonstrated an upregulated immune response toward the silk ligatures compared to non-ligated controls. Silk and cotton ligatures provoke foreign body reactions of soft tissue encapsulation type and bone resorption around implants in the absence of plaque.

Keywords: ligature induced peri-implantitis; dental implant; marginal bone loss; osseointegration; aseptic loosening

1. Introduction

Dental implant therapy is a well-documented treatment for edentulism with an overall success rate of approximately 95% after 10 years [1]. A small degree of marginal bone resorption can often be observed during the first year of implant loading, probably due to tissue adaptation to the foreign material. Even though it is self-limiting in most cases, the marginal bone resorption sometimes progresses to the extent that the osseointegration becomes threatened. In a systematic review on implants with different surface types, Doornewaard et al., reported a 5% overall rate of implants with ≥3 mm of marginal bone loss after at least 5 years of function. They further indicated that smoking and a history of periodontitis yielded more bone loss [2]. With regards to treatment need, Albrektsson et al. reported that 2.7% of modern, moderately rough implants were either removed or subjected to other surgical procedures due to progressive marginal bone resorption during 7 to 16 years of follow up. [3].

In severe cases, continuous marginal bone loss may be locally detrimental to patients due to significant peri-implant bone defects that may impede future implant revision. Hence, animal models have been developed to study the onset and progression of marginal bone loss [4]. Such models have generally been based on the theory of peri-implantitis, which defines all marginal bone loss after osseointegration as solely a bacterial infection if coupled with bleeding from the peri-implant pocket in response to pocket probing [5].

The infectious peri-implantitis theory has been criticized for being narrow and exclusive of other potential causes for marginal bone resorption, such as poor implants, traumatic implantation or change of marginal conditions over time in response to wear products [6–8]. Furthermore, the marginal bone level has been shown to both increase and decrease around some implants over time, indicating a dynamic foreign body response to implants that may not require treatment, rather than a progressive infectious condition that demands intervention [9]. It has also been well-established that other types of endosseous implants that function in presumably sterile environments, such as hip and knee arthroplasties are equally susceptible to progressive bone loss and long-term failure (>10 years), as are transmucosal dental implants [10,11]. Aseptic loosening, caused by an immunological response to increasing amounts of wear debris at the bone-implant interface over time is believed to be the main cause of such late prosthetic joint failures [12,13].

In animal studies, undisturbed peri-implant plaque accumulation has resulted in negligible or absent marginal bone loss [14–16]. In order to speed up the process, a large majority of previous experimental peri-implantitis studies have therefore utilized sub-marginal ligatures of cotton, silk or other materials. Sub-marginal ligation has commonly resulted in significant bone loss after a few months, especially when the ligatures were replaced or added to in number every few weeks [17]. The ligature method aims to mimic infectious, clinical peri-implantitis and several authors have claimed that the utilized ligatures merely act as carriers of bacteria, without capacity to induce bone resorption by themselves [4,18,19]. In one of the very first ligature studies on implants, Lindhe et al. referred to a study that used silk ligatures in the periodontal tissues (natural teeth not implants) of germ free and conventional rats from 1966 to support this claim; however, none of the rats in either group lost any bone in that study [20]. The validity of the claim was further questioned in a recent systematic review by our group, in which we failed to identify any attempts to prove that ligatures cannot induce peri-implant bone resorption by themselves. Along with previous reviews on the method, we concluded that it remains unknown whether bone resorption can be induced by a foreign body reaction to the ligature materials themselves or the tissue trauma that results from their insertion [17,21,22]. An eventual capacity for ligatures to induce bone resorption in absence of bacteria would cast serious doubt on the clinical value of the method, especially when considering that ligation is an artificial manipulation that does not mimic any clinical condition, with the possible exception if someone unintentionally leaves a retraction chord in a peri-implant pocket, which, however, must be regarded a most unusual clinical error. Hence, a validation of the infectious model of explanation provided for the ligature method is warranted.

The aim of the current study was to evaluate the capacity of aseptic ligatures to induce peri-implant bone resorption in rabbits. We chose silk ligatures due to their common use in other small animals, i.e., rodents, as well as existing, relevant real time polymerase chain reaction (qPCR) data from one of these studies [23] and an ongoing aseptic silk ligature trial on rats, by another group at our faculty. The hard and soft tissue reactions against the silk ligatures were evaluated for tibial implants, with histological methods and also selected qPCR markers in order investigate the immunological activity of adjacent cells, as well as the local bone reactions. Furthermore, since no comparisons of different ligature materials have been published previously according to our knowledge, a histological comparison of silk and cotton ligatures was also performed on femoral implants. Our null hypothesis was that marginal ligatures should not be able to induce marginal bone loss in the absence of a bacterial plaque, as repeatedly claimed in previous ligature induced peri-implantitis studies [4,18,19].

2. Experimental Section

2.1. Implants

The implants used (Ospol Regular, Malmö, Sweden) were turned/machined (diameter 4 mm and length 8 mm) from rods of commercially pure titanium (grade 4) followed by an anodising process.

Surface Roughness

The implant surface roughness was characterized by white light interferometry, GBS, mbH, Ilmenau, Germany and MountainsMap Imaging Topography software (version 7.0, Digital Surf, Besancon, France). Three implants were measured on nine sites each: three tops, three valleys and three flanks. Each measurement had a size of 350 × 224 µm. Errors of form and waviness were removed with a Gaussian filter size of 50 × 50µm. Three parameters were selected to describe the surface, one height descriptive parameter (Sa), one spatial parameter (Sds) and one hybrid parameter (Sdr).

Sa is the average height deviation over the surface calculated from a mean plane. Calculated in µm.

Sds is the density of summits, expressed in number/mm^2.

Sdr is the increase in surface area compared to a completely flat area reference. Expressed in %.

2.2. Animal Model and Surgical Procedure

Ten male Swedish lop-eared rabbits with weight between 3.65 to 4.95 Kg were used in this experiment, with ethical approval (number 188-15) from the Regional Ethics Committee for Animal Research of Malmö/Lund, Sweden. All experiments were carried out in accordance with the rules and regulations of the Swedish Board of Agriculture. The number of the animals included in the study was selected after power analysis performed with G*Power software (version 3.1.9.4, Department of Psychology, University of Düsseldorf, Düsseldorf, Germany) to achieved a statistical power of 80%, given an α-error of 0.05 and an effect size of 0.8.

General anesthesia was induced by intramuscular injection of ketamin (Ketaminol; Intervet, Stockholm, Sweden) and dexmedetomidine (Dexdomitor; Orion Pharma Animal Health, Danderyd, Sweden) followed by subcutaneous injection of buprenorfin (Temgesic; Indivior, Berkshire, Great Britain).

The surgical site was shaved and cleaned with chlorhexidine ethanol solution 0.5 mg/mL (Klorhexidinsprit; Fresenius Kabi, Uppsala, Sweden) and covered with a sterile surgical drape. After injection of lidokain 10 mg/mL (Xylocain; Aspen Nordic, Ballerup, Denmark) at the surgical sites, the femoral and tibial metaphyseal plates were exposed by incision and dissection of covering tissue layers, including skin, muscle and periosteum on the medial side. A total of 60 implants ($n = 60$) were inserted according to Figure 1; one in each condylar metaphyseal plate and two in each tibial metaphyseal plate, with a center to center implant distance of 10 mm.

The implant insertion and ligature application technique are depicted in Figure 2. Osteotomies were performed with burrs of increasing diameter up to 3.5 mm under constant irrigation with physiological saline solution. After inserting the implants halfway, a single ligature loop of sterile 3-0 braided silk (Ethicon, Cincinnati, OH, USA) were tied with a surgical knot around the neck of the (i) right femoral, (ii) right proximal and (iii) left distal tibia implants of all rabbits. The ligature was then compressed between the implant neck and marginal bone, by finishing the fixture insertion. With an identical procedure, the left femoral implants were ligated with non-impregnated cotton gingival retraction cord (GingiKNIT non-impregnated; Kerr Dental, Bioggio, Switzerland). The right distal and left proximal implants were inserted without ligatures and used as controls. Multi-layered wound closure was performed with resorbable sutures in fascia and skin (Vicryl 3-0, Ethicon, Cincinatti, OH, USA) at all sites in order to ensure a submerged and non-contaminated healing environment for all implants.

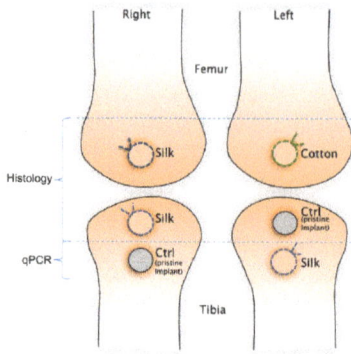

Figure 1. Schematic drawing of implant and ligature placement.

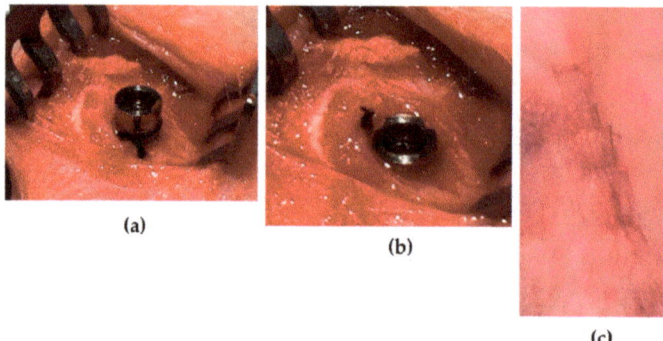

Figure 2. (a) Ligature tied around the implant neck after half-way insertion of the implant. (b) Ligature compressed against the bone by finishing the implant insertion. (c) Wound closure with interrupted resorbable sutures in a layered fashion.

At 8 weeks, the rabbits were sacrificed with a lethal injection of intra peritoneal pentobarbital (Euthasol; Virbac, Kolding, Denmark). Femoral- ($n = 20$) and proximal tibial ($n = 20$) implants were resected en bloc and directly immersed in 4% buffered formaldehyde (Merck, Darmstadt, Germany) for three days.

The distal tibia samples (tissues and implants) were harvested for gene expression analysis in the following way:

(i) The soft tissue that adhered to the implant margin was removed by a 6 mm punch after removing the cutis.
(ii) The implants were then unscrewed and the marginal bone trephined out using a 6 mm trephine.

These respective tissues were placed in RNA-later store in +4 °C overnight and then −20 °C until processing.

2.3. Histology

2.3.1. Histological Sample Preparation

Following the formalin fixation, the femoral ($n = 20$) and distal tibia ($n = 20$) samples were rinsed in tap water and then dehydrated in increasing concentrations of ethanol from 70% up to 99.9% (Solveco, Rosersberg, Sweden). The next steps involved pre-infiltration in diluted resin and pure resin followed by embedment in light-curing resin (Technovit 7200 VLC; Heraeus Kultzer, Wehrheim, Germany). All samples were divided in a similar direction i.e., in the center of the implant (in a longitudinal manner of the implant) using the cutting and grinding system, i.e., the ExaktR equipment (Exakt Apparatebau, Norderstedt, Germany). A central section of about 150–200 µm were cut. The samples were ground with Silicon carbide wet grinding papers of 800–1200 grit (Struers ApS, Ballerup, Denmark) to a final thickness of about 15 µm. The section surfaces were cleaned and dried prior to histological staining in toluidine blue mixed with pyronin G.

Finally, the sections were glass cover-slipped using a routine glue (Pertex, Histolab Products AB, Göteborg). The sample preparation related to the cutting and grinding procedure followed the routine laboratory-guidelines as deduced by Donath et al. [24] and Johansson and Morberg [25,26]

2.3.2. Histological Analysis: Qualitative and Quantitative

The histological sections were qualitatively and quantitatively investigated in a light microscope (L.M., Eclipse Nikon ME600, Nikon, Tokyo, Japan) by two of the authors: C.J. and D.R. Measurements were performed with the NIS-Elements D 64-bit software (version 3.2, Nikon Metrology, SARL, Lisses, France) using a 10× objective. Light microscopic (LM) images of the histological features were obtained with a Nikon DS-Ri1 camera (Nikon Instruments Inc. Meville, NY, USA). The first implant-bone contact was ascertained with a 40× objective.

The distance from the implant top to first bone contact was measured on both sides of each implant (anterior and posterior) sides. The difference between the distances for control versus test (silk ligatures) samples in the proximal tibia and for the cotton versus silk samples in the femur, were analyzed using non-parametric Wilcoxon Signed Rank with the pair considered as the control and test samples from the same rabbit. Statistical significance was set for $p < 0.05$. A level of 0.05 was selected for the α-error and the statistical significance was set for $p < 0.025$ after Bonferroni's adjustment for multiple calculations. A qualitative investigation of the marginal hard and soft tissues was also performed.

2.4. Gene Expression Analysis—qPCR

The samples for the gene expression analysis originated from the soft tissues that were in direct contact with the implant heads in the distal tibias and bone tissue that was adherent to the implants in distal tibia and constituted four study groups (soft tissues specimens from implants with and without ligature and bone specimens from implants with and without ligatures). A total of 32 samples (20 soft tissues and 12 bone tissue) were analyzed. The soft tissues were cut with sterile, disposable tissue punches of 6 mm diameter (1 punch per specimen) and dissected from the implant surface with a curette (Miltex, Inc. York, PA, USA).

The specimens were immediately placed in separate sterile plastic tubes containing RNA*later* solution (Ambion, Inc., Austin, TX, USA), for fixation. The samples were then stored at 4 °C overnight and further stored at −20 °C until processing.

2.4.1. mRNA Isolation

(This step is performed to purify the mRNA from the samples.)

mRNA isolation and qPCR amplification were performed at TATAA Biocenter, Gothenburg, Sweden.

Before mRNA isolation and extraction, the samples were thawed on ice. The samples were extracted using Qiazol (Cat.No 79306) and the RNeasy mini kit (Cat.No 74104) (Qiagen GmbH, Venlo, Netherlands) according to manufacturer's instructions.

Sample concentrations where determined using spectrophotometry (Dropsense, Trinean, Pleasanton, CA, USA) and RNA integrity was analyzed using capillary electrophoresis (Fragment Analyzer, Thermo Fisher Scientific, Waltham, MA, USA).

After extraction, the RNA was cleaned of inhibitory factors using the RNeasy MinElute Clean up kit (Qiagen GmbH, Venlo, Netherlands, Cat no. 74204).

2.4.2. Reverse Transcription (RT)

(This step produces complementary DNA (cDNA) to the mRNA isolated from the respective samples.)

RNA was reverse transcribed in single 20 µL reactions on all 32 samples.

Samples where first normalized to 33.33 ng/µL to reach a quantity of 500 ng RNA per tube that was loaded into the reaction. The RT was performed according to manufacturer's instructions with TATAA Grandscript cDNA synthesis kit Cat.No A103 (TATAA Biocenter AB, Gothenburg, Sweden), with the following concentration: 1 µL RT enzyme, 4 µL reaction mix, 15 µL normalized sample RNA.

2.4.3. Assays Design and Validation

(This step is performed to create short DNA fragments that are later used to determine each specific region of DNA to be copied, in this case the regions that encode the proteins of interest for the study.)

Eleven assays where designed and validated by TATAA (according to SOP 009 ver 1.2 SOP 001 ver1.4) (Validation plan qPCR assay validation). A list of all assays can be found in Table 1. For validation, a control genomic DNA (gDNA) from male rabbit (Zyagen) and a pool of all the cDNA samples was used. Seven-point standard curves in 10-fold dilutions were run for all the assays, in quadruplicates. The annealing temperature was set to 60 °C for all assays. PCR products; gDNA, cDNA, selected standard point and NTC were then run on Fragment Analyzer using the DNF-910-33-DNA 35-1500bp kit (Thermo Fisher Scientific, Waltham, MA, USA) to check the product lengths and primer specificity. The qPCR data for the assay validation was analysed with GenEx software (version 6, MultiD Analyses AB, Göteborg, Sweden) to calculate the efficiencies and performance of the assays with a confidence interval of 95%.

Table 1. Gene sequences and biological entity.

Primer	Forward Sequence	Reverse Sequence	Accession Number	Biological Entity
ACTβ	GAGATGCCATGTGACGGAAG	TTACACAAATGCGATGCTGC	NM_001101683.1	Reference gene
ALPL	ACTGTGGACTACCTCTTG	GGTCAGTGATGTGTTCC	XM_017346489	Bone mineralization
ARG1	GGATCATTGGAGCCCCTTTCTC	TCAAGCAGACCAGCCTTTCTC	NM_001082108.1	M2 macrophage
C5aR1	ACGTCAACTGCTGCATCAACC	AGGCTGGGAGAGACTTGC	NM_017338812.1	The complement system
CD11β	TTCAACCTGGAGACTGAGAACAC	TCAAACTGGACCACGCTCTG	XM_008248697.2	M1 macrophage
CD19	GGATGTATGTCTGCGCCGT	AAGCAAAGCCACAACTGGAA	NM_002711879.3	B lymphocytes
CD4	CAACTGGAAACATGCGAACCA	TTGATGACCAGGGGAAAGA	NM_008254148.2	T lymphocytes
CD8	GGCGTCTACTTCTGCATGACC	GAACGGCACACTCTCTCT	NM_008254148.2	T lymphocytes
GAPDH	CCGAGACACGATGGTGAAGG	TGTAGACCATGTAGTGGAGGTCA	NM_001082253.1	Reference gene
IL8	CTTTTTGCCCTGACCATGCC	TCCTTCACAAGCGAGACCAC	NM_001171082.1	Macrophage
LDHA	ACAAGTGCACAAACAAGTGGT	AGAGCCCCTTAAGCATGGTG	NM_001082277	Reference gene
MCP1	GCTCATAGACGTGCCCTTCA	CATGAAGATCACAGCTTCTTTGCC	NM_001082294	Macrophage fusion
NCF1	TTCATCCGCCACATTGCCC	GTCCTGCCACTTCACCAAGA	XM_001082102.1	Neutrophil
OC	AGAGTCTGGCAGAGGCTCAG	TCGCTTCACCACCTCGCT	XM_002715383	Bone mineralization
CTSK	ACTCTGAAGATGCCTACCCCT	TTCAGGGCTTTCTCATTCCCC	NM_001082641	Bone resorption
FGF2	ATCTACACTGTGAGCTTGCAG	TCATGCGGTCACACACTTCC	XM_002711077	Fibroblast
IL1β	TCCTTGGTGTCTGTGCAC	GGCCACAGGTATCTTGTCGTT	NM_001082201	M1 macrophage
IL6	GAGGAAAGAGATGTGACCAT	AGCATCCGTCTTCTCTATCAG	NM_001082064	M1 macrophage
VEGFα	CTGGGTGCATTGGAGCCTT	CTTCACCACTTCGTGGGGTTTA	XM_017345155	Endothelial cells
TNFα	CTCTTCCTGCTCGTGCCTG	GGAGGTTGTTTGGGGACTCTT	NM_001082263	M1 Macrophage
TRAP	CTGGGTTTGCAGGAGTTG	TTGAAGACAGCGACAGA	NM_001081988	Bone resorption

ACTβ, β-actin (reference gene); ALPL, alkaline phosphatase; ARG1, arginase 1; C5aR1, complement C5a Receptor 1; CD11β, macrophage marker CD11β; CD19, B-lymphocyte surface protein CD19; CD4, T-cell surface glycoprotein CD4; CD8, T-cell transmembrane glycoprotein CD8; GAPDH, glyceraldehyde 3-phosphate dehydrogenase (reference gene); IL8, interleukin 8 receptor alpha; LDHA, lactate dehydrogenase A (reference gene); MCP1, monocyte chemotactic and activating factor; NCF1, neutrophil cytosolic factor; OC, osteocalcin; CTSK, Cathepsin K; FGF2, fibroblast growth factor 2; IL1β, interleukin 1 beta; IL6, interleukin 6; VEGFα, vascular endothelial growth factor alpha; TNFα, tumor necrosis factor alpha; TRAP, Triiodothyronine receptor auxiliary protein.

2.4.4. Real-Time Quantitative Polymerise Chain Reaction (RT-qPCR)

(This final step monitors the amplification of the selected DNA segments in real time and enables the researcher to quantify the amount of each DNA segment at the start of the reaction.)

The cDNA samples were diluted 10× to have enough volume and were then analyzed using TATAA SYBR GrandMaster® Mix Cat. No. TA01-625 (TATAA Biocenter AB, Gothenburg, Sweden). Five µl of TATAA SYBR Green Master Mix, 0.4 µL of Primer (forward & reverse), 2.6 µL of nuclease-free water and 2 µL of cDNA templates were used for each reaction mix. All pipetting was performed by a pipetting robot (EpMotion 5070, Eppendorf, Germany). Duplicate NTCs were included for all the assays and cDNA samples were run in duplicate reactions. Universal ValidPrime assay, Cat No. A107P (TATAA Biocenter AB, Göteborg, Sweden) was used to compensate for possible gDNA contamination.

The quantification was performed using the LightCycler 480 (Roche, Basel, Switzerland) and detection was performed in the SYBR channel. Cq values were based on the second derivative maximum threshold method. Inter-plate calibrator, IPC Cat. No. IPC250 (TATAA Biocenter AB, Göteborg, Sweden) was run on each plate to be able to correct for inter-run differences. qPCR raw data were pre-processed and analyses with GenEx software (version 6, MultiD Analyses AB, Gothenburg, Sweden) and were thereafter imported in Qbase+ software (version 3.1, Biogazelle, Zwijnaarde, Belgium) for calibrated normalized relative quantification of the gene expression. Three assays were used as reference genes (ACTB, GAPDH and LDHA) and their quality as reference genes was assessed with the GeNorm algorithm.

2.4.5. Statistical Analysis

The gene expression results were reported as calibrated normalized relative quantities (CNRQ). Mean and 95% confidence intervals were reported for each assay for each group.

The difference in mean between the test (silk ligated implants) and the control (pristine Ti-implant) groups in the soft tissue samples and between the test and control groups in the bone samples were analyzed using non-parametric Wilcoxon Signed Rank. The test and control samples from the same rabbit were considered as paired. The level of α-error was set to 0.05 and statistical significance was adjusted according to Bonferroni´s method for multiple testing; therefore, it was set to $p < 0.0027$.

3. Results

3.1. Clinical Appearance at Sacrifice

The tissue harvesting procedure is shown in Figure 3. Uneventful healing and primary wound closure were achieved in all cases. Dissection of the tissues revealed no pus or other signs of infection around the implants. Exposure of the bone adjacent to the implants revealed small saucerization-like defects around most ligated implants and sometimes callus formation lateral to the ligatures. Some control implants presented with callus formation lateral to the implants, but no saucerization-like bone defects were noted.

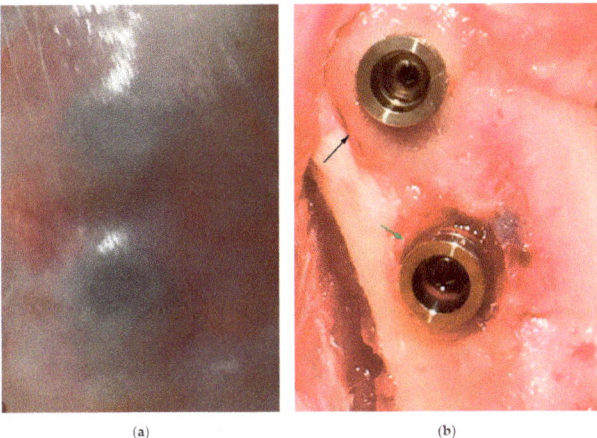

Figure 3. (**a**) The soft tissue covering a tibial control implant (superior) and test implant (inferior) after removal of skin and subcutaneous tissues. (**b**) A small saucerization-like defect (green arrow) visible after removal of the silk ligature around the inferior implant and callus formation (black arrow) around the superior control implant.

3.2. Histological Results

3.2.1. Histomorphometrical Results

One implant with a cotton ligature was excluded from the histomorphometrical analysis due to a superior displacement of the ligature and unfavorable implant location that engaged the dorsal femoral bone plate and showed non-union of the implant on that side. The distance from the implant top to first bone contact was significantly longer for test implants ligated with silk compared to controls ($p = 0.007$) (Figure 4). This difference was due to the combined effect of bone resorption inferior to the ligatures in the test implants and also bone gain due to callus formation adjacent to protrusive implant tops in some control implants. The difference between implants ligated with silk or cotton was not statistically significant ($p = 0.37$).

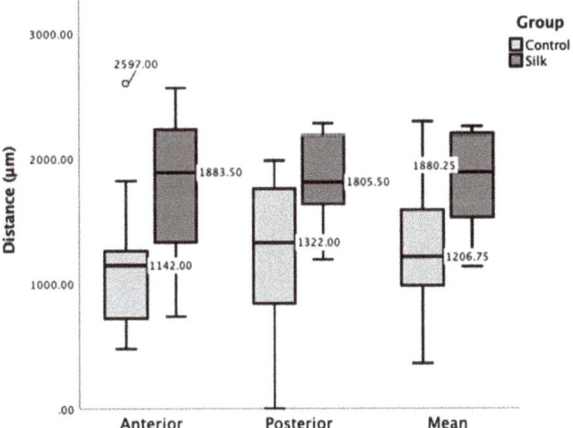

Figure 4. Box-plot showing the distance from implant top to first bone-to-implant contact for implants with silk ligatures (Silk) and pristine implants (Control).

3.2.2. Qualitative Histological Results

Control Implants (No Ligature Involved)

Control samples are shown in Figure 5. The control samples demonstrated both periosteal and endosteal new bone formation. The old cortical bone surfaces, observed in regions close to the implant, were undergoing remodeling with bone forming and bone resorption areas present. Most control sections demonstrated that the implant interface regions consisted of new formed bone with various amounts of bone-to-implant contact (BIC) and active bone forming regions (bone tissue covered by osteoid with osteoblasts visible) close to the implant. In some sections, multinucleated giant cells (MNGCs) of various sizes could be observed in close vicinity to metal oxide debris and particles (most likely detached from the bulk implant being anodized).

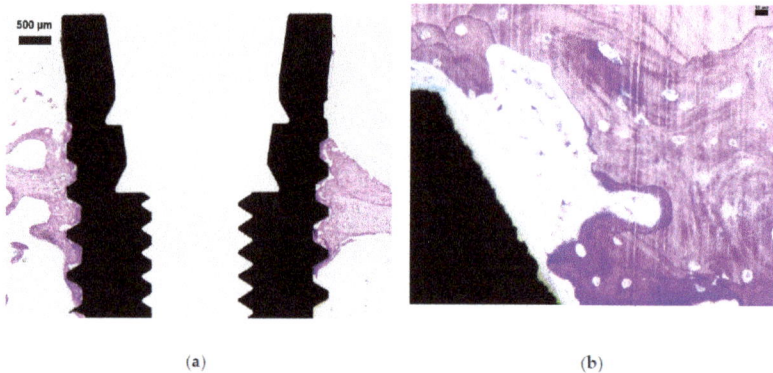

Figure 5. (**a**) A typical example of a control sample (no ligature involved) with darker stained periosteal and endosteal new bone formation. (**b**) This figure illustrates seemingly an ongoing bone remodeling region with clear demarcation between old bone (lighter stained) and younger bone (larger osteocytes and a bit darker stained bone tissue). Possibly some macrophages can be observed in the region closer to the implant.

Test Implants (Ligated with Silk or Cotton)

Silk samples are shown in Figure 6. The silk samples demonstrated soft tissue encapsulation of the material with capsules of varying thickness and sometimes also distant bony encapsulation. The capsules appeared both as a "loose" and a "tight" formation with macrophages of various sizes as the dominating cell type. Possibly some plasma-cells were also part of the cell population in such regions. One section demonstrated loosened single silk fibers in the soft tissue region appearing as being encapsulated by a rather thick formation of macrophages of various sizes and shapes. The silk material was not in contact with bone and a capsule formation separating bone and silk could sometimes be observed. In five samples, MNGCs could be seen as long elongated rims that captured the silk material (i.e., foreign body reaction). This rim of cells was involved in a soft tissue space that separated the bone from the silk. The bone surfaces, at some distance away, showed signs of resorption but no osteoclasts could be observed. Macrophages of various sizes and shapes were observed in the soft tissue regions close to the implant surface. The silk material was most often located "above" the bone surface, seemingly glued onto the implant, compared to cotton being "spread out". One silk sample demonstrated a shell/dome-like bone formation with marrow tissue at the periosteal side.

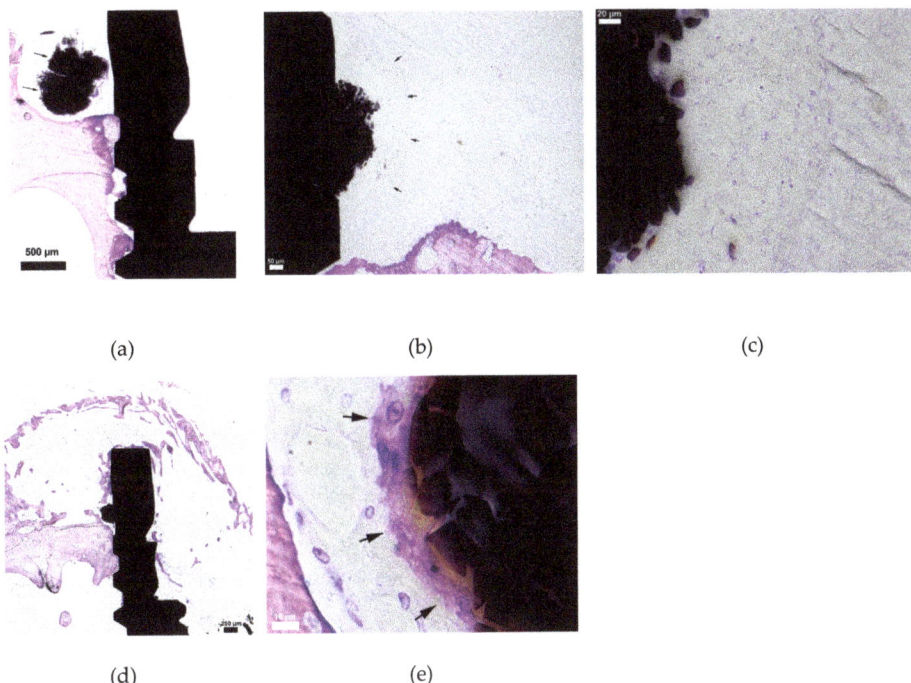

Figure 6. Sample figures from different silk sections. (**a**) Survey figure of a typical section with a silk ligature (arrows) above a partly resorbed cortical bone surface in the periosteal region. (**b**) In some cases, the silk ligatures (in close contact to the implant) were surrounded by a thick cellular infiltrate layer (arrows) dominated by macrophages of various sizes and shapes. Outside this formation, loose connective tissue was formed. (**c**) The same section in higher resolution. (**d**) This figure illustrates a rather large "dome-like" callus formation of the periosteal bone and it seems like the implant part above the silk ligature is almost covered by new formed bone. (**e**) The arrows illustrate a large, elongated multinucleated giant cell (MNGC) in intimate contact with the silk.

Cotton samples are shown in Figure 7. The majority of the sections of the cotton material could be observed as "huge loosened regions" with the material encapsulated by soft tissue situated above the periosteal bone surface. The capsule itself was often surrounded by bone trabecula and the interface between the periosteal bone surface and soft tissue seemed to undergo resorption, with regions of "mouse-eaten" bone; however, no osteoclasts could be observed. Cotton demonstrated a larger diameter of the material than silk, with several separate "cotton rolls" visible both at a distance from the implant and in close contact, compared to the silk. No active bone forming surface (i.e., osteoid rim with osteoblasts) could be observed close to the soft tissue. Although the bone surface, in general, seemed to be resorbed ("mouse-eaten" surface) no osteoclasts were visible, except in one cotton-section. In higher magnification MNGCs could be observed in close vicinity to cotton. Macrophages were also visible but seemingly in less amount (albeit not counted) compared to silk. Cotton seemed to have a greater soft tissue area surrounding the material compared to silk, which possibly indicated a higher degree of encapsulation of cotton compared to silk.

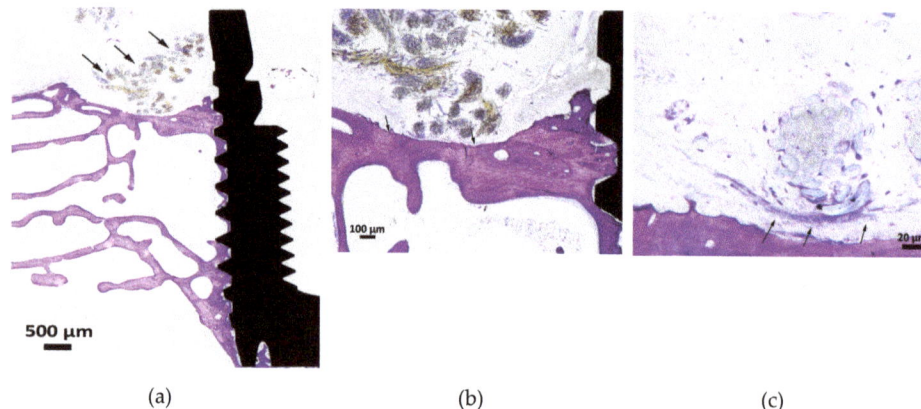

(a) (b) (c)

Figure 7. Three images from one cotton section with arrows showing the cotton ligature. (**a**) An illustration of a typical section with cotton suture situated above the periosteal bone. (**b**) The periosteal bone surface is separated from the cotton ligature by a soft tissue layer and the bone surface appears to be resorbed (arrows), although no osteoclasts could be observed. (**c**) The amount of macrophages in the soft tissue between the bone and the cotton seemed to be less compared to the silk sections. However, macrophages were visible as being more spread out and "darker" compared to silk samples. None of the cotton samples demonstrated a typical MNGC formation and the "encapsulation" of cotton was often loosely arranged (arrows).

3.3. Gene Expression Results

The expression of a panel of genes in the soft tissue around titanium implants either left pristine (control) or treated with a silk ligature placed around the implant neck (test) was evaluated with RT-qPCR. The relative expressions of the selected markers are presented in Table 2 and Figure 8 for soft tissue and in Table 3 and Figure 9 for bone tissue.

Table 2. Relative expression of the selected gene targets in the soft tissues around implants with silk ligature versus the soft tissues around controls (no ligature involved).

Target Gene	Relative Expression in Test versus Control	95% CI Low	95% CI High	p-Value
NCF1	4.9	1.9	12.4	0.008
CD11β	2.8	1.5	5.4	0.016
CD4	2.3	1.7	3.1	0.016
VEGFα	1.6	1.0	2.5	0.05
TNFα	1.7	0.9	2.9	0.08
ARG1	2.4	0.9	6.5	0.11
IL8	0.5	0.2	1.2	0.11
FGF2	0.8	0.5	1.2	0.11
CD8	3.9	0.5	27.4	0.22
CD19	2.1	0.5	12.3	0.22
OC	1.7	0.7	4.2	0.25
C5aR1	1.3	0.9	2.0	0.31
TRAP	1.7	0.5	5.4	0.37
IL1β	0.7	0.2	2.5	0.58
IL6	0.8	0.3	2.5	0.58
ALPL	1.2	0.5	3.1	0.64
MCP1	0.9	0.3	2.8	0.84
CTSK	1.0	0.7	1.5	0.84

CI = confidence interval. p-value was calculated with Wilcoxon Signed Rank test, significance level was set to $p \leq 0.0027$ after Bonferroni's adjustment for multiple testing. No gene showed significant difference in expression.

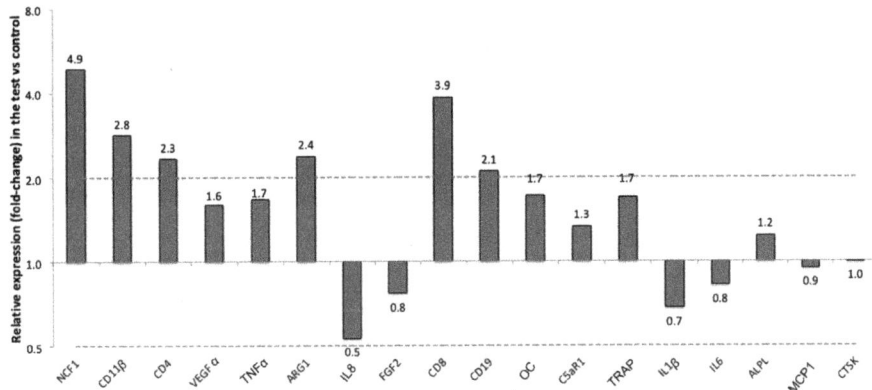

Figure 8. Up and down regulation of the selected markers in the soft tissues around implants with silk ligatures versus controls (no ligature).

Table 3. Relative expression of the selected gene targets in the bone around implants with silk ligature versus the bone around controls (no ligature).

Target Gene	Relative Expression in Test versus Control	95% CI Low	95% CI High	p-Value
IL6	0.1	0.0	0.9	0.04
CTSK	0.7	0.5	1.0	0.04
OC	0.6	0.4	1.1	0.07
NCF1	3.5	0.8	15.2	0.07
MCP1	2.2	0.8	5.9	0.08
CD19	2.7	0.6	12.3	0.13
CD11β	2.6	0.6	12.2	0.14
TNFα	0.4	0.1	2.3	0.19
FGF2	0.6	0.2	1.6	0.19
IL1β	2.1	0.5	8.8	0.19
IL8	0.5	0.1	2.4	0.26
C5aR1	1.9	0.4	9.3	0.28
CD4	2.6	0.3	25.0	0.28
CD8	1.4	0.4	5.2	0.42
TRAP	2.2	0.1	40.0	0.46
VEGFα	1.8	0.2	20.4	0.49
ALPL	0.8	0.2	4.4	0.76

CI = confidence interval. p-value calculated with Wilcoxon Signed Rank test, significance level was set to $p \leq 0.0027$ after Bonferroni's adjustment for multiple testing. No gene showed significant difference in expression.

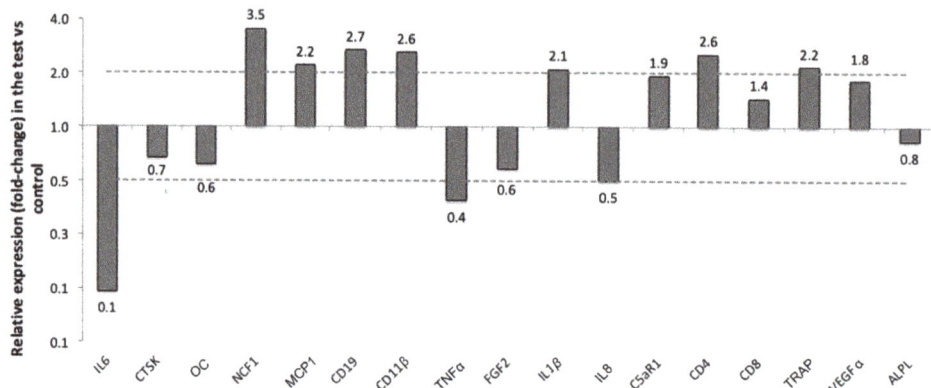

Figure 9. Up and down regulation of the selected markers in the bone around implants with silk ligatures versus controls (no ligature).

In the soft tissues near the silk ligature, several genes mediating reactions of immune cells were more than two-folds up-regulated compared to the controls. Those were NCF1 (CNRQ 4.9), which is specific for neutrophils, CD8 (CNRQ 3.9), which is a marker for T-lymphocytes, CD11β (CNRQ 2.8), a M1 macrophages marker, ARG1 (CNRQ 2.4), a marker for M2 macrophages, CD4 (CNRQ 2.3), which is another gene specific for T-lymphocytes, and CD19 (CNRQ 2.1), which is associated with B-lymphocytes. One gene, IL8, related to macrophages was two-folds down-regulated in the tests versus the controls. None of the markers reached a level of significance of $p \leq 0.0025$ in expression between the tests and the controls, which was the adjusted p-value (Table 2, Figure 8).

In the bone surrounding the implants ligated with silk, six genes related to the immune response were expressed more than two-folds compared to the bone surrounding pristine implants. Of those, four were the same that were overexpressed in the soft tissues near the ligatures: NCF1 (CNRQ 3.5), CD19 (CNRQ 2.7), CD11β (CNRQ 2.6) and CD4 (CNRQ 2.6). Other genes up-regulated in the bone of the test samples were MCP1 (CNRQ 2.2), which is related to macrophage fusion, ILβ1 (CNRQ 2.1) which is another gene related to M1 macrophages, and Triiodothyronine receptor auxiliary protein (TRAP) (CNRQ 2.2), which is an osteoclast marker for bone resorption.

Three genes were instead two-folds or more down-regulated in the bone around the test implants compared to the controls. They were IL6 (CNRQ 0.1), which is a cytokine related to inflammation, but also to bone formation [1], TNFα (CNRQ 0.4), another cytokine related to inflammation, and IL8 (CNRQ 0.5), which is related to macrophages and that was down-regulated also in the soft tissues of the test implants. None of these investigated genes in the bone reached a level of significant difference in expression for $p \leq 0.0025$ (Table 3, Figure 9).

4. Discussion

The current study described marginal peri-implant bone and soft tissue reactions to marginal silk and cotton ligatures without plaque accumulation. Our findings present clear criticism to the present interpretation of ligature models that they verify bacteria to be the initiating problem behind marginal bone loss. In reality, previous claims that ligatures induce bone loss solely by plaque accumulation and not by themselves are incorrect [4,18,26]. The present findings also raise questions as to what extent potential clinical provocations may also induce bone loss. Consider for example apically displaced cementum residues, unsuitable, lose or ill-fitting abutments or increasing amounts of wear debris in peri-implant tissues over time. Indeed, wear particles of both cementum and titanium has been found in abundance in human biopsies of peri-implantitis lesions [27]. Furthermore, the possible role of sterile Ti debris in the development of soft tissue inflammation and marginal bone resorption was recently demonstrated by Wang et al., who showed marginal bone resorption around submerged titanium implants in Sprauge Dawley rats and also demonstrated a role of M1 macrophages in that process. [28]. Future studies may strive to provide more knowledge about potential aseptic causes for marginal bone resorption, with the ultimate goal to prevent and treat such conditions.

As described by Donath et al., the body will always strive to alienate an implanted material by rejection, dissolution, resorption, demarcation (i.e., fibrous or bony encapsulation) or a combination of these reactions [29]. The type and extent of the immunological response has been shown to depend on multiple factors, such as material type, surface characteristics, type of receiving tissue, degree of surgical trauma, micromovement between material and host and other factors [7,29]. From studies on osteoimmunology we know that focal bone loss is achieved by osteoclasts when activated by adjacent inflammation, and that TNFα is likely the most significant inflammatory cytokine necessary to activate the osteoclasts [30]. TNFα is expressed in the acute inflammatory response against many types of provocations, such as surgical trauma or presence of infectious microorganisms, necrotic tissue or certain foreign materials. Hence, bone resorption can be expected to occur from almost any type of adjacent, pro-inflammatory provocation of a certain magnitude and may also be continuous if the provocation is sustained or repeated. In experimental peri-implantitis, this is well-exemplified by the rapid marginal bone loss that often occurs when ligatures are frequently exchanged and new ligatures are pushed apically towards the bone, as compared to the frequent self-containing resorption that often occurs from non-exchanged ligatures [17].

The extensive, macrophage-dominated infiltrates adjacent to the silk and cotton ligatures in the present study demonstrates a stronger inflammatory reaction to the ligatures compared to non-ligated control implants, which may likely explain the resorbed bone defects frequently found adjacent to the ligatures. Macrophages can initiate bone resorption in different ways: indirectly by secretion of pro-inflammatory cytokines that stimulate osteoclast generation and activation as described above [30] or directly by the secretion of certain matrix metalloproteinases that can degrade bone matrix [31]. However, the present study demonstrated a late stage foreign body reaction, with fibrous encapsulation of the ligatures, lack of up-regulation of the pro-inflammatory cytokine markers for TNFα, IL1β and IL6 in the soft tissues around them and seemingly arrested bone resorption as evident by the lack of osteoclasts in the resorbed bone defects adjacent to them. This late stage reaction was likely due to the long healing time of 8 weeks and is consistent with the previous findings of Setzen et al., who reported a quite extensive inflammatory response to black braided silk sutures during the first few weeks, followed by the thickest fibrous capsule formation compared to 10 other suture types inserted subcutaneously in rabbits [32]. Recent findings by Nguyen et al. suggested that active bone resorption occurs much earlier, even when plaque accumulation is allowed. In their recent experimental peri-implantitis study in mice, high expression levels of TNFα and IL1 were observed during the first 2 weeks after application of plaque accumulating 5-0 silk-ligatures, followed by a subsequent decrease back to baseline levels after 4 weeks. Simultaneously, the number of osteoclasts and rate of marginal bone resorption both decreased towards the end of the study at 4 weeks [23]. The tissue reactions to strictly bacterial assaults also share many similarities, and is perhaps best exemplified by the closed confines of the periapical bone, when provoked by endodontic pathogens. As explained by Nair et al., the endodontic pathogens typically trigger an acute inflammatory reaction with simultaneous active bone resorption, followed by a chronic stage, or equilibrium, with arrested bone resorption and a dense fibrous capsule that shields off the inflammatory infiltrate from the bone while it continues to hold back the infection [33]. New acute episodes may then be triggered years later, in response to changed local or systemic circumstances.

In contrast to the complex combined assault of repeated mechanic tissue trauma, hostile ligatures and hostile bacteria provided by classical experimental peri-implantitis, the present study demonstrated the isolated capacity of silk and cotton ligature to initiate bone loss. While the distance from the implant top to the first bone contact point varied significantly between silk and controls, the difference between silk and cotton was not significant. However, the fact that the soft tissue capsules that separated the ligatures from the bone were thicker around cotton than silk, may indicate a more consistent bone resorption against cotton. Future studies could benefit from a histomorphometrical method, which unfortunately cannot be performed successfully on non-decalcified, resin-embedded, cut-and-ground sections. The difference in bone loss between similar study subjects (the rabbits in our study) conforms to the findings of traditional ligature induced peri-implantitis studies, where the time to achieve a certain amount of bone loss has also varied greatly [34,35]. These differences are likely due to both immunological differences between animals, as indicated by recent knock out models [36], as well as methodological aspects such as possible variations in the distance between ligature and bone at the time of ligation. The choice of a rabbit model in the present study makes it difficult to compare the present results to those of previous studies that used different mammals as experimental models, considering the great differences in the resulting bone loss for different animal species [17]. For example, Beagle dogs have shown >3 mm of bone loss after 10-weeks with ligatures [37], while monkeys have sometimes required a year of regularly exchanged ligatures to induce 1 mm of bone loss [15].

Another important difference between the present and previous studies was the simultaneous implant and ligature insertion, as opposed to the few months of implant healing before ligation utilized in the majority of previous studies. Jovanovic et al. demonstrated that the amount of marginal bone loss and configuration of peri-implant pockets did not differ from ligation at implant placement compared to a preceding 3 months implant healing time [38].

Although the impact of the ligature has often been overlooked in ligature induced peri-implantitis studies, as evident from the fact that some authors have not specified any details about the type of material used [39,40], information about the ligature materials can be found from other research fields. The most commonly used ones are the organic materials cotton and silk. In surgery, cotton gauze sponges are used to soak up fluids and maintain the surgical field, but are then carefully removed from the tissues due to their capacity to provoke extensive foreign body reactions. When extensive, these foreign body reactions can manifest themselves as tumor-like lesions referred to as cotton-ballomas or gossypibomas. In some cases, these lesions have induced significant bone resorption and may then mimic an osteolytic tumour such as a sarcoma [41,42]. A study on mice also showed that even microscopic remnants of sterile cotton may induce foreign body reactions when left in a surgical wound [43].

Silk, on the other hand, has been used as a suture material for over a century, and the black, braided silk sutures used in the present study are made from fibroin, extracted from virgin Bombyx mori silk in a process that separates the fibroin from a second, glue-like protein called sericin [44]. In addition to fibroin, the utilized suture type also contains a beeswax coating. It is unknown to what extent this particular coating affects the immunological response, but it should be noted that beeswax is the main ingredient of bone wax, a product used to stop osseous bleeding during surgery and well known to arrest bone healing and induce significant foreign body reactions [45]. Older pre-1980s silk sutures contained both fibroin and sericin and were known to induce considerable acute and chronic inflammatory responses, as well as frequent late allergic reactions. Modern fibroin type silk sutures very rarely induce allergy, but still elicit a relatively strong acute inflammatory reaction in the early healing phase. Silk also undergoes slow proteolytic degradation, even though the sutures are defined as non-resorbable [44,46]. Spelzini et al., compared two types of fibroin silk implants with a polypropylene implant for fascial repair in mice and reported a somewhat stronger acute inflammatory reaction to the silk implants, followed by a much stronger chronic inflammatory response with progressive accumulation of chronic inflammatory cells up until 30 days that remained virtually unchanged after 90 days. They also reported a high initial presence of polymorphnuclear neutrophil (PMN) cells, which subsequently dropped in numbers with time but still remained in smaller numbers after 90 days [46].

The clinical significance of the PCR results of the present study must be considered in light of the histological sections and the evident late healing stage and arrested bone resorption described above. It must also be kept in mind that the PCR results only demonstrate the difference between test (silk ligature) and control (no ligature) implants, and hence do not show the immunological reaction to the Ti-implants that were identical for tests and controls. For example, CD11β was 2.8 times upregulated in the present study but 13 times upregulated in response to Ti compared to sham after 28 days in a previous rabbit study, which suggests a pronounced immunological reaction dominated by macrophages to Ti that was masked in the present study design [47]. Additional biopsies at baseline or from untouched distant tissues at sacrifice may facilitate the interpretation in future studies. Regarding the bone specimens, the small differences between tests and controls may in part be due to the harvesting technique, considering that the entire implants + surrounding bone were harvested and analyzed, while only a very small marginal portion of them was ever in contact with the ligatures.

With the above factors in mind, the more than two-fold upregulation of the soft tissue markers NCF1, CD11β, and CD4, ARG1, CD8 and CD19 for silk ligated test implants compared to pristine implants demonstrated a greater activation of the immune response in the test compared to the controls that corresponded to the chronic inflammatory cell infiltrates present around the ligatures. The upregulation of CD11β and ARG1 indicate a mixed M1/M2 phenotype of the macrophages in this tissue. CD4 and CD8 upregulation indicate T-cell presence. T-cells play a key role in antigen specific defense, but are also involved in foreign body reactions in absence of known antigens [48]. Their increased presence in the present study may correspond to the larger number of adherent macrophages and MNGCs on the silk ligatures as compared to controls (Ti), as demonstrated by Brodbeck et al., who described that lymphocytes (mainly CD8+ T-cells and CD4+ T-cells) "rosetted around" biomaterial-adherent macrophages and MNGCs in a co-cell culture study [48]. The authors further demonstrated that the presence of lymphocytes augmented macrophage adherence to biomaterials as well as MNGC-fusion, when both cell types were present from the start of the in vitro experiment [48]. However, a later study on T-cell deficient mice demonstrated a seemingly normal foreign body response with adhesion and fusion of macrophages to an implanted material even in absence of T-cells, which indicates that, while present, T-cells are probably not necessary for a normal foreign body reaction to occur [49]. The prolonged neutrophil presence in soft tissue indicated by upregulation of NCF1 further indicates a more pronounced foreign body reaction to the silk ligatures than controls (no ligature involved). Recent studies demonstrate a long-term role of neutrophils in foreign body reactions, as well as a capacity for them to regulate the long term reaction toward an implant [50]. Jhunjhunwala et al., recently demonstrated a 30-500-fold increased neutrophil presence in the peritoneal lavage of mice in response to sterile implanted microcapsules after 2 weeks, which is much longer than the hours or few days they have previously been thought to survive at a wound site. Jhunjhunwala et al. further demonstrated that the neutrophils became activated in response to the implant, resulting in the secretion of different immunomodulatory cytokines and chemokines and formation of extracellular traps (NETs) on the material surface [51]. The increasing knowledge about the pivotal role of neutrophils in the regulation of foreign body reactions suggests that a strong acute inflammation, associated with the implantation, can predispose an equally strong chronic inflammation orchestrated by neutrophils and characterized by prolonged neutrophil presence and frustrated phagocytosis in the very long run [50]. Beside the impact of material properties on the long-term neutrophil response indicated in the present study, the eventual influence of other factors, such as traumatic surgery and pre-existing disorders that influence the inflammatory response, such as diabetes, may be considered in future studies [52–54].

The immunological reactions to aseptic provocations of dental implants remains largely unexplored and future studies may focus on investigating the details in the immune response to different provocations at different time points throughout the healing phase, as well as refining the methods for such investigation.

5. Conclusions

Within the limitations of the present study, it was demonstrated that aseptic marginal ligatures made of silk and cotton triggered an immunological reaction in the peri-implant tissue of rabbits, with abundant numbers of inflammatory cells in contact with the ligatures. Marginal bone resorption was also evident adjacent to the ligatures, which rejected our null-hypothesis that ligatures cannot induce bone resorption in the absence of a bacterial plaque. Future studies may aim to describe the tissue reactions at both earlier and later time points, as well as further elucidate the details of the immunological events responsible for bone resorption adjacent to aseptic marginal ligatures.

Author Contributions: Conceptualization, D.R., S.G., T.A., P.T. and A.W.; Data curation, S.G., P.H.J. and A.W.; Formal analysis, D.R., P.H.J. and A.W.; Funding acquisition, A.W.; Investigation, D.R., S.G., T.A., P.H.J. and A.W.; Methodology, D.R., S.G., T.A., P.T., C.B.J. and P.H.J.; Project administration, T.A., and A.W.; Supervision, T.A., P.T., C.B.J. and A.W.; Validation, C.B.J.; Visualization, D.R., S.G., C.B.J. and P.H.J.; Writing—Original Draft, D.R., S.G., C.B.J. and P.H.J.; Writing—Review & Editing, D.R., S.G., T.A., P.T., C.B.J. and A.W.

Funding: This study was funded by the Swedish Research Council grant number 2015-02971.

Conflicts of Interest: The authors declare no conflict of interest.

References

1. Moraschini, V.; Poubel, L.A.; Ferreira, V.F.; Barboza Edos, S. Evaluation of survival and success rates of dental implants reported in longitudinal studies with a follow-up period of at least 10 years: A systematic review. *Int. J. Oral Maxillofac Surg.* **2015**, *44*, 377–388. [CrossRef] [PubMed]
2. Doornewaard, R.; Christiaens, V.; De Bruyn, H.; Jacobsson, M.; Cosyn, J.; Vervaeke, S.; Jacquet, W. Long-Term Effect of Surface Roughness and Patients' Factors on Crestal Bone Loss at Dental Implants. A Systematic Review and Meta-Analysis. *Clin. Implant. Dent. Relat. Res.* **2017**, *19*, 372–399. [CrossRef] [PubMed]
3. Albrektsson, T.; Buser, D.; Sennerby, L. Crestal bone loss and oral implants. *Clin. Implant. Dent. Relat Res.* **2012**, *14*, 783–791. [CrossRef] [PubMed]
4. Lindhe, J.; Berglundh, T.; Ericsson, I.; Liljenberg, B.; Marinello, C. Experimental breakdown of peri-implant and periodontal tissues. A study in the beagle dog. *Clin. oral implant res.* **1992**, *3*, 9–16. [CrossRef]
5. Zitzmann, N.U.; Berglundh, T. Definition and prevalence of peri-implant diseases. *J. Clin. Periodontol.* **2008**, *35*, 286–291. [CrossRef] [PubMed]
6. Albrektsson, T.; Dahlin, C.; Jemt, T.; Sennerby, L.; Turri, A.; Wennerberg, A. Is marginal bone loss around oral implants the result of a provoked foreign body reaction? *Clin. Implant Dent. Relat. Res.* **2014**, *16*, 155–165. [CrossRef]
7. Albrektsson, T.; Chrcanovic, B.; Ostman, P.O.; Sennerby, L. Initial and long-term crestal bone responses to modern dental implants. *Periodontology 2000* **2017**, *73*, 41–50. [CrossRef]
8. Frydman, A.; Simonian, K. Review of models for titanium as a foreign body. *C.D.A. J.* **2014**, *42*, 829–833.
9. Jemt, T.; Sunden Pikner, S.; Grondahl, K. Changes of Marginal Bone Level in Patients with "Progressive Bone Loss" at Branemark System(R) Implants: A Radiographic Follow-Up Study over an Average of 9 Years. *Clin. Implant Dent. Relat. Res.* **2015**, *17*, 619–628. [CrossRef]
10. Albrektsson, T.; Becker, W.; Coli, P.; Jemt, T.; Molne, J.; Sennerby, L. Bone loss around oral and orthopedic implants: An immunologically based condition. *Clin. Implant Dent. Relat. Res.* **2019**. [CrossRef]
11. Harris, W. *Vanishing Bone—Conquering a Stealth Disease Caused by Total Hip Replacements*; Oxford Press: Oxford, UK, 2018.
12. Landgraeber, S.; Jäger, M.; Jacobs, J.J.; Hallab, N.J. The pathology of orthopedic implant failure is mediated by innate immune system cytokines. *Mediators Inflamm.* **2014**, *2014*, 185150. [CrossRef] [PubMed]
13. Jiang, Y.; Jia, T.; Wooley, P.H.; Yang, S.Y. Current research in the pathogenesis of aseptic implant loosening associated with particulate wear debris. *Acta. Orthop. Belg.* **2013**, *79*, 1–9. [PubMed]
14. Abrahamsson, I.; Berglundh, T.; Lindhe, J. Soft tissue response to plaque formation at different implant systems. A comparative study in the dog. *Clin. Oral Implants Res.* **1998**, *9*, 73–79. [CrossRef] [PubMed]
15. Lang, N.P.; Bragger, U.; Walther, D.; Beamer, B.; Kornman, K.S. Ligature-induced peri-implant infection in cynomolgus monkeys. I. Clinical and radiographic findings. *Clin. Oral Implants Res.* **1993**, *4*, 2–11. [CrossRef] [PubMed]

16. Watzak, G.; Zechner, W.; Tangl, S.; Vasak, C.; Donath, K.; Watzek, G. Soft tissue around three different implant types after 1.5 years of functional loading without oral hygiene: A preliminary study in baboons. *Clin. Oral Implants Res.* **2006**, *17*, 229–236. [CrossRef] [PubMed]
17. Reinedahl, D.; Chrcanovic, B.; Albrektsson, T.; Tengvall, P.; Wennerberg, A. Ligature-Induced Experimental Peri-Implantitis-A Systematic Review. *J. Clin. Med.* **2018**, *7*. [CrossRef] [PubMed]
18. Moest, T.; Wrede, J.; Schmitt, C.M.; Stamp, M.; Neukam, F.W.; Schlegel, K.A. The influence of different abutment materials on tissue regeneration after surgical treatment of peri-implantitis—A randomized controlled preclinical study. *J. Craniomaxillofac. Surg.* **2017**, *45*, 1190–1196. [CrossRef] [PubMed]
19. Carcuac, O.; Abrahamsson, I.; Albouy, J.P.; Linder, E.; Larsson, L.; Berglundh, T. Experimental periodontitis and peri-implantitis in dogs. *Clin. Oral Implants Res.* **2013**, *24*, 363–371. [CrossRef]
20. Rovin, S.; Costich, E.R.; Gordon, H.A. The influence of bacteria and irritation in the initiation of periodontal disease in germfree and conventional rats. *J. Periodontal Res.* **1966**, *1*, 193–204. [CrossRef]
21. Martins, O.; Ramos, J.C.; Baptista, I.P.; Dard, M.M. The dog as a model for peri-implantitis: A review. *J. Investig. Surg.* **2014**, *27*, 50–56. [CrossRef]
22. Baron, M.; Haas, R.; Dortbudak, O.; Watzek, G. Experimentally induced peri-implantitis: A review of different treatment methods described in the literature. *Int. J. Oral Maxillofac. Implants* **2000**, *15*, 533–544.
23. Nguyen Vo, T.N.; Hao, J.; Chou, J.; Oshima, M.; Aoki, K.; Kuroda, S.; Kaboosaya, B.; Kasugai, S. Ligature induced peri-implantitis: Tissue destruction and inflammatory progression in a murine model. *Clin. Oral Implants Res.* **2017**, *28*, 129–136. [CrossRef]
24. Donath, K.; Breuner, G. A method for the study of undecalcified bones and teeth with attached soft tissues. The Sage-Schliff (sawing and grinding) technique. *J. Oral Pathol.* **1982**, *11*, 318–326. [CrossRef]
25. Johansson, C.B.; Morberg, P. Importance of ground section thickness for reliable histomorphometrical results. *Biomaterials* **1995**, *16*, 91–95. [CrossRef]
26. Johansson, C.B.; Morberg, P. Cutting directions of bone with biomaterials in situ does influence the outcome of histomorphometrical quantifications. *Biomaterials* **1995**, *16*, 1037–1039. [CrossRef]
27. Wilson, T.G.; Valderrama, P.; Burbano, M.; Blansett, J.; Levine, R.; Kessler, H.; Rodrigues, D.C. Foreign bodies associated with peri-implantitis human biopsies. *J. Periodontol.* **2015**, *86*, 9–15. [CrossRef]
28. Wang, X.; Li, Y.; Feng, Y.; Cheng, H.; Li, D. Macrophage polarization in aseptic bone resorption around dental implants induced by Ti particles in a murine model. *J. Periodontal Res.* **2019**. [CrossRef]
29. Donath, K.; Laass, M.; Günzl, H.J. The histopathology of different foreign-body reactions in oral soft tissue and bone tissue. *Virchows. Arch. A* **1992**, *420*, 131–137. [CrossRef]
30. Mbalaviele, G.; Novack, D.V.; Schett, G.; Teitelbaum, S.L. Inflammatory osteolysis: A conspiracy against bone. *J. Clin. Invest.* **2017**, *127*, 2030–2039. [CrossRef]
31. Paiva, K.B.S.; Granjeiro, J.M. Matrix Metalloproteinases in Bone Resorption, Remodeling, and Repair. *Prog Mol. Biol. Transl. Sci.* **2017**, *148*, 203–303. [CrossRef]
32. Setzen, G.; Williams, E.F., 3rd. Tissue response to suture materials implanted subcutaneously in a rabbit model. *Plast. Reconstr. Surg.* **1997**, *100*, 1788–1795. [CrossRef]
33. Nair, P.N. Pathogenesis of apical periodontitis and the causes of endodontic failures. *Crit. Rev. Oral Biol. Med.* **2004**, *15*, 348–381. [CrossRef]
34. You, T.M.; Choi, B.H.; Zhu, S.J.; Jung, J.H.; Lee, S.H.; Huh, J.Y.; Lee, H.J.; Li, J. Treatment of experimental peri-implantitis using autogenous bone grafts and platelet-enriched fibrin glue in dogs. *Oral Surg. Oral Med. Oral Pathol. Oral Radiol. Endod.* **2007**, *103*, 34–37. [CrossRef]
35. Schou, S.; Holmstrup, P.; Jorgensen, T.; Stoltze, K.; Hjorting-Hansen, E.; Wenzel, A. Autogenous bone graft and ePTFE membrane in the treatment of peri-implantitis. I. Clinical and radiographic observations in cynomolgus monkeys. *Clin. Oral Implants Res.* **2003**, *14*, 391–403. [CrossRef]
36. Yu, X.; Hu, Y.; Freire, M.; Yu, P.; Kawai, T.; Han, X. Role of toll-like receptor 2 in inflammation and alveolar bone loss in experimental peri-implantitis versus periodontitis. *J. Periodontal Res.* **2018**, *53*, 98–106. [CrossRef]
37. Albouy, J.P.; Abrahamsson, I.; Berglundh, T. Spontaneous progression of experimental peri-implantitis at implants with different surface characteristics: An experimental study in dogs. *J.Clin. Periodontol.* **2012**, *39*, 182–187. [CrossRef]
38. Jovanovic, S.A.; Kenney, E.B.; Carranza, F.A., Jr.; Donath, K. The regenerative potential of plaque-induced peri-implant bone defects treated by a submerged membrane technique: An experimental study. *Int. J. Oral Maxillofac. Implants* **1993**, *8*, 13–18.

39. Hayek, R.R.; Araujo, N.S.; Gioso, M.A.; Ferreira, J.; Baptista-Sobrinho, C.A.; Yamada, A.M.; Ribeiro, M.S. Comparative study between the effects of photodynamic therapy and conventional therapy on microbial reduction in ligature-induced peri-implantitis in dogs. *J. Periodontol.* **2005**, *76*, 1275–1281. [CrossRef]
40. Machtei, E.E.; Kim, D.M.; Karimbux, N.; Zigdon-Giladi, H. The use of endothelial progenitor cells combined with barrier membrane for the reconstruction of peri-implant osseous defects: An animal experimental study. *J. Clin. Periodontol.* **2016**, *43*, 289–297. [CrossRef]
41. Abdul-Karim, F.W.; Benevenia, J.; Pathria, M.N.; Makley, J.T. Case report 736: Retained surgical sponge (gossypiboma) with a foreign body reaction and remote and organizing hematoma. *Skeletal Radiol.* **1992**, *21*, 466–469.
42. Puvanesarajah, V.; Fayad, L.M.; Rao, S.S.; McCarthy, E.F.; Morris, C.D. Extremity gossypiboma mimicking sarcoma: Case report and review. *Skeletal Radiol.* **2019**, *48*, 629–635. [CrossRef]
43. Sari, A.; Basterzi, Y.; Karabacak, T.; Tasdelen, B.; Demirkan, F. The potential of microscopic sterile sponge particles to induce foreign body reaction. *Int. Wound J.* **2006**, *3*, 363–368. [CrossRef]
44. Altman, G.H.; Diaz, F.; Jakuba, C.; Calabro, T.; Horan, R.L.; Chen, J.; Lu, H.; Richmond, J.; Kaplan, D.L. Silk-based biomaterials. *Biomaterials* **2003**, *24*, 401–416. [CrossRef]
45. Nooh, N.; Abdullah, W.A.; Grawish Mel, A.; Ramalingam, S.; Javed, F.; Al-Hezaimi, K. The effects of surgicel and bone wax hemostatic agents on bone healing: An experimental study. *Indian J. Orthop.* **2014**, *48*, 319–325. [CrossRef]
46. Spelzini, F.; Konstantinovic, M.L.; Guelinckx, I.; Verbist, G.; Verbeken, E.; De Ridder, D.; Deprest, J. Tensile strength and host response towards silk and type i polypropylene implants used for augmentation of fascial repair in a rat model. *Gynecol. Obstet. Invest.* **2007**, *63*, 155–162. [CrossRef]
47. Trindade, R.; Albrektsson, T.; Galli, S.; Prgomet, Z.; Tengvall, P.; Wennerberg, A. Osseointegration and foreign body reaction: Titanium implants activate the immune system and suppress bone resorption during the first 4 weeks after implantation. *Clin. Implant. Dent. Relat. Res.* **2018**, *20*, 82–91. [CrossRef]
48. Brodbeck, W.G.; Macewan, M.; Colton, E.; Meyerson, H.; Anderson, J.M. Lymphocytes and the foreign body response: Lymphocyte enhancement of macrophage adhesion and fusion. *J. Biomed. Mater. Res. A* **2005**, *74*, 222–229. [CrossRef]
49. Rodriguez, A.; Macewan, S.R.; Meyerson, H.; Kirk, J.T.; Anderson, J.M. The foreign body reaction in T-cell-deficient mice. *J. Biomed. Mater. Res. A* **2009**, *90*, 106–113. [CrossRef]
50. Selders, G.S.; Fetz, A.E.; Radic, M.Z.; Bowlin, G.L. An overview of the role of neutrophils in innate immunity, inflammation and host-biomaterial integration. *Regen. Biomater.* **2017**, *4*, 55–68. [CrossRef]
51. Jhunjhunwala, S.; Aresta-DaSilva, S.; Tang, K.; Alvarez, D.; Webber, M.J.; Tang, B.C.; Lavin, D.M.; Veiseh, O.; Doloff, J.C.; Bose, S.; et al. Neutrophil Responses to Sterile Implant Materials. *PLoS ONE* **2015**, *10*, e0137550. [CrossRef]
52. Laffey, J.G.; Boylan, J.F.; Cheng, D.C. The systemic inflammatory response to cardiac surgery: Implications for the anesthesiologist. *Anesthesiology* **2002**, *97*, 215–252. [CrossRef]
53. Chrcanovic, B.R.; Albrektsson, T.; Wennerberg, A. Diabetes and oral implant failure: A systematic review. *J. Dent. Res.* **2014**, *93*, 859–867. [CrossRef]
54. Chrcanovic, B.R.; Albrektsson, T.; Wennerberg, A. Reasons for failures of oral implants. *J. Oral Rehabil.* **2014**, *41*, 443–476. [CrossRef]

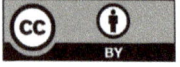

© 2019 by the authors. Licensee MDPI, Basel, Switzerland. This article is an open access article distributed under the terms and conditions of the Creative Commons Attribution (CC BY) license (http://creativecommons.org/licenses/by/4.0/).

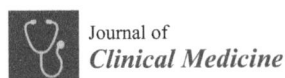

Article

Bone Immune Response to Materials, Part I: Titanium, PEEK and Copper in Comparison to Sham at 10 Days in Rabbit Tibia

Ricardo Trindade [1,*], Tomas Albrektsson [2,3], Silvia Galli [3], Zdenka Prgomet [4], Pentti Tengvall [2] and Ann Wennerberg [1]

1. Department of Prosthodontics, Faculty of Odontology, The Sahlgrenska Academy, University of Gothenburg, 405 30 Gothenburg, Sweden; ann.wennerberg@odontologi.gu.se
2. Department of Biomaterials, Institute of Clinical Sciences, University of Gothenburg, 405 30 Gothenburg, Sweden; tomas.albrektsson@biomaterials.gu.se (T.A.); pentti.tengvall@gu.se (P.T.)
3. Department of Prosthodontics, Faculty of Odontology, Malmö University, 205 06 Malmö, Sweden; silvia.galli@mau.se
4. Department of Oral Pathology, Faculty of Odontology, Malmö University, 205 06 Malmö, Sweden; zdenka.prgomet@mau.se
* Correspondence: ricardo.bretes.trindade@gu.se

Received: 9 November 2018; Accepted: 5 December 2018; Published: 7 December 2018

Abstract: Bone anchored biomaterials have become an indispensable solution for the restoration of lost dental elements and for skeletal joint replacements. However, a thorough understanding is still lacking in terms of the biological mechanisms leading to osseointegration and its contrast, unwanted peri-implant bone loss. We have previously hypothesized on the participation of immune mechanisms in such processes, and later demonstrated enhanced bone immune activation up to 4 weeks around titanium implants. The current experimental study explored and compared in a rabbit tibia model after 10 days of healing time, the bone inflammation/immunological reaction at mRNA level towards titanium, polyether ether ketone (PEEK) and copper compared to a Sham control. Samples from the test and control sites were, after a healing period, processed for gene expression analysis (polymerase chain reaction, (qPCR)) and decalcified histology tissue analysis. All materials displayed immune activation and suppression of bone resorption, when compared to sham. The M1 (inflammatory)/M2 (reparative) -macrophage phenotype balance was correlated to the proximity and volume of bone growth at the implant vicinity, with titanium demonstrating a M2-phenotype at 10 days, whereas copper and PEEK were still dealing with a mixed M1- and M2-phenotype environment. Titanium was the only material showing adequate bone growth and proximity inside the implant threads. There was a consistent upregulation of (T-cell surface glycoprotein CD4) CD4 and downregulation of (T-cell transmembrane glycoprotein CD8) CD8, indicating a CD4-lymphocyte phenotype driven reaction around all materials at 10 days.

Keywords: osseointegration; immune system; biomaterials; foreign body reaction; in vivo study

1. Introduction

Recent evidence suggests that biomaterials induce an immunomodulatory interaction with the host, and materials such as titanium or bone substitutes seem not at all inert upon contact with host bone [1]. The ultimate outcome of biomaterial implantation depends on the extent of the ensuing foreign body reaction (FBR) and related immune and inflammatory mechanisms; current scientific efforts are focusing on understanding this complex host reaction, in order to improve the behavior of implanted biomaterials [2]. However, the precise mechanisms of osseointegration are today not fully understood, especially the long-term immune recognition of implants.

The present authors have explored some immunological mechanisms in a previously published review [3], following the hypothesis that osseointegration is nothing but a special type of immune driven foreign body reaction to the implanted material, ending up in bone demarcation at or near the surface [4]. The main hypothesis was that implants are not biologically inert, meaning that the immune/inflammatory system, in this case with emphasis on the immune system, is activated when titanium interacts with host bone—A hypothesis that later was tested and verified in a recent 4 week experimental pilot animal study, where immunological markers representing macrophages, complement, neutrophils, lymphocytes and bone resorption markers were compared in osteotomy sites, with and without the presence of titanium implants [5]: Titanium sites, showed significant up-/or down-regulation of immune (and inflammatory) markers after 28 days, i.e., at a time point well into the bone remodeling phase The immune system was apparently activated through the complement system, displayed M1 (inflammatory) - and M2 (reparative) -macrophages phenotypes, neutrophil cytosolic factor 1 (NCF-1), and down regulation of markers related to osteoclastic activity. Comparatively, at an earlier stage (10 days) only the M2-macrophage (reparative) phenotype was identified around titanium, when compared to the sham site. From earlier studies immune complement is known to become activated at a very early time point around titanium, and materials are then recognized as foreign objects by inflammatory cells [6]. During bone healing, and after the acute inflammatory phase, macrophages and their classically described polarization into M1 (inflammatory) and M2 (reparative) phenotypes dominate, and are considered to be central in the host reaction to implanted biomaterials [7,8], but the precise in vivo mechanisms are still in need of a thorough clarification. Macrophages are also intimately related to bone biology, interacting closely with osteoblasts during bone formation (these macrophages are named Osteomacs), and also fusing into either osteoclasts or material related multinucleated giant cells (named Foreign Body Giant Cells), determining a further important role for macrophages when considering bone borne biomaterials [9].

In the earlier review [3], and pertaining the current manuscript, it was further hypothesized that the reason why different materials may or not achieve osseointegration is probably related, to some extent, to a persistent immune patrolling resulting in a modified inflammatory reaction around the different materials. These two concepts—That materials are not biologically inert and that a specific persistent immune-inflammatory balance or patrolling around different materials largely dictates whether osseointegration occurs or not—Are fundamental to our understanding of longer-term host reactions to materials in bone.

The aim of the present exploratory in vivo study is to test the hypothesis that different materials trigger different early immune/inflammatory responses upon implantation in rabbit bone, and that these different responses may be important for the establishment of osseointegration, or the ultimate lack of it.

2. Materials and Methods

The current study consists of an experiment in the rabbit proximal tibia (metaphysis), comparing bone healing on sites where osteotomies were performed and then either left to heal without the placement of a material (sham site- Sh), or had one of the three test materials placed for comparison: titanium (Ti), copper (Cu) or polyether ether ketone (PEEK). Each rabbit received one site of each group (two sites per tibia): Sh, Ti, Cu and PEEK. Ti and PEEK were placed on the right tibia and a Sham site was produced and Cu was introduced in the other osteotomy on the left tibia. All implants were machined with a turning process, with a threaded 0.6 mm pitch height, 3.75 mm width Branemark MkIII design. The Ti implants were made of commercially pure titanium grade IV. Implant manufacturers: Ti and PEEK implants were produced by Carlsson and Möller, Helsingborg, Sweden; Copper implants were produced by TL Medical Company, Molndal, Sweden.

The sham site also provokes an inflammatory reaction, which is still present at 10 days and is used as a baseline to compare with the immune reaction elicited by each of the different materials.

2.1. Surgical Procedure

This study was performed on 6 mature, female New Zealand White Rabbits ($n = 6$, weight 3 to 4 Kg), with the ethical approval from the Ethics Committee for Animal Research (number 13-011) of the École Nationale Vétérinaire D'Alfors, Maisons-Alfors, Val-de-Marne, France. All care was taken to minimize animal pain or discomfort during and after the surgical procedures. For the surgical procedures, the rabbits were placed under general anesthesia using a mixture of medetomidine (Domitor, Zoetis, Florham Park, NJ, USA), ketamine (Imalgène 1000, Merial, Lyon, France) and diazepam (Valium, Roche, Basel, Switzerland) for induction, then applying subcutaneous buprenorphine (Buprecare, Animalcare, York, UK) and intramuscular Meloxicam (Metacam; Boehringer Ingelheim Vetmedica, Inc., Ridgefield, CT, USA). A single incision was performed in the internal knee area on each side and the bone exposed for osteotomies and insertion of implants in the sites mentioned above. The surgical site was sutured with a resorbable suture (Vicryl 3-0, Ethicon, Cincinnati, OH, USA) and hemostasis achieved. Following surgery, Fentanyl patches (Duragesic, Janssen Pharmaceutica, Beerse, Belgium) were applied.

The osteotomies were produced with a sequence of increasing diameter twist drills, from 2 mm to 3.15 mm width, and a final countersink bur prepared the cortical part of the bone. The implants used were 3.75 mm in diameter.

The rabbits were housed in separate cages and were allowed to move and eat freely. At 10 days, the rabbits were sacrificed with a lethal injection of sodium pentobarbital (Euthasol, Virbac, Fort Worth, TX, USA). The 6 animals had the implants removed through unscrewing. On 4 of those animals, bone was collected with a 2 mm twist drill from the periphery of the Sh, Ti, Cu and PEEK sites on the most distal portion, and then processed for Gene Expression Analysis through quantitative polymerase chain reaction (qPCR). The 6 animals had the test sites then removed en bloc for histological processing.

2.2. Gene Expression Analysis—qPCR

The bone samples for gene expression analysis were collected from the distal side of the osteotomies of all four groups (following the removal of the implant from the implant sites), with a 2 mm twist drill that removed both cortical and marrow bone in the full length of the osteotomy, to enable the study of the 2 mm peri-implant bone area of each of the Sh, Ti, Cu and PEEK sites. The samples were immediately transferred to separate sterile plastic recipients containing RNA*later* medium (Ambion, Inc., Austin, TX, USA), for preservation. The samples were then refrigerated first at 4 °C and then stored at -20 °C until processing.

2.3. mRNA Isolation

Samples were homogenized using an ultrasound homogenizer (Sonoplus HD3100, Brandelin, Berlin, Germany) in 1 mL PureZOL and total RNA was isolated via column fractionalization using the Aurum^{TM} Total RNA Fatty and Fibrous Tissue Kit (Bio-Rad Laboratories Inc., Hercules, CA, USA) following the manufacturer's instructions. All the samples were DNAse treated using an on-column DNAse I contained in the kit to remove genomic DNA. The RNA quantity for each sample was analyzed in the NanoDrop 2000 Spectrophotometer (Thermo Scientific, Wilmington, NC, USA). BioRad iScript cDNA synthesis kit (Bio-Rad Laboratories Inc., Hercules, CA, USA) was then used to convert mRNA into cDNA, following the manufacturer's instructions.

qPCR primers (Tataa Biocenter, Gothenburg, Sweden) were designed following the National Center of Biotechnology Information (NCBI) Sequence database, including the local factors chosen in order to characterize the immune, inflammatory and bone metabolic pathways (Tables 1 and 2). All primers had an efficiency between 90 and 110%.

J. Clin. Med. **2018**, *7*, 526

Table 1. Gene sequences.

Primer	Forward Sequence	Reverse Sequence	Accession nr/Transcript ID
NCF-1	TTCATCCGCCACATTGCCC	GTCCTGCCACTTCACCAAGA	NM_001082102.1
CD68	TTTCCCCAGCTCTCCACCTC	CGATGATGAGGGGCACCAAG	ENSOCUT00000010382
CD11b	TTCAACCTGGAGACTGAGAACAC	TCAAACTGGACCACGCTCTG	ENSOCUT00000001589
CD14	TCTGAAAATCCTGGGCTGGG	TTCATTCCCGCGTTCCGTAG	ENSOCUT00000004218
ARG1	GGATCATTGGAGCCCCTTTCTC	TCAAGCAGACCAGCCTTTCTC	NM_001082108.1
IL-4	CTACCTCCACCACAAGGTGTC	CCAGTGTAGTCTGTCTGGCTT	ENSOCUT00000024099
IL-13	GCAGCCTCGTATCCCCAG	GGTTGACGCTCCACACCA	ENSOCUT00000000154
M-CSF	GGAACTCTCGCTCAGGCTC	ACATTCTTGATCTTCTCCAGCAAC	ENSOCUT00000030714
OPG	TGTGTGAATGCGAGGAAGGG	AACTGTATTCCGCTCTGGGG	ENSOCUT00000011149
RANKL	GAAGGTTCATGGTTCGATCTGG	CCAAGAGGACAGGCTCACTTT	ENSOCUT00000024354
TRAP	TTACTTCAGTGGCGTGCAGA	CGATCTGGGCTGAGACGTTG	NM_001081988.1
CathK	GGAACCGGGGCATTGACTCT	TGTACCCTCTGCATTTGGCTG	NM_001082641.1
PPAR-γ	CAAGGCGAGGGCGATCTT	ATGCGGATGGCGACTTCTTT	NM_001082148.1
C3	ACTCTGTCGAGAAGGAACGGG	CCTTGATTTGTTGATGCTGGCTG	NM_001082286.1
C3aR1	CATGTCAGTCAACCCCTGCT	GCGAATGGTTTTGCTCCCTG	ENSOCUT00000007435
CD46	TCCTGCTGTTCACTTTCTCGG	CATGTTCCCATCCTTGTTTACACTT	ENSOCUT00000033915
CD55	TGGTGTTGGGTGGAGTGACC	AGAGTGAAGCCTCTGTTGCATT	ENSOCUT00000031985
CD59	ACCACTGTCTCCTCCCAAGT	GCAATCTTCATACCGCCAACA	NM_001082712.1
C5	TCCAAAACTCTGCAACCTTAACA	AAATGCTTTGACACAACTTCCA	ENSOCUT00000005683
C5aR1	ACGTCAACTGCTGCATCAACC	AGGCTGGGGAGAGACTTGC	ENSOCUT00000029180
CD3	CCTGGGGACAGGAAGATGATGAC	CAGCACCACGGGTTCCA	NM_001082001.1
CD4	CAACTGGAAACATGCGAACCA	TTGATGACCAGGGGAAAGA	NM_001082313.2
CD8	GGCGTCTACTTCTGCATGACC	GAACCGGCACACTCTCTTCT	ENSOCUT00000009383
CD19	GGATGTATGTCTGTCGCCGT	AAGCAAAGCCACAACTGGAA	ENSOCUT00000028895
GAPDH	GGTGAAGGTCGGAGTGAACGG	CATGTAGACCATGTAGTGGAGGTCA	NM_001082253.1
ACT-β	TCATTCCAAATATCGTGAGATGCC	TACACAAATGCGATGCTGCC	NM_001101683.1
LDHA	TGCAGACAAGGAACAGTGGA	CCCAGGTAGTGTAGCCCTT	NM_001082277.1

NCF-1, neutrophil cytosolic factor 1; CD68, macrosialin; CD11b, macrophage marker; CD14, monocyte differentiation antigen CD14; ARG1, Arginase 1; IL-4, Interleukin 4; IL-13, Interleukin 13; M-CSF, colony stimulating factor-macrophage; OPG, osteoprotegerin; RANKL, Receptor activator of nuclear factor kappa-B ligand; TRAP, tartrate resistant acid phosphatase; CathK, cathepsin K; PPAR-γ, peroxisome proliferator activated receptor gamma; C3, complement component 3; C3aR1, complement component 3a receptor 1; CD46, complement regulatory protein; CD55, decay accelerating factor for complement; CD59, complement regulatory protein; C5, complement component 5; C5aR1, complement component 5a receptor 1; CD3, T-cell surface glycoprotein CD3; CD4, T-cell surface glycoprotein CD4; CD8, T-cell transmembrane glycoprotein CD8; CD19, B-lymphocyte surface protein CD19; GAPDH, glyceraldehyde-3-phosphate dehydrogenase; ACT-β, actin beta; LDHA, lactate dehydrogenase A.

Table 2. Correspondence between studied gene expression and biological entities.

Biological Entity	Gene
Neutrophil	NCF-1
Macrophage	CD68, CD11b, CD14, ARG1
Macrophage fusion	IL-4, IL-13, M-CSF
Bone resorption	OPG, RANKL, TRAP, CathK, PPAR-γ
Complement	Activation: C3, C3aR1, C5, C5aR1 Inhibition: CD46, CD55, CD59
T-lymphocytes	CD3, CD4, CD8
B-lymphocytes	CD19
Reference genes	GAPDH, ACT-β, LDHA

2.4. Amplification Process

Five µL of SsoAdvanced SYBR™ Green Supermix (Bio-Rad Laboratories Inc., Hercules, CA, USA) and 1 µL of cDNA template together with 0.4 µM of forward and reverse primer were used in the qPCR reaction. Each cDNA sample was performed on duplicates. The thermal cycles were performed on the CFX Connect Real-Time System (Bio-Rad Laboratories Inc., Hercules, CA, USA). The CFX Manager Software 3.0 (Bio-Rad, Hercules, CA, USA) was used for the data analysis.

Three genes (GAPDH, ACT-β, LDHA) were selected as reference genes using the geNorm algorithm integrated in the CFX Manager Software. A quantification cycle (Cq) value of the chosen reference genes (Tables 1 and 2) was used as control; hence the mean Cq value of each target gene (Table 1) was normalized against the reference gene's Cq, giving the genes' relative expression.

For calculation of fold change, the ΔΔCq was used, comparing mRNA expressions from the different groups. Significance was set at $p < 0.05$ and the regulation threshold at ×2-fold change.

2.5. Decalcified Bone Histology

After removal of the implants from the studied Sh, Ti, Cu and PEEK sites on the 6 subjects, bone was removed en bloc and preserved in 10% formalin (4% buffered formaldehyde, VWR international, Leuven, Belgium) during 48 h for fixation. Samples were decalcified in ethylene diamine tetra-acetic acid (10% unbuffered EDTA; Milestone Srl, Sorisole, Italy) for 4 weeks, with weekly substitution of the EDTA solution, dehydrated and embedded in paraffin (Tissue-Tek TEC, Sakura Finetek Europe BV, Leiden, The Netherlands). Samples were sectioned (4 μm thick) with a microtome (Microm HM355S, Thermo Fischer Scientific, Walldorf, Germany) and stained with hematoxylin-eosin (HE) for histological analysis.

2.6. Statistical Analysis

The gene expression statistical analysis was performed using the *t* test built in the algorithm of the CFX Manager Software 3.0 package (BioRad, Hercules, CA, USA). The gene expression analysis was made pair wise, each material being evaluated against the Sham in each animal.

2.7. Surface Roughness

The surface roughness of each material was measured (following Wennerberg and Albrektsson guidelines (2000)) [10], with a white light 3D optical Profilometer, gbs, smart WLI extended (Gesellschaft für Bild und Signal verarbeitung mbH, Immenau, Germany) using a 50× objective. MountainsMap®Imaging Topography 7.4 (Digital Surf, Besancon, France) software was used to evaluate the data. Surface roughness parameters were calculated after removing errors of form and waviness. A gaussian filter with a size of 50 × 50 μm was used. The measuring area was 350 × 220 μm for all measurements, 3 copper, 3 titanium and 3 PEEK implants were measured, each implant on 9 sites (3 tops, 3 valleys and 3 flanks).

In order to characterize the surface in height, spatial and surface enlargement aspects 4 parameters were selected; S_a that describes the average height distribution measured in μm, S_{ds} which is a measure of the density of summits over the measured area, measured in $1/\mu m^2$, Ssk (skewness) a parameter that describes the asymmetry of the surface deviation from the mean plane and S_{dr} which describes the surface enlargement compared to a totally flat reference area, measured in %.

3. Results

3.1. Gene Expression Analysis

Each material (Ti, Cu and PEEK) was compared against the Sh site for gene expression regarding the immunological reaction after 10 days of healing- and considering that the Sh site itself, also produces an immune-inflammatory reaction. The results show that when comparing Ti sites with Sh sites (Table 3 and Figure 1), ARG1 (M2-macrophage) is statistically significantly and almost 2-fold upregulated, while CD4 (T helper lymphocytes) is 2-fold upregulated and close to statistical significance. This indicates an activation of the immune system already at 10 days around Ti, when compared to Sh. On the other hand, the downregulation of both C3aR1 (complement component 3a receptor 1) and CD8 (T cytotoxic lymphocytes) was more than 2-fold and at a statistically significant level around Ti compared to Sh, which further supports the notion of an immunological involvement in the host response towards titanium, as it probably represents a biological feedback effect following activation of complement factor C3 and T cells at an earlier stage. Furthermore, peroxisome proliferator-activated receptor gamma (PPAR-γ) is significantly downregulated, while RANKL (Receptor activator of nuclear factor kappa-B ligand) and OPG (osteoprotegerin) showed a non-significant downregulation, indicating an environment around Ti where bone resorption is apparently suppressed. Macrophage colony-stimulating factor (M-CSF) is significantly downregulated, indicating suppression of cell (macrophage) fusion around Ti at 10 days, into either osteoclasts or foreign body giant cells (FBGCs).

Table 3. Gene expression Ti vs. Sham.

Marker	Down-Regulation	p-Value
ARG1	1.82	0.0254
CD4	2.03	0.0598
Marker	Down-Regulation	p-Value
M-CSF	−2.23	0.0004
PPAR-G	−3.07	0.0008
RANKL	−2.24	0.0678
OPG	−1.85	0.5711
C3aR1	−3.55	0.0137
CD8b	−2.80	0.0195

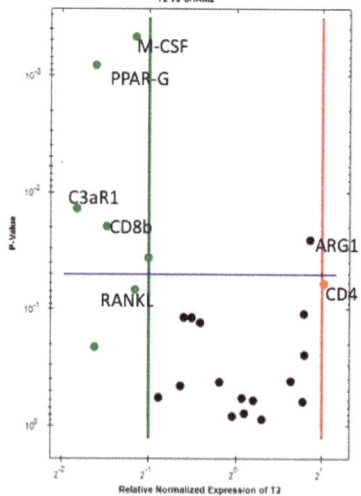

Figure 1. Volcano plot comparing the gene expression of Ti versus Sh at 10 days. Downregulation (vertical green line) and Upregulation (vertical red line) set a ×2 regulation. Statistical significance (horizontal blue line) set at $p < 0.05$—Marker is significant when above blue line.

When comparing PEEK sites with Sh sites (Table 4 and Figure 2), even if not significantly, ARG1 (M2-macrophages), NCF-1 (neutrophils), CD68 (M1-macrophages) and CD4 (T helper cells) are upregulated 2-fold or more around PEEK when compared to Sh sites, indicating early immune activation around PEEK. Downregulation of CD8 (T cytotoxic cell—Significant), complement factors (C3aR1, CD55, CD59 and C5- the last two statistically significant), strongly adds to the notion of immune system involvement in the host reaction towards PEEK implants. The downregulation of PPAR-gamma, RANKL, OPG, TRAP (all statistically significant) and CATHK demonstrates the suppression of bone resorption around PEEK implants after 10 days of insertion in the bone.

Table 4. Gene expression PEEK vs. Sham.

Marker	Down-Regulation	p-Value
ARG1	3.11	0.1091
CD68	2.00	0.4304
NCF1	2.61	0.1556
CD4	1.95	0.0771

Marker	Down-Regulation	p-Value
PPAR-G	−4.81	0.0009
RANKL	−3.16	0.0286
OPG	−3.13	0.0210
TRAP	−1.91	0.0109
CATHK	−1.75	0.0985
C5	−2.73	0.0044
CD59	−1.87	0.0181
CD55	−1.81	0.0578
C3aR1	−2.84	0.0601
CD8b	−2.86	0.0044

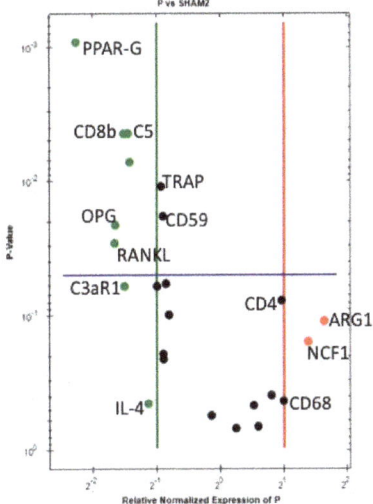

Figure 2. Volcano plot comparing the gene expression of PEEK versus Sh at 10 days. Downregulation (vertical green line) and Upregulation (vertical red line) set a ×2 regulation. Statistical significance (horizontal blue line) set at $p < 0.05$—Marker is significant when above blue line.

Around Copper (Cu) implants, when compared to Sh (Table 5 and Figure 3) at 10 days, ARG1 (M2 macrophage), NCF1 (neutrophils) and CD4 (T helper cells) are statistically significantly upregulated. Furthermore, even if not reaching the statistical significance level of $p < 0.05$, CD19 (B cells), C5aR1 (complement C5 receptor 1), CD68, CD14 and CD11b (the latter three are M1-macrophage markers) are upregulated. These results demonstrate a strong immune activation around Cu upon contact with host bone tissue.

C5, CD59, CD55, CD46 and C3aR1 (complement factors) are downregulated, suggesting a feedback effect following complement activation (which is confirmed by C5aR1 upregulation).

CD8 (T cytotoxic cell) shows a tendency for downregulation around Cu.

The statistically significant downregulation of M-CSF, with the tendency for downregulation of IL-4, even if both not reaching a 2-fold change, suggests that at 10 days of implantation, macrophage fusion into either osteoclasts or FBGCs is suppressed around Cu—Similar to what was observed above around Ti. Additionally, as for Ti and PEEK, bone resorption is suppressed around Cu at 10 days, when compared to Sh, since PPAR-gamma is statistically significantly downregulated and the other bone resorption markers (RANKL, OPG, TRAP and CATHK) show a tendency for downregulation.

Table 5. Gene expression Cu vs. Sham.

Marker	Up-Regulation	p-Value
ARG1	25.74	0.0072
NCF1	3.41	0.0234
CD4	3.11	0.0178
CD19	1.88	0.3768
C5aR1	2.03	0.1021
CD68	1.80	0.4153
CD11b	1.79	0.5131
CD14	1.61	0.6120
Marker	**Down-Regulation**	**p-Value**
PPAR-G	−5.28	0.0001
RANKL	−1.71	0.1301
OPG	−3.74	0.2815
TRAP	−2.25	0.0676
C5	−1.66	0.0007
CD59	−2.01	0.3376
C3aR1	−2.14	0.2071
CD8b	−2.09	0.0906

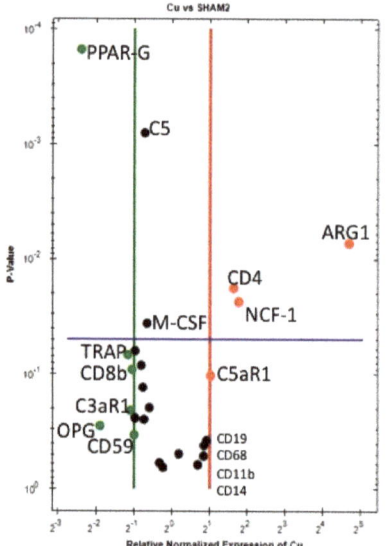

Figure 3. Volcano plot comparing the gene expression of Cu versus Sh at 10 days. Downregulation (vertical green line) and Upregulation (vertical red line) set a ×2 regulation. Statistical significance (horizontal blue line) set at $p < 0.05$—Marker is significant when above blue line.

3.2. Decalcified Bone Histology

Decalcified histological sections of the four groups (Sham and the three different materials) were analyzed at a tissue level. The Sh sites display some bone formation around the osteotomy site, which is decreasing in size after 10 days, as the new bone fills in the osteotomy defect (Figure 4). Ti sites show new bone formation and bone remodeling in the thread areas (Figure 5). Cu sites display no bone formation at the interface of the implant site, showing a division (from the implant area) of a first layer of inflammatory cells with signs of cell lysis and some foreign body giant cells, followed by a proliferative area with parallel aligned fibers to the implant site, which in turn is followed outwards by an area of bone remodeling, more noticeable in areas closer to cortical bone, where osteoblasts and osteoclasts can be observed remodeling the old bone (Figure 6). PEEK sites present very little new bone formation/remodeling areas close to the implant interface, confined to areas in cortical bone proximity, whereas most of the interface presents only a thin proliferative area parallel to the implant site, mostly consisting of fibrous tissue and with very few calcified islands (Figure 7). The cellular components have all been clearly identified, neutrophils, macrophages, osteoclasts, osteoblasts, and also foreign body giant cells. However, quantification has not been performed, as it is not within the scope of the present study.

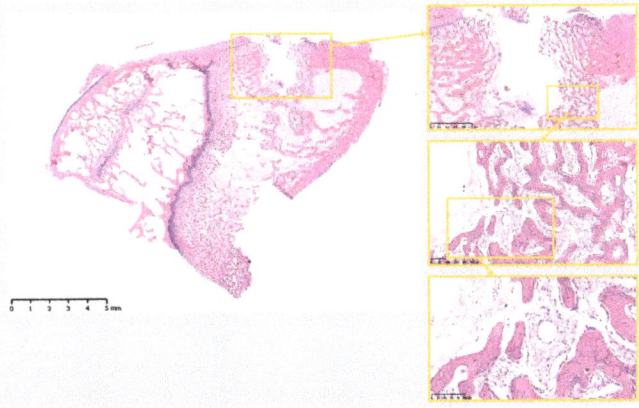

Figure 4. The 10 days Sh site. Bone remodeling with new bone formation around the osteotomy site. Defect is isolated from the marrow space. Scale bars, clockwise: 5 mm, 1 mm, 250 µm and 100 µm.

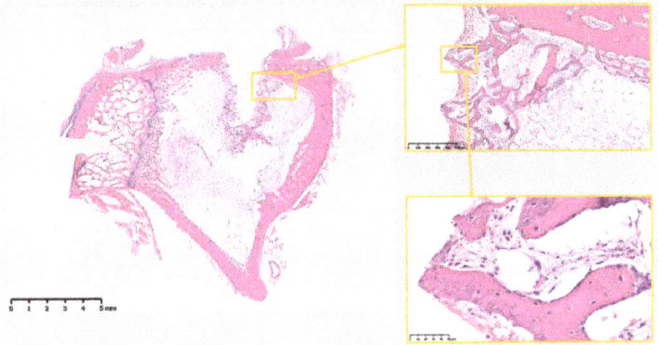

Figure 5. The 10 days Ti site. Bone remodeling and new bone formation around the implant site, isolating it from the marrow space. Scale bars, clockwise: 5 mm, 500 µm and 50 µm.

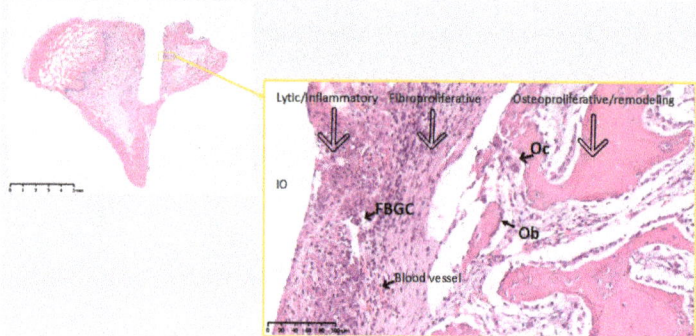

Figure 6. The 10 days Cu site. No bone on the immediate implant vicinity. FBGC, foreign body giant cells; Oc, osteoclast actively remodeling old bone; Ob, Seam of osteoblasts producing new bone (part of the remodeling); IO, Implant/Osteotomy. Reaction to Cu divided in 3 zones, representing the 3 phenomena around implant materials in the bone: From the implant surface Lytic/Inflammatory area, Fibroproliferative area and Osteoproliferative area. The latter two represent an attempt to isolate the material from the marrow cavity. No osseointegration is viable at this time point. Theoretically, around Ti the same phenomena exist, but at a different balance, allowing for osseointegration, through direct bon-to-implant contact. Inflammatory area is highly vascularized. Scale bars 5 mm (left) and 100 µm (right).

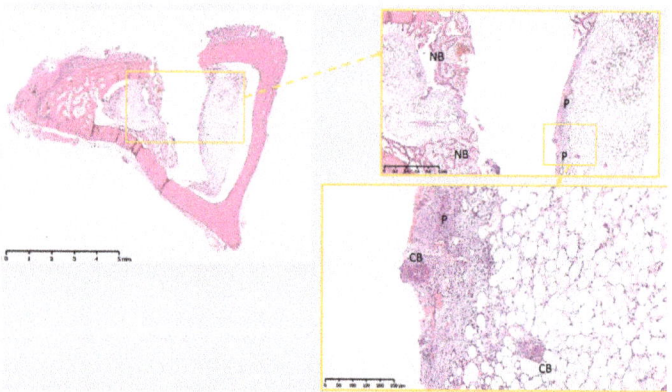

Figure 7. The 10 days PEEK. NB, new bone; forming only in the areas adjacent to cortical bone, while most other interfacial tissue shows no bone formation. P, proliferative area; no visible calcified tissue formation, but for some isolated calcified bone areas (CB, calcified bone). Scale bars, clockwise: 5 mm, 1 mm and 250 µm.

3.3. Surface Roughness

Table 6 shows the results on each material surface roughness analysis. The surface enlargement, which is depending on both height and the density of the surface irregularities, was smallest for the copper implants mostly depending on the lower height deviation compared to titanium and PEEK. Titanium and PEEK had a frequency distribution close to zero, while copper implants had slightly more peaks than pits. In terms of height deviation, titanium demonstrated the roughest surface.

Table 6. Surface roughness analysis.

Surface Roughness	S_a μm Mean	S_{sk} Mean	S_{ds} 1/μm² Mean	S_{dr} % Mean
Copper	0.40	1.2	0.28	47
Titanium	0.75	−0.02	0.25	66
PEEK	0.56	−0.23	0.31	69

S_a, describes the average height distribution measured in μm; S_{ds}, a measure of the density of summits over the measured area, measured in 1/μm²; S_{sk} (skewness), a parameter that describes the asymmetry of the surface deviation from the mean plane; S_{dr}, describes the surface enlargement compared to a totally flat reference area, measured in %.

4. Discussion

The present results demonstrate the immune system activation around Ti, PEEK and Cu once in contact with host bone, after 10 days of implantation- this demonstrates that, eventually, all materials render an immune activation, when in contact with bone.

Macrophage polarization, between M1-macrophage and M2-macrophage phenotypes, has been highlighted as a determining factor in the foreign body reaction, i.e., how host tissues interact with biomaterials [7,8]. M1-macrophages present a pro-inflammatory phenotype, while M2-macrophages have been identified as anti-inflammatory cells, participating in wound healing—Namely in the healing phase of acute inflammation—And also in chronic inflammation associated with immunological diseases, such as Rheumatoid Arthritis and Psoriasis [11]. M1-macrophages are described as induced by interferon-gamma (IFN-γ), while M2 macrophages are described as induced by e.g., IL-4 and IL-13 [8].

One of the main findings in this study is the importance of the M1/M2-macrophage (M1/M2) immunological balance in osseointegration already at this early stage: Titanium displays a reparative/anti-inflammatory M2-macrophage (M2) phenotype (ARG1), whereas Cu and PEEK are still dealing with a mixed pro-inflammatory M1-macrophage (M1) and M2 anti-inflammatory type of reaction (CD68, CD14 and CD11b; ARG1, respectively). The early preferential polarization towards a M2 phenotype around Ti, in the M1/M2 balance, probably explains the event of osseointegration being successful around Ti and not around the other materials—A fact already hypothesized in our previous work [3] and further discussed below.

Another important, and unpredicted, finding is the tilting towards the CD4 T-cell phenotype and suppression of the CD8 T-cell phenotype around all materials, opening a window to further understanding the immune reaction to biomaterials in the bone, by demonstrating the participation of T-cells and indicating an early specific T-cell phenotype (discussed below).

The current results confirm the present authors' previously published results comparing Ti and Sh immune responses, where immune activation around Ti implants was demonstrated in a femur study at 10 days and even more so at 28 days after implantation, i.e., outside the major inflammatory period [12].

For the present experiment, Ti was chosen as an already studied material, and the results of the previous study were confirmed, while PEEK was chosen for its perceived bio-inertness [13] and Cu for its known induction of a stronger inflammatory reaction when in contact with tissues—As demonstrated by Suska et al. 2008 in a rat soft tissue model [14]. As already mentioned, Ti displays mostly a reparative type-2 phenotype (ARG1 and CD4), whereas around Cu (ARG1, NCF1, CD11b, CD68, CD14, C5aR1, CD19) and PEEK (ARG1, CD68, NCF1, CD4) there is still a mixed environment, with pro-inflammatory and anti-inflammatory/reparative elements, which may explain the different bone tissue reaction towards the different materials at a tissue level (supported by the histological findings in this study). Even if some of these markers are not expressed with a statistically significant difference in value, most pass the ×2 threshold in regulation fold-change or are very close to that value; hence, their interpretation is crucial to understand the biological events and the osteoimmunology in relation to the studied materials.

The three materials have shown up-regulation of ARG1, indicating a reparative type-2 anti-inflammatory reaction (M2- macrophages and ILC-2). PEEK and Cu also show a M1-macrophage pro-inflammatory type of reaction, meaning that at 10 days the host tissue is not yet tilting the balance towards a full reparative mode around Cu and PEEK, which may explain, at least in part, the results at tissue level. Hence, the present results confirm the notion of macrophages being central in host reaction to biomaterials, with a decisive role already at 10 days- it would be interesting to study how the biological immune process develops at a later time point, whether it resolves, maintains or increases around Cu and PEEK.

Furthermore, the results show activation of CD4+ T-cells around all materials at 10 days, whereas the CD8+ T-cell phenotype is suppressed. These findings demonstrate the participation of T-cells in the bone healing process around solid biomaterials, although it is not known whether solely an innate or also an adaptive type of immune reaction is present—Classically, the host reaction to biomaterials is perceived as an innate immunological process [5], hence indicating T-cell activity through cytokines, rather than an antigen-antibody interaction. Furthermore, ARG1, which shows a tendency for upregulation in the three materials compared to Sh, is also expressed by type-2 innate lymphoid-cells (ILC-2) [15], supporting an innate immune mechanism. T-helper cells (CD4+) are involved in the regulation of immune responses at many levels, such as interaction with macrophages and the recruitment of neutrophils [16]. Regulatory T-cells (Treg) are also CD4+, and are responsible for suppressing immune inflammatory responses to allow reparative processes, being important, for instance, in halting some forms of autoimmune diseases [17]; hence, upregulation of CD4 most probably indicates an immunologically driven reaction towards tissue repair and proliferation around the studied materials, which has also been suggested by other authors [18].

The statistically significant upregulation of NCF1 around Cu and a similar upregulation around PEEK (even if not statistically significant) already at 10 days, highlights the role of neutrophils in the host-biomaterial interaction; however, in our previous study [5], Ti showed a statistically significant upregulation of NCF1 only after 28 days of healing, which implies a stronger inflammatory reaction around Cu and PEEK at an early stage that may further help dictate a soft tissue formation around these materials, not enabling bone deposition at the implant surface. At an earlier stage in the healing response, neutrophils participate in the inflammatory reaction, although changing phenotype at a later stage in this response, which may be the result of either macrophages inhibiting neutrophil apoptosis for continued neutrophil local performance, or the possible participation in the reparative process, mainly through an enhancing effect on vascularization [19,20]. Vascularization is of particular importance for the early development of tissue around the implants in an attempt to isolate these from the marrow compartment during the foreign body reaction; this is especially important considering that bone is a hypoxic tissue [21].

Complement factors seem mostly suppressed around all of the materials studied, at 10 days. The complement system, however, is complex and self-regulated [22]. The results show that the complement components are mostly downregulated, probably reflecting an inhibitory reaction to an earlier complement activation during the initial healing phase- thus indicating the possible involvement of the complement system from an early time point in the host reaction to implanted materials in the bone.

Furthermore, bone resorption markers were downregulated around all three materials at 10 days, when compared to Sh sites. This demonstrates a bone resorption suppression in the immediate implant environment from an early stage, when compared to our previous study, where this was mostly perceived at a later time point (28 days) around Ti [5]. Hence, a bone forming environment is already being developed around materials from an early healing stage and within the inflammatory period.

Further studies including protein identification techniques are recommended to confirm the gene expression outcomes presented here and rule out possible post-transcriptional or post-translational changes in the biological response.

Copper presents with extensive apoptosis around the surface; one would attribute this to the toxicity of Copper ions, but the surface topography may play an important role in determining the phenotype of Macrophages here: Copper compared to Sham shows an upregulation of ARG1, indicating M2-macrophages already at 10 days (25 times up regulated in Cu, while Ti and PEEK show a less pronounced increase in ARG1, even if also relevant). A possible conclusion is that the chemical aspect of Copper surface is likely a major factor, given the apoptosis seen, but that the surface topography also has to be considered, given that current evidence on M1/M2-macrophage polarization has a clear link to surface topography [8], which relates to our results both on surface analysis and gene expression analysis. Further studies are hence necessary to understand the role of both surface topography and chemistry, which likely differs between different materials. The surface may play a role in the macrophage phenotype, however, in the present study, Cu did not demonstrate an exceptional roughness, rather similar to commercial Ti implants produced with grade 4 Ti. Therefore, the topography may have had an influence but not likely a major one. Recent in vitro studies have shown the effect of surface chemistry and topography in macrophage polarization. Zhang H et al. have demonstrated the surface chemistry immunomodulatory effect of amine silanized titanium, which reduced inflammation and promoted M2 polarization of macrophages [23], while Gao L et al. have demonstrated a M1- to M2-macrophage switch, through surface release of IL-4 [24]. Regarding surface topography, Shayan M et al. have demonstrated both in vitro and in a soft tissue in vivo study, that implant surface nanopatterning is able to selectively polarize macrophages towards M2, hence modulating the immune response to the selected biomaterial [25]. These studies concur with the current bone tissue in vivo experimental results, which demonstrated that different materials modulate the host immune response through the polarization of macrophages, where Ti promotes an early shift to a M2-macrophage phenotype- with the inherent consequences observed at the tissue level, and which may explain the clinical osseointegration seen around Ti implants in bone.

Decalcified histology of specimens from the four groups shows that only Ti develops a structured thread infill of new bone, at 10 days. All the groups form an area of several cell layers clearly isolating the implant material (or osteotomy site in Sh), although Cu and PEEK fail to produce an adequate volume of osseous tissue, showing mostly soft tissue in the interfacial zone. In fact, the present histological results support the published work by Osborne and Newesley (1980), indicating contact osteogenesis around "well tolerated" biomaterials and distance osteogenesis around "less well tolerated" biomaterials [26]. This difference can be explained by the above gene expression analysis, where Ti shows a more reparative environment at such an early stage, when compared to PEEK and Cu.

5. Conclusions/Summary

1. All three materials display immune/inflammatory system activation at 10 days;
2. A more favourable macrophage M1/M2 balance likely leads to a better osseointegration of Ti, as compared to Cu and PEEK:
3. A clearer M2 anti-inflammatory/reparative regulation around Ti at 10 days;
4. A mixture of M1 and M2 (pro- and anti-inflammatory, respectively) regulation around Cu and PEEK (more pronounced around Cu);
5. T-lymphocytes participate in the foreign body reaction to biomaterials at an early stage;
6. T-cells may act through a CD4+ phenotype (T_{helper}/T_{reg}), suppressing the CD8+ $T_{cytotoxic}$ type of reaction at 10 days;
7. The up-regulation of the neutrophil specific factor NCF-1 around Cu and PEEK, indicates a higher inflammatory activity and may in part contribute to an inferior osseointegration on materials other than Ti;
8. Complement system seems predominantly downregulated around materials at 10 days, when compared to the Sh;

9. Bone forming environment (suppression of bone resorption) develops around all three implanted materials at an early stage, and within the inflammatory period;
10. At tissue level, only Ti seems to lead to osseointegration; PEEK and Cu show little or no implant related bone formation (respectively)—Which probably reflects the slightly more pronounced immune activation around the latter materials at this early stage;
11. Surface topography may play a role in macrophage phenotype and on the ultimate tissue level reaction to biomaterials, but further studies are needed.

The present results indicate that Ti osseointegration likely arises from a material-specific inflammatory/immune process leading to a shorter pro-inflammatory period and earlier reparative process, starting still within the inflammatory period and promoting bone apposition on Ti implant surfaces. It is further confirmed that all materials trigger an immune activation, even by materials like PEEK, previously considered as bio-inert. Different materials thus display different inflammatory balances in their vicinity, partly controlled by the immune system. Longer-term studies are necessary to better comprehend the immunobiology and tissue performance beyond the inflammatory period around established and new biomaterials.

Author Contributions: Conceptualization, R.T., T.A., P.T. and A.W.; Methodology, R.T., T.A., P.T. and A.W.; Software, R.T., Z.P., A.W. and S.G.; Validation, R.T. and P.T.; Formal Analysis, R.T. and A.W.; Investigation, R.T. and A.W.; Resources, R.T., P.T., T.A. and A.W.; Data Curation, R.T.; Writing—Original Draft Preparation, R.T. and A.W.; Writing—Review & Editing, P.T., T.A. and A.W.; Visualization, R.T., S.G. and Z.P.; Supervision, A.W., T.A. and P.T.; Project Administration, R.T.; Funding Acquisition, A.W.

Funding: This study was financially supported by: Swedish Research Council grant nr 2015-02971, Sweden; Swedish Research Council grant nr 621-2014-3700, Sweden; Odontology Research Region Skane nr 509641, Sweden; King Gustaf V and Queen Victoria Foundation, Swedish Order of Freemasons; RT supported by TePe Stipendium grant 2016, Sweden.

Conflicts of Interest: The authors declare no conflict of interest.

References

1. Chen, Z.; Wu, C.; Gu, W.; Klein, T.; Crawford, R.; Xiao, Y. Osteogenic differentiation of bone marrow MSCs by β-tricalcium phosphate stimulating macrophages via BMP2 signalling pathway. *Biomaterials* **2014**, *35*, 1507–1518. [CrossRef] [PubMed]
2. Vishwakarma, A.; Bhise, N.S.; Evangelista, M.B.; Rouwkema, J.; Dokmeci, M.R.; Ghaemmaghami, A.M.; Khademhosseini, A. Engineering immunomodulatory biomaterials to tune the inflammatory response. *Trends Biotechnol.* **2016**, *34*, 470–482. [CrossRef] [PubMed]
3. Trindade, R.; Albrektsson, T.; Tengvall, P.; Wennerberg, A. Foreign body reaction to biomaterials: On mechanisms for buildup and breakdown of osseointegration. *Clin. Implant. Dent. Relat. Res.* **2016**, *18*, 192–203. [CrossRef] [PubMed]
4. Albrektsson, T.; Dahlin, C.; Jemt, T.; Sennerby, L.; Turri, A.; Wennerberg, A. Is marginal bone loss around oral implants the result of a provoked foreign body reaction? *Clin. Implant. Dent. Relat. Res.* **2014**, *16*, 155–165. [CrossRef] [PubMed]
5. Trindade, R.; Albrektsson, T.; Galli, S.; Prgomet, Z.; Tengvall, P.; Wennerberg, A. Osseointegration and foreign body reaction: Titanium implants activate the immune system and suppress bone resorption during the first 4 weeks after implantation. *Clin. Implant. Dent. Relat. Res.* **2018**, *20*, 82–91. [CrossRef] [PubMed]
6. Arvidsson, S.; Askendal, A.; Tengvall, P. Blood plasma contact activation on silicon, titanium and aluminium. *Biomaterials* **2007**, *28*, 1346–1354. [CrossRef]
7. Anderson, J.M.; Jones, J.A. Phenotypic dichotomies in the foreign body reaction. *Biomaterials* **2007**, *28*, 5114–5120. [CrossRef]
8. Sridharan, R.; Cameron, A.R.; Kelly, D.J.; Kearney, C.J.; O'Brien, F.J. Biomaterial based modulation of macrophage polarization: A review and suggested design principles. *Mater. Today (Kidlington)* **2015**, *18*, 313–325. [CrossRef]
9. Miron, R.J.; Bosshardt, D.D. OsteoMacs: Key players around bone biomaterials. *Biomaterials* **2016**, *82*, 1–19. [CrossRef]

10. Wennerberg, A.; Albrektsson, T. Suggested guidelines for the topographic evaluation of implant surfaces. *Int. J. Oral Maxillofac. Implants* **2000**, *15*, 331–344.
11. Porcheray, F.; Viaud, S.; Rimaniol, A.C.; Léone, C.; Samah, B.; Dereuddre-Bosquet, N.; Domont, D.; Gras, G. Macrophage activation switching: An asset for the resolution of inflammation. *Clin. Exp. Immunol.* **2005**, *142*, 481–489. [CrossRef] [PubMed]
12. Anderson, J.M.; Rodriguez, A.; Chang, D.T. Foreign body reaction to biomaterials. *Semin. Immunol.* **2008**, *20*, 86–100. [CrossRef]
13. Johansson, P.; Jimbo, R.; Kjellin, P.; Currie, F.; Chrcanovic, B.R.; Wennerberg, A. Biomechanical evaluation and surface characterization of a nano-modified surface on PEEK implants: A study in the rabbit tibia. *Int. J. Nanomed.* **2014**, *9*, 3903–3911. [CrossRef]
14. Suska, F.; Emanuelsson, L.; Johansson, A.; Tengvall, P.; Thomsen, P. Fibrous capsule formation around titanium and copper. *J. Biomed. Mater. Res. A* **2008**, *85*, 888–896. [CrossRef]
15. Monticelli, L.A.; Buck, M.D.; Flamar, A.L.; Saenz, S.A.; Tait Wojno, E.D.; Yudanin, N.A.; Osborne, L.C.; Hepworth, M.R.; Tran, S.V.; Rodewald, H.R.; et al. Arginase 1 is an innate lymphoid-cell-intrinsic metabolic checkpoint controlling type 2 inflammation. *Nat. Immunol.* **2016**, *17*, 656–665. [CrossRef] [PubMed]
16. Zhu, J.; Paul, W.E. CD4 T cells: Fates, functions, and faults. *Blood* **2008**, *112*, 1557–1569. [CrossRef] [PubMed]
17. Hori, S.; Nomura, T.; Sakaguchi, S. Control of regulatory T cell development by the transcription factor Foxp3. *Science* **2003**, *299*, 1057–1061. [CrossRef]
18. Julier, Z.; Park, A.J.; Briquez, P.S.; Martino, M.M. Promoting tissue regeneration by modulating the immune system. *Acta Biomater.* **2017**, *53*, 13–28. [CrossRef]
19. Soehnlein, O.; Steffens, S.; Hidalgo, A.; Weber, C. Neutrophils as protagonists and targets in chronic inflammation. *Nat. Rev. Immunol.* **2017**, *17*, 248–261. [CrossRef]
20. Christoffersson, G.; Vagesjo, E.; Vandooren, J.; Liden, M.; Massena, S.; Reinert, R.B.; Brissova, M.; Powers, A.C.; Opdenakker, G.; Phillipson, M. VEGF-A recruits a proangiogenic MMP-9-delivering neutrophil subset that induces angiogenesis in transplanted hypoxic tissue. *Blood* **2012**, *120*, 4653–4662. [CrossRef]
21. Taylor, C.T.; Colgan, S.P. Regulation of immunity and inflammation by hypoxia in immunological niches. *Nat. Rev. Immunol.* **2017**, *17*, 774–785. [CrossRef]
22. Ignatius, A.; Schoengraf, P.; Kreja, L.; Liedert, A.; Recknagel, S.; Kandert, S.; Brenner, R.E.; Schneider, M.; Lambris, J.D.; Huber-Lang, M. Complement C3a and C5a modulate osteoclast formation and inflammatory response of osteoblasts in synergism with IL-1β. *J. Cell. Biochem.* **2011**, *112*, 2594–2605. [CrossRef]
23. Zhang, H.; Wu, X.; Wang, G.; Liu, P.; Qin, S.; Xu, K.; Tong, D.; Ding, H.; Tang, H.; Ji, F. Macrophage polarization, inflammatory signaling, and NF-κB activation in response to chemically modified titanium surfaces. *Colloids Surf. B Biointerfaces.* **2018**, *166*, 269–276. [CrossRef]
24. Gao, L.; Li, M.; Yin, L.; Zhao, C.; Chen, J.; Zhou, J.; Duan, K.; Feng, B. Dual-inflammatory cytokines on TiO_2 nanotube-coated surfaces used for regulating macrophage polarization in bone implants. *J. Biomed. Mater. Res. A* **2018**, *106*, 1878–1886. [CrossRef]
25. Shayan, M.; Padmanabhan, J.; Morris, A.H.; Cheung, B.; Smith, R.; Schroers, J.; Kyriakides, T.R. Nanopatterned bulk metallic glass-based biomaterials modulate macrophage polarization. *Acta Biomater.* **2018**, *75*, 127–138. [CrossRef]
26. Osborn, J.F.; Newesly, H. Dynamic aspects of the implant-bone interface. In *Dental Implants, Materials and Systems*; Heimke, G., Ed.; Hanser Verlag: München, Germany, 1980; pp. 111–123, ISBN 978-3446132122.

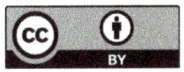 © 2018 by the authors. Licensee MDPI, Basel, Switzerland. This article is an open access article distributed under the terms and conditions of the Creative Commons Attribution (CC BY) license (http://creativecommons.org/licenses/by/4.0/).

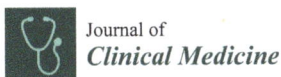

Article

Bone Immune Response to Materials, Part II: Copper and Polyetheretherketone (PEEK) Compared to Titanium at 10 and 28 Days in Rabbit Tibia

Ricardo Trindade [1,*], Tomas Albrektsson [2,3], Silvia Galli [3], Zdenka Prgomet [4], Pentti Tengvall [2] and Ann Wennerberg [1]

1. Department of Prosthodontics, Institute of Odontology, The Sahlgrenska Academy, University of Gothenburg, 405 30 Gothenburg, Sweden; ann.wennerberg@odontologi.gu.se
2. Department of Biomaterials, Institute of Clinical Sciences, University of Gothenburg, 405 30 Gothenburg, Sweden; tomas.albrektsson@biomaterials.gu.se (T.A.); pentti.tengvall@gu.se (P.T.)
3. Department of Prosthodontics, Faculty of Odontology, Malmö University, 205 06 Malmö, Sweden; silvia.galli@mau.se
4. Department of Oral Pathology, Faculty of Odontology, Malmö University, 205 06 Malmö, Sweden; zdenka.prgomet@mau.se
* Correspondence: ricardo.bretes.trindade@gu.se; Tel.: +46-31-786-0000

Received: 20 May 2019; Accepted: 5 June 2019; Published: 7 June 2019

Abstract: Osseointegration is likely the result of an immunologically driven bone reaction to materials such as titanium. Osseointegration has resulted in the clinical possibility to anchor oral implants in jaw bone tissue. However, the mechanisms behind bony anchorage are not fully understood and complications over a longer period of time have been reported. The current study aims at exploring possible differences between copper (Cu) and polyetheretherketone (PEEK) materials that do not osseointegrate, with osseointegrating cp titanium as control. The implants were placed in rabbit tibia and selected immune markers were evaluated at 10 and 28 days of follow-up. Cu and PEEK demonstrated at both time points a higher immune activation than cp titanium. Cu demonstrated distance osteogenesis due to a maintained proinflammatory environment over time, and PEEK failed to osseointegrate due to an immunologically defined preferential adipose tissue formation on its surface. The here presented results suggest the description of two different mechanisms for failed osseointegration, both of which are correlated to the immune system.

Keywords: biomaterial; bone; osseointegration; immune; implant; healing; titanium; PEEK; Cu

1. Introduction

Osseointegration [1] is a central event for oral implant function. This specific bone reaction has been described and studied at length for titanium and other materials. Technical innovations have led to improvements of bone reactions, such as material surface topographical changes [2–4] that have been vastly adopted by the oral implant industry, as well as different forms of chemical surface modulations [5,6]. Such surface related innovations have resulted in improved clinical results and widening of clinical indications [7,8]. However, the specific bone related control mechanisms that lead to osseointegration are still in need of scientific analyses, as are the reasons for marginal bone resorption. Generally speaking, the foreign body reaction (FBR) is accepted as the series of host events that follow the introduction of a material into tissues. The host–biomaterial interaction [9] depends on the type of material, clinical handling and on the tissue where the implant is placed (e.g., bone, skin, and blood vessel), as well as the host specific conditions. The immune system has a central role in the FBR [10–12] where the M1/M2-macrophage phenotype balance has been identified as one of the main controlling factors at the cellular level [13]. Macrophages are thus able to shift between an M1-phenotype (proinflammatory) and an M2-phenotype (reparative/anti-inflammatory), with obvious consequences for tissue reaction to biomaterials, and experimental modulation of this balance has been studied to direct a favorable pathway for bone regeneration [14]. The current authors have demonstrated an early M1/M2 shift around titanium, at 10 days of follow-up towards a dominant M2 macrophage phenotype [15], in contrast to other materials such as polyetheretherketone (PEEK) and Copper (Cu) that present mixed M1/M2 phenotypes at the same short term of follow-up. Osseointegration is thus seen as the result of an FBR which in the long run may achieve a foreign body equilibrium allowing for long term loading of implants [16]. However, the basis for the control of bone metabolism around implants in health and disease remains largely unclear [17]. Particularly the events taking place after the inflammatory period of initial healing and a possible immunological regulation of bone metabolism are examples of important fields for further studies. Our group has demonstrated that titanium activates the immune system when compared to a sham site at 10 and 28 days of follow-up [12]. In Part I of this series of studies (where the current work is Part II), the importance of the specific immune response around different materials when compared to a sham site was demonstrated at an early stage of 10 days [15]. The current study aims at comparing materials that do not osseointegrate, i.e., test materials copper (known to induce a pronounced FBR in soft tissues [18]) and PEEK (considered a bioinert material [19]), to a material that osseointegrates, cp titanium (control) at 10 and 28 days, in order to investigate and compare the respective immune modulation reactions between the inflammatory (10 days) and postinflammatory (28 days) stages of bone healing.

2. Materials and Methods

The current study consists of an experiment in the rabbit proximal tibia (metaphysis), comparing bone healing on sites where osteotomies were performed and one of three test materials were placed for comparison: titanium (Ti), copper (Cu), or polyether ether ketone (PEEK), where Ti was a control.

All implants were turned with a threaded 0.6 mm pitch height, 3.75 mm width, and Branemark MkIII design (Figure 1). The Ti implants were made of commercially pure titanium grade IV (98.55% Ti, with specified maximum traces of elements Fe, O, N, H, and C for the remaining 1.45%).

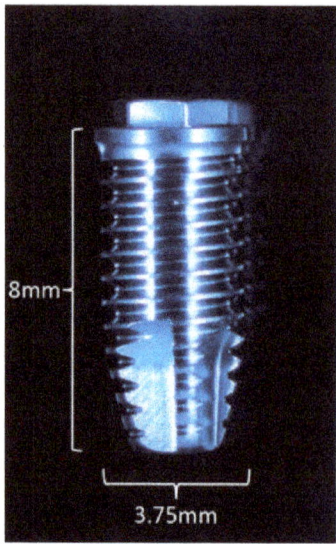

Figure 1. Implant design with 3.75mm width and 8mm length. Representative image of titanium (Ti) implant; copper (Cu) and polyetheretherketone (PEEK) implants with the same design.

2.1. Surgical Procedure

This study was performed on 12 mature, female New Zealand White Rabbits ($n = 6$ for each time point, 10 and 28 days, weight 3 to 4 Kg), with the ethical approval from the Ethics Committee for Animal Research (No. 13-011) of the École Nationale Vétérinaire D'Alfors, Maisons-Alfors, Val-de-Marne, France. The 6 animals at 10 days are the same used for Part I of this series of studies [12]. All care was taken to minimize animal pain or discomfort during and after the surgical procedures. For the surgical procedures, the rabbits were placed under general anesthesia using a mixture of medetomidine (Domitor; Zoetis, Florham Park, NJ, USA), ketamine (Imalgène 1000; Merial, Lyon, France), and diazepam (Valium; Roche, Basel, Switzerland) for induction, then applying subcutaneous buprenorphine (Buprecare; Animalcare, York, UK) and intramuscular meloxicam (Metacam; Boehringer Ingelheim Vetmedica, Inc., Ridgefield, CT, USA). A single incision was performed in the internal knee area on each side and the bone exposed for osteotomies and insertion of implants in the sites mentioned above. The surgical site was sutured with a resorbable suture (Vicryl 3/0; Ethicon, Cincinnati, OH, USA) and hemostasis achieved. Following surgery, Fentanyl patches (Duragesic; Janssen Pharmaceutica, Beerse, Belgium) were applied.

The osteotomies were produced with a sequence of increasing diameter twist drills, from 2 mm to 3.15 mm width, and a final countersink bur prepared the cortical part of the bone. The implants used were 3.75 mm in diameter, placed in an underprepared osteotomy to achieve primary (mechanical) stability.

The rabbits were housed in separate cages and were allowed to move and eat freely.

At 10 and 28 days, the rabbits were sacrificed with a lethal injection of sodium pentobarbital (Euthasol; Virbac, Fort Worth, TX, USA). The 6 animals at each time point had the implants removed through unscrewing. On 4 animals at 10 days and 5 animals at 28 days, bone was collected with a 2 mm twist drill from the periphery of the Ti, Cu, and PEEK sites on the most distal portion, and then processed through quantitative-polymerase chain reaction (qPCR). After this, at each time point, the implant sites were removed en bloc for histological processing on the 6 animals.

2.2. Gene Expression Analysis—qPCR

The bone samples for gene expression analysis at 10 or 28 days were collected from the distal side of the osteotomies of all three groups (following the removal of the implant from the implant sites), with a 2 mm twist drill that removed both cortical and marrow bone in the full length of the osteotomy, to enable the study of the 2 mm peri-implant bone area of each of the Ti, Cu, and PEEK sites. The samples were immediately transferred to separate sterile plastic recipients containing RNA*later* medium (AmbionInc, Austin, TX, USA) for preservation. The samples were then refrigerated first at 4 °C and then stored at −20 °C until processing.

2.2.1. mRNA Isolation

Samples were homogenized using an ultrasound homogenizer (Sonoplus HD3100, Brandelin) in 1 ml PureZOL and total RNA was isolated via column fractionalization using the Aurum^{TM} Total RNA Fatty and Fibrous Tissue Kit (Bio-Rad Laboratories Inc.; Hercules, CA, USA) following the manufacturer's instructions. All the samples were DNAse treated using an on-column DNAse I contained in the kit to remove genomic DNA. The RNA quantity for each sample was analyzed in the NanoDrop 2000 Spectrophotometer (Thermo Scientific; Wilmington, DE, USA). BioRad iScript cDNA synthesis kit (Bio-Rad Laboratories Inc.; Hercules, CA, USA) was then used to convert mRNA into cDNA, following the manufacturer's instructions.

qPCR primers (Tataa Biocenter; Gothenburg, Sweden) were designed following the NCBI Sequence database, including the local factors chosen in order to characterize the immune, inflammatory, and bone metabolic pathways (Tables 1 and 2). All primers had efficiency between 90% and 110%.

Table 1. Gene sequences.

Primer	Forward Sequence	Reverse Sequence	Accession No./Transcript ID
NCF-1	TTCATCCGCCACATTGCCC	GTCCTGCCACTTCACCAAGA	NM_001082102.1
CD68	TTTCCCCAGCTCTCCACCTC	CGATGATGAGGGGCACCAAG	ENSOCUT00000010382
CD11b	TTCAACCTGGAGACTGAGAACAC	TCAAACTGGACCACGCTCTG	ENSOCUT00000001589
CD14	TCTGAAAATCCTGGGCTGGG	TTCATTCCCGCGTTCCGTAG	ENSOCUT00000004218
ARG1	GGATCATTGGAGCCCCTTTCTC	TCAAGCAGACCAGCCTTTCTC	NM_001082108.1
IL-4	CTACCTCCACCACAAGGTGTC	CCAGTGTAGTCTGTCTGGCTT	ENSOCUT00000024099
IL-13	GCAGCCTCGTATCCCCAG	GGTTGACGCTCCACACCA	ENSOCUT00000000154
M-CSF	GGAACTCTCGCTCAGGCTC	ACATTCTTGATCTTCTCCAGCAAC	ENSOCUT00000030714
OPG	TGTGTGAATGCGAGGAAGGG	AACTGTATTCCGCTCTGGGG	ENSOCUT00000011149
RANKL	GAAGGTTCATGGTTCGATCTGG	CCAAGAGGACAGGCTCACTTT	ENSOCUT00000024354
TRAP	TTACTTCAGTGGCGTGCAGA	CGATCTGGGCTGAGACGTTG	NM_001081988.1
CathK	GGAACCGGGGCATTGACTCT	TGTACCCTCTGCATTTGGCTG	NM_001082641.1
PPAR-γ	CAAGGCGAGGGCGATCTT	ATGCGGATGGCGACTTCTTT	NM_001082148.1
C3	ACTCTGTCGAGAAGGAACGGG	CCTTGATTTGTTGATGCTGGCTG	NM_001082286.1
C3aR1	CATGTCAGTCAACCCCTGCT	GCGAATGGTTTTGCTCCCTG	ENSOCUT00000007435
CD46	TCCTGCTGTTCACTTTCTCGG	CATGTTCCCATCCTTGTTTACACTT	ENSOCUT00000033915
CD55	TGGTGTTGGGTGGAGTGACC	AGAGTGAAGCCTCTGTTGCATT	ENSOCUT00000031985
CD59	ACCACTGTCTCCTCCCAAGT	GCAATCTTCATACCGCCAACA	NM_001082712.1
C5	TCCAAAACTCTGCAACCTTAACA	AAATGCTTTGACACAACTTCCA	ENSOCUT00000005683
C5aR1	ACGTCAACTGCTGCATCAACC	AGGCTGGGGAGAGACTTGC	ENSOCUT00000029180
CD3	CCTGGGGACAGGAAGATGATGAC	CAGCACCACAGGGTTCCA	NM_001082001.1
CD4	CAACTGGAAACATGCGAACCA	TTGATGACCAGGGGGAAAGA	NM_001082313.2
CD8	GGCGTCTACTTCTGCATGACC	GAACCGGCACACTCTCTTCT	ENSOCUT00000009383
CD19	GGATGTATGTCTGTCGCCGT	AAGCAAAGCCCACAACTGAA	ENSOCUT00000028895
GAPDH	GGTGAAGGTCGGAGTGAACGG	CATGTAGACCATGTAGTGGAGGTCA	NM_001082253.1
ACT-β	TCATTCCAAATATCGTGAGATGCC	TACACAAATGCGATGCTGCC	NM_001101683.1
LDHA	TGCAGACAAGGAACAGTGGA	CCCAGGTAGTGTAGCCCTT	NM_001082277.1

NCF-1 (neutrophil cytosolic factor 1); CD68 (macrosialin); CD11b (MAC-1, macrophage marker); CD14 (monocyte differentiation antigen CD14); ARG1 (Arginase 1); IL-4 (Interleukin 4); IL-13 (Interleukin 13); M-CSF (colony stimulating factor-macrophage); OPG (osteoprotegerin); RANKL (Receptor activator of nuclear factor kappa-B ligand); TRAP (tartrate resistant acid phosphatase); CathK (cathepsin K); PPAR-γ (peroxisome proliferator activated receptor gamma); C3 (complement component 3); C3aR1 (complement component 3a receptor 1); CD46 (complement regulatory protein); CD55 (decay accelerating factor for complement); CD59 (complement regulatory protein); C5 (complement component 5); C5aR1 (complement component 5a receptor 1); CD3 (T cell surface glycoprotein CD3); CD4 (T cell surface glycoprotein CD4); CD8 (T cell transmembrane glycoprotein CD8); CD19 (B-lymphocyte surface protein CD19); GAPDH (glyceraldehyde-3-phosphate dehydrogenase); ACT-β (actin beta); LDHA (lactate dehydrogenase A).

Table 2. Correspondence between studied gene expression and biological entities.

Biological Entity	Gene
Neutrophil	NCF-1
Macrophage	CD68, CD11b, CD14, ARG1
Macrophage fusion	IL-4, IL-13, M-CSF
Bone resorption	OPG, RANKL, TRAP, CathK, PPAR-γ
Complement	Activation: C3, C3aR1, C5, C5aR1; Inhibition: CD46, CD55, CD59
T lymphocytes	CD3, CD4, CD8
B-lymphocytes	CD19
Reference genes	GAPDH, ACT-β, LDHA

NCF-1 (neutrophil cytosolic factor 1); CD68 (macrosialin); CD11b (MAC-1, macrophage marker); CD14 (monocyte differentiation antigen CD14); ARG1 (Arginase 1); IL-4 (Interleukin 4); IL-13 (Interleukin 13); M-CSF (colony stimulating factor-macrophage); OPG (osteoprotegerin); RANKL (Receptor activator of nuclear factor kappa-B ligand); TRAP (tartrate resistant acid phosphatase); CathK (cathepsin K); PPAR-γ (peroxisome proliferator activated receptor gamma); C3 (complement component 3); C3aR1 (complement component 3a receptor 1); CD46 (complement regulatory protein); CD55 (decay accelerating factor for complement); CD59 (complement regulatory protein); C5 (complement component 5); C5aR1 (complement component 5a receptor 1); CD3 (T cell surface glycoprotein CD3); CD4 (T cell surface glycoprotein CD4); CD8 (T cell transmembrane glycoprotein CD8); CD19 (B-lymphocyte surface protein CD19); GAPDH (glyceraldehyde-3-phosphate dehydrogenase); ACT-β (actin beta); LDHA (lactate dehydrogenase A).

2.2.2. Amplification Process

Five microliters of SsoAdvanced SYBR™ Green Supermix (Bio-Rad Laboratories Inc.; Hercules, CA, USA) and 1 µL of cDNA template together with 0.4 µM of forward and reverse primer were used in the qPCR reaction. Each cDNA sample was performed on duplicates. The thermal cycles were performed on the CFX Connect Real-Time System (Bio-Rad Laboratories Inc.; Hercules, CA, USA). The CFX Manager Software 3.0 (Bio-Rad, Hercules, CA, USA) was used for the data analysis.

Three genes (*GAPDH*, *ACT-beta*, and *LDHA*) were selected as reference genes using the geNorm algorithm integrated in the CFX Manager Software. A quantification cycle (Cq) value of the chosen reference genes (Tables 1 and 2) was used as control; hence the mean Cq value of each target gene (Table 1) was normalized against the reference gene's Cq, giving the gene's relative expression. For calculation of fold-change, the $^{\Delta\Delta}$Cq was used, comparing mRNA expressions from the different groups. Significance was set at $p < 0.05$ and the regulation threshold at ×2 fold-change.

2.3. Decalcified Bone Histology

After removal of the implants from the studied Ti, Cu, and PEEK sites on the 6 subjects of each time point, bone was removed en bloc and preserved in 10% formalin (4% buffered formaldehyde; VWR international, Leuven, Belgium) during 48 h for fixation. Samples were decalcified in Ethylene diamine tetra-acetic acid (10% unbuffered EDTA; Milestone srl, BG, Italy) for 4 weeks, with weekly substitution of the EDTA solution, dehydrated and embedded in paraffin (Tissue-Tek TEC; Sakura Finetek Europe BV, Leiden, NL, USA). Samples were sectioned (4-μm-thick) with a microtome (Microm HM355S; Microm International GmbH, Thermo Fischer Scientific, Walldorf, Germany) and stained with Haematoxylin-Eosin (HE) for histological analysis.

2.4. Statistical Analysis

The gene expression statistical analysis was performed using the *t*-test built in the algorithm of the CFX Manager Software 3.0 package (BioRad, Hercules, CA, USA).

3. Results

3.1. Gene Expression Analysis

3.1.1. Days

The gene expression analysis results at 10 days, comparing Cu and PEEK against Ti (control), are displayed in the volcano plots (Figures 2 and 3) and data given in corresponding tables (Tables 3 and 4) with the numerical results expressed in fold-change (regulation, x-axis) and significance (*p* value, y-axis). Data from 10 days have been published in Part I [15] of this study, if with another control.

At 10 days, Cu (vs. Ti, Figure 2 and Table 3) triggered an increased expression of *ARG1* gene (around 14× fold-change). This probably translates to a much higher presence of M2 macrophages (reparative phenotype) around Cu. *NCF1* showed close to a 2× fold upregulation for Cu, and elicited an increased participation of neutrophils at this early stage. Less increased markers, with approximately ×1.5 fold-change were observed for Complement (*C3aR1*), M1-macrophages (*CD14*) [20,21], B-lymphocytes (*CD19*) and Th/Treg-lymphocytes (*CD4*). On the other hand, Cu displayed a downregulation in *TRAP*, *PPAR-gamma* and *OPG*.

At 10 days PEEK (vs. Ti, Figure 3 and Table 4) showed less downregulation of the same bone remodeling markers as Cu, *TRAP*, *OPG*, and *PPAR-gamma*, as well as the B cell marker *CD19* and macrophage fusion marker *IL-4*. Increased expression of *NCF1* was observed for PEEK, probably translating to an increased presence of neutrophils around this material (as also observed for Cu).

Table 3. Gene expression analysis of Cu compared to Ti (10 days).

Marker	Regulation	*p* Value
PPAR-G	−1.72	0.087477
TRAP	−1.98	0.137344
OPG	−2.03	0.539750

Table 3. Cont.

Marker	Regulation	p Value
CD3	−1.52	0.411951
IL-4	−1.71	0.185082
ARG1	14.17	0.006031
NCF1	1.96	0.125414
C3aR1	1.66	0.154634
CD14	1.50	0.414019
CD4	1.53	0.431624
CD19	1.64	0.279592

Minus values: downregulation; plus values: upregulation.

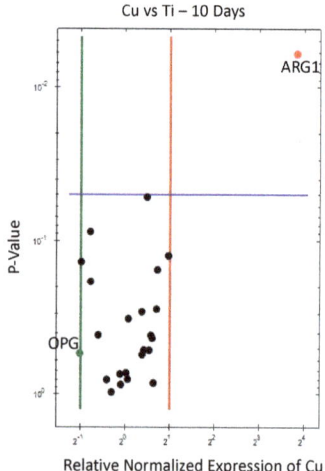

Figure 2. Volcano plot for gene expression of Cu compared to Ti (10 days). Downregulation (vertical green line) and upregulation (vertical red line) set at ×2 regulation. Statistical significance (set at $p < 0.05$) when marker above horizontal blue line.

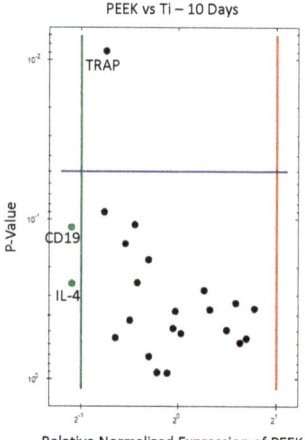

Figure 3. Volcano plot for gene expression of PEEK compared to Ti (10 days). Downregulation (vertical green line) and upregulation (vertical red line) set at ×2 regulation. Statistical significance (set at $p < 0.05$) when marker above horizontal blue line.

Table 4. Gene expression analysis of PEEK compared to Ti (10 days).

Marker	Regulation	p Value
PPAR-G	−1.57	0.550176
TRAP	−1.68	0.008821
OPG	−1.70	0.089695
CD19	−2.14	0.111496
IL-4	−2.14	0.251881
ARG1	1.71	0.361937
NCF1	1.50	0.333874
CD68	1.62	0.556273

Minus values: downregulation; plus values: upregulation.

3.1.2. 28 Days

At 28 days, Cu against Ti (Figure 4 and Table 5), showed upregulation around Cu of *CD68* and *CD14*, as well as *ARG1* (macrophages of both M1-and M2- phenotypes), with M2 far more significant, indicating an overall higher macrophage activation for Cu vs. Ti at 28 days, when compared to 10 days. Complement markers *C3aR1* and *C5aR1* are also upregulated around Cu, as well as *IL-13* (a macrophage fusion marker). On the other hand, there was downregulation of bone remodeling markers *TRAP*, *CATHK*, *PPAR-gamma*, and *RANKL*, as well as *CD3* and *CD4* (T lymphocytes), *C3* complement factor, *CD59* (complement inhibitor), and *IL-4* (the other macrophage fusion marker).

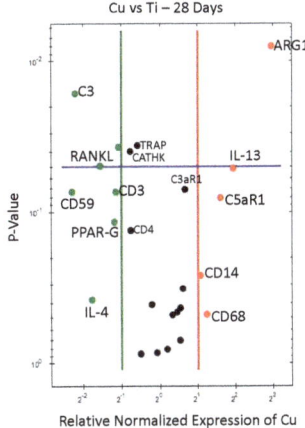

Figure 4. Volcano plot for gene expression analysis of Cu compared to Ti (28 days). Downregulation (vertical green line) and upregulation (vertical red line) set at ×2 regulation. Statistical significance (set at $p < 0.05$) when marker above horizontal blue line.

PEEK vs. Ti at 28 days (Figure 5 and Table 6), showed upregulation of most markers used, with the exception of *TRAP* and *CATHK*, which are effector bone resorption markers that were downregulated. This excessive upregulation indicates a wide and strong immune activation around PEEK compared to Ti at 28 days. However, these results had a limitation in that only two out of the five rabbits used in the study allowed enough mRNA extraction on PEEK samples for gene expression analysis (see Discussion). Nevertheless, both subjects' results were analysed separately for regulation (fold-change) and showed similar responses compatible with that presented in the overall results. However, the significance (*p* value) should not be taken in consideration here, since the low number of subjects (only 2) renders impossible a statistical analysis.

Table 5. Gene expression analysis of Cu compared to Ti (28 days).

Marker	Regulation	p-Value
C3	−4.64	0.016332
CD59	−4.93	0.073238
RANKL	−2.96	0.049318
PPAR-G	−2.29	0.115578
TRAP	−1.49	0.036164
CATH-K	−1.70	0.039611
CD3	−2.22	0.073334
CD4	−1.69	0.132057
IL-4	−3.43	0.379695
ARG1	7.69	0.007955
CD14	2.09	0.260868
CD68	2.35	0.473322
C5aR1	3.03	0.080240
C3aR1	2.25	0.084210
IL-13	3.84	0.051296

Minus values: downregulation; plus values: upregulation.

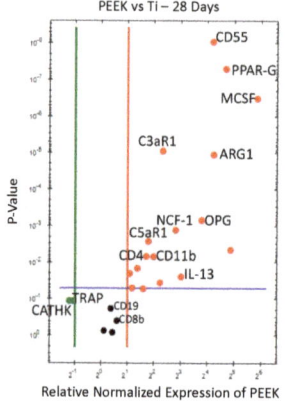

Figure 5. Volcano plot for gene expression analysis of PEEK compared to Ti (28 days). Only 2 subjects to be interpreted with caution. Downregulation (vertical green line) and upregulation (vertical red line) set at ×2 regulation. Statistical significance (set at $p < 0.05$) when marker above horizontal blue line.

Table 6. Gene expression analysis of PEEK compared to Ti (28 days).

Marker	Regulation	p-Value
TRAP	−2.09	0.112708
CATHK	−2.31	0.111423
CD55	18.29	0.000000
C3aR1	8.31	0.000818
C5aR1	3.46	0.002609
CD46	4.68	0.035842
TRAP	−2.09	0.112708
CATHK	−2.31	0.111423
CD55	18.29	0.000000
C3aR1	8.31	0.000818
C5aR1	3.46	0.002609
CD46	4.68	0.035842
CD59	3.03	0.052696
ARG1	18.72	0.000011
CD11b	3.95	0.006903

Table 6. Cont.

Marker	Regulation	p-Value
CD14	2.14	0.020201
NCF-1	7.04	0.001291
CD3	2.60	0.014589
CD4	3.28	0.006753
CD8b	1.53	0.393394
CD19	1.30	0.182925
MCSF	57.55	0.000000
IL-13	8.11	0.024702
PPAR-G	25.54	0.000000
OPG	13.77	0.000687

Only 2 subjects to be interpreted with caution. Minus values: downregulation; plus values: upregulation.

It is interesting to note that T_{helper}/T_{reg} (*CD4*) was upregulated for Cu at 10 days, but downregulated at 28 days, which could indicate a shift in the presence of T lymphocytes between the two time points and these cells' participation in the biomaterial-associated healing process.

3.2. Comparative Analysis of Gene Expression: 10 vs. 28 Days

The comparison between Cu and PEEK when compared to Ti was divided by respective outcome (Figures 6 and 7): macrophage, complement, neutrophils, lymphocytes, macrophage fusion and bone metabolism. Data from 10 days have been published in Part I [15] of this study, if with another control.

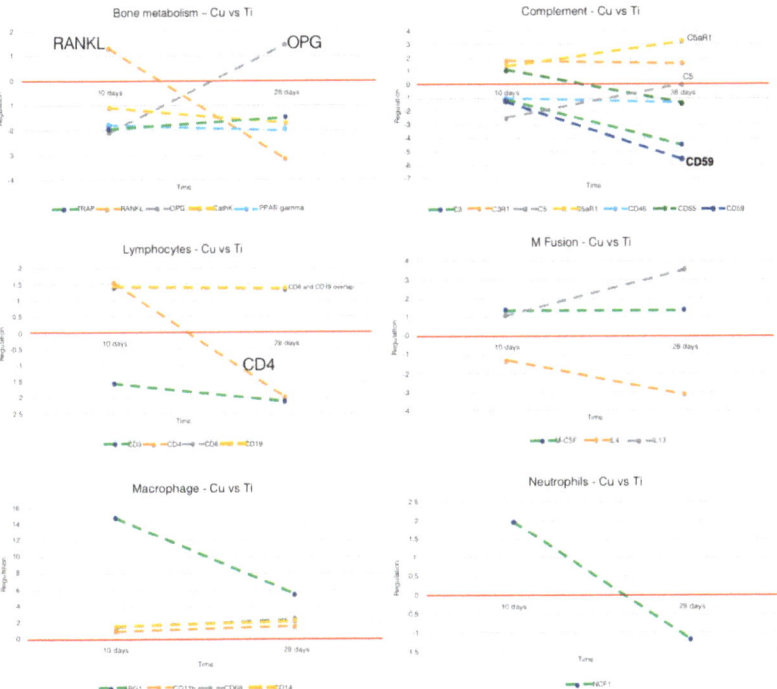

Figure 6. Comparative analysis of gene expression between 10 and 28 days for Cu vs. Ti. Horizontal red line: zero regulation mark; x-axis: time; y-axis: gene marker regulation (10 or 28 days). Intermittent lines do not represent actual results at time points other than 10 or 28 days, but only highlight trend from 10 to 28 days.

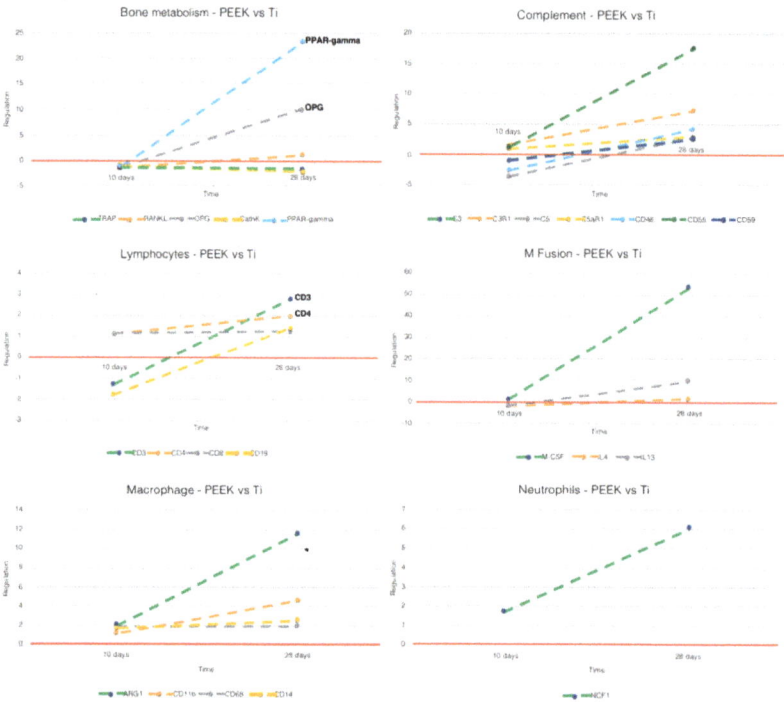

Figure 7. Comparative analysis of gene expression between 10 and 28 days for PEEK vs. Ti. Horizontal red line: zero regulation mark; x-axis: time; y-axis: gene marker regulation (10 or 28 days). Intermittent lines: do not represent actual results at time points other than 10 or 28 days, but only highlight trend from 10 to 28 days.

3.2.1. Cu vs. Ti (Figure 6)

Macrophages: The immune activation was clearly higher around Cu than Ti at both time points. The M2-macrophage phenotype (*ARG1*) was reduced around Cu, but still upregulated when compared to Ti. The M1 markers (combination of *CD68*, *CD11b* and *CD14*) were upregulated slightly around Cu at both 10 and 28 days, i.e., Cu sustained a proinflammatory environment after the acute inflammatory and beginning of the bone remodeling period.

Complement: The results show that *C5* expression increased around Cu from 10 to 28 days, when compared to Ti (both *C5aR1* and *C5* suffered a sharp increase in regulation while the *CD59* (a *C5* inhibitor) was sharply downregulated over time).

Neutrophils: There was a shift observed for *NCF1* from upregulation at 10 days to downregulation at 28 days. This likely indicates a change (reduction) in the presence of neutrophils around Cu.

Lymphocytes: The *CD4* reduction (from up- to downregulated) at 28 days around Cu may indicate a decrease in T_{helper}/T_{reg} function, whereas effector $T_{cytotoxic}$ (*CD8*) and B cells (*CD19*) remain slightly upregulated.

Macrophage fusion: More pronounced *IL4* downregulation and *IL13* upregulation from 10 to 28 days.

Bone metabolism: The *RANKL/OPG* shunt reveals an obvious shift around Cu between 10 and 28 days. *RANKL* changes from upregulated to downregulated and the opposite for *OPG*, which becomes upregulated at 28 days, meaning a suppression of osteoclastogenesis from 10 to 28 days.

3.2.2. PEEK vs. Ti (Figure 7)

It should be noted at 28 days that the results for PEEK should be read with caution since it was only possibility to retrieve mRNA from two of the five samples at 28 days. The possible reasons for this will be discussed below. Data from 10 days have been published in Part I [15] of this study, if with another control.

Macrophages: The macrophage activation around PEEK observed at 10 days and 28 days showed increase in both M1 and M2 markers. This confirms that there was an elevated M1 activation at 28 days, as well as a strong increase in M2-phenotype.

Complement: The results indicate, after 28 days, a continued immune activation around PEEK, especially pronounced for *C3*-related markers (*C3*, *C3aR1*, *CD46*, and *CD55*), and with slight upregulation for *C5*-related markers.

Neutrophils: *NCF1*, the specific neutrophil marker, was at both time points upregulated for PEEK, but showed a sharp increase at 28 days.

Lymphocytes: All lymphocyte markers increased from 10 to 28 days around PEEK. This was especially evident for *CD4+* T$_{h/reg}$ and *CD19+* B cells.

Macrophage fusion: The results indicate a sharp increase in macrophage fusion markers around PEEK, also with a possible contribution to a M2-macrophage phenotype (*IL13*- confirmed by the above mentioned *ARG1* upregulation at 28 days). *M-CSF* also contributes to bone/adipose tissue balance in the osseous tissue, an important finding for PEEK and osseointegration in general, as discussed below.

Bone metabolism: The results suggest formation of adipose-like tissue around PEEK, as expressed by the extreme upregulation of *PPAR-gamma* and by the upregulation of *M-CSF*. Suppression of bone resorption was sustained over time—RANKL still shows at 28 days some upregulation, but was overtaken by a sharp upregulation of *OPG*.

3.3. Histological Analysis

The histological analysis was performed at tissue level. At 10 days (Figures 8–10), Ti presents with initial bone formation within the threads, represented by unorganized collagen proliferation, whereas Cu presents mostly a lytic and cell infiltrate area on the implant surface, followed by a fibrous layer and finally a new bone formation, away from the surface. At 10 days, PEEK demonstrated very little initial bone tissue formation in some threads, but mostly adipose tissue surrounding the implant. Data from 10 days have been published in Part I [15] of this study, if with another control.

At 28 days (Figures 11–13), Ti shows the bone within the threads maturing, while Cu demonstrates a reduction of the cell infiltrate, but still a bone formation away from the implant surface, whereas PEEK presents with mostly adipose tissue around the implant and the little bone tissue formed has not matured (unlike Ti) and shows little calcification.

J. Clin. Med. **2019**, *8*, 814

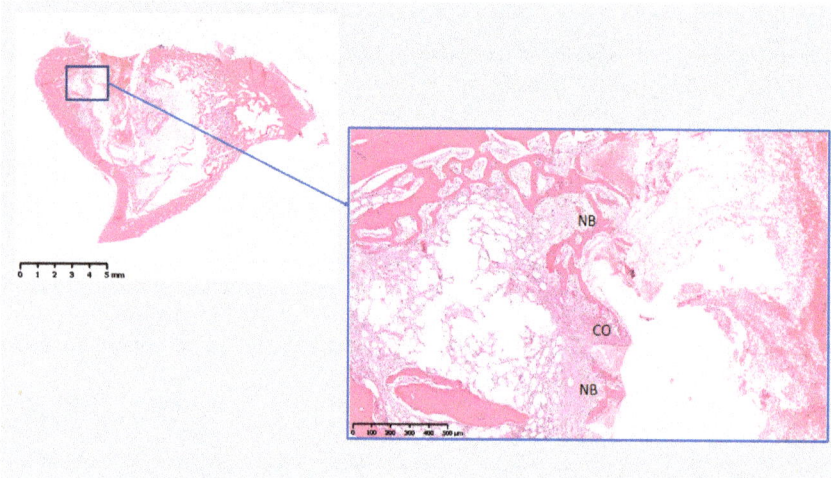

Figure 8. Histological analysis of Ti (10 days). NB: New bone; CO: Contact osteogenesis. Collagen proliferation and some initial calcification to form new bone in the threads. Scale bars: 5 mm and 500 µm.

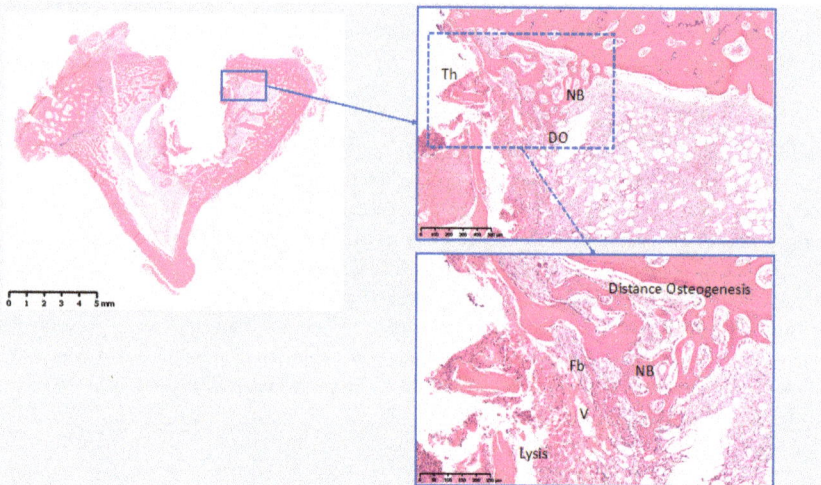

Figure 9. Histological analysis of Cu (10 days). Lytic area next to the implant; Fb: fibroproliferative; NB: New bone; DO: distance osteogenesis; Th: implant thread; V: blood vessel. New bone forming away from the implant surface. Scale bars: 5 mm, 500 µm, and 250 µm clockwise from left.

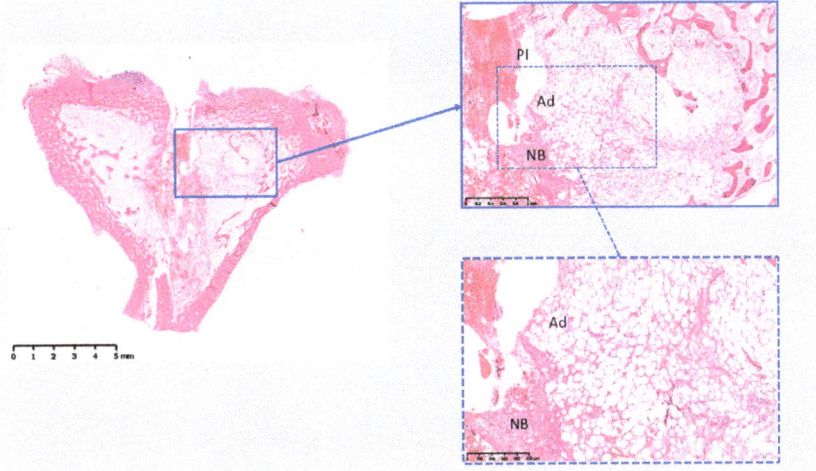

Figure 10. Histological analysis of PEEK (10 days). PI: PEEK implant; NB: New bone; Ad: Adipose tissue. Some collagen proliferation in one thread, adipose tissue also on the implant surface. Scale bars: 5 mm, 1 mm, and 500 µm.

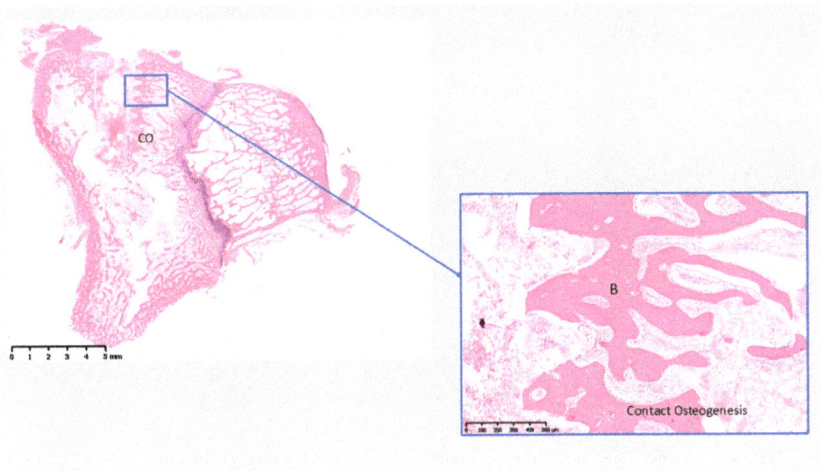

Figure 11. Histological analysis of Ti 28 (days). CO: contact osteogenesis. B: Bone. Formation of mature bone within the implant threads. Scale bars: 5 mm and 500 µm.

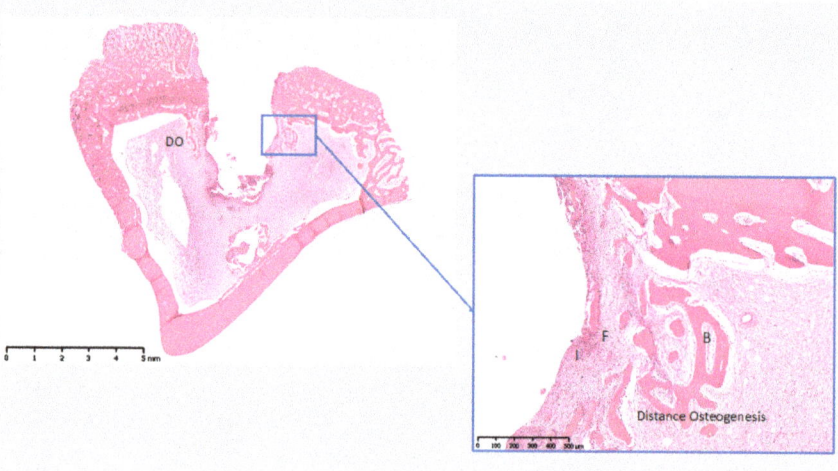

Figure 12. Histological analysis of Cu (28 days). DO: Distance osteogenesis; I: Inflammatory infiltrate; F: fibrous tissue; B: Bone. Formation of bone away from the implant surface, with a reduction of the infiltrate on the implant surface compared to 10 days. Scale bars: 5 mm and 500 μm.

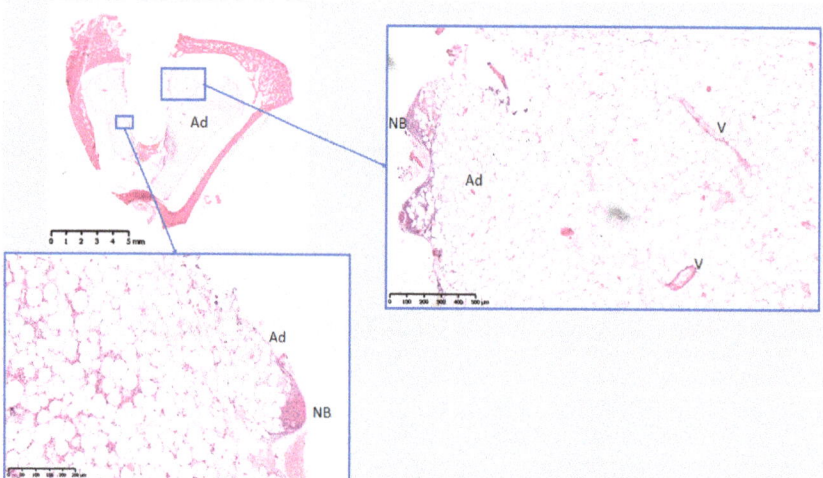

Figure 13. Histological analysis of PEEK (28 days). Ad: Adipose tissue; V: blood vessels; NB: New bone. Mostly adipose tissue proliferation and the bone tissue in the threads has not matured, nor calcified substantially. Scale bars: 5 mm, 500 μm, and 250 μm.

4. Discussion

The osseointegration of materials for biomedical purposes has led to significant advances in patient treatment. Oral implants have become common in clinical practice, and by large base their success on osseointegration of materials such as titanium. Previous studies from the present authors have demonstrated the activation of the immune system around a material placed in bone [12,15], and it was hypothesized that the immune system has a regulatory function on the achievement of osseointegration [11]. In the present experimental study, the bone immune reaction around the materials polyetheretherketone (PEEK) and copper (Cu) was compared to titanium (Ti) as a control, at 10 and 28 days of implantation in rabbit tibia. The current study design aimed at comparing the immune modulation of two materials with poor osseointegration (Cu and PEEK) against a material that osseointegrates (Ti). The comparison between 10 and 28 days is important to understand the evolution of the reaction between the inflammatory period (10 days) and the postinflammatory period (28 days) of healing. Data from 10 days have been published in Part I [15] of this study, but with a Sham (no biomaterial) site as a control.

At 10 days, both PEEK and Cu showed upregulation of markers indicating a higher and different macrophage activity than was found around Ti (confirming the previous study [15]), namely predominantly an M2-phenotype, but also an elevated M1-phenotype. This was more pronounced around Cu than PEEK. At day 10, PEEK did not differ much from Ti, if with higher activation of the immune system (neutrophils and macrophages). This was however observed for Cu, with a higher overall immune activation. Both PEEK and Cu displayed some inhibition of bone resorption when compared to Ti. It is worth noting that PEEK, commonly referred to as a bioinert material [22,23], shows a higher immune activation than Ti at 10 days.

After 28 days of implantation the scenario changes for both PEEK and Cu. Cu shows, as expected, a higher upregulation of the immune markers when compared to Ti, in all its innate components (complement, neutrophils, and macrophages of both M1- and M2-phenotypes). However, the macrophage fusion markers *IL-4* and *IL-13* expressions provide some contradictory indications since *IL-13* was upregulated and *IL-4* downregulated. This could be hypothesized as a stage for initial fusion into foreign body giant cells (FBGCs), but needs confirmation through further studies. Such macrophage fusion is not likely to be guided towards osteoclastogenesis, since bone resorption markers were widely downregulated, hence the macrophage behavior was probably directed towards the formation of FBGCs. However, *IL-13*, also known to induce the M2-phenotype [24] and combined with *ARG1* upregulation, confirms, at 28 days, the elevated M2 phenotype activity around Cu and PEEK compared to Ti, meaning a more pronounced host reparative effort for both materials, even if proinflammatory markers are simultaneously upregulated. The downregulation of bone resorption markers highlights the probable effort around Cu at 28 days, to build bone tissue around the implant for a bony delimitation that, as the histology shows, clearly develops away from the surface of the Cu implant.

PEEK, on the other hand, seems to suffer a vast transformation at 28 days, into a high immune activation in the bone environment surrounding the implant, or rather fails to reduce that immune activation when compared to Ti. Reasons for the high immune upregulation around PEEK at 28 days are not well understood, although the current study results may offer an explanation regarding the bone/adipose tissue balance, as developed below. As mentioned in the results section, the 28 days results for PEEK should be read with caution, since only two subjects out of the five used for gene expression analysis actually enabled collection of enough mRNA to perform the PCR analysis. The difficulty to extract sufficient mRNA from the tissues surrounding PEEK implants was probably due to a low bone tissue formation adjacent to PEEK implants. Furthermore, the reasons behind the classical claim of a supposed bioinertness of PEEK is either that only in vitro studies of it have been presented or that in vivo studies have failed to analyze the immunological response; in contrast, the present results indicate immune activation around PEEK that may persist over extended periods of time.

Regarding the comparison between the two time points of 10 and 28 days, for Cu, the *CD4* expression shifting over time from up- to downregulation, and the maintained upregulation of *CD8* and *CD19* at 28 days, demonstrates a shift in T_{helper}/T_{reg} function whereas effector $T_{cytotoxic}$ and B cells remain slightly upregulated over time. B cells, not only osteoblasts, are known to produce *OPG* in humans [25], which correlates with the increased gene expression of OPG at 28 days and adds another regulatory mechanism of the immune system on bone effector cells, and consequently on the ultimate anabolic/catabolic balance outcome of bone metabolism around implanted materials. It is important to mention that this B cell mechanism is known to be regulated by T cells, and the production of *OPG* by

B/plasma cells can reach 64% of total *OPG* in some mammals [26], thus the present results highlight the immune regulation of bone metabolism around implanted materials.

The notion that Cu starts to enter the remodeling phase and bone production at 28 days, even if at a distance as seen from the histological analysis, is further supported by the results for the above mentioned bone metabolism, with a sharp shift in *RANKL* (upregulated at 10 days and downregulated at 28 days) and in *OPG* (displaying the exact opposite trend) since *RANKL* induces osteoclastogenesis and *OPG* is the decoy molecule that stops this process, the results indicate a shift to a bone reparative environment around Cu at 28 days (through inhibition of the bone resorption inducive mechanisms).

As for the results of the two time point comparisons between PEEK and Ti, the M1-macrophage activation at 28 days may impair bone formation at the PEEK implant surface, with a preferred fatty tissue deposition during repair, as indicated by the upregulation of *PPAR-gamma*, which is produced by differentiated macrophages [27] and in turn triggers the differentiation of adipocytes [28] at 28 days. The upregulation of complement around PEEK, the sharp increase in *NCF1* and the increase in regulation from 10 to 28 days around PEEK for Th/reg and B cells demonstrates that over time a higher immune activity is maintained around PEEK than Ti. This goes beyond the inflammatory period and is most likely proinflammatory.

The upregulation at 28 days of macrophage fusion markers around PEEK indicates also other possible interpretations, such as the M2-phenotype connection of *IL-13* and the fact that *M-CSF*, besides its role in macrophage fusion into either osteoclasts or FBGCs, is intimately related to adipose tissue hyperplasia and growth (through proliferation) [29]. In the present study, the preferential adipose tissue growth observed on PEEK surface is supported at 28 days by the concomitant sharp upregulation of *PPAR-gamma* and *M-CSF*, and downregulation of *TRAP* and *Cathepsin-K* (bone resorption effectors), clearly indicating a sharp imbalance towards adipose tissue formation instead of bone formation around PEEK. It is important to note that in our previous study where Ti was compared to a Sham site at 28 days, no significant differences regarding *PPAR-gamma* or *M-CSF* were observed between the test and control [12], reinforcing the difference observed between PEEK and Ti at 28 days. Fat cell degeneration has previously been described in bone tissue after trauma upon overheating [30]. Such bone/adipose tissue imbalance, tilting towards more adipose tissue formation, has also been demonstrated in osteoporosis studies [31]. The present results after 28 days around PEEK support the description of this new-found mechanism for bone biomaterials. The orchestration of this process by the immune system has also been shown in literature [24], indicating a M1-macrophage chronic inflammation presence in proliferating adipose tissue [32], as well as $CD4+$ $T_{helper/reg}$ and $CD19$ B cells, as demonstrated in our results with a shift from downregulation at 10 days to upregulation at 28 days. The *PPAR-gamma* and *M-CSF* upregulation reaction likely overrules the OPG upregulation that would suppress bone resorption and increase osteoblast differentiation around PEEK; it is known that bone marrow mesenchymal stem cells (BMMSC) may either differentiate into osteoblasts or adipocytes [33], and PEEK, as demonstrated by the current results, seems to induce immune regulated adipocyte formation and proliferation in its vicinity.

5. Conclusions

Overall, at 10 and 28 days after implantation in rabbit tibia, both Cu and PEEK show a higher immune activation than Ti. This more pronounced and extended immune reaction translates into a prolonged inflammatory phase of the healing period, and may be the cause for the bone tissue failing to form a layer in direct contact with these materials, as shown in the histological sections.

The current results demonstrate that, over time, different materials elicit a different immune regulation of bone metabolism around implanted materials.

From a clinical orofacial perspective, it is fair to state that a fibrous tissue encapsulation or adipose instead of bone tissue formation could also occur around clinically placed titanium implants, should less ideal host conditions be present.

The results from the current study suggest that osseointegration may fail by at least two immunologically regulated mechanisms: (1) soft tissue encapsulation or (2) an imbalance in bone/adipose tissue formation around the implanted material.

Author Contributions: Conceptualization, R.T., T.A., P.T., and A.W.; Methodology, R.T., T.A., P.T., and A.W.; Software, R.T., Z.P., A.W., and S.G.; Validation, R.T. and P.T.; Formal Analysis, R.T. and A.W.; Investigation, R.T. and A.W.; Resources, R.T., P.T., T.A., and A.W.; Data Curation, R.T.; Writing—Original Draft Preparation, R.T. and A.W.; Writing—Review & Editing, P.T., T.A., and A.W.; Visualization, R.T., S.G., and Z.P.; Supervision, A.W., T.A., and P.T.; Project Administration, R.T.; Funding Acquisition, A.W.

Funding: This study was financially supported by Swedish Research Council grant nr 2015-02971, Sweden; Swedish Research Council grant nr 621-2014-3700, Sweden; Odontology Research Region Skane No. 509641, Sweden; and King Gustaf V and Queen Victoria Foundation, Swedish Order of Freemasons. RT supported by TePe Stipendium grant 2016, Sweden.

Conflicts of Interest: The authors declare no conflicts of interest.

References

1. Albrektsson, T.; Brånemark, P.-I.; Hansson, H.-A.; Lindström, J. Osseointegrated titanium implants: Requirements for ensuring a long-lasting, direct bone-to-implant anchorage in man. *Acta Orthop. Scand.* **1981**, *52*, 155–170. [CrossRef] [PubMed]
2. Wennerberg, A.; Albrektsson, T. On implant surfaces: A review of current knowledge and opinions. *Int. J. Oral Maxillofac. Implants* **2010**, *25*, 63–74. [PubMed]
3. Wennerberg, A.; Albrektsson, T.; Andersson, B. Bone tissue response to commercially pure titanium implants blasted with fine and coarse particles of aluminum oxide. *Int. J. Oral Maxillofac. Implants* **1996**, *11*, 38–45. [PubMed]
4. Wennerberg, A.; Albrektsson, T.; Lausmaa, J. Torque and histomorphometric evaluation of c.p. titanium screws blasted with 25- and 75-μm-sized particles of Al2O3. *J. Biomed. Mater. Res.* **1996**, *30*, 251–260. [CrossRef]
5. Buser, D.; Broggini, N.; Wieland, M.; Schenk, R.K.; Denzer, A.J.; Cochran, D.L.; Hoffmann, B.; Lussi, A.; Steinemann, S.G. Enhanced bone apposition to a chemically modified SLA titanium surface. *J. Dent. Res.* **2004**, *83*, 529–533. [CrossRef] [PubMed]
6. Ellingsen, J.E.; Johansson, C.B.; Wennerberg, A.; Holmén, A. Improved retention and bone-to-implant contact with fluoride-modified titanium implants. *Int. J. Oral Maxillofac. Implants* **2004**, *19*, 659–666. [PubMed]
7. Chrcanovic, B.R.; Kisch, J.; Albrektsson, T.; Wennerberg, A. A retrospective study on clinical and radiological outcomes of oral implants in patients followed up for a minimum of 20 years. *Clin. Implant Dent. Relat. Res.* **2018**, *20*, 199–207. [CrossRef] [PubMed]
8. Friberg, B.; Gröndahl, K.; Lekholm, U.; Brånemark, P.-I. Long-term follow-up of severely atrophic edentulous mandibles reconstructed with short brånemark implants. *Clin. Implant Dent. Relat. Res.* **2000**, *2*, 184–189. [CrossRef]
9. Anderson, J.M.; Rodriguez, A.; Chang, D.T. Foreign body reaction to biomaterials. *Semin. Immunol.* **2008**, *20*, 86–100. [CrossRef]
10. Goodman, S.B. Wear particles, periprosthetic osteolysis and the immune system. *Biomaterials* **2007**, *28*, 5044–5048. [CrossRef]
11. Trindade, R.; Albrektsson, T.; Tengvall, P.; Wennerberg, A. Foreign body reaction to biomaterials: On mechanisms for buildup and breakdown of osseointegration. *Clin. Implant Dent. Relat. Res.* **2016**, *18*, 192–203. [CrossRef] [PubMed]
12. Trindade, R.; Albrektsson, T.; Galli, S.; Prgomet, Z.; Tengvall, P.; Wennerberg, A. Osseointegration and foreign body reaction: Titanium implants activate the immune system and suppress bone resorption during the first 4 weeks after implantation. *Clin. Implant Dent. Relat. Res.* **2018**, *20*, 82–91. [CrossRef] [PubMed]
13. Anderson, J.M.; Jones, J.A. Phenotypic dichotomies in the foreign body reaction. *Biomaterials* **2007**, *28*, 5114–5120. [CrossRef] [PubMed]
14. Lin, T.H.; Kohno, Y.; Huang, J.F.; Romero-Lopez, M.; Maruyama, M.; Ueno, M.; Pajarinen, J.; Nathan, K.; Yao, Z.; Yang, F.; et al. Preconditioned or IL4-secreting mesenchymal stem cells enhanced osteogenesis at different stages. *Tissue Eng.* **2019**. [CrossRef] [PubMed]

15. Trindade, R.; Albrektsson, T.; Galli, S.; Prgomet, Z.; Tengvall, P.; Wennerberg, A. Bone immune response to materials, part I: Titanium, PEEK and copper in comparison to sham at 10 days in rabbit tibia. *J. Clin. Med.* **2018**, *7*, 526. [CrossRef] [PubMed]
16. Albrektsson, T.; Dahlin, C.; Jemt, T.; Sennerby, L.; Turri, A.; Wennerberg, A. Is marginal bone loss around oral implants the result of a provoked foreign body reaction? *Clin. Implant Dent. Relat. Res.* **2014**, *16*, 155–165. [CrossRef]
17. Insua, A.; Monje, A.; Wang, H.-L.; Miron, R.J. Basis of bone metabolism around dental implants during osseointegration and peri-implant bone loss. *J. Biomed. Mater. Res.* **2017**, *105*, 2075–2089. [CrossRef]
18. Suska, F.; Emanuelsson, L.; Johansson, A.; Tengvall, P.; Thomsen, P. Fibrous capsule formation around titanium and copper. *J. Biomed. Mater. Res.* **2008**, *85*, 888–896. [CrossRef]
19. Johansson, P.; Jimbo, R.; Kjellin, P.; Currie, F.; Chrcanovic, B.R.; Wennerberg, A. Biomechanical evaluation and surface characterization of a nano-modified surface on PEEK implants: A study in the rabbit tibia. *Int. J. Nanomed.* **2014**, *9*, 3903–3911. [CrossRef]
20. Da Silva, T.A.; Zorzetto-Fernandes, A.L.V.; Cecílio, N.T.; Sardinha-Silva, A.; Fernandes, F.F.; Roque-Barreira, M.C. CD14 is critical for TLR2-mediated M1 macrophage activation triggered by N-glycan recognition. *Sci. Rep.* **2017**, *7*. [CrossRef]
21. McNally, A.K.; Anderson, J.M. Foreign body-type multinucleated giant cells induced by interleukin-4 express select lymphocyte costimulatory molecules and are phenotypically distinct from osteoclasts and dendritic cells. *Exp. Mol. Pathol.* **2011**, *91*, 673–681. [CrossRef] [PubMed]
22. Wenz, L.M.; Merritt, K.; Brown, S.A.; Moet, A.; Steffee, A.D. In vitro biocompatibility of polyetheretherketone and polysulfone composites. *J. Biomed. Mater. Res.* **1990**, *24*, 207–215. [CrossRef] [PubMed]
23. Katzer, A.; Marquardt, H.; Westendorf, J.; Wening, J.V.; von Foerster, G. Polyetheretherketone—Cytotoxicity and mutagenicity in vitro. *Biomaterials* **2002**, *23*, 1749–1759. [CrossRef]
24. Vishwakarma, A.; Bhise, N.S.; Evangelista, M.B.; Rouwkema, J.; Dokmeci, M.R.; Ghaemmaghami, A.M.; Khademhosseini, A. Engineering immunomodulatory biomaterials to tune the inflammatory response. *Trend. Biotechnol.* **2016**, *34*, 470–482. [CrossRef] [PubMed]
25. Yun, T.J.; Chaudhary, P.M.; Shu, G.L.; Kimble Frazer, J.; Ewings, M.K.; Schwartz, S.M.; Pascual, V.; Hood, L.E.; Clark, E.A. OPG/FDCR-1, a TNF receptor family member, is expressed in lymphoid cells and is up-regulated by ligating CD40. *J. Immunol.* **1998**, *161*, 6113–6121.
26. Weitzmann, M.N.; Ofotokun, I. Physiological and pathophysiological bone turnover—Role of the immune system. *Nat. Rev. Endocrinol.* **2016**, *12*, 518–532. [CrossRef]
27. Chinetti, G.; Griglio, S.; Antonucci, M.; Torra, I.P.; Delerive, P.; Majd, Z.; Fruchart, J.-C.; Chapman, J.; Najib, J.; Staels, B. Activation of proliferator-activated receptors α and γ induces apoptosis of human monocyte-derived macrophages. *J. Biol. Chemist.* **1998**, *273*, 25573–25580. [CrossRef]
28. Jiang, C.; Ting, A.T.; Seed, B. PPAR-γ agonists inhibit production of monocyte inflammatory cytokines. *Nature* **1998**, *391*, 82–86. [CrossRef]
29. Levine, J.A.; Jensen, M.D.; Eberhardt, N.L.; O'Brien, T. Adipocyte macrophage colony-stimulating factor is a mediator of adipose tissue growth. *J. Clin. Invest.* **1998**, *101*, 1557–1564. [CrossRef]
30. Eriksson, A.; Albrektsson, T.; Magnusson, B. Assessment of bone viability after heat trauma: A histological, histochemical and vital microscopic study in the rabbit. *Scand. J. Plast. Reconstr. Surg.* **1984**, *18*, 261–268. [CrossRef]
31. Ambrosi, T.H.; Scialdone, A.; Graja, A.; Gohlke, S.; Jank, A.-M.; Bocian, C.; Woelk, L.; Fan, H.; Logan, D.W.; Schurmann, A.; et al. Adipocyte accumulation in the bone marrow during obesity and aging impairs stem cell-based hematopoietic and bone regeneration. *Cell Stem Cell* **2017**, *20*, 771–784. [CrossRef] [PubMed]
32. Kawanishi, N.; Yano, H.; Yokogawa, Y.; Suzuki, K. Exercise training inhibits inflammation in adipose tissue via both suppression of macrophage infiltration and acceleration of phenotypic switching from M1 to M2 macrophages in high-fat-diet-induced obese mice. *Exerc. Immunol. Rev.* **2016**, *16*, 105–118.
33. Bianco, P.; Riminucci, M.; Gronthos, S.; Robey, P.G. Bone marrow stromal stem cells: Nature, biology, and potential applications. *Stem Cells* **2001**, *19*, 180–192. [CrossRef] [PubMed]

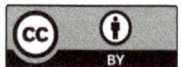

© 2019 by the authors. Licensee MDPI, Basel, Switzerland. This article is an open access article distributed under the terms and conditions of the Creative Commons Attribution (CC BY) license (http://creativecommons.org/licenses/by/4.0/).

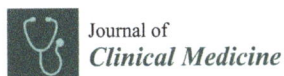

Article

Cytokine Profile in Patients with Aseptic Loosening of Total Hip Replacements and Its Relation to Metal Release and Metal Allergy

Rune J. Christiansen [1,2,*], Henrik J. Münch [3], Charlotte M. Bonefeld [2], Jacob P. Thyssen [4], Jens J. Sloth [5], Carsten Geisler [2], Kjeld Søballe [3], Morten S. Jellesen [1] and Stig S. Jakobsen [3,*]

1. Department of Mechanical Engineering, Technical University of Denmark, DK-2800 Kgs. Lyngby, Denmark
2. Department of Immunology and Microbiology, University of Copenhagen, DK-2200 Copenhagen, Denmark
3. Institute of Clinical Medicine—Orthopedic Surgery, Aarhus University, DK-8000 Aarhus C, Denmark
4. Institute of Clinical Medicine, Copenhagen University, Gentofte Hospital, DK-2900 Hellerup, Denmark
5. National Food Institute, Research Group on Nanobio Science, Technical University of Denmark, DK-2860 Søborg, Denmark
* Correspondence: rujuch@mek.dtu.dk (R.J.C.); Stig.Jakobsen@ki.au.dk (S.S.J.); Tel.: +45-61680969 (R.J.C.); +45-40976165 (S.S.J.)

Received: 19 July 2019; Accepted: 9 August 2019; Published: 20 August 2019

Abstract: Metal release from total hip replacements (THRs) is associated with aseptic loosening (AL). It has been proposed that the underlying immunological response is caused by a delayed type IV hypersensitivity-like reaction to metals, i.e., metal allergy. The purpose of this study was to investigate the immunological response in patients with AL in relation to metal release and the prevalence of metal allergy. THR patients undergoing revision surgery due to AL or mechanical implant failures were included in the study along with a control group consisting of primary THR patients. Comprehensive cytokine analyses were performed on serum and periimplant tissue samples along with metal analysis using inductive coupled plasma mass spectrometry (ICP-MS). Patient patch testing was done with a series of metals related to orthopedic implant. A distinct cytokine profile was found in the periimplant tissue of patients with AL. Significantly increased levels of the proinflammatory cytokines IL-1β, IL-2, IL-8, IFN-γ and TNF-α, but also the anti-inflammatory IL-10 were detected. A general increase of metal concentrations in the periimplant tissue was observed in both revision groups, while Cr was significantly increased in patient serum with AL. No difference in the prevalence of metal sensitivity was established by patch testing. Increased levels of IL-1β, IL-8, and TNF-α point to an innate immune response. However, the presence of IL-2 and IFN-γ indicates additional involvement of T cell-mediated response in patients with AL, although this could not be detected by patch testing.

Keywords: arthroplasty; replacement; hip; hypersensitivity; contact; allergy and immunology; cytokines; Interleukin-8

1. Introduction

1.1. Background

Aseptic loosening (AL) of implants is the most common reason for revision surgeries in patients with total hip replacements (THRs), representing close to 75% of all cases, with serious consequences for patients and healthcare systems [1,2]. Although the etiology of AL is multifactorial and yet to be fully understood, evidence suggest that the predominant cause of AL is due to a macrophage-driven chronic inflammatory response initiated by implant wear [1,3–5]. This adverse tissue reaction is associated with the innate immune system and can lead to the bone degrading state of osteolysis, subsequently resulting in implant failure by AL.

Cytokines are small messenger molecules that coordinate the immune response by regulating inflammation and modulating cellular activities such as growth, differentiation and survival [6]. Key mediators of osteolysis have been identified as pro-inflammatory cytokines like interleukin (IL)-1β, IL-6, IL-8 and tumor necrosis factor (TNF)-α secreted by activated macrophages. In turn, these cytokines are capable of inducing the differentiation of osteoclast precursor cells into mature, bone resorbing, osteoclasts [1,7–11]. Interferon (IFN)-γ is another important immune regulatory cytokine implicated in bone resorption but also in inflammation progression and cell mediated immunity [12,13].

Macrophages have been established as important mediators of ostolysis, but several other cell types have also been identified in the periimplant tissue of failed implants, including lymphocytic T cells [9,14–16]. T helper (Th) cells, a subtype of T cells, are important regulators of macrophage function and the adaptive immune response, which given rise to the concept of implant-related metal sensitivity. This concept is evolved around a delayed type IV T cell mediated hypersensitivity (DTH), exemplified by allergic contact dermatitis to metal ions (metal allergy). Due to their small size, metal ions are considered to be incomplete antigens, referred to as haptens, and must interact with peptides or proteins to form an antigen able to mount DTH.

In support of the concept above, findings of elevated levels of metal particles and ions have been shown to correlate with an increased prevalence of metal allergy in patients with failing implants [17–21]. Furthermore, some of the most commonly applied alloys for THR like stainless steel (FeCrNiMo), cobalt chromium (CoCrMo) and titanium alloys (Ti6Al4V) contain known sensitizing metals [22].

Immunological studies of AL in THRs, have suggested the involvement of a Th1 cell response, crucial for DTH, due to increased levels of Th1 cell specific cytokines like IFN-γ and IL-2 [4,23]. Previous studies also suggest the involvement of a Th2 and Th17 cell response in AL, which are respectively characterized by the production of IL-4, IL-17 and granulocyte-macrophage colony-stimulating factor (GM-CSF) [24–26]. However, the causal relationship between immune reactions, metal release from implants, and AL is still uncertain.

1.2. Aim

The aim of the present study was to determine and compare levels of THR relevant metals and cytokine profiles from periimplant tissue and blood serum, and to investigate the prevalence of metal allergy in patients undergoing revision surgery due AL, mechanical failure or undergoing primary THR surgery. Periimplant tissue obtained from patients with AL showed a significantly different cytokine profile suggesting the involvement of both innate and adaptive immunity in AL. No prevalence of metal allergy was established in patients with failed implants despite elevated levels of metal ions in the periimplant tissue.

2. Experimental Section

2.1. Patients and Samples

We conducted a prospective case study including three patient groups. This study was approved by the Central Denmark Region Committee on Biomedical Research Ethics (Journal number: 1-10-72-90-13). All patients gave their written informed consent before entering the study.

Criteria for inclusion in the AL (+) group were: revision (entirely or partial) due to aseptic loosening, osteolysis, or unexplainable pain that could not be treated conservatively. The AL (−) group; revision (entirely or partial) due to fracture, dislocation, or component failure. The Control group; patients received a primary THR. Implant components are listed in Table 1.

Table 1. Implant overview. Implant types and materials used for femoral, head, liner and acetabular components are given for patients in the revision groups. In addition to the implant bulk material, model names and surface finish is also listed. cpTi relates to commercially pure titanium and PS to plasma sprayed coatings. FeCrNiMn is also referred to as Orthinox stainless steel.

Patient #	Type	Femoral	Head	Liner	Acetabular
1 AL (+)	MoP	Ti-6Al-4V, ZMR®, uncemented, porous coating	CoCrMo	PE	Ti-6Al-4V, Trilogy®, uncommented, cpTi fiber mesh.
2 AL (+)	MoP	FeCrNiMn, Exeter®, cemented, polished.	CoCrMo	PE	cpTi, Duraloc®, uncemented, porous coating.
3 AL (+)	MoP	CoCrMo, Lubinus®, cemented polished.	CoCrMo	PE	PE, Lubinus®, cemented, all-polycup
4 AL (+)	MoP	FeCrNiM, Exeter®, cemented, polished.	CoCrMo	PE	Ti-6Al-4V, Mallory Head, uncemented, PS.
5 AL (+)	MoP	Ti-6Al-4V, Bi-metric®, uncemented, grit blasted.	CoCrMo	PE	Ti-6Al-4V, Mallory®Head, uncemented, PS.
6 AL (+)	MoM	Ti-6Al-4V, Bi-metric®, uncemented, grit blasted.	CoCrMo	CoCrMo	CoCrMo, ReCap®, uncemented, cpTI PS.
1 AL (−)	MoP	Ti-6Al-7Nb, CLS spotorno®, uncemented, grit blasted.	CoCrMo	PE	Ti-6Al-4V, Trilogy®, uncemented, cpTi fiber mesh.
2 AL (−)	MoP	Ti-6Al-7Nb, CLS spotorno®, uncemented, grit blasted.	CoCrMo	PE	Ti-6Al-4V, Trilogy®, uncemented, cpTi fiber mesh.
3 AL (−)	CoP	Ti-6Al-4V, Biocontact®, uncemented, grit blasted.	Ceramic	PE	Ti-6Al-4V, Plasmacup®, uncemented, plasmapore PS.
4 AL (−)	MoP	FeCrNiMn, Exeter®, cemented, polished.	CoCrMo	PE	cpTi, Pinnacle®, uncemented porocoat, porous coating.
5 AL (−)	MoP	FeCrNiMn, Exeter®, cemented, polished	CoCrMo	PE	Ti-6Al-4V, Trilogy®, uncemented, cpTi fiber mesh.
6 AL (−)	MoP	FeCrNiMn, Exeter®, cemented, polished	CoCrMo	PE	cpTi, Pinnacle®, uncemented porocoat, porous coating.

Criteria for exclusion: infection (positive Kamme-Lindberg biopsies [27]), use of immunomodulating medication, occupational metal exposure, known metal allergies towards implanted metals or secondary osteoarthritis (fracture, inflammation). The mean age for the AL (+) group was 60.8 years with a gender distribution of 4/2 (M/W). For the AL (−) group, the mean age was 73 years, and the distribution was 4/2 (M/W). The control group had a mean age of 62 years and a distribution of 5/3 (M/W). Tissue samples for cytokine and ICP-MS analysis were snap-frozen in liquid nitrogen and stored at −80 °C for later use. Serum obtained from patients blood samples were taken before the operation and stored at −80 °C for later cytokine and ICP-MS analysis.

2.2. Cytokine Profile Analysis

Snap frozen tissue samples from group AL (+), group AL (−) and the control group were mechanically disrupted and homogenized (Precellys®24 and Cryolys®—Bertin Technologies, Bie & Berntsen A/S 2730, Herlev, Denmark) at 4 °C for 4 × 20 s in lysis buffer containing protease inhibitor cocktail (REF 11836145001, Roche Diagnostics, Indianapolis, IN, USA). Homogenized tissue samples were then spun for 10 min at 10,000 × G at 4 °C (Microcentrifuge 157MP—Ole Dich Instrumentmakers ApS, Hvidovre, Denmark) and the protein concentration in the supernatant was estimated by Bradford protein assay [28] using Coomassie blue (#1610436. Bio-Rad Laboratories, Inc., Hercules, CA, USA). Prior to cytokine analysis, total protein concentrations of the samples were adjusted to 0.5 mg/mL. Cytokine analysis was performed using a validated V-PLEX electrochemiluminescence immunoassays (Meso Scale Discovery, Rockville, MD, USA). A total of 11 cytokines divided on two separate kits were analyzed. Proinflammatory Panel 1 contained; IL-1β, IL-2, IL-4, IL-6, IL-8, IL-10, IFN-γ and TNF-α (catalog # K15049D-1), and cytokine panel 1 kit contained; IL-15, IL-17A, GM-CSF (catalog # K15050D-1). Samples were analyzed in triplicates (MESO QuickPlex SQ 120—Meso Scale Discovery). Calibration curves used to calculate cytokine concentrations were established by fitting to a 4 parameters logistic model with a $1/Y^2$ weighting. Cytokine concentrations were calculated using the Discovery workbench

4.0.12 software (Meso Scale Discovery). Serum samples were analyzed undiluted using the same cytokine kits as used for the tissue.

2.3. Patch Testing

A special patch test series, provided by Smart Practice®(Phoenix, AZ, USA), was used in this study. The patch contained prefabricated panels with metallic compounds associated with orthopedic prostheses on Scanpor tape. Standard metal allergens included; nickel (II) sulphate $NiSO_4$ (1.0 wt.%), potassium dichromate (VI) $K_2Cr_2O_7$ (0.054 wt.%) and cobalt (II) chloride $CoCl_2$ (0.02 wt.%). In addition, a customized panel with the following metals and corresponding titrations were included; vanadium (IV) oxide sulfate hydrate $VOSO_4 \cdot H_2O$ (0.36, 0.18, 0.06, 0.02 wt.%), vanadium (III) chloride VCl_3 (0.24, 0.12, 0.013, 0.04 wt.%), manganese (II) chloride $MnCl_2 \cdot 4H_2O$ (0.24, 0.08, 0.06, 0.0057 wt.%), aluminum (III) chloride $AlCl_3 \cdot 6H_2O$ (0.72, 0.38, 0.039 wt.%), ammonium molybdate (VI) $(NH_4)_6Mo_7O_{24}\ 4H_2O$ (0.12, 0.013, 0.04 wt.%), titanium (IV) oxalate hydrate $TiC_4O_8 \cdot H_2O$ (0.32, 0.16, 0.08, 0.04 wt.%), titanium (IV) dioxide TiO_2 (0.24 wt.%), potassium titanium (II) oxide oxalate $C_4K_2O_9Ti \cdot 2H_2O$ (2.4, 1.2, 0.6 wt.%), ammonium titanium (II) lactate, solution Ti $[(C_3H_4O_3)_2(NH_4OH)_2]$ (0.16, 0.08, 0.04 wt.%), ammonium titanium (IV) peroxocitrate $(NH_4)_4[Ti_2(C_6H_4O_7)_2(O_2)_2] \cdot 4H_2O$ (0.32, 0.16, 0.08, 0.04 wt.%). methyl methacrylate $C_5H_8O_2$ (2 wt.%), gentamycin sulfate (20 wt.%) and ferrous chloride $FeCl_2$ (2 wt.%) were tested by manually loading of a Finn chamber on Scanpor tape. Patches were applied on the upper back and were occluded for 48 h. Readings were completed 96 h after application [29]. The patients were instructed to remove the panels after 48 h, and not to shower, scratch or expose to sunlight. Reactions were scored using the International Contact Dermatitis Research Group's (ICDRG) criteria [30]. Only definite +1, +2 and +3 reactions were regarded as positive.

2.4. ICP-MS (Serum)

Blood samples were sent to Vejle Hospital, Department of Clinical Biochemistry, Denmark, for determination of chromium and cobalt levels before the surgery. The samples were analyzed by ICP-MS instrument (iCAPq, Thermo Fisher Scientific Inc., Waltham, MA, USA). The samples were diluted with 0.5% HNO_3, gallium was added as an internal standard prior to analysis. The detection limit was 10 nmol/L equivalent to 0.59 ppb (cobalt) and 0.52 ppb (chromium).

2.5. ICP-MS (Tissue and Serum)

Elemental analysis of tissues and titanium (Ti) analysis of blood was performed at the National Food Institute at the Technical University of Denmark.

Elemental analysis in tissues: Tissue samples (0.1–0.5 g) were digested with a mixture of concentrated nitric acid (4 mL; PlasmaPure, SCPScience, Courtaboeuf, France) and hydrogenperoxide (1 mL; Merck, Darmstadt, Germany) in a microwave oven (Multiwave 3000, Anton Paar, Graz, Austria). The concentration of aluminum (Al), vanadium (V), chromium (Cr), cobalt (Co) and nickel (Ni) was determined using ICPMS (iCAPq, Thermo Fisher Scientific, Waltham, MA, USA) using rhodium as an internal standard and external calibration. The ICPMS instrument was run in the kinetic energy discrimination (KED) mode using helium as a collision cell gas. The limit of detection was estimated at 100 µg/kg for all elements.

Determination of Ti in tissue and blood: The acid digests of tissues were also subjected to Ti analysis. Serum subsamples (200 µL) were diluted with 4.8 mL diluent solution consisting of 0.5% Triton X-100, 10% ethanol (both Merck) and 1% nitric acid (SCPScience) prior to the analysis of the concentration of Ti using a triple quadrupole ICPMS (Agilent 8800 ICP-QQQ, Agilent Technologies, Yokogawa, Japan) and using ammonia as a cell gas with determination of Ti after MS/MS mass shift from $m/z\ 48 \geq m/z\ 150$ with scandium (Sc) as internal standard and external calibration. The data quality of Ti analysis was assessed by the analysis of the reference material Seronorm (Sero, Oslo, Norway). The obtained value 7.2 µg/L was in good agreement with the reference value 6.8 µg/L. The limit of detection was estimated at 1 µg/L in serum samples and 20 µg/kg in tissues. All calibration standards and internal standards were produced from certified single-element stock solutions (SCPScience).

2.6. Statistical Analysis

For group comparison the Kruskal-Wallis test was used, and if statistically significant, the Mann-Whitney U test was used to compare between individual groups. By convention, to calculate group medians, metal concentrations below the detection limit were assigned a value of one-half the detection limit. Comparisons were made using the Mann-Whitney test. Contingency tables (patch test) were analyzed using Fisher's exact test. A significance level of $p < 0.05$ was considered statistically significant. Matlab R2014a (8.3.0.532) with statistical toolbox (MathWorks Inc. Natick, MA, USA) was used for statistical analysis. For graphical representation Prism 6.0 (GraphPad Software, San Diego, CA, USA) was used.

3. Results

3.1. Cytokine Profile Analysis

3.1.1. Analysis of Cytokine Levels in Periimplant Tissue

Cytokine levels were measured in periimplant tissue obtained from revision or primary surgery to identify a potential local immune response (Figure 1).

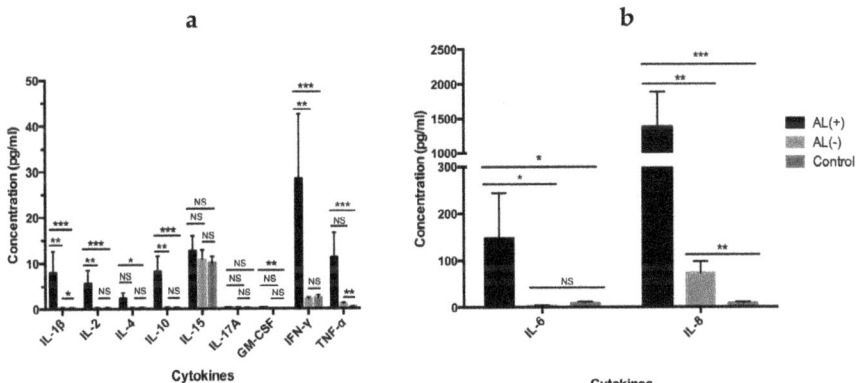

Figure 1. Cytokine profiles of periimplant tissue. Cytokines are shown in graph (**a**) and (**b**) with different concentration scales. Except from IL-15 and IL-17, patients with aseptic loosening AL (+) showed a statistically significant increase in the cytokine levels when compared with the control group. Out of the statistically significant cytokines, IL-4 and TNF-α did not show any statistical significance (NS) when comparing the two revision groups. IL-8 was found to be highly increased in patients with AL. Results are expressed as the mean (±SEM). The Mann-Whitney U test was used for the statistical analysis with a significance level of 0.05. p values are given by * $p < 0.05$, ** $p \leq 0.01$, *** $p \leq 0.001$.

Altogether, 10 cytokines (IL-1β, IL-2, IL-4, IL-6, IL-8, IL-10, IL-15, IL-17A, IFN-γ and TNF-α) and growth factor GM-CSF were analyzed (Figure 1a/b). We found a highly increased cytokine profile in patients with AL, with a statistical significant increase of IL-1β, IL-2, IL-4, IL-6, IL-8, IL-10, GM-CSF, IFN-γ and TNF-α when compared to the AL (+) and the control group. When compared to the AL (−) group we found a statistically significant increase for all cytokines except from IL-4, IL-15, GM-CSF, and TNF-α. Of note, IL-8 was highly increased and the most strongly associated cytokine with AL.

3.1.2. Analysis of Cytokine Levels in Serum

An identical cytokine profile analysis was performed in serum to investigate a corresponding systemic response (Figure 2). Cytokine levels in serum appeared 10–100 fold lower and although IL-8 and IFN-γ seemed increased in the AL (+) group, no statistical differences could be established. Together these results show a general increase of the investigated cytokine profile, in periimplant tissue obtained from patients with AL, but also that cytokine levels in periimplant tissue are not necessarily reflected in blood serum. Among other increased cytokines, IL-8 was established as the most potent marker of AL.

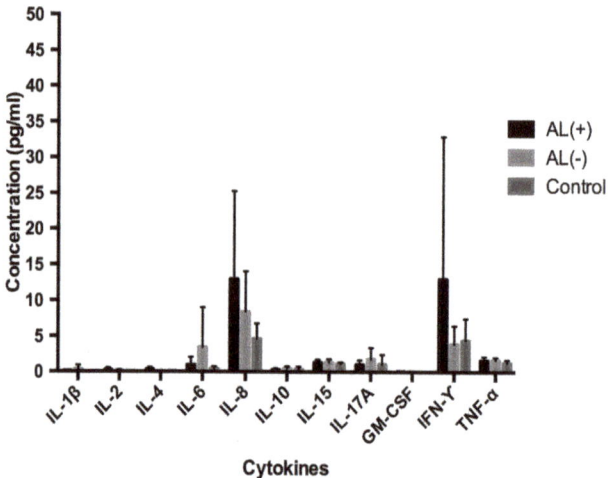

Figure 2. Cytokine profiles in serum. Patients with aseptic loosening are represented as AL (+), patients with dislocations are represented as AL (−) and the controls. Increased IL-8 and IFN-γ levels appeared for the AL (+) group. Results are expressed as the mean concentration (±SEM). No statistically significant differences could be established between the groups using the Mann-Whitney U test with a significance level of 0.05.

3.2. Patch Test

All patient groups were subjected to a comprehensive patch test containing orthopedically relevant metals and methyl methacrylate, the monomer of poly (methyl methacrylate) (PMMA) used as bone cement in THR (Table 2). Positive and doubtful reactions to these metals are summarized in Table 2. No statistical significant differences between either of the groups could be established. Few positive test reaction were observed even for the metals used in the standard series (Cr, Co and Ni), only one reaction to Ni and one to Cr were observed in all three groups. However, three positive reactions for Ti and two positive skin reactions to V were observed in the (AL+) group. In fact, the two positive reactions to V were observed in the same patient who had a positive reaction to Cr (Figure 3).

Table 2. Skin reactions. Positive (+) and doubtful (+?) skin reactions to different metals and methyl methacrylate. Patch test reactions were scored using the International Contact Dermatitis Research Group's (ICDRG) criteria [30]. Only definite +1, +2 and +3 reactions were regarded as positive. No reactions were categorized as +2 and +3 reactions in this study and only compounds with either positive (+1) or doubtful (+?) reactions are listed in the table. Prevalence of positive reactions was tested against the control group using Fisher's exact test with two tailed p values. No statistical significant differences were found.

	AL (+) (n = 6)	AL (−) (n = 6)	Control (n = 8)
	Reactions		
Metal compound (concentration)	+ (+?)	+ (+?)	+ (+?)
Al(III), $AlCl_3$ (0.72%)	0 (0)	0 (0)	0 (1)
Ti(IV), TiC_4O_8 (0.32%)	0 (0)	1 (0)	2 (0)
Ti(II), $C_4K_2O_9Ti$ (2.4%)	0 (0)	0 (0)	0 (0)
V(III), VCl_3 (0.24%)	1 (2)	0 (3)	0 (3)
V(III), VCl_3 (0.12%)	1 (0)	0 (1)	0 (3)
V(III), VCl_3 (0.013%)	0 (0)	0 (1)	0 (0)
V(III), VCl_3 (0.04%)	0 (0)	0 (1)	0 (0)
V(IV), $VOSO_4$ (0.36%)	0 (1)	0 (1)	0 (2)
V(IV), $VOSO_4$ (0.18%)	0 (1)	0 (1)	0 (0)
Cr(VI), $K_2Cr_2O_7$ (0.054%)	1 (0)	0 (0)	0 (0)
Mn(II), $MnCl_2$ (0.24%)	0 (1)	1 (2)	0 (2)
Ni(II), $NiSO_4$ (5.0%)	0 (0)	0 (0)	1 (1)
Methyl Methacrylate, $C_5H_8O_2$ (2%)	0 (0)	0 (0)	0 (1)
Total reactions	3 (4)	2 (8)	3 (12)

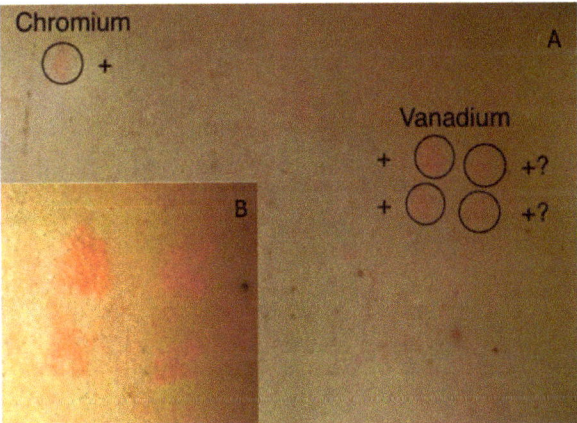

Figure 3. Patch test. (**A**) Example of a positive (+) and a doubtful skin reactions (+?) to vanadium and chromium in a patient from the AL (+) group. (**B**) Enlarged photograph of the skin reaction to vanadium.

3.3. ICP-MS Analysis

3.3.1. Metal Concentrations in Periimplant Tissue

Periimplant tissue was analyzed for Al, Ti, V, Cr, Co and Ni by ICP-MS (Table 3). Raised median concentrations of most metals could be observed in both revision groups, AL (+) and AL (−) as shown in Table 3. Metals found at highest concentrations were, Al, Ti and Cr, although no statistically significant differences could be established between the AL (+) and AL (−) group, however, a difference was observed when compared to the control group. Despite the raised concentrations of Cr observed in the

AL (+) group compared to the control group no statistical significant increase could be determined ($p = 0.074$). These results clearly demonstrate the presence of metal release in the two revision groups.

Table 3. Elemental analysis. Metal concentrations (ppb) measured by ICP-MS in periimplant tissue and blood serum. Titanium, chromium and cobalt were measured in blood serum. Values are shown as group medians with interquartile range below. Statistics are based on medians using the Wilcoxon-Mann-Whitney test with a significance level of 0.05. * Indicate significantly increased values compared to the control group. Elemental analysis for Al, V and Ni was only carried out on tissue samples and are therefore indicated as not available (N/A) for serum samples.

Metal	AL (+) n = 6		AL (−) n = 6		Control n = 10	
	Tissue	Serum	Tissue	Serum	Tissue	Serum
Al	7186 * (1905–29,019)	N/A	3407 * (845–26,709)	N/A	1258 (352–2615)	N/A
Ti	1610 * (891–13,328)	0.65 (0.60–2.95)	12978 * (588–47,078)	1.45 (0.60–3.98)	716.5 (504–1152)	0.60 (0.60–1.00)
V	210 (128–920)	N/A	381 (151–573)	N/A	160 (133–209)	N/A
Cr	3648 (358–21,075)	0.98 * (0.26–3.4)	499 (151–6235)	0.26 (0.26–0.26)	484 (184–1868)	0.26 (0.26–0.26)
Co	210 (128–2724)	0.30 (0.30–1.93)	167 (118–2549)	0.30 (0.30–0.74)	160 (133–209)	0.30 (0.30–0.30)
Ni	772 * (355–2027)	N/A	328 (151–1589)	N/A	212 (162–326)	N/A

3.3.2. Metal Concentrations in Serum

Serum samples were analyzed for Ti, Co and Cr by ICP-MS (Table 3). A statistical significant increase of Cr concentrations in the AL (+) group was found, compared to the control group. No statistical significant increase was observed between the two revision groups ($p = 0.105$). Nevertheless, the highest concentrations of both Co and Cr was found in the AL (+) group. One patient in the control group showed a high concentration of Ti and despite reanalysis, this sample still showed a high Ti concentration, preventing it from being regarded as an outlier. All other Ti concentrations in the control group were at the detection limit of the ICP-MS method. Furthermore, the results show that local metal concentrations in the periimplant tissue can be highly increased compared to serum levels.

4. Discussion

The possibility of metal allergy leading to aseptic loosening has been debated in the literature for many years [21,31–33]. Still, the long-term effect of internally released metals remains unknown and so does the underlining immunological response lead to AL and implant failure [22]. In this study we investigated the correlations between the immunological profile, metal allergy and metal released from implants, in THR patients with AL.

We found that patients with AL had a cytokine profile with statistically significant increased levels of the pro-inflammatory cytokines IL-1β, IL-6, and IL-8, but also Th1 associated cytokines, IL-2 and IFN-γ, and the anti-inflammatory cytokine IL-10, when compared to patients with implant failures due to mechanical causes. Despite a statistically significant and substantial metal exposure both locally and systemically in THR patients, we were not able to prove any systemic effect by cytokine analysis of serum or by positive patch testing. Based on the present study, a systemic effect cannot be ruled out due to the low number of patients enrolled in this study. The findings are, however, in line with the clinical observations, where the adverse effect to implants is predominantly observed locally rather than systemically. A further limitation of this study was the clinical approach, where polyethylene (PE) debris derived from the acetabular liner is most likely contributing the innate part of the cytokine profile observed in the periimplant tissue.

Cytokines play an important role in AL, not only as regulators of osteolysis, but also as important identifiers of the occurring immune response. In our cytokine analysis we included IL-1β IL-2, IL-4, IL-6, IL-8, IL-10, IL-15, IL-17A, GM-CSF, IFN-γ and TNF-α due to their implication in innate and adaptive immunity and their function as osteolytic mediators (Figures 1 and 2). In addition to being involved in the innate immune response, IL-1β, IL-6, IL-8, GM-CSF, and TNF-α have previously been identified as mediators of osteolysis [14,34]. In accordance with these observations, we found elevated levels of these cytokines in the periimplant tissue from the AL (+) group when compared to the control group. When comparing the two revision groups, AL (+) and AL (−), no statistically significant difference was seen for GM-CSF and TNF-α. However, levels of GM-CSF were very low and might be considered without any biological effect. TNF-α is well-known as a strong inducer of osteolysis and is the first proinflammatory cytokine produced in response to many wear particles and stimulates macrophage production of IL-1β and IL-6 [35]. Although no statistically significance is seen for TNF-α between the two revision groups, both IL-1β and IL-6 still showed a statistically significant increase in the AL (+) group. In comparison, other investigators have found low levels of IL-1β and TNF-α in periimplant tissue from patients with failed THRs due to osteolysis [36]. Moreover, they found that IL-6 and IL-8 were consistent with failed implants, suggesting that IL-6 and IL-8 might be the primary drivers of end-stage osteolysis, while IL-1β and TNF-α are critical mediators in the acute phase of inflammation. Interestingly, these observations did indeed correspond well to our findings of IL-6 and notably IL-8, which we found to be the strongest predictor of AL.

The main IL-8 secreting cells are macrophages, osteoblasts and osteoclasts. Studies have shown that IL-8 holds multiple functions in AL and has been found to affect both neutrophils, T cells, monocyte/macrophages and osteoclasts [37,38]. It has been demonstrated that wear particle stimulation of osteoblasts and macrophages promotes IL-8 production, which in turn can lead to both macrophage activation and induce phagocytosis [39]. Interleukin-8 also possess chemotactic properties on neutrophils and T cells and could conceivably play a role in attracting such cells to the periimplant tissue [37,40]. Moreover, IL-8 is shown to promote osteoclastogenesis and the formation of osteoclasts that are capable of secreting IL-8 on their own. Thus, the high levels of IL-8 observed in patients with AL is probably not only caused by an innate immune response but also in part by the osteolytic process taking place in the patients with AL, which could explain the differences in IL-8 observed between the AL (+) and the AL (−) group [40].

As indicators of DTH, IL-2 and IFN-γ levels were statistical significantly increased in the AL (+) group compared to the AL (−), supporting the involvement of a Th1 cell response in AL. This is consistent with other studies, showing lymphocyte reactivity to implant related metals and production of Th1-specific cytokines (IFN-γ and IL-2), and even the generation of metal specific T cells [41,42]. Macrophages are capable of producing IFN-γ but abundant evidence suggests that T cells and natural killer (NK) cells are the major sources of IFN-γ [3,43,44]. Accompanied by the increased levels of IL-2, the increased IFN-γ levels found in patients with AL further support the involvement of a Th1 cell response. Interferon-gamma possess both pro- and anti-inflammatory activities with the functional outcome being dependent on secretion levels, pathogenesis and disease severity [13,44]. Some studies show a protective effect of IFN-γ on osteolysis, possible by inhibiting the early differentiation of osteoclasts, whereas others have shown that IFN-γ promotes osteoclast formation [13]. How IFN-γ affects the progression of AL in this study is difficult to decipher but low levels of IFN-γ does not exert the inhibitory effect on osteoclasts and seems to be limited to the early stage of osteoclast differentiation. Furthermore, IFN-γ can promote osteoclast maturation in the late state of osteoclast formation leading to a shift from the inhibitory effect towards a state of bone resorption [45].

In addition to the Th1 signature cytokines, we also observed an increase of IL-4, along with a statistically significant increase of IL-10 when comparing the two revision groups.

Although the production of these cytokines are related to Th2 cells, IL-10 is also produced by monocytes and regulatory T cells, acting as an anti-inflammatory cytokine, which could regulate cell-mediated reactions involved in AL [46–48]. We were not able to detect any consistent cytokine profile at a systemic level in serum, underlining the difficulty of detecting AL based on the systemic levels of cytokines. In fact, cytokines have a short half-life in serum due to their potent nature as signaling molecules, which makes cytokines very challenging to use as biomarkers in serum [49].

In our analysis of Ti, Co and Cr in serum, we found a statistically significant increase of Cr in the AL (+) group and Ti in the Al (−) group (Table 3). Furthermore, we did detect a correlation between raised Ti concentrations in serum from patients with a stem component made from a Ti containing alloy, which corresponds to the findings of other studies applying the ICP-MS method [50]. Metal release, has previously been shown to increase in patients with poorly functioning implants [17]. From a corrosion point of view, this could be explained by increased micro-motions of the implant leading to fretting corrosion [20,51]. Fretting of the Ti6Al4V and the Orthinox SS alloys could contribute to the statistically significant raise in Al, Ti, and Ni observed in the revision groups (Table 4) [52,53]. Highest concentrations of Co and Cr were detected in the AL (+) group. One patient in this group had a MoM implant but no markedly increased in Co or Cr concentrations were detected in either periimplant tissue or serum from this specific patient. Interestingly, relative low concentrations of Co were found in tissue and blood samples compared to Cr concentrations. This observation has previously been explained by a faster elimination of Co from both the tissue and blood than that of Cr [54]. No upper limits are currently employed to describe critical metal release from implants, but an upper limit of 7 ppb for Co and Cr in blood is often used as an action level for MoM implants [55]. Serum concentrations of this magnitude were not detected in this study. In general, our results confirm previous metal concentrations reported in serum and periimplant tissue from patients with poorly functioning implants [17]. A correlation between the metal content in periimplant tissue but not that of serum has recently been made to a lymphocyte dominated response [56]. This emphasizes the importance of the periimplant environment, in which we found highly raised metal concentrations.

Table 4. Alloy composition. Elemental composition of the different implant alloys found patient groups, based on the ASTM international standard.

Implant Alloy	CoCrMo ASTM-(F75)	Orthinox SS ASTM-(F1586)	cpTi ASTM-(F67)	Ti6Al7Nb ASTM-(F1295)	Ti6Al4V ASTM-(F136)
Element	Composition, wt.%				
Aluminum (Al)	0.10	-	0.03	5.50–6.50	5.5–6.50
Carbon (C)	0.35	0.08	0.08	0.08	0.08
Chromium (Cr)	27–30	19.5–22	-	-	-
Cobalt (Co)	Balance	-	-	-	-
Copper (Cu)	-	0.25	0.10	-	-
Iron (Fe)	0.75	Balance	0.50	0.25	0.25
Manganese (Mn)	1	2–4.25	-	-	-
Molybdenum (Mo)	5–7	2–3	-	-	-
Nickel (Ni)	0.50	9.0–11.0	-	-	-
Niobium (Nb)	-	0.25–0.8	0.015	6.50–7.50	-
Nitrogen (N)	0.25	0.25–0.5	0.15	0.05	0.05
Oxygen (O)	-	-	0.40	0.20	0.13
Tantalum (Ta)	-	-	Balance	0.50	-
Titanium (Ti)	0.10	-	-	Balance	Balance
Tungsten (W)	0.20	-	-	-	-
Vanadium (V)	-	-	-	-	3.5–4.5

In this study implants with different fixation strategies was used i.e. cemented implants and different surface treatments for optimizing stability and osseointegration. Metal release and implant performance is highly dependent on the micro/nano topography of the implant surface [57,58]. Cemented implants have been proved to increased initial stability and minimize micro-motions of cemented parts leading to long survival rates [59]. The downside of this approach is the possible formation of a crevice between the cement and implant, which can provide a highly corrosive environment and lead to accelerated corrosion and subsequently implant failure by AL [60,61]. All uncemented implants in this study had some form of increased roughness applied to their surfaces for optimal osseointegration (Table 1). One of the costs of increasing the surface roughness on implant is an increased functional surface area, which in turn will increase metal release. Especially titanium release has recently become a subject of concern and not only in implants used for THRs [62–65]. Another debated strategy of improving osseointegration is the use of hydroxyapatite (HA) coatings, simulating the bone chemistry and structure. However, recent studies suggest that the long-term effects are not improved compared to other porous coatings or rough sandblasted surfaces [66,67].

Patch testing showed a diverse profile of test reactions across all groups making results difficult to interpret (Table 2). Metals salts are well-known skin irritants and skin reactions may therefore, in reality, be an irritant rather than an allergic reaction. On the other hand, a positive reaction can only occur if the metal reaches the viable layers of the epidermis, and this might be a challenge for some metals [68]. One patient in the AL (+) group had a positive reaction to Cr, which is higher than expected considering that less than 1% of the general population are allergic to Cr [69]. Surprisingly, we found positive reactions to Ti (IV) in the control group, which had not been exposed to Ti containing implants. Although Ti allergy is considered very limited in THRs, in vitro studies of Ti particles suggest that these can initiate innate and adaptive Th2 cell response [68,70]. Within the field of odontology there is a growing concern of the innate immune response associated with Ti, which is believed to cause osteolysis through macrophage secretion of IL1β, IL6, and TNFα [6,71]. A relative high number of skin reactions to V were observed, although most of these were scored as doubtful, true allergy cannot be ruled out. While larger cohort studies have found an increased prevalence of metal allergy in THR patients our study was not powered to examine a possible association [21,72]. Nonetheless, our findings indicate that metal allergy, as tested by patch test, is not likely to be a key driver of AL in most patients.

5. Conclusions

Aseptic loosening of implants is a complex tissue response influenced by various factors. Metal release from implants may generate DTH response capable of accelerating aseptic loosening of implants. In this study, we report a distinct cytokine profile in periimplant tissues between patients with implant failure due to AL, compared to mechanical causes, with statistically significant increased levels of IL-1β, IL-2, IL-4, IL-6, IL-8, IL-10, GM-CSF, IFN-γ and TNF-α. In addition, raised metal concentrations were found in blood and periimplant tissue from patients with failed THRs. Despite these observations, we failed to detect any correlation between the prevalence of metal allergy and failed THRs or AL. This work contributes to a better understanding of the immunologic nature of aseptic loosening and suggests that the immunological events involved in AL are of both innate and adaptive character.

Author Contributions: Composer of manuscript, study design, acquisition of cytokine data, analysis and interpretation of data obtained from ICP-MS and patch test, R.J.C. Research design, acquisition of patch test data, patient recruitment and sample collection from patients and critical revising of manuscript draft, H.J.M. Research design, interpretation of cytokine data, critical revising of manuscript draft and final approval of manuscript, C.M.B. Interpretation of patch test results and critical revising of manuscript draft, J.P.T. Acquisition of ICP-MS data and interpretation of these, J.J.S. Critical revising of manuscript draft, on allergy and cytokine data, C.G. Study design, critical revising and approval of final approval of manuscript, K.S. Interpretation of ICP-MS data and critical revising on corrosion/metal release from implants and final approval of manuscript, M.S.J. Study design, patient recruitment and sample collection from patients and critical revising of manuscript draft and final approval of manuscript, S.S.J.

Funding: This research was funded by The Danish Council for Independent Research, Technology and Production Sciences, as part of the METIMP project (0602-02401B FTP).

Conflicts of Interest: The authors declare no conflict of interest. The funders had no role in the design of the study; in the collection, analyses, or interpretation of data; in the writing of the manuscript, or in the decision to publish the results.

References

1. Camuzard, O.; Breuil, V.; Carle, G.F.; Pierrefite-Carle, V. Autophagy Involvement in Aseptic Loosening of Arthroplasty Components. *J. Bone Jt. Surg.* **2019**, *101*, 466–472. [CrossRef] [PubMed]
2. Ulrich, S.D.; Seyler, T.M.; Bennett, D.; Delanois, R.E.; Saleh, K.J.; Thongtrangan, I.; Kuskowski, M.; Cheng, E.Y.; Sharkey, P.F.; Parvizi, J.; et al. Total Hip Arthroplasties: What Are the Reasons for Revision? *Int. Orthop.* **2008**, *32*, 597–604. [CrossRef] [PubMed]
3. Cobelli, N.; Scharf, B.; Crisi, G.M.; Hardin, J.; Santambrogio, L. Mediators of the Inflammatory Response to Joint Replacement Devices. *Nat. Rev. Rheumatol.* **2011**, *7*, 600–608. [CrossRef] [PubMed]
4. Gallo, J.; Goodman, S.B.; Konttinen, Y.T.; Raska, M. Particle Disease: Biologic Mechanisms of Periprosthetic Osteolysis in Total Hip Arthroplasty. *Innate Immun.* **2013**, *19*, 213–224. [CrossRef] [PubMed]
5. Holt, G.; Murnaghan, C.; Reilly, J.; Meek, R.M.D.; Features, S. The Biology of Aseptic Osteolysis. *Clin. Orthop. Relat. Res.* **2007**, *460*, 240–252. [CrossRef] [PubMed]
6. Eger, M.; Sterer, N.; Liron, T.; Kohavi, D.; Gabet, Y. Scaling of Titanium Implants Entrains Inflammation-Induced Osteolysis. *Sci. Rep.* **2017**, *7*, 39612. [CrossRef] [PubMed]
7. Dyskova, T.; Gallo, J.; Kriegova, E. The Role of the Chemokine System in Tissue Response to Prosthetic By-Products Leading to Periprosthetic Osteolysis and Aseptic Loosening. *Front. Immunol.* **2017**, *8*. [CrossRef]
8. Hallab, N.J.; Jacobs, J.J. Chemokines Associated with Pathologic Responses to Orthopedic Implant Debris. *Front. Endocrinol.* **2017**, *8*, 5. [CrossRef]
9. Nich, C.; Takakubo, Y.; Pajarinen, J.; Ainola, M.; Salem, A.; Sillat, T.; Rao, A.J.; Raska, M.; Tamaki, Y.; Takagi, M.; et al. Macrophages-Key Cells in the Response to Wear Debris from Joint Replacements. *J. Biomed. Mater. Res. A* **2013**, *101*, 3033–3045. [CrossRef]
10. Stea, S.; Visentin, M.; Granchi, D.; Ciapetti, G.; Donati, M.; Sudanese, A.; Zanotti, C.; Toni, A. Cytokines and Osteolysis Around Total Hip Prostheses. *Cytokine* **2000**, *12*, 1575–1579. [CrossRef]
11. Wolfe, J.; Goldberg, J.; Harris, H. Production of Cytokines around Loosened Cemented Acetabular Components. *J. Bone Jt. Surg.* **1993**, *75*, 663–879.
12. Fiorillo, L.; Cervino, G.; Herford, A.; Lauritano, F.; D'Amico, C.; Lo Giudice, R.; Laino, L.; Troiano, G.; Crimi, S.; Cicciù, M. Interferon Crevicular Fluid Profile and Correlation with Periodontal Disease and Wound Healing: A Systemic Review of Recent Data. *Int. J. Mol. Sci.* **2018**, *19*, 1908. [CrossRef] [PubMed]
13. Tang, M.; Tian, L.; Luo, G.; Yu, X. Interferon-Gamma-Mediated Osteoimmunology. *Front. Immunol.* **2018**, *9*. [CrossRef] [PubMed]
14. Goodman, S.B.; Huie, P.; Song, Y.; Schurman, D.; Maloney, W.; Woolson, S.; Sibley, R. Cellular Profile and Cytokine Production at Prosthetic Interfaces. Study of Tissues Retrieved from Revised Hip and Knee Replacements. *J. Bone Joint Surg. Br.* **1998**, *80*, 531–539. [CrossRef] [PubMed]
15. Kadoya, Y.; Revell, P.A.; Al-Saffar, N.; Kobayashi, A.; Scott, G.; Freeman, M.A.R. Bone Formation and Bone Resorption in Failed Total Joint Arthroplasties: Histomorphometric Analysis with Histochemical and Immunohistochemical Technique. *J. Orthop. Res.* **1996**, *14*, 473–482. [CrossRef] [PubMed]
16. Büdinger, L.; Hertl, M. Immunologic Mechanisms in Hypersensitivity Reactions to Metal Ions: An Overview. *Allergy* **2000**, *55*, 108–115. [CrossRef]
17. Hallab, N.J.; Mikecz, K.; Vermes, C.; Skipor, A.; Jacobs, J.J. Orthopaedic Implant Related Metal Toxicity in Terms of Human Lymphocyte Reactivity to Metal-Protein Complexes Produced from Cobalt-Base and Titanium-Base Implant Alloy Degradation. *Mol. Cell. Biochem.* **2001**, *222*, 127–136. [CrossRef] [PubMed]
18. Sundfeldt, M.; Carlsson, L.V.; Johansson, C.B.; Thomsen, P.; Gretzer, C. Aseptic Loosening, Not Only a Question of Wear: A Review of Different Theories. *Acta Orthop.* **2006**, *77*, 177–197. [CrossRef]
19. Grosse, S.; Haugland, H.K.; Lilleng, P.; Ellison, P.; Hallan, G.; Høl, P.J. Wear Particles and Ions from Cemented and Uncemented Titanium-Based Hip Prostheses-A Histological and Chemical Analysis of Retrieval Material. *J. Biomed. Mater. Res. Part B Appl. Biomater.* **2015**, *103*, 709–717. [CrossRef]
20. McGrath, L.R.; Shardlow, D.L.; Ingham, E.; Andrews, M.; Ivory, J.; Stone, M.H.; Fisher, J. A Retrieval Study of Capital Hip Prostheses with Titanium Alloy Femoral Stems. *J. Bone Jt. Surg. Ser. B* **2001**, *83*, 1195–1201. [CrossRef]
21. Frigerio, E.; Pigatto, P.D.; Guzzi, G.; Altomare, G. Metal Sensitivity in Patients with Orthopaedic Implants: A Prospective Study. *Contact Dermat.* **2011**, *64*, 273–279. [CrossRef]

22. Hallab, N. Metal Sensitivity in Patients with Orthopedic Implants. *J. Clin. Rheumatol.* **2001**, *7*, 215–218. [CrossRef]
23. Schmidt, M.; Goebeler, M. Immunology of Metal Allergies. *JDDG J. Der Dtsch. Dermatol. Ges.* **2015**, *13*, 653–659. [CrossRef]
24. Summer, B.; Paul, C.; Mazoochian, F.; Rau, C.; Thomsen, M.; Banke, I.; Gollwitzer, H.; Dietrich, K.; Mayer-Wagner, S.; Ruzicka, T.; et al. Nickel (Ni) Allergic Patients with Complications to Ni Containing Joint Replacement Show Preferential IL-17 Type Reactivity to Ni. *Contact Dermat.* **2010**, *63*, 15–22. [CrossRef] [PubMed]
25. Arora, A.; Song, Y.; Chun, L.; Huie, P.; Trindade, M.; Smith, R.L.; Goodman, S. The Role of the TH1 and TH2 Immune Responses in Loosening and Osteolysis of Cemented Total Hip Replacements. *J. Biomed. Mater. Res. A* **2003**, *64*, 693–697. [CrossRef]
26. Looney, R.J.; Schwarz, E.M.; Boyd, A.; O'Keefe, R.J. Periprosthetic Osteolysis: An Immunologist's Update. *Curr. Opin. Rheumatol.* **2006**, *18*, 80–87. [CrossRef] [PubMed]
27. Kamme, C.L.L. Aerobic and Anaerobic Bacteria in Deep Infections after Total Hip Arthroplasty: Differential Diagnosis between Infectious and Non-Infectious Loosening. *Clin. Orthop. Relat. Res.* **1981**, *154*, 201–207. [CrossRef]
28. Bradford, M.M. A Rapid and Sensitive Method for the Quantitation of Microgram Quantities of Protein Utilizing the Principle of Protein-Dye Binding. *Anal. Biochem.* **1976**, *72*, 248–254. [CrossRef]
29. Todd, D.J.; Hasdlev, J.; Metwali, M.; Allen, G.E.; Burrows, D. Day 4 Is Better than Day 3 for a Single Patch Test Reading. *Contact Dermat.* **1996**, *34*, 402–404. [CrossRef]
30. Wilkinson, D.S.; Fregert, S.; Magnusson, B.; Bandmann, H.J.; Calnan, C.D.; Cronin, E.; Hjort, N.; Maibach, H.J.; Malten, K.E.; Meneghini, C.L.; et al. Terminology of Contact Dermatitis. *Acta Derm. Venereol.* **1970**, *50*, 287–292.
31. Krecisz, B.; Kieć-Swierczyńska, M.; Bakowicz-Mitura, K. Allergy to Metals as a Cause of Orthopedic Implant Failure. *Int. J. Occup. Med. Environ. Health* **2006**, *19*, 178–180. [CrossRef]
32. Thyssen, J.P.; Jakobsen, S.S.; Engkilde, K.; Johansen, J.D.; Søballe, K.; Menné, T. The Association between Metal Allergy, Total Knee Arthroplasty, and Revision. *Acta Orthop.* **2015**, *86*, 378–383. [CrossRef]
33. Granchi, D.; Cenni, E.; Giunti, A.; Baldini, N. Metal Hypersensitivity Testing in Patients Undergoing Joint Replacement. *J. Bone Jt. Surg. Br.* **2012**, *94-B*, 1126–1134. [CrossRef]
34. Konttinen, Y.; Xu, J.W.; Pätiälä, H.; Imai, S.; Waris, V.; Li, T.F.; Goodman, S.; Nordsletten, L.; Santavirta, S. Cytokines in Aseptic Loosening of Total Hip Replacement. *Curr. Orthop.* **1997**, *11*, 40–47. [CrossRef]
35. Hirayama, T.; Tamaki, Y.; Takakubo, Y.; Iwazaki, K.; Sasaki, K.; Ogino, T.; Goodman, S.B.; Konttinen, Y.T.; Takagi, M. Toll-like Receptors and Their Adaptors Are Regulated in Macrophages after Phagocytosis of Lipopolysaccharide-Coated Titanium Particles. *J. Orthop. Res.* **2011**, *29*, 984–992. [CrossRef]
36. Shanbhag, A.S.; Kaufman, A.M.; Hayata, K.; Rubash, H.E. Assessing Osteolysis with Use of High-Throughput Protein Chips. *J. Bone Jt. Surg. Am.* **2007**, *89*, 1081–1089. [CrossRef]
37. Baggiolini, M.; Loetscher, P.; Moser, B. Interleukin-8 and the Chemokine Family. *Int. J. Immunopharmacol.* **1995**, *17*, 103–108. [CrossRef]
38. Bendre, M.S.; Montague, D.C.; Peery, T.; Akel, N.S.; Gaddy, D.; Suva, L.J. Interleukin-8 Stimulation of Osteoclastogenesis and Bone Resorption Is a Mechanism for the Increased Osteolysis of Metastatic Bone Disease. *Bone* **2003**, *33*, 28–37. [CrossRef]
39. Fritz, E.A.; Jacobs, J.J.; Roebuck, A. Chemokine IL-8 Induction by Particulate Wear Debris in Osteoblasts Is Mediated by NF-ΚB. *J. Orthop. Res.* **2005**, *23*, 1249–1257. [CrossRef]
40. Qin, S.; Larosa, G.; Campbell, J.J.; Smith-heath, H.; Kassam, N.; Zeng, L.; Butcher, E.C.; Mackay, C.R. Expression of Monocyte Chemoattractant Protein-1 and Interleukin-8 Receptors on Subsets of T Cells: Correlation with Transendothelial Chemotactic Potential. *Eur. J. Immunol.* **1996**, *26*, 640–647. [CrossRef]
41. Chan, E.; Cadosch, D.; Gautschi, O.P.; Sprengel, K.; Filgueira, L. Influence of Metal Ions on Human Lymphocytes and the Generation of Titanium-Specific T-Lymphocytes. *J. Appl. Biomater. Biomech.* **2011**, *9*, 137–143. [CrossRef]
42. Hallab, N.J.; Anderson, S.; Stafford, T.; Glant, T.; Jacobs, J.J. Lymphocyte Responses in Patients with Total Hip Arthroplasty. *J. Orthop. Res.* **2005**, *23*, 384–391. [CrossRef]

43. Valladares, R.D.; Nich, C.; Zwingenberger, S.; Li, C.; Swank, K.R.; Gibon, E.; Rao, A.J.; Yao, Z.; Goodman, S.B. Toll-like Receptors-2 and 4 Are Overexpressed in an Experimental Model of Particle-Induced Osteolysis. *J. Biomed. Mater. Res. Part A* **2014**, *102*, 3004–3011. [CrossRef]
44. Lees, J.R. Interferon Gamma in Autoimmunity: A Complicated Player on a Complex Stage. *Cytokine* **2015**, *74*, 18–26. [CrossRef]
45. Kim, J.W.; Lee, M.S.; Lee, C.H.; Kim, H.Y.; Chae, S.U.; Kwak, H.B.; Oh, J. Effect of Interferon-γ on the Fusion of Mononuclear Osteoclasts into Bone-Resorbing Osteoclasts. *BMB Rep.* **2012**, *45*, 281–286. [CrossRef]
46. Couper, K.; Blount, D.; Riley, E. IL-10: The Master Regulator of Immunity to Infection. *J. Immunol.* **2008**, *180*, 5771–5777. [CrossRef]
47. Van Roon, J.A.G.; Van Roy, J.L.A.M.; Gmelig-Meyling, F.H.J.; Lafeber, F.P.J.G.; Bijlsma, J.W.J. Prevention and Reversal of Cartilage Degradation in Rheumatoid Arthritis by Interleukin-10 and Interleukin-4. *Arthritis Rheum.* **1996**, *39*, 829–835. [CrossRef]
48. Perretti, M.; Szabó, C.; Thiemermann, C. Effect of Interleukin-4 and Interleukin-10 on Leucocyte Migration and Nitric Oxide Production in the Mouse. *Br. J. Pharmacol.* **1995**, *116*, 2251–2257. [CrossRef]
49. Tarrant, J.M. Blood Cytokines as Biomarkers of In Vivo Toxicity in Preclinical Safety Assessment: Considerations for Their Use. *Toxicol. Sci.* **2010**, *117*, 4–16. [CrossRef]
50. Sarmiento-González, A.; Marchante-Gayón, J.M.; Tejerina-Lobo, J.M.; Paz-Jiménez, J.; Sanz-Medel, A. High-Resolution ICP–MS Determination of Ti, V, Cr, Co, Ni and Mo in Human Blood and Urine of Patients Implanted with a Hip or Knee Prosthesis. *Anal. Bioanal. Chem.* **2008**, *391*, 2583–2589. [CrossRef]
51. Revell, P.A. The Combined Role of Wear Particles, Macrophages and Lymphocytes in the Loosening of Total Joint Prostheses. *J. R. Soc. Interface* **2008**, *5*, 1263–1278. [CrossRef]
52. Pound, B.G. Corrosion Behavior of Metallic Materials in Biomedical Applications. I. Ti and Its Alloys. *Corros. Rev.* **2014**, *32*, 1–20. [CrossRef]
53. Pellier, J.; Geringer, J.; Forest, B. Fretting-Corrosion between 316L SS and PMMA: Influence of Ionic Strength, Protein and Electrochemical Conditions on Material Wear. Application to Orthopaedic Implants. *Wear* **2011**, *271*, 1563–1571. [CrossRef]
54. Merritt, K.; Brown, S.A. Distribution of Cobalt Chromium Wear and Corrosion Products and Biologic Reactions. *Clin. Orthop. Relat. Res.* **1996**, *329*, 233–243. [CrossRef]
55. Hart, A.J.; Sabah, S.A.; Bandi, A.S.; Maggiore, P.; Tarassoli, P.; Sampson, B.; Skinner, J.A. Sensitivity and Specificity of Blood Cobalt and Chromium Metal Ions for Predicting Failure of Metal-on-Metal Hip Replacement. *J. Bone Jt. Surg. Br. Vol.* **2011**, *93-B*, 1308–1313. [CrossRef]
56. Lohmann, C.H.; Meyer, H.; Nuechtern, J.V.; Singh, G.; Schmotzer, H.; Morlock, M.M. Periprosthetic Tissue Metal Content but Not Serum Metal Content Predicts the Type of Tissue Response in Failed Small-Diameter Metal-on-Metal Total Hip Arthroplasties. *J. Bone Jt. Surg.* **2013**, *95*, 1561–1568. [CrossRef]
57. Cicciù, M.; Fiorillo, L.; Herford, A.S.; Crimi, S.; Bianchi, A.; D'Amico, C.; Laino, L.; Cervino, G. Bioactive Titanium Surfaces: Interactions of Eukaryotic and Prokaryotic Cells of Nano Devices Applied to Dental Practice. *Biomedicines* **2019**, *7*, 12. [CrossRef]
58. Cervino, G.; Fiorillo, L.; Iannello, G.; Santonocito, D.; Risitano, G.; Cicciù, M. Sandblasted and Acid Etched Titanium Dental Implant Surfaces Systematic Review and Confocal Microscopy Evaluation. *Materials (Basel)* **2019**, *12*, 1763. [CrossRef]
59. Howell, J.R. Cemented Hip Arthroplasty: Why I Do It. *Orthop. Trauma* **2018**, *32*, 13–19. [CrossRef]
60. Thomas, S.R.; Shukla, D.; Latham, P.D. Corrosion of Cemented Titanium Femoral Stems. *J. Bone Jt. Surg. Br.* **2004**, *86-B*, 974–978. [CrossRef]
61. Cohen, J. Current Concepts Review. Corrosion of Metal Orthopaedic Implants. *J. Bone Jt. Surg. Am.* **1998**, *80*, 1554. [CrossRef]
62. Cadosch, D.; Sutanto, M.; Chan, E.; Mhawi, A.; Gautschi, O.P.; von Katterfeld, B.; Simmen, H.P.; Filgueira, L. Titanium Uptake, Induction of RANK-L Expression, and Enhanced Proliferation of Human T-Lymphocytes. *J. Orthop. Res.* **2010**, *28*, 341–347. [CrossRef]
63. Dmd, R.T.; Albrektsson, T.; Dds, S.G.; Prgomet, Z.; Tengvall, P.; Dds, A.W. Osseointegration and Foreign Body Reaction: Titanium Implants Activate the Immune System and Suppress Bone Resorption during the First 4 Weeks after Implantation. *Clin. Implant Dent. Relat. Res.* **2018**, *2017*, 82–91. [CrossRef]

64. Cadosch, D.; Chan, E.; Gautschi, O.P.; Meagher, J.; Zellweger, R.; Filgueira, L. Titanium IV Ions Induced Human Osteoclast Differentiation and Enhanced Bone Resorption in Vitro. *J. Biomed. Mater. Res. A* **2009**, *91*, 29–36. [CrossRef]
65. Nuevo-Ordóñez, Y.; Montes-Bayón, M.; Blanco-González, E.; Paz-Aparicio, J.; Raimundez, J.D.; Tejerina, J.M.; Peña, M.A.; Sanz-Medel, A. Titanium Release in Serum of Patients with Different Bone Fixation Implants and Its Interaction with Serum Biomolecules at Physiological Levels. *Anal. Bioanal. Chem.* **2011**, *401*, 2747–2754. [CrossRef]
66. Lazarinis, S.; Mäkelä, K.T.; Eskelinen, A.; Havelin, L.; Hallan, G.; Overgaard, S.; Pedersen, A.B.; Kärrholm, J.; Hailer, N.P. Does Hydroxyapatite Coating of Uncemented Cups Improve Long-Term Survival? An Analysis of 28,605 Primary Total Hip Arthroplasty Procedures from the Nordic Arthroplasty Register Association (NARA). *Osteoarthr. Cartil.* **2017**, *25*, 1980–1987. [CrossRef]
67. Hailer, N.P.; Lazarinis, S.; Mäkelä, K.T.; Eskelinen, A.; Fenstad, A.M.; Hallan, G.; Havelin, L.; Overgaard, S.; Pedersen, A.B.; Mehnert, F.; et al. Hydroxyapatite Coating Does Not Improve Uncemented Stem Survival after Total Hip Arthroplasty! *Acta Orthop.* **2015**, *86*, 18–25. [CrossRef]
68. Fage, S.W.; Muris, J.; Jakobsen, S.S.; Thyssen, J.P. Titanium: A Review on Exposure, Release, Penetration, Allergy, Epidemiology, and Clinical Reactivity. *Contact Dermat.* **2016**, *74*, 323–345. [CrossRef]
69. Thyssen, J.P.; Jensen, P.; Carlsen, B.C.; Engkilde, K.; Menné, T.; Johansen, J.D. The Prevalence of Chromium Allergy in Denmark Is Currently Increasing as a Result of Leather Exposure. *Br. J. Dermatol.* **2009**, *161*, 1288–1293. [CrossRef]
70. Mishra, P.K.; Wu, W.; Rozo, C.; Hallab, N.J.; Benevenia, J.; Gause, W.C. Micrometer-Sized Titanium Particles Can Induce Potent Th2-Type Responses through TLR4-Independent Pathways. *J. Immunol.* **2011**, *187*, 6491–6498. [CrossRef]
71. Eger, M.; Hiram-Bab, S.; Liron, T.; Sterer, N.; Carmi, Y.; Kohavi, D.; Gabet, Y. Mechanism and Prevention of Titanium Particle-Induced Inflammation and Osteolysis. *Front. Immunol.* **2018**, *9*. [CrossRef]
72. Thomas, P.; Braathen, L.R.; Dörig, M.; Aubock, J.; Nestle, F.; Werfel, T.; Willert, H.G. Increased Metal Allergy in Patients with Failed Metal-on-Metal Hip Arthroplasty and Peri-Implant T-Lymphocytic Inflammation. *Allergy Eur. J. Allergy Clin. Immunol.* **2009**, *64*, 1157–1165. [CrossRef]

 © 2019 by the authors. Licensee MDPI, Basel, Switzerland. This article is an open access article distributed under the terms and conditions of the Creative Commons Attribution (CC BY) license (http://creativecommons.org/licenses/by/4.0/).

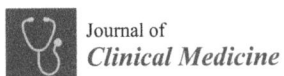

Review

Etiology and Measurement of Peri-Implant Crestal Bone Loss (CBL)

Adrien Naveau [1,2], Kouhei Shinmyouzu [3,4], Colman Moore [5], Limor Avivi-Arber [6], Jesse Jokerst [5,7,8] and Sreenivas Koka [9,10,11],*

1. Department of Prosthodontics, Dental Science Faculty, University of Bordeaux, 33000 Bordeaux, France; Adrien.naveau@laposte.net
2. Dental and Periodontal Rehabilitation Unit, Saint Andre Hospital, Bordeaux University Hospital, 33000 Bordeaux, France
3. Department of Oral Implants, Kyushu Dental University, Kitakyushu, Fukuoka 803-8580, Japan; k.shinmyouzu@spice.ocn.ne.jp
4. Tanpopo Dental Clinic, Nerima ward, Tokyo 178-0062, Japan
5. Department of NanoEngineering, University of California San Diego, La Jolla, CA 92093, USA; cam081@eng.ucsd.edu (C.M.); jjokerst@eng.ucsd.edu (J.J.)
6. Faculty of Dentistry, University of Toronto, Toronto M5G1G6, ON M5G 1G6, Canada; Limor.Avivi-Arber@dentistry.utoronto.ca
7. Materials Science Program, University of California San Diego, La Jolla, CA 92093, USA
8. Department of Radiology, University of California San Diego, La Jolla, CA 92093, USA
9. Private practice, Koka Dental Clinic, San Diego, CA 92111, USA
10. Advanced Prosthodontics, Loma Linda University School of Dentistry, Loma Linda, CA 92350, USA
11. Advanced Prosthodontics, University of California Los Angeles School of Dentistry, Los Angeles, CA 90095, USA
* Correspondence: skoka66@gmail.com; Tel.: +1-858-268-5020

Received: 31 December 2018; Accepted: 24 January 2019; Published: 1 February 2019

Abstract: The etiology of peri-implant crestal bone loss is today better understood and certain factors proposed in the past have turned out to not be of concern. Regardless, the incidence of crestal bone loss remains higher than necessary and this paper reviews current theory on the etiology with a special emphasis on traditional and innovative methods to assess the level of crestal bone around dental implants that will enable greater sensitivity and specificity and significantly reduce variability in bone loss measurement.

Keywords: Crestal bone loss; osseosufficiency; osseoseparation; peri-implantitis; photoacoustic ultrasound; brain–bone axis; foreign body reaction; overloading; radiography; CBCT (cone beam computerized tomography)

---

1. Introduction

Crestal bone loss (CBL) was relatively uncommon and non-progressing with the commercially pure titanium implants with a machined surface introduced by Per-Ingvar Branemark. It was accepted in the late 1980s and 1990s that 1 mm of CBL could be expected in the first year after implant placement and then 0.2 mm of CBL on average might occur after that. In fact, an adage took hold that with these implants, CBL to between the first and second thread is common after which time bone levels remained remarkably stable for years.

Predictably, as the application of the initial wave of implants was so successful, an expansion of clinical scenarios amenable to dental implant therapy took place. Following on, an expansion of the clinical provider pool considered appropriate to place and restore implants took place. Finally, "innovations" to the dental implant systems with the goal of fostering the expansion of clinical scenarios and provider pool also took place. Unfortunately, despite the noblest of intentions, and indeed some not so noble, the number of complications associated with dental implant therapy reported today is high. Indeed, it is far higher than necessary, and puts patients at unnecessary, and hence unjustifiable, risk for suboptimal clinical outcomes including implant loss, biological tissue loss, financial loss, and psychological trauma.

Koka and Zarb first proposed the concept of osseosufficiency to describe the role of the interplay between clinician, patient, and implant system inasmuch as promoting and perpetuating osseointegration [1]. In this model, if the combination of the ingredients that clinician (skill, knowledge, experience), patient (genetic, environmental, behavioral), and implant system (design, material) are "enough" to promote and perpetuate osseointegration, a state of osseousufficiency is attained. If the combination of ingredients is "not enough", a state of osseoinsufficiency results. Although it is commonplace to attribute implant loss as representing "implant failure", this is clearly not the case in most instances where implants are retrieved from jawbones, the main exception being when an implant body fractures. To state that an implant failed implies that the implant was at fault for its retrieval and assigns blame for the undesirable outcome to the one ingredient in the osseointegration recipe that is the most predictable and by far, compared to patient and clinician, the least variable. Conveniently, it is also the one element that is unable to defend itself in conversations about why an implant was retrieved. Clearly, albeit an uncomfortable state of affairs, most complications in implant therapy are clinician-dependent (inexperience, incompetence, or ignorance) and the remainder are patient-dependent or a combination of clinician and patient factors. Therefore, throughout this manuscript, the term "implant failure" will not be used. In the place of "implant failure", terms like "implant retrieval", "implant removal", or "implant loss" will be used to more accurately describe the clinical outcome and to avoid inaccurate assignment of blame.

One manifestation of osseoinsufficiency that has significant clinical ramifications is peri-implant CBL because it can lead to implant retrieval, osseous deformation, soft tissue deformation, esthetic compromise, and a dissatisfied/upset patient who loses confidence in their clinical provider. Clearly, prevention is better than cure when it comes to peri-implant CBL as effective and predictable methods to restore lost bone remain elusive.

Crestal bone loss has been postulated to have a multi-factorial etiology [2] and can be considered to occur early or late in the lifetime of a dental implant. Here, early means within the first year after placement and CBL observed is a consequence of bone remodeling subsequent to surgical and restorative procedures and early loading challenges undertaken by an implant and its associated prosthesis [2,3]. Given the role of adaptive bone remodeling, early CBL is not necessarily influenced by infection from oral microflora. Over the longer term, the cumulative effect of chronic etiological factors that are immunological (foreign body reaction), environmental, including patient factors such as motivation, smoking, bruxism, and infection/inflammation, and the influence of clinician (surgeon/prosthodontist) may influence late CBL [2–5]. Given that other manuscripts in this volume will address different etiological factors of CBL, in Section A, this manuscript will provide a summary of current knowledge related to two common etiological factors, mechanical overloading and periodontopathogens/perimplantopathogens/bacteria. It will also discuss the role of the immune system through the foreign body reaction mechanisms that lie at the heart of osseointegration, and describe how adverse immune reactions and a tantalizing new potential mechanism involving the brain–bone axis may lead to CBL. In Section B, it will focus on a key and related issue of how CBL is currently measured and how it can be improved in the future.

2. Section A. Selected Etiological Factors in Crestal Bone Loss

2.1. Overloading

After an implant body osseointegrates and is exposed to functional loading, Esposito et al. reported that overload of the implant prosthesis may lead to implant loss. Furthermore, the report suggests that overload contributes to peri-implantitis and is one of the major determinants of late implant retrieval [6].

There are a wide variety of experimental reports about overloading and implant therapy including computer simulations, such as finite element analysis, and in vivo and in vitro experiment. However, the results are inconclusive regarding the strength and validity of the evidence clearly linking overloading to CBL. Here, we consider the clinical significance of overloading in peri-implant CBL.

What is 'overloading'? 'Overloading' is difficult to describe but could be considered to be the force level and/or nature of force application that exceeds the permissible or tolerable range of the prosthetic and biological resistance to CBL. Each patient presents with a unique prosthetic and biological resistance profile and reference ranges of permissibility are, as yet, unknown. Hence, predicting who will be more or less susceptible to the effects of overloading is difficult. Most reports draw a conclusion of overloading based on the findings of a complication (fracture of the prosthesis, marginal bone loss etc.) as a post hoc event. Nevertheless, the complication is a result of distortion between implant and marginal bone interface caused by stress applied to the structural components of the implant prosthesis instead of the occlusal bite force itself.

Notationally, 0.1% deformation in volume is transcribed to 1000 με (microstrain). Frost et al. divided the reaction of bone as a result of strain application into four phases or "windows" according to the amount of distortion between bone and implant (Figure 1). (i) Disuse atrophy window (50–100 με). Bone resorption may result in this phase where the net effect of bone formation and resorption is negative; (ii) Steady state window (100–1500 με). Here, the net volume of the bone remains steady; (iii) Mild overload window (1500–3000 με). Here, the net effect of bone formation and resorption is positive and bone volume increases; (iv) Fatigue failure window (>3000 με). Here, bone resorption and destruction occur [6].

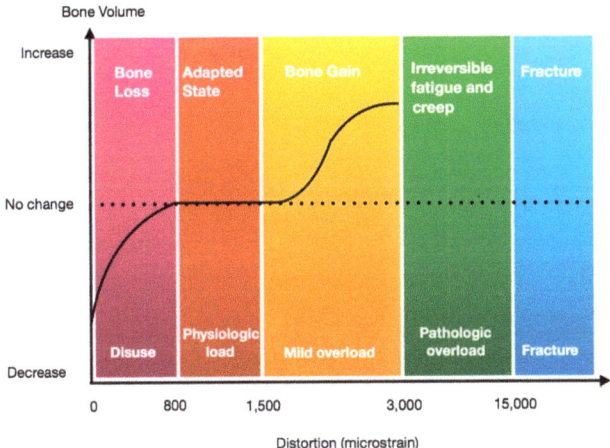

Figure 1. Diagram showing clinical effect on bone relative to strain level applied.

Theoretically, when we classify the reaction of bone to force application/distortion at the implant–bone interface, we can use Frost's definition of overload, the fatigue failure window. However, Naert et al. noted that the definition of overload in implant dentistry is more complex, open to interpretation and they suggested the range of distortion represented by Frost's fatigue failure window does not accurately represent the over load in the clinical situation [7].

Past reports focused on overload and CBL are presented in Table 1. Isidor et al. reported on crestal bone reaction following excessive occlusal load or plaque accumulation in monkeys. In this report, 6 months after insertion of implants, a fixed partial prosthesis was mounted and there were two experimental groups: Excessive occlusal over load and plaque accumulation. A loss of osseointegration and/or CBL was observed 4.5 months to 15.5 months after overloading was initiated. None of the implants with plaque accumulation experienced CBL [8]. Miyata et al. reported the influence of controlled occlusal overload on peri-implant tissue, again in monkeys and in this model, supra-occlusal contact was applied for four weeks to implants starting fourteen weeks after insertion. Neither inflammation nor CBL was observed when supra-occlusal contact was of approximately 100 microns. In contrast, CBL was observed in the group with supra-occlusal contact was over 180 microns. The authors concluded that peri-implant CBL occurred with 180 microns or more of supra-occlusion [9]. Esaki et al. reported the relationship between the magnitude of immediate loading and peri-implant osteogenesis in a canine model [10]. In this report, immediate load (0 N, 10 N, 50 N) using a cyclic loading device was applied to implants placed in healed sites. In the 10 N group, newly formed bone was observed over a wide area from the implant neck toward the tip. In contrast, in the 50 N group, newly formed bone was rarely observed around the neck and signs of infection were seen. The authors suggested there is a certain load that is beneficial and promotes osteogenesis and an overload threshold that is detrimental. Heitz-Mayfield et al. evaluated the effect of excessive occlusal load following placement of implants in dog [11]. After six months of healing after implant insertion, supra-occlusal crowns were placed. At eight months, all implants were osseointegrated with no statistically difference between test and control implants observed with regard to osseous response.

Table 1. Animal experiments about biological complications related to implant loading.

Year	Animal Model	Loading Pattern	Bone Resorption	Healing Period	Loading Period	Implant System
Isidor [9]	Monkey mandible	10–300 N330 N/s for 5 days	Yes	6 months	4–15 months	Astra
Miyata et al. [10]	Monkey mandible	Supra-occlusal contact	Yes	3.5 months	4 weeks	Intra-mobile element (IMZ)
Heitz-Mayfield et al. [12]	Dog mandible	Supra-occlusal contact	No	6 months	8 months	Straumann
Esaki et al. [11]	Dog mandible	Immediate load	Yes	None	3 weeks	Branemark

Although each of the experiments described above employed different experimental models, taken together, it is clear that certain dynamic force applications influence CBL and bone formation around implants. Managing occlusal loading to achieve desirable effects and prevent undesirable effects is an important consideration during treatment planning and treatment.

In recent years, attention has been paid to osseous activity at the molecular level when force is applied to bone. As a result of technological advances of technology, the role of the osteocyte has become better understood.

Osteocytes are most abundant bone cell in the adult skeleton and function as mechanosensors directing osteoblast and osteoclast function in order to maintain the optimal integrity of load bearing bone. Early histologists upon observing enlarged osteocyte lacunae in bone sections proposed that mature osteocytes could remove their perilacunar matrix, a term called "osteocytic osteolysis". New insights into this process have occurred during the last decade using novel technology thereby providing a means to identify molecular mechanisms responsible for osteocytic osteolysis [12].

Dendritic osteocytes connect to the vasculature, to each other and to periosteal bone surface cells creating a broad communication network within bone tissue. Osteocytes lie in a fluid-filled interstitium of lacunae and canaliculi and are capable of sensing when mechanical load that applied to the skeleton [13]. In response to force application, osteocytes react to and transmit information via secretion of molecules with a signaling function such as sclerostin and receptor activator of nuclear factor kappa-B ligand (RANKL) which then regulate bone matrix turnover by osteoblasts and osteoclasts [14,15]. Due to the recently discovered multi-functionality of osteocytes, ranging from phosphate homeostasis to interaction with distant organs, the regulation of the osteoblast–osteoclast axis is one mechanism by which the osteocyte network contributes to mechanosensory response to loading and may lead to osteocyte apoptosis and targeted bone resorption by osteoclasts [16]. As a result of this mechanosensing communication stream, bone resorption and targeted bone remodeling, in the absence of bacterial inflammation, may change peri-implant crestal bone contours.

2.2. Peri-Implant CBL and Periodontal Pathogens

The success of implant therapy ad modum Branemark in experiencing minimal CBL led to the proposal of optimistic criteria for success of implant therapy by Albrektsson et al. in 1986 [1]. These criteria were quickly accepted as clinicians and scholars worldwide were able to achieve the criteria proposed based on $\leq$1–2 mm of CBL in the first year after placement and $\leq$0.2 mm mean CBL bone loss in subsequent years. The fact that these criteria were based on clinical outcomes from implant therapy in edentulous patients/subjects was appreciated and concern remained that implants placed in partially edentulous patients with their dental reservoirs of periodontopathogens would not be able to duplicate the excellent crestal bone response seen in edentulous patients. These concerns were laid to rest by Van Steenberghe et al. who, from multi-center study findings published in 1993, clearly demonstrated that implant therapy ad modum Branemark in partially edentulous patients also exhibited the same excellent resistance to CBL as observed in edentulous patients [17].

Nevertheless, in the relatively uncommon cases of CBL seen, the concurrent peri-implant mucosal inflammation and bacterial cultures yielding traditional periodontopathogens spawned an erroneous belief system that peri-implant CBL was fashioned after the same etiology as periodontitis. This despite that nowhere else in the human body is an artificial substitute considered to be the same as the original biological tissue: A man-made substance is yet to be fabricated that is identical to natural tissue (see next section). Today, one comes across people who simultaneously claim that bone created from an allograft is different to native bone and yet who argue that periodontal bone loss is the same as peri-implant CBL and should be prevented, diagnosed, and treated similarly. The use of the term peri-implantitis has merely cemented the error of association in the minds of clinicians and scholars despite the fact that, to date, there is no clear and compelling evidence that peri-implant CBL is primarily a consequence of bacterial insult. Of course, many of the same bacteria are found in diseased periodontal and peri-implant sites, more a consequence of anaerobic environments that lend themselves to colonization and propagation of these bacteria [18]. The osseosufficiency model presents the patient as an important element of the path towards successful implant therapy. Yet, it is critical to recognize that is the host response of the patient that is important, not the presence or absence or site concentration of specific bacterial species that prevails and the host response to an artificial implant substitute is markedly different than the host response to a natural tooth. Once peri-implant CBL or inflammation is observed, addressing the bacterial component may alleviate the symptoms and signs, but it will not address the root cause of the problem which is more likely to be improper diagnosis, treatment planning and treatment by the unaware clinician that then leads to peri-implant CBL.

Further erroneous implications are engendered when research models used to study periodontitis are applied to the dental implant ecosystem, most notably, the use of ligature-induced peri-implantitis canine model that creates an artificial scenario by which bacterial inflammation is induced around implants in order to study the degree of CBL. Clinically irrelevant periods of oral hygiene cessation, sometimes 4 months in duration, are combined with the introduction of plaque-attracting sulcular ligatures in order to create a scenario that bears no resemblance to clinical practice and which, therefore, have no clinical meaning [19,20].

2.3. Bone and the Immune System—Foreign Body Reaction

Any foreign-body implant that is placed in contact with vital tissues can activate the immune/inflammatory systems whereby under normal conditions the defense cells, including neutrophils, lymphocytes, reactive pro-inflammatory macrophages (i.e., M1 and OsteoMac), and osteoclasts are activated and engulf and then digest the foreign body. The repair cells, such as fibroblasts, osteoblasts as well as macrophages (M2 and OsteoMacs) are also activated and assist in tissue repair and remodeling, and protection of the tissues from further destruction. However, when a foreign body is too large to be engulfed or digested by the immune cells, a fibrous (granuloma) or osseous encapsulation of the foreign body is formed around the foreign body. This encapsulation isolates the foreign body from the surrounding tissue and is characterized by a chronic presence of macrophages and multinucleated foreign body giant cells (i.e., Langerhan's cells) at the foreign-body surface. These foreign-body giant cells are the result of fusion of monocytes and macrophages activated upon adherence to the foreign-body surface during the earlier inflammation and tissue-repair stages. While these giant cells may present throughout the foreign-body life-time, it is unclear whether they remain active or become inactive with time. Another possible immune reaction to a foreign-body occurs when the immune response is too vigorous or too prolonged, or its function is disrupted. In such situations, the defense/repair balance may shift towards chronic inflammation and chronic tissue destruction [21–24].

In the case of dental implants (see above), it is well established that when titanium implants are placed in the jaw-bone, an evoked inflammatory reaction is followed by formation of new bone in close approximation around the implant. Subsequently, a long-lasting (i.e., implant lifetime) steady state bone remodeling activity is established which maintains the bone around the implant including the marginal bone level height. This process has been named by Branemark 'osseointegration', whereby titanium has been considered an immunologically inert material that supports the bone healing process. It was Donath et al [25] who first suggested that in fact, this reaction of bone-tissue engulfing a dental implant is consistent with a protective foreign body immune response whereby the bone formed around the implant isolates it and thus protects the surrounding bone marrow tissue (Figure 2). This hypothesis has been further investigated and subsequently supported by the Wennerberg and Albrektsson group and others who have further suggested that once new bone is formed around the implant, maintenance of a balance between bone resorption and bone formation (i.e., 'foreign-body equilibrium') can maintain the osseointegration and the marginal bone height around the implants [4,21,22,26–33]. Albrektsson and colleagues have proposed a revised definition of osseointegration to state that "osseointegration is a foreign body reaction where interfacial bone is formed as a defense reaction to shield off the implant from the tissues [34] and further elucidated the importance of host response in long-term osseointegration outcomes [35]. However, the majority of the studies on foreign-body response are in vitro studies or studies that have utilized titanium or other biomaterial implants placed in limb bones or other body tissues. In vitro studies have shown that titanium can activate macrophages [30], and that complement factors in blood plasma binds to titanium implant surface which suggests that during the early stage of inflammation following titanium implant placement, the implant surfaces can be recognized by the immune cells through complement factors in the blood [36]. In the recent study in rabbits, it has been shown that the formation and subsequent maintenance of new bone around titanium implants placed in a femur bone are associated with time-dependent immune responses. These responses were manifested first (10 days) as up-regulation of immune defense cells (i.e., macrophages), and subsequently (at 28 days) by up-regulation of immune repair cells (macrophages, lymphocytes, neutrophils, and the complement system), plus down-regulation of bone-resorbing cells (osteoclasts) around the implants [33]. In addition, similar to foreign-body host response in other body parts, multinucleated giant cells are present at the dental implant–bone interface [25,37], and while these giant cells can be present throughout the implant life-time, it is unclear whether they become inactive with time, or remain active, or become active under certain conditions leading to marginal bone resorption.

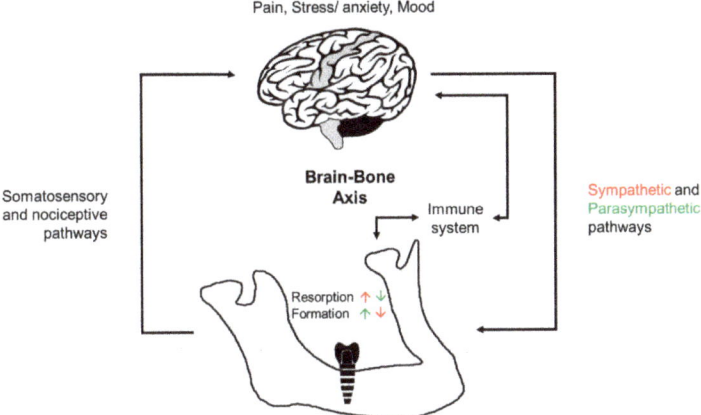

Figure 2. A diagram illustrating brain–bone axis involving the sympathetic and parasympathetic nervous systems that act through direct and direct neuronal innervation of bone tissue (black arrows). Centrally modulated sympathetic activity inhibits osteoblasts and bone formation and enhances osteoclast activity and bone resorption (red), while centrally modulated parasympathetic activity enhances osteoblast activity and bone formation and inhibits osteoclasts and bone resorption (green). Somatosensory and nociceptive inputs from the bone to the brain as well as pain, stress, and mood responses can impact bone formation and resorption either directly through the autonomic nervous system or indirectly through activation of the immune system that can also be activated directly by bone injury.

Considering the intimate relations between the immune system and bone healing and remodeling, when the immune response to titanium implants is coupled with certain factors or health conditions that impact the immune system or the immune response, the balance between osteoblast and osteoclast activity can shift during the healing phase from a net bone apposition to a net bone resorption resulting in osseointegration failure or unwarranted CBL. Moreover, since osseointegration is a dynamic state of bone remodeling, these factors or health conditions may also impact the osseointegration after it had already been established. These factors or conditions include genetic factors, immunosuppressed diseases, smoking, poorly controlled surgery, excess cement, and medications [26,38–42]. Therefore, patient examination and medical history taking should be evaluated not only prior to implant placement, but also on a regular basis as part of the postoperative follow-up appointments. Other possible causes for impaired bone healing or marginal bone loss could be titanium ion leakage, titanium particles detachment and implant surface contamination with metal or organic particles that are residues of the implant manufacturing, implant cleaning and handling, surgical placement or prosthetic installation processes, as well as prosthetic materials [43,44]. Such particles in the bone surrounding the dental implants can induce chronic inflammatory reaction and immune response which include activation of immune cell mediators such as cytokines (e.g., tumor necrosis factor-alpha (TNF-α)) that can influence the activities of osteoblasts and osteoclasts and thereby impact on bone healing and bone turnover around the implants [29,45–47]. On the other hand, if osseointegration had already occurred, considering osseointegration is dynamic, the above-mentioned factors can also impact bone homeostasis and shift bone turnover into a net bone resorption manifested as aseptic osseoseparation and/or marginal bone resorption (see above). This condition is considered aseptic since its initiation does not involve the oral microbiota however, this does not rule out the possibility of a secondary bacterial infection or a bacterial-derived marginal bone resorption in individual cases [4,22,26,27,29,34,35,47,48].

2.4. The Role of the Brain in Modulating Osseointegration: Brain–Bone Axis

Novel evidence suggests that the brain and the nervous system in general play vital roles in long-bone healing and remodeling processes [49–51]. Complex neural networks exist between the central nervous system and the bones, and nerve fibers of sympathetic, parasympathetic, and somatic origin innervate long bones [52,53]. Furthermore, nerve-derived neuropeptides [e.g., neuropeptide Y, endocannabinoids (CB)], and neurotransmitters (e.g., norepinephrine, dopamine, serotonin, and calcitonin gene-related peptide) were found in the vicinity of long-bone cells that express receptors for these neuropeptides (e.g., β2-adrenergic, Y1 (the name of the receptor) and Y2 (the name of the receptor), CB1 and CB2) and neurotransmitters (e.g., dopamine, and serotonin). These neuropeptides, neurotransmitters and receptors can in turn contribute to the regulatory mechanisms underlying bone remodeling [49,54]. In addition, the central nervous system can integrate internal (e.g., glycemia, menstruation hormones) and external signals that can impact brain control of bone formation and remodeling [51]. For example, experimental denervation of sensory and sympathetic nerve fibers can impact bone development and remodeling [55,56]. While nerve fibers of sympathetic, parasympathetic, and somatic origin also innervate jaw-bones including extraction sockets and peri-implant tissues [53,57–61], no information is available on the role of the nervous system in the healing and remodeling of jaw bones.

Recent studies have also shown important functional links between the central nervous system and the immune system that as we have discussed above plays a key role in peri-implant bone healing. Immune organs, such as lymphoid organs (e.g., lymph nodes, spleen) are innervated by sympathetic and parasympathetic nerve fibers of the autonomic nervous system which can in turn control bone remodeling [52,62]. The notion that the brain can modulate the immune response is also supported by studies showing the effects of mental and physical stress on the general health and immunity [63]. Moreover, usage of central nervous system medications (e.g., opioids, antidepressants, anticonvulsants) as well as depression conditions are associated with low bone mass and increased risk of osteoporosis and fractures [64]. It is interesting to note that recent studies have shown that impaired osseointegration and failures of dental implants are higher in patients treated with antidepressant drugs (selective serotonin reuptake inhibitors) [65–67]. However, it is unclear if the increased loss of osseointegration is produced by the drug or by the mental health condition itself and the impaired communication between the nervous system, immune system and bone healing and remodeling and thus, more robust research is required to identify the exact cause of osseointegration loss.

Another evidence for the role of the brain in bone growth in general comes from the effects of growth hormones in regulating bones growth during development, and bone remodeling throughout life. Growth hormones are secreted from the cerebral pituitary gland under the control of the cerebral hypothalamus. In fact, growth hormones can induce proliferation and activation of both osteoblasts and osteoclasts with an overall net effect of either bone growth, bone resorption or homeostasis [68]. Furthermore, growth hormones play a crucial role in fracture healing, and novel therapeutic approaches utilizing growth hormones (and other growth factors) to improve long bone healing are currently under investigation and development [69].

Altogether, the clinical significance of these studies on brain–bone axis (Figure 2) lies in them providing novel potential therapeutic targets for modulating bone remodeling. Thus, research is needed to gain a better understanding of the possible role of brain–immune system interaction also on jaw-bone remodeling and peri-implant bone healing and CBL.

3. Section B. Methods of Measuring Crestal Bone Loss

3.1. Current Methods

The need for measuring CBL has come with the spectrum of osseoseparation and peri-implantitis. A "lifetime" treatment for a patient requires osseosufficiency, i.e., the harmonious relationship between the host, the implant, and the clinician [3]. The rise of osseointegration science (and related expectations) led to the preservation of crestal bone height after implant placement in the context of quantitative success criteria for implant osseointegration. Monitoring changes in the bony anchorage routinely, at regular intervals, was advocated [1]. In this context, X-ray imaging techniques naturally emerged as a convenient tool for characterizing the marginal bone loss.

Change in bone height (loss or gain) represents the difference in bone levels at the same site at separate time-points. The initial reference bone level value is subtracted from each of the later values, usually but not always, resulting in a negative measurement representing loss of crestal bone. The initial reference is often recorded either right after implant placement (post-operative value) or once the implant becomes functionally loaded (prosthetic loading). These calculations compare the vertical distance between the crestal bone level at the implant contact and a reference point on the implant (implant platform for example), and as a consequence, should be referred as "distance to bone" values than to "bone level" values. Clinical routine measurements are often reported at the tenth of millimeter, while experimental ones may exhibit more accuracy.

To be consistent, the use of a single technique for both measurements is recommended (same imaging materials, same settings and same measure method). Then the known implant diameter, platform diameter, implant length or distance between two threads of screw-type implants may be used for calibration [70].

In the scientific literature, various imaging techniques have been used for measuring CBL, such as standardized intraoral radiographs (SIR), panoramic radiographs, computerized tomography scans, and cone beam computerized tomography (CBCT) scans [71]. The accuracy of the measurements have usually been assessed on jaws from animals or human cadavers, and those studies have repeatedly showed that panoramic radiographs lack reproducibility and resolution due to structure distortions and superimpositions, while computed tomography scans are affected by metal artifacts combined with an excessive exposure dose [71]. Today, SIR and CBCT appear to be the appropriate methods for routine assessment of crestal bone levels on living patients.

3.1.1. Standardized Intraoral Radiographs (SIR)

Standardized intraoral (or periapical) radiographs have historically been, and remain to be, the most commonly used method for longitudinal assessment of peri-implant bone loss. For limiting distortion, the long cone paralleling technique is preferred to the intra-oral bisecting angle technique [72,73]. This technique, routinely used in periodontology, consists in holding the radiographic film parallel to the long axis of the implant and placing the X-ray beam perpendicularly to the receptor [74]. This paralleling technique requires the use of a film holder for routine clinical care, but for research purpose, a customized occlusal bite jig may be also fabricated to standardize the procurement of the implant image at different time points. The bite jig improves comparative measurements by limiting the parallax effect (apparent displacement of bony structures when radiographs are taken from different angles). The bite jig, typically fabricated from silicone, wax, or resin, is a repositioning key that fits to the film holder and can be stored by the dentist until next use. In some clinical studies, the bite jig is clipped on the attachment (locator, ball) or screwed into the implant. However, bone level interventions are not advocated as they may predispose to the bone loss. Some interesting devices have been described for the assessment of functional implants, such as a bite jig designed to be perpendicular to the initial implant placement driver [75].

Periapical radiographs used to be obtained on conventional films; however, the use of digital radiography is expanding in dental practice. When routine measurements are performed on conventional films, a magnifying lens can be used. Nowadays however, most research protocols incorporate high-resolution digitalization of a conventionally-obtained radiograph film. When routine measurements are performed directly with digital radiography, a sliding gauge tool can be used with most of the currently-available radiograph-related software to assess the distance between the crestal bone and the implant reference-point chosen. For research purposes, a method called the digital subtraction technique has been developed to directly measure bone loss by superimposing two serial radiographic images before subtracting them to isolate/quantify bone changes using specially-designed software [72].

Accuracy

Measurement accuracy is the closeness of agreement between measured and the true bone level. The accuracy relies not only on the resolution and sharpness of the radiographic material, but also on many clinical parameters, such as the degree of CBL, the jaw anatomy and configuration, the delay between placement and function, and the quantity of serial radiographs on the same implant [76].

When using a magnifying lens, e.g. ×10, with conventional SIR, inter- and intra-observer variability were shown to be approximately 0.14 mm and 0.08 mm respectively [76]. Conventional film and digital radiography exhibit the same accuracy [77]. Digitized conventional films may exhibit more noise artifacts and may lose density range but still provide comparable measurements [77,78].

Sensitivity and Specificity

In our context, the sensitivity of a radiographic technique consists in detecting the presence of crestal bone, while its specificity is about correctly detecting the bone (or defect) absence. These parameters have been tested in animals or in cadaver studies, when bone level estimations can be compared to the physical measurements. In a recent meta-analysis pooling the results of 5 studies, the SIR exhibited clinically acceptable sensitivity (60% when pooled; 56–100%) and specificity (59% when pooled; 51–98%) [71]. SIR detected more precisely large defects (around 3 mm) than small ones (1–2 mm) [71,79,80]. As a consequence, many authors reported the proximal bone loss to be underestimated by SIR measurements [81–83].

Pros and Cons

The primary advantages of SIR are the low exposure dose and being the least invasive of all the radiographic techniques. Combined with its low cost, the reliability of linear distance measurements, easy access and easy handling for dentists, this technique remains the gold standard for routine clinical measurements.

However, only the mesial and distal CBL can be assessed with this technique. Furthermore, in the context of peri-implantitis, proximal bone levels were often shown to be more apical than the radiographically measured ones [81–83]. The tangential measurements can be affected by geometric distortions and anatomical superimpositions, especially since a strict parallel projection is difficult to obtain in some clinical situations [84]. In addition, SIR do not allow identification of the 3D morphology of a bone defect (intra-bony and supracrestal components) that influences diagnosis, prognosis and treatment planning [83,85,86].

3.1.2. Cone Beam Computerized Tomography (CBCT)

The use of CBCT, also called digital volume tomography, to assess peri-implant bone level is more recent as this technology emerged in dentistry only 20 years ago. Compared with traditional CT, the lower irradiation dose and less severe metallic artifacts raised opportunities for new dental applications.

In comparison with SIRs, CBCT image quality relies mainly on the technological performance of the material. Some of the most influencing parameters are the voxel size and the field of view. Indeed, image resolution is related to the size of volume elements, called voxels, which are often cubes (with edge ranging from 0.08–0.3 mm in research studies on peri-implant defects). However, small voxels come with additional noise [87]. Also, the field of view defines the volume of interest undergoing examination (cube ranging from 4×4 to 8×8 cm) and influences accuracy. This technological parameter is determined by the available detector, beam projection geometry and beam collimation. Small voxels and small fields of view improve measurements; but seeking the most precise peri-implant morphology when combining these two parameters will still deliver high radiation levels [80,88]. Image reconstruction parameters and filter software (used to lower metal artifacts) also influence the performance quality of the peri-implant measurements [89,90].

Accuracy

As previously mentioned, CBCT accuracy is defined by the field of view size, but also by the device scan mode and arc of rotation [91–93]. Indeed, the full-scan mode (360°) provides a higher diagnostic accuracy for peri-implant defects [90]. A recent systematic review concluded that large defects are more accurately detected than small ones, and that circumferential and fenestration peri-implant defects are more accurately detected than dehiscence defects [94].

Experimental measurements of peri-implant defects showed very low deviation when compared with direct measurement (0.18 ± 0.12 mm) and the proximal values were comparable to those obtained with periapical radiographs [95,96]. The spatial resolution can reach around 150–200 µm [72,97].

Sensitivity and Specificity

In a recent meta-analysis pooling the results of 9 studies, the CBCT exhibited clinically acceptable sensitivity (59% when pooled; 28–97%) and specificity (67% when pooled; 25–97%) [71]. Sensitivity globally increases with small voxels but remains challenged by small defects [90]. On the other hand, some authors suggested that specificity may increase with bigger voxels [80]. Filters can improve the detection of true positive or negative values [90].

Pros & Cons

When compared with SIR, CBCT delivers more radiation to patients, is more expensive for the patient and for the medical team, and has relatively limited availability. Metal artifacts (streaking, beam hardening, or scatter) increase with CBCT low energy settings and may add some false-positive bone on the vestibular side and false-negative bone on the other sides [96].

Both SIR and CBCT are interesting and validated imaging techniques for measuring peri-implant CBL. Their accuracy, sensitivity, and specificity are clinically acceptable [71,98]. On one hand, SIR provides only proximal values, but the data obtained often are sufficient to confirm changes in peri-implant CBL. On the other hand, CBCT exposes the patient to higher cost and radiation dose but offers a 3D characterization of the peri-implant defect. For these reasons, SIR remains the gold standard for routine assessment of bone level changes and for helping in peri-implantitis diagnosis, while CBCT is still confined to providing clear 3D images of diagnosed peri-implantitis that require a treatment plan [71,94,99]. In the future, CBL assessment may not be in X-ray imaging but rather in non-invasive 3D procedures such as ultrasound [100].

3.2. Novel Method: Photoacoustic Ultrasound as an Innovative Method to Measure Peri-Implant Pocket Depths and Bone Loss over Time

Ultrasound is the most widely used clinical imaging modality in medicine but has limited deployment in dental and periodontal practices [101]. In recent years, however, the number of preclinical dental applications of ultrasound has been increasing [102]. The advantages of ultrasound include the ability to image soft tissues in real-time without ionizing radiation at a relatively low cost.

One of the drawbacks of ultrasound is its limited contrast (signal from target versus signal from background). Contrast in conventional ultrasound is a function in differences in the acoustic impedance of different tissue types. Photoacoustic imaging is a hybrid form of ultrasound that can overcome this limitation and increase the contrast of ultrasound (Figure 3) [103]. It has a rapidly growing number of applications and uses optical—rather than acoustic—excitation to harness the photoacoustic effect. Photoacoustic imaging converts the incident light into sound following absorption and thermoelastic expansion of a target material [104]. It combines the good spatial and temporal resolution of ultrasound with the contrast and spectral imaging capabilities of optics. Typically, the optical excitation source (5–50 ns pulses at ~ 5 Hz) is a pulsed near-infrared laser (Nd:YAG/OPO) but low-power LED sources can also be used [105]. These pulses are absorbed by tissue, and the energy is released acoustically and detected by ultrasound transducers with center frequencies in the MHz range. The coupling of fiber optics with ultrasound transducers allows simultaneous ultrasound and photoacoustic imaging [106]. A variety of algorithms can be used for image reconstruction to maximize contrast, resolution, and signal-to-noise [107–110].

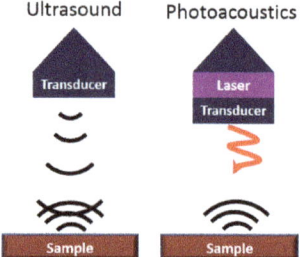

Figure 3. Acoustic Modalities. Ultrasound uses echoes to create contrast ("sound in/sound out"). Photoacoustics is "light in/sound out" and is based on thermal expansion of the target tissue or contrast agent.

The most common uses of photoacoustic imaging are image-guided therapies [111], diagnosis of disease states [112,113], surgeries [114,115], and drug delivery [116,117]. These applications can be achieved through either endogenous or exogenous contrast. Endogenous contrast is based on the optical absorption of naturally occurring targets such as oxygenated/deoxygenated hemoglobin, melanin, lipids, and water [118]. Exogenous contrast mechanisms leverage the absorption of materials such as small-molecule dyes, fluorophores, and nanoparticles that originate from outside of the body [119]. In both cases, because photoacoustic intensity is proportional to optical absorption, light sources with specific wavelengths can be used for spectral differentiation between materials according to their absorption spectra.

Imaging the Periodontal Pocket with Photoacoustic Ultrasound

Assessment of periodontal disease uses physical measurements (e.g., attachment level, probing depth, bone loss, mobility, recession, and degree of inflammation) [120]. Periodontal probing offers a numerical metric that reflects the extent of apical epithelial attachment relative to the gingival margin [121] but suffers from poor reproducibility due to variation in probing force [122]. Indeed, a recent meta-analysis showed a wide range of probing forces (51 to 995 N/cm^2)—a variation of ~20-fold [123]. Other error sources include variation in the insertion point, probe angulation, the patient's overall gingival health (weakly inflamed tissue), and the presence of calculus [121,124]. Thus, the exam is subject to large errors with inter-operator variation as high as 40% with r values between technicians <0.80 [125]. These errors can hamper clinical decision-making and epidemiological studies ultimately resulting in poor patient outcomes [126]. Furthermore, many patients find probing to be uncomfortable or painful—this can prevent patients from seeking care [127,128]. Moreover, the periodontal probing is time consuming for the practitioners. It is perhaps not surprising that periodontal examination was not performed in 50–90% of the audited dental records offices [129–131]. Finally, the benefit of traditional periodontal probing around implants is abrogated due to implant threads that impede probe penetration along the implant surface [132,133]. This limits the clinical assessment of these tissues, potentially leading to peri-implantitis [134,135].

The first study to use photoacoustic imaging for visualizing pocket depths was conducted by Lin et al. in 2017 [136]. A commercially available tomographic system (Visualsonics Vevo LAZR) was used for imaging porcine jaws extracted from frozen cadavers. A food-grade contrast agent containing melanin nanoparticles derived from cuttlefish ink was used to increase the photoacoustic signal of the pockets. This material acted as a safe, highly absorbing material capable of filling the gingival sulcus following oral irrigation. It had broad absorbance and photoacoustic signal.

This technique was recently expanded to a healthy young adult case [137]. The same imaging system was adapted so that a subject could be scanned while seated (Figure 4A). Here, ultrasound gel was used for coupling and a medical head immobilizer and cheek retractors were used to minimize movements from the subject; 40 MHz ultrasound was used throughout. Again, the procedure began with irrigation of the pocket followed by laser pulsing and imaging, removal of the contrast agent, and image processing. The pocket depth could be visualized for a given sagittal plane (Figure 4B–D) after administration of the agent. Because these experiments used ultrasound gel for coupling, it was common during scanning for the agent to nonspecifically coat the surface of tooth. However, this nonspecific signal could be removed in post-processing by using the ultrasound-only images to locate the gingival margin. Any signal originating from tooth surface occlusal to the margin was ignored allowing a final mapping of the pocket to be manually generated (Figure 4E). In the future, this processing step will be automated.

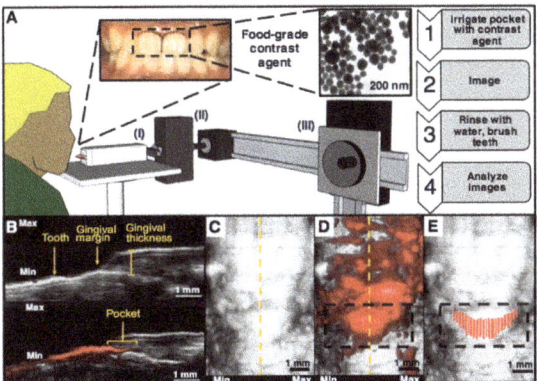

Figure 4. Representative human data of photoacoustic-ultrasound imaging for pocket depth measurements. (**A**) Overview of the imaging setup and methodology. The subject was seated in front of the transducer (I) and ultrasound gel was used for coupling. The stepper motor (II) was used for scanning the transducer and the sliding frame allowed positioning (III). First, the teeth of interest were irrigated with the contrast agent followed by imaging, removal of the agent, and image analysis. (**B**) A sagittal cross-section (dashed yellow line in Panel C) of a mandibular central incisor before (top) and after (before) irrigation with the contrast agent, revealing the pocket depth, measured from the gingival margin to the edge of photoacoustic signal. Nonspecific signal from the tooth, caused by the movement of coupling gel during scanning, did not contribute to the measurement. (**C**) A frontal view of the same tooth before (**D**) and after (**E**) irrigation. Nonspecific signal from contrast agent was removed during image processing by measuring the pocket from each sagittal plane as in Panel B and overlaying each measurement on the ultrasound-only image.

In the case of implants, physical probing is typically hindered by threads that impede probe penetration along the implant surface [132,133]. This limits the ability for clinical assessment of these tissues potentially leading to peri-implantitis [134,135]. We note that photoacoustic ultrasound has not been explicitly tested yet for imaging the pockets around implants. However, because it relies on the flow of contrast agent into the pocket rather than the physical penetration of a metal probe, the presence of implant threads should not affect measurements. For this reason, we believe photoacoustic imaging is promising for patients with implants that obstruct manual probing. Of course, additional work remains to improve the clinical feasibility of the technique including development of a mouthpiece transducer and the implementation of more affordable and stable excitation sources, such as LEDs or laser diodes.

4. Summary

New ways of appreciating CBL are blending traditional etiologies with novel mechanisms that better reconcile what was originally thought to be taking place during osseointegration with actual long-term clinical outcomes. Today, the ability to look back on osseointegration outcomes at the implant level, the prosthesis level, the patient level and even the clinician level allow us to recognize that osseointegration likely represents a form of foreign body reaction and focuses our attention on elements that, therefore, influence the immune response or the consequence of a patient's immune response. In this way, traditional etiologies such as inflammation from infection and overloading can be viewed as modulators of the immune response and the effect of immune response through neuroimmunomodulation opens up new and exciting avenues for future research.

Clinically, measuring crystal bone loss remains at the mercy of the constraints of radiographic imaging. Nevertheless, new methodologies and digital technologies portend the introduction of non-invasive methods that may be more sensitive and specific with regard to measurement of crestal bone position and changes in crestal bone position over time. Here too, innovations in imaging will allow us to better assess the effect of new techniques, products, protocols and materials.

Author Contributions: For this paper, individuals contributed to the following activities: Conceptualization, S.K.; writing—original draft preparation, A.N., K.S., C.M., L.A.-A., J.J., and S.K.; project administration, S.K.

Conflicts of Interest: The authors declare no conflict of interest.

References

1. Koka, S.; Zarb, G.A. On osseointegration: The healing adaptation principle in the context of osseosufficiency, osseoseparation, and dental implant failure. *Int. J. Prosthodont.* **2012**, *25*, 48–52. [PubMed]
2. Bryant, S.R. Oral Implant Outcomes Predicted by Age- and Site-Specific Aspects of Bone Condition. Ph.D. Thesis, University of Toronto, Toronto, ON, Canada, 2001.
3. Linkevicius, T.; Puisys, A.; Vindasuite, E.; Linkeviciene, L.; Apse, P. Does residual cement around implant-supported restorations cause peri-implant disease? A retrospective case analysis. *Clin. Oral Implants Res.* **2013**, *24*, 1179–1184. [CrossRef] [PubMed]
4. Roos-Jansaker, A.M. Long time follow up of implant therapy and treatment of peri-implantitis. *Swed. Dent. J. Suppl.* **2007**, *188*, 7–66.
5. Fransson, C.; Lekholm, U.; Jemt, T.; Berglundh, T. Prevalence of subjects with progressive bone loss. *Clin. Oral Implants Res.* **2005**, *16*, 440–446. [CrossRef] [PubMed]
6. Esposito, M.; Hirsch, J.M.; Lekholm, U.; Thomsen, P. Biological factors contributing to failures of osseointegrated oral implants. (I). Success criteria and epidemiology. *Eur. J. Oral Sci.* **1998**, *106*, 527–551. [CrossRef] [PubMed]
7. Frost, H.M. A 2003 update of bone physiology and Wolff's Law for clinicians. *Angle Orthod.* **2004**, *74*, 3–15. [PubMed]
8. Naert, I.; Duyck, J.; Vandamme, K. Occlusal overload and bone/implant loss. *Clin. Oral Implants Res.* **2012**, *23* (Suppl. 6), 95–107. [CrossRef]
9. Isidor, F. Loss of osseointegration caused by occlusal load of oral implants. *Clin. Oral Implants Res.* **1996**, *7*, 143–152. [CrossRef]
10. Miyata, T.; Kobayashi, Y.; Araki, H.; Ohto, T.; Shin, K. The influence of controlled occlusal overload on peri-implant tissue. Part 3: A histologic study in monkeys. *Int. J. Oral Maxillofac. Implants* **2000**, *15*, 425–431.
11. Esaki, D.; Matsushita, Y.; Ayukawa, Y.; Sakai, N.; Sawae, Y.; Koyano, K. Relationship between magnitude of immediate loading and peri-implant osteogenesis in dogs. *Clin. Oral Implants Res.* **2012**, *23*, 1290–1296. [CrossRef]
12. Heitz-Mayfield, L.J.; Schmid, B.; Weigel, C.; Gerber, S.; Bosshardt, D.D.; Jonsson, J.; Lang, N.P.; Jönsson, J. Does excessive occlusal load affect osseointegration? *Exp. Study Dog Clin. Oral Implants Res.* **2004**, *15*, 259–268. [CrossRef] [PubMed]
13. Tsourdi, E.; Jahn, K.; Rauner, M.; Busse, B.; Bonewald, L.F. Physiological and pathological osteocytic osteolysis. *J. Musculoskelet. Neuronal Interact.* **2018**, *18*, 292–303. [PubMed]

14. Klein-Nulend, J.; van der Plas, A.; Semeins, C.M.; Ajubi, N.E.; Frangos, J.A.; Nijweide, P.J.; Burger, E.H. Sensitivity of osteocytes to biomechanical stress in vitro. *FASEB J.* **1995**, *9*, 441–445. [CrossRef] [PubMed]
15. Van Bezooijen, R.L.; Roelen, B.A.; Visser, A.; van der Wee-Pals, L.; de Wilt, E.; Karperien, M.; Hamersma, H.; Papapoulos, S.E.; ten Dijke, P.; Löwik, C.W. Sclerostin is an osteocyte-expressed negative regulator of bone formation, but not a classical BMP antagonist. *J. Exp. Med.* **2004**, *199*, 805–814. [CrossRef] [PubMed]
16. Nakashima, T.; Hayashi, M.; Fukunaga, T.; Kurata, K.; Oh-Hora, M.; Feng, J.Q.; Bonewald, L.F.; Kodama, T.; Wutz, A.; Wagner, E.F.; et al. Evidence for osteocyte regulation of bone homeostasis through RANKL expression. *Nat. Med.* **2011**, *17*, 1231–1234. [CrossRef] [PubMed]
17. Dallas, S.L.; Prideaux, M.; Bonewald, L.F. The osteocyte: An endorine cell ... and more. *Endocr. Rev.* **2013**, *34*, 658–690. [CrossRef] [PubMed]
18. Van Steenberghe, D.; Klinge, B.; Lindén, U.; Quirynen, M.; Herrmann, I.; Garpland, C. Periodontal indices around natural and titanium abutments: A longitudinal multicenter study. *J. Periodontol.* **1993**, *64*, 538–541. [CrossRef]
19. Charalampakis, G.; Abrahamsson, I.; Carcuac, O.; Dahlén, G.; Berglundh, T. Microbiota in experimental periodontitis and peri-implantitis in dogs. *Clin. Oral Implants Res.* **2014**, *25*, 1094–1098. [CrossRef]
20. Berglundh, T.; Gotfredsen, K.; Zitzmann, N.U.; Lang, N.P.; Lindhe, J. Spontaneous progression of ligature induced peri-implantitis at implants with different surface roughness: An experimental study in dogs. *Clin. Oral Implants Res.* **2007**, *18*, 655–661. [CrossRef]
21. Carcuac, O.; Abrahamsson, I.; Albouy, J.P.; Linder, E.; Larsson, L.; Berglundh, T. Experimental periodontitis and peri-implantitis in dogs. *Clin. Oral Implants Res.* **2013**, *24*, 363–371. [CrossRef]
22. Anderson, J.M. Inflammation, wound healing, and the foreign-body response. In *Biomaterials Science: An Introduction to Materials*, 3rd ed.; Academic Press: Cambridge, UK, 2013; pp. 503–512.
23. Anderson, J.M.; Rodriguez, A.; Chang, D.T. Foreign body reaction to biomaterials. *Semin. Immunol.* **2008**, *20*, 86–100. [CrossRef] [PubMed]
24. Miron, R.J.; Zohdi, H.; Fujioka-Kobayashi, M.; Bosshardt, D.D. Giant cells around bone biomaterials: Osteoclasts or multi-nucleated giant cells? *Acta Biomater.* **2016**, *46*, 15–28. [CrossRef] [PubMed]
25. Sheikh, Z.; Sima, C.; Glogauer, M. Bone replacement materials and techniques used for achieving vertical alveolar bone augmentation. *Materials* **2015**, *8*, 2953–2993. [CrossRef]
26. Donath, K.; Laass, M.; Gunzl, H.J. The histopathology of different foreign-body reactions in oral soft tissue and bone tissue. *Virchows Archiv. A* **1992**, *420*, 131–137. [CrossRef]
27. Albrektsson, T.; Chrcanovic, B.; Molne, J.; Wennerberg, A. Foreign body reactions, marginal bone loss and allergies in relation to titanium implants. *Eur. J. Oral Implantol.* **2018**, *11* (Suppl. 1), S37–S46.
28. Albrektsson, T.; Dahlin, C.; Jemt, T.; Sennerby, L.; Turri, A.; Wennerberg, A. Is marginal bone loss around oral implants the result of a provoked foreign body reaction? *Clin. Implant Dent. Relat. Res.* **2014**, *16*, 155–165. [CrossRef] [PubMed]
29. Bielemann, A.M.; Marcello-Machado, R.M.; Del Bel Cury, A.A.; Faot, F. Systematic review of wound healing biomarkers in peri-implant crevicular fluid during osseointegration. *Arch. Oral Biol.* **2018**, *89*, 107–128. [CrossRef]
30. Kzhyshkowska, J.; Gudima, A.; Riabov, V.; Dollinger, C.; Lavalle, P.; Vrana, N.E. Macrophage responses to implants: Prospects for personalized medicine. *J. Leukoc. Biol.* **2015**, *98*, 953–962. [CrossRef]
31. Takayanagi, H. Osteoimmunology: Shared mechanisms and crosstalk between the immune and bone systems. *Nat. Rev. Immunol.* **2007**, *7*, 292–304. [CrossRef]
32. Takayanagi, H. New developments in osteoimmunology. *Nat. Rev. Rheumatol.* **2012**, *8*, 684–689. [CrossRef]
33. Trindade, R.; Albrektsson, T.; Galli, S.; Prgomet, Z.; Tengvall, P.; Wennerberg, A. Osseointegration and foreign body reaction: Titanium implants activate the immune system and suppress bone resorption during the first 4 weeks after implantation. *Clin. Implants Dent. Relat Res.* **2018**, *20*, 82–91. [CrossRef] [PubMed]
34. Trindade, R.; Albrektsson, T.; Tengvall, P.; Wennerberg, A. Foreign body reaction to biomaterials: On mechanisms for buildup and breakdown of osseointegration. *Clin. Implants Dent. Relat. Res.* **2016**, *18*, 192–203. [CrossRef] [PubMed]
35. Albrektsson, T.; Chrcanovic, B.; Jacobsson, M.; Wennerberg, A. Osseointegration of implants—A biological and clinical overview. *JSM Dent. Surg* **2017**, *2*, 1022–1027.

36. Albrektsson, T.; Jämt, T.; Molne, J.; Tengvall, P.; Wennerberg, A. On inflammation-immunological balance theory—A critical apprehension of disease concepts around implants: Mucositis and marginal bone loss may represent normal conditions and not necessarily a state of disease. *J. Clin. Implant Dent. Relat. Res.* **2019**, in press. [CrossRef] [PubMed]
37. Chappuis, V.; Cavusoglu, Y.; Gruber, R.; Kuchler, U.; Buser, D.; Bosshardt, D.D. Osseointegration of zirconia in the presence of multinucleated giant cells. *Clin. Implants Dent. Relat. Res.* **2016**, *18*, 686–698. [CrossRef] [PubMed]
38. Avivi-Arber, L.; Avivi, D.; Perez, M.; Arber, N.; Shapira, S. Impaired bone healing at tooth extraction sites in cd24-deficient mice: A pilot study. *PLoS ONE* **2018**, *13*, e0191665. [CrossRef] [PubMed]
39. Berglundh, T.; Giannobile, W.V. Investigational clinical research in implant dentistry: Beyond observational and descriptive studies. *J. Dent. Res.* **2013**, *92* (Suppl. 12), 107s–108s. [CrossRef]
40. Brånemark, P.I.; Zarb, G.A.; Albrektsson, T. *Tissue-Integrated Prostheses. Osseointegration in Clinical Dentistry*; Quintessence: Chicago, IL, USA, 1985.
41. Nishimura, I. Genetic networks in osseointegration. *J. Dent. Res.* **2013**, *92* (Suppl. 12), 109s–118s. [CrossRef]
42. Wennerberg, A.; Ide-Ektessabi, A.; Hatkamata, S.; Sawase, T.; Johansson, C.; Albrektsson, T.; Martinelli, A.; Sodervall, U.; Odelius, H. Titanium release from implants prepared with different surface roughness. *Clin. Oral Implants Res.* **2004**, *15*, 505–512. [CrossRef]
43. Delgado-Ruiz, R.; Romanos, G. Potential causes of titanium particle and ion release in implant dentistry: A systematic review. *Int J. Mol. Sci.* **2018**, *19*, 3585. [CrossRef]
44. Franchi, M.; Bacchelli, B.; Martini, D.; Pasquale, V.D.; Orsini, E.; Ottani, V.; Fini, M.; Giavaresi, G.; Giardino, R.; Ruggeri, A. Early detachment of titanium particles from various different surfaces of endosseous dental implants. *Biomaterials* **2004**, *25*, 2239–2246. [CrossRef] [PubMed]
45. Trindade, R.; Albrektsson, T.; Galli, S.; Prgomet, Z.; Tengvall, P.; Wennerberg, A. Bone Immune Response to Materials, Part I: Titanium, PEEK and Copper in Comparison to Sham at 10 Days in Rabbit Tibia. *J. Clin. Med.* **2018**, *7*, 526. [CrossRef] [PubMed]
46. Lechner, J.; Noumbissi, S.; von Baehr, V. Titanium implants and silent inflammation in jawbone-a critical interplay of dissolved titanium particles and cytokines tnf-alpha and rantes/ccl5 on overall health? *EPMA J.* **2018**, *9*, 331–343. [CrossRef] [PubMed]
47. Noronha Oliveira, M.; Schunemann, W.V.H.; Mathew, M.T.; Henriques, B.; Magini, R.S.; Teughels, W.; Souza, J.C.M. Can degradation products released from dental implants affect peri-implant tissues? *J. Periodontal. Res.* **2018**, *53*, 1–11. [CrossRef] [PubMed]
48. Christiansen, R.J. Metal Release from Implants and Its Effect on the Immune System. Ph.D. Thesis, Technical University of Denmark, DTU Mechanical Engineering, Lyngby, Denmark, 2016.
49. Elefteriou, F. Regulation of bone remodeling by the central and peripheral nervous system. *Arch. Biochem. Biophys.* **2008**, *473*, 231–236. [CrossRef] [PubMed]
50. Kim, J.G.; Sun, B.H.; Dietrich, M.O.; Koch, M.; Yao, G.Q.; Diano, S.; Insogna, K.; Horvath, T.L. AGRP neurons regulate bone mass. *Cell Rep.* **2015**, *13*, 8–14. [CrossRef] [PubMed]
51. Takeda, S.; Ducy, P. Regulation of bone remodeling by central and peripheral nervous signals. In *Principles of Bone Biology*; Bilezekian, J., Raisz, L.G., Martin, T.J., Eds.; Academic Press: Cambridge, MA, USA, 2008; pp. 1059–1068.
52. Bajayo, A.; Bar, A.; Denes, A.; Bachar, M.; Kram, V.; Attar-Namdar, M.; Zallone, A.; Kovacs, K.J.; Yirmiya, R.; Bab, I. Skeletal parasympathetic innervation communicates central il-1 signals regulating bone mass accrual. *Proc. Natl. Acad. Sci. USA* **2012**, *109*, 15455–15460. [CrossRef]
53. Ysander, M.; Branemark, R.; Olmarker, K.; Myers, R.R. Intramedullary osseointegration: Development of a rodent model and study of histology and neuropeptide changes around titanium implants. *J. Rehabil. Res. Dev.* **2001**, *38*, 183–190.
54. Elefteriou, F. Neuronal signaling and the regulation of bone remodeling. *Cell. Mol. Life Sci.* **2005**, *62*, 2339–2349. [CrossRef]
55. Chenu, C. Role of innervation in the control of bone remodeling. *J. Musculoskelet. Neuronal Interact.* **2004**, *4*, 132–134.
56. Jiang, S.D.; Jiang, L.S.; Dai, L.Y. Mechanisms of osteoporosis in spinal cord injury. *Clin. Endocrinol.* **2006**, *65*, 555–565. [CrossRef] [PubMed]

57. Corpas Ldos, S.; Lambrichts, I.; Quirynen, M.; Collaert, B.; Politis, C.; Vrielinck, L.; Martens, W.; Struys, T.; Jacobs, R. Peri-implant bone innervation: Histological findings in humans. *Eur J. Oral Implants* **2014**, *7*, 283–292.
58. Fujii, N.; Ohnishi, H.; Shirakura, M.; Nomura, S.; Ohshima, H.; Maeda, T. Regeneration of nerve fibres in the peri-implant epithelium incident to implantation in the rat maxilla as demonstrated by immunocytochemistry for protein gene product 9.5 (pgp9.5) and calcitonin gene-related peptide (cgrp). *Clin. Oral Implants Res.* **2003**, *14*, 240–247. [CrossRef] [PubMed]
59. Mason, A.G.; Holland, G.R. The reinnervation of healing extraction sockets in the ferret. *J. Dent. Res.* **1993**, *72*, 1215–1221. [CrossRef] [PubMed]
60. Wada, S.; Kojo, T.; Wang, Y.H.; Ando, H.; Nakanishi, E.; Zhang, M.; Fukuyama, H.; Uchida, Y. Effect of loading on the development of nerve fibers around oral implants in the dog mandible. *Clin. Oral Implants Res.* **2001**, *12*, 219–224. [CrossRef] [PubMed]
61. Wang, Y.-H.; Kojo, T.; Ando, H.; Nakanishi, E.; Yoshizawa, H.; Zhang, M.; Fukuyama, H.; Wada, S.; Uchida, Y. Nerve regeneration after implantation in peri-implant area. A histological study on different implant materials in dogs. In *Osseoperception*; Jacobs, R., Ed.; Catholic University Leuven: Leuven, Belgium, 1998; pp. 3–11.
62. Elefteriou, F.; Campbell, P.; Ma, Y. Control of bone remodeling by the peripheral sympathetic nervous system. *Calcif. Tissue Int.* **2014**, *94*, 140–151. [CrossRef] [PubMed]
63. Schneiderman, N.; Ironson, G.; Siegel, S.D. Stress and health: Psychological, behavioral, and biological determinants. *Annu. Rev. Clin. Psychol.* **2005**, *1*, 607–628. [CrossRef] [PubMed]
64. Kinjo, M.; Setoguchi, S.; Schneeweiss, S.; Solomon, D.H. Bone mineral density in subjects using central nervous system-active medications. *Am. J. Med.* **2005**, *118*, 1414.e7–1414.e12. [CrossRef]
65. Chrcanovic, B.R.; Kisch, J.; Albrektsson, T.; Wennerberg, A. Factors influencing early dental implant failures. *J. Dent. Res.* **2016**, *95*, 995–1002. [CrossRef]
66. Gupta, B.; Acharya, A.; Pelekos, G.; Gopalakrishnan, D.; Kolokythas, A. Selective serotonin reuptake inhibitors and dental implant failure-a significant concern in elders? *Gerodontology* **2017**, *34*, 505–507. [CrossRef]
67. Wu, X.; Al-Abedalla, K.; Rastikerdar, E.; Abi Nader, S.; Daniel, N.G.; Nicolau, B.; Tamimi, F. Selective serotonin reuptake inhibitors and the risk of osseointegrated implant failure: A cohort study. *J. Dent. Res.* **2014**, *93*, 1054–1061. [CrossRef] [PubMed]
68. Olney, R.C. Regulation of bone mass by growth hormone. *Med. Pediatric Oncol.* **2003**, *41*, 228–234. [CrossRef] [PubMed]
69. Giannoudis, P.V. Bone healing the diamond concept. In *European Instructional Lectures: 15th EFORT Congress, London, United Kingdom*; Bentley, G., Ed.; Springer: Berlin/Heidelberg, Germany, 2014. [CrossRef]
70. Malloy, K.A.; Wadhwani, C.; McAllister, B.; Wang, M.; Katancik, J.A. Accuracy and reproducibility of radiographic images for assessing crestal bone height of implants using the precision implant X-ray locator (pixrl) device. *Int J. Oral Maxillofac. Implants* **2017**, *32*, 830–836. [CrossRef] [PubMed]
71. Bohner, L.O.L.; Mukai, E.; Oderich, E.; Porporatti, A.L.; Pacheco-Pereira, C.; Tortamano, P.; De Luca Canto, G. Comparative analysis of imaging techniques for diagnostic accuracy of peri-implant bone defects: A meta-analysis. *Oral Surg. Oral Med. Oral Pathol. Oral Radiol.* **2017**, *124*, 432.e5–440.e5. [CrossRef] [PubMed]
72. Wakoh, M.; Harada, T.; Otonari, T.; Otonari-Yamamoto, M.; Ohkubo, M.; Kousuge, Y.; Kobayashi, N.; Mizuta, S.; Kitagawa, H.; Sano, T. Reliability of linear distance measurement for dental implant length with standardized periapical radiographs. *Bull. Tokyo Dent. Coll.* **2006**, *47*, 105–115. [CrossRef] [PubMed]
73. Daros, P.; Carneiro, V.C.; Siqueira, A.P.; de-Azevedo-Vaz, S.L. Diagnostic accuracy of 4 intraoral radiographic techniques for misfit detection at the implant abutment joint. *J. Prosthet. Dent.* **2018**, *120*, 57–64. [CrossRef] [PubMed]
74. Duckworth, J.E.; Judy, P.F.; Goodson, J.M.; Socransky, S.S. A method for the geometric and densitometric standardization of intraoral radiographs. *J. Periodontol.* **1983**, *54*, 435–440. [CrossRef]
75. Lin, K.C.; Wadhwani, C.P.; Cheng, J.; Sharma, A.; Finzen, F. Assessing fit at the implant-abutment junction with a radiographic device that does not require access to the implant body. *J. Prosthet. Dent.* **2014**, *112*, 817–823. [CrossRef]
76. Grondahl, K.; Sunden, S.; Grondahl, H.G. Inter- and intraobserver variability in radiographic bone level assessment at Branemark fixtures. *Clin. Oral Implants Res.* **1998**, *9*, 243–250. [CrossRef]

77. Morner-Svalling, A.C.; Tronje, G.; Andersson, L.G.; Welander, U. Comparison of the diagnostic potential of direct digital and conventional intraoral radiography in the evaluation of peri-implant conditions. *Clin. Oral Implants Res.* **2003**, *14*, 714–719. [CrossRef]
78. Kamburoglu, K.; Gulsahi, A.; Genc, Y.; Paksoy, C.S. A comparison of peripheral marginal bone loss at dental implants measured with conventional intraoral film and digitized radiographs. *J. Oral Implants* **2012**, *38*, 211–219. [CrossRef] [PubMed]
79. Sewerin, I.P.; Gotfredsen, K.; Stoltze, K. Accuracy of radiographic diagnosis of peri-implant radiolucencies–an in vitro experiment. *Clin. Oral Implants Res.* **1997**, *8*, 299–304. [CrossRef] [PubMed]
80. Dave, M.; Davies, J.; Wilson, R.; Palmer, R. A comparison of cone beam computed tomography and conventional periapical radiography at detecting peri-implant bone defects. *Clin. Oral Implants Res.* **2013**, *24*, 671–678. [CrossRef] [PubMed]
81. Tonetti, M.S.; Pini Prato, G.; Williams, R.C.; Cortellini, P. Periodontal regeneration of human infrabony defects. Iii. Diagnostic strategies to detect bone gain. *J. Periodontol.* **1993**, *64*, 269–277. [CrossRef] [PubMed]
82. Eickholz, P.; Hausmann, E. Accuracy of radiographic assessment of interproximal bone loss in intrabony defects using linear measurements. *Eur. J. Oral Sci.* **2000**, *108*, 70–73. [CrossRef] [PubMed]
83. Garcia-Garcia, M.; Mir-Mari, J.; Benic, G.I.; Figueiredo, R.; Valmaseda-Castellon, E. Accuracy of periapical radiography in assessing bone level in implants affected by peri-implantitis: A cross-sectional study. *J. Clin. Periodontol.* **2016**, *43*, 85–91. [CrossRef]
84. Hermann, J.S.; Schoolfield, J.D.; Nummikoski, P.V.; Buser, D.; Schenk, R.K.; Cochran, D.L. Crestal bone changes around titanium implants: A methodologic study comparing linear radiographic with histometric measurements. *Int. J. Oral Maxillofac. Implants* **2001**, *16*, 475–485.
85. Schwarz, F.; Herten, M.; Sager, M.; Bieling, K.; Sculean, A.; Becker, J. Comparison of naturally occurring and ligature-induced peri-implantitis bone defects in humans and dogs. *Clin. Oral Implants Res.* **2007**, *18*, 161–170. [CrossRef]
86. Schwarz, F.; Sahm, N.; Schwarz, K.; Becker, J. Impact of defect configuration on the clinical outcome following surgical regenerative therapy of peri-implantitis. *J. Clin. Periodontol.* **2010**, *37*, 449–455. [CrossRef]
87. Demirturk Kocasarac, H.; Helvacioglu Yigit, D.; Bechara, B.; Sinanoglu, A.; Noujeim, M. Contrast-to-noise ratio with different settings in a cbct machine in presence of different root-end filling materials: An in vitro study. *Dentomaxillofac. Radiol.* **2016**, *45*, 20160012. [CrossRef]
88. Sirin, Y.; Horasan, S.; Yaman, D.; Basegmez, C.; Tanyel, C.; Aral, A.; Guven, K. Detection of crestal radiolucencies around dental implants: An in vitro experimental study. *J. Oral Maxillofac. Surg.* **2012**, *70*, 1540–1550. [CrossRef] [PubMed]
89. Fienitz, T.; Schwarz, F.; Ritter, L.; Dreiseidler, T.; Becker, J.; Rothamel, D. Accuracy of cone beam computed tomography in assessing peri-implant bone defect regeneration: A histologically controlled study in dogs. *Clin. Oral Implants Res.* **2012**, *23*, 882–887. [CrossRef] [PubMed]
90. De-Azevedo-Vaz, S.L.; Alencar, P.N.; Rovaris, K.; Campos, P.S.; Haiter-Neto, F. Enhancement cone beam computed tomography filters improve in vitro periimplant dehiscence detection. *Oral Surg. Oral Med. Oral Pathol. Oral Radiol.* **2013**, *116*, 633–639. [CrossRef] [PubMed]
91. Neves, F.S.; Vasconcelos, T.V.; Campos, P.S.; Haiter-Neto, F.; Freitas, D.Q. Influence of scan mode (180 degrees/360 degrees) of the cone beam computed tomography for preoperative dental implant measurements. *Clin. Oral Implants Res.* **2014**, *25*, e155–e158. [CrossRef] [PubMed]
92. Pinheiro, L.R.; Scarfe, W.C.; Augusto de Oliveira Sales, M.; Gaia, B.F.; Cortes, A.R.; Cavalcanti, M.G. Effect of cone-beam computed tomography field of view and acquisition frame on the detection of chemically simulated peri-implant bone loss in vitro. *J. Periodontol.* **2015**, *86*, 1159–1165. [CrossRef] [PubMed]
93. Al-Nuaimi, N.; Patel, S.; Foschi, F.; Mannocci, F. The detection of simulated periapical lesions in human dry mandibles with cone-beam computed tomography: A dose reduction study. *Int. Endod. J.* **2016**, *49*, 1095–1104. [CrossRef] [PubMed]
94. Pelekos, G.; Acharya, A.; Tonetti, M.S.; Bornstein, M.M. Diagnostic performance of cone beam computed tomography in assessing peri-implant bone loss: A systematic review. *Clin. Oral Implants Res.* **2018**, *29*, 443–464. [CrossRef]
95. Mengel, R. Kruse, B. Flores-de-Jacoby, L. Digital volume tomography in the diagnosis of peri-implant defects: An in vitro study on native pig mandibles. *J. Periodontol.* **2006**, *77*, 1234–1241. [CrossRef]

96. Ritter, L.; Elger, M.C.; Rothamel, D.; Fienitz, T.; Zinser, M.; Schwarz, F.; Zoller, J.E. Accuracy of peri-implant bone evaluation using cone beam ct, digital intra-oral radiographs and histology. *Dentomaxillofac. Radiol.* **2014**, *43*, 20130088. [CrossRef]
97. Fleiner, J.; Hannig, C.; Schulze, D.; Stricker, A.; Jacobs, R. Digital method for quantification of circumferential periodontal bone level using cone beam ct. *Clin. Oral Investig.* **2013**, *17*, 389–396. [CrossRef]
98. Kuhl, S.; Zurcher, S.; Zitzmann, N.U.; Filippi, A.; Payer, M.; Dagassan-Berndt, D. Detection of peri-implant bone defects with different radiographic techniques—A human cadaver study. *Clin. Oral Implants Res.* **2016**, *27*, 529–534. [CrossRef] [PubMed]
99. Tyndall, D.A.; Price, J.B.; Tetradis, S.; Ganz, S.D.; Hildebolt, C.; Scarfe, W.C. Position statement of the American Academy of Oral and Maxillofacial Radiology on selection criteria for the use of radiology in dental implantology with emphasis on cone beam computed tomography. *Oral Surg. Oral Med. Oral Pathol. Oral Radiol.* **2012**, *113*, 817–826. [CrossRef] [PubMed]
100. Chan, H.L.; Sinjab, K.; Li, J.; Chen, Z.; Wang, H.L.; Kripfgans, O.D. Ultrasonography for noninvasive and real-time evaluation of peri-implant tissue dimensions. *J. Clin. Periodontol.* **2018**, *45*, 986–995. [CrossRef] [PubMed]
101. Bloch, S.H.; Dayton, P.A.; Ferrara, K.W. Targeted imaging using ultrasound contrast agents. *IEEE Eng. Med. Biol. Mag.* **2004**, *23*, 18–29. [CrossRef] [PubMed]
102. Marotti, J.; Heger, S.; Tinschert, J.; Tortamano, P.; Chuembou, F.; Radermacher, K.; Wolfart, S. Recent advances of ultrasound imaging in dentistry—A review of the literature. *Oral Surg. Oral Med. Oral Pathol. Oral Radiol.* **2013**, *115*, 819–832. [CrossRef] [PubMed]
103. Wang, L.V.; Hu, S. Photoacoustic Tomography: In Vivo Imaging from Organelles to Organs. *Science* **2012**, *335*, 1458–1462. [CrossRef] [PubMed]
104. Xu, M.; Wang, L.V. Photoacoustic imaging in biomedicine. *Rev. Sci. Instrum.* **2006**, *77*, 041101. [CrossRef]
105. Hariri, A.; Lemaster, J.; Wang, J.; Jeevarathinam, A.S.; Chao, D.L.; Jokerst, J.V. The characterization of an economic and portable LED-based photoacoustic imaging system to facilitate molecular imaging. *Photoacoustics* **2018**, *9*, 10–20. [CrossRef]
106. Asao, Y.; Hashizume, Y.; Suita, T.; Nagae, K.-I.; Fukutani, K.; Sudo, Y.; Matsushita, T.; Kobayashi, S.; Tokiwa, M.; Yamaga, I.; et al. Photoacoustic mammography capable of simultaneously acquiring photoacoustic and ultrasound images. *J. Biomed. Opt.* **2016**, *21*, 116009. [CrossRef]
107. Mozaffarzadeh, M.; Hariri, A.; Moore, C.; Jokerst, J.V. The double-stage delay-multiply-and-sum image reconstruction method improves imaging quality in a LED-based photoacoustic array scanner. *Photoacoustics* **2018**, *12*, 22–29. [CrossRef]
108. Hoelen, C.; de Mul, F.; Pongers, R.; Dekker, A. Three-dimensional photoacoustic imaging of blood vessels in tissue. *Opt. Lett.* **1998**, *23*, 648–650. [CrossRef] [PubMed]
109. Köstli, K.P.; Beard, P.C. Two-dimensional photoacoustic imaging by use of Fourier-transform image reconstruction and a detector with an anisotropic response. *Appl. Opt.* **2003**, *42*, 1899–1908. [CrossRef] [PubMed]
110. Xu, M.; Wang, L.V. Universal back-projection algorithm for photoacoustic computed tomography. *Phys. Rev. E* **2005**, *71*, 016706. [CrossRef] [PubMed]
111. Lovell, J.F.; Liu, T.W.; Chen, J.; Zheng, G. Activatable photosensitizers for imaging and therapy. *Chem. Rev.* **2010**, *110*, 2839–2857. [CrossRef] [PubMed]
112. Hariri, A.; Wang, J.; Kim, Y.; Jhunjhunwala, A.; Chao, D.L.; Jokerst, J.V. In vivo photoacoustic imaging of chorioretinal oxygen gradients. *J. Biomed. Opt.* **2018**, *23*, 036005. [CrossRef] [PubMed]
113. Luke, G.P.; Emelianov, S.Y. Label-free Detection of Lymph Node Metastases with US-guided Functional Photoacoustic Imaging. *Radiology* **2015**, *277*, 435–442. [CrossRef] [PubMed]
114. Kircher, M.F.; de la Zerda, A.; Jokerst, J.V.; Zavaleta, C.L.; Kempen, P.J.; Mittra, E.; Pitter, K.; Huang, R.; Campos, C.; Habte, F.; et al. A Brain Tumor Molecular Imaging Strategy Using A New Triple-Modality MRI-Photoacoustic-Raman Nanoparticle. *Nat. Med.* **2012**, *18*, 829–834. [CrossRef]
115. Guan, T.; Shang, W.; Li, H.; Yang, X.; Fang, C.; Tian, J.; Wang, K. From Detection to Resection: Photoacoustic Tomography and Surgery Guidance with Indocyanine Green Loaded Gold Nanorod@liposome Core–Shell Nanoparticles in Liver Cancer. *Bioconjugate Chem.* **2017**, *28*, 1221–1228. [CrossRef]
116. Wang, J.; Chen, F.; Arconada-Alvarez, S.J.; Hartanto, J.; Yap, L.-P.; Park, R.; Wang, F.; Vorobyova, I.; Dagliyan, G.; Conti, P.S. A Nanoscale Tool for Photoacoustic-based Measurements of Clotting Time and Therapeutic Drug Monitoring of Heparin. *Nano Lett.* **2016**, *16*, 6265–6271. [CrossRef]

117. Cash, K.J.; Li, C.; Xia, J.; Wang, L.V.; Clark, H.A. Optical Drug Monitoring: Photoacoustic Imaging of Nanosensors to Monitor Therapeutic Lithium in Vivo. *ACS Nano* **2015**, *9*, 1692–1698. [CrossRef]
118. Zackrisson, S.; van de Ven, S.; Gambhir, S. Light in and sound out: Emerging translational strategies for photoacoustic imaging. *Cancer Res.* **2014**, *74*, 979–1004. [CrossRef] [PubMed]
119. Luke, G.P.; Yeager, D.; Emelianov, S.Y. Biomedical applications of photoacoustic imaging with exogenous contrast agents. *Ann. Biomed. Eng.* **2012**, *40*, 422–437. [CrossRef] [PubMed]
120. Mariotti, A.; Hefti, A.F. Defining periodontal health. *BMC Oral Health* **2015**, *15*, S6. [CrossRef] [PubMed]
121. Perry, D.A.; Beemsterboer, P.; Essex, G. *Periodontology for the Dental Hygienist*, 4th ed.; Elsevier/Saunders: St. Louis, MO, USA, 2014.
122. Araujo, M.W.; Benedek, K.M.; Benedek, J.R.; Grossi, S.G.; Dorn, J.; Wactawski-Wende, J.; Genco, R.J.; Trevisan, M. Reproducibility of probing depth measurements using a constant-force electronic probe: Analysis of inter-and intraexaminer variability. *J. Periodontol.* **2003**, *74*, 1736–1740. [CrossRef]
123. Larsen, C.; Barendregt, D.S.; Slot, D.E.; van der Velden, U.; van der Weijden, F. Probing pressure, a highly undervalued unit of measure in periodontal probing: A systematic review on its effect on probing pocket depth. *J. Clin. Periodontol.* **2009**, *36*, 315–322. [CrossRef]
124. Biddle, A.J.; Palmer, R.M.; Wilson, R.F.; Watts, T.L. Comparison of the validity of periodontal probing measurements in smokers and non-smokers. *J. Clin. Periodontol.* **2001**, *28*, 806–812. [CrossRef] [PubMed]
125. Listgarten, M.A. Periodontal probing: What does it mean? *J. Clin. Periodontol.* **1980**, *7*, 165–176. [CrossRef]
126. Holtfreter, B.; Albandar, J.M.; Dietrich, T.; Dye, B.A.; Eaton, K.A.; Eke, P.I.; Papapanou, P.N.; Kocher, T. Standards for reporting chronic periodontitis prevalence and severity in epidemiologic studies: Proposed standards from the Joint EU/USA Periodontal Epidemiology Working Group. *J. Clin. Periodontol.* **2015**, *42*, 407–412. [CrossRef]
127. Karadottir, H.; Lenoir, L.; Barbierato, B.; Bogle, M.; Riggs, M.; Sigurdsson, T.; Crigger, M.; Egelberg, J. Pain experienced by patients during periodontal maintenance treatment. *J. Periodontol.* **2002**, *73*, 536–542. [CrossRef]
128. Van Wijk, A.; Hoogstraten, J. Experience with dental pain and fear of dental pain. *J. Dent. Res.* **2005**, *84*, 947–950. [CrossRef]
129. Cole, A.; McMichael, A. Audit of dental practice record-keeping: A PCT-coordinated clinical audit by Worcestershire dentists. *Prim. Dent. Care* **2009**, *16*, 85–93. [CrossRef] [PubMed]
130. McFall, W.T., Jr.; Bader, J.D.; Rozier, R.G.; Ramsey, D. Presence of periodontal data in patient records of general practitioners. *J. Periodontol.* **1988**, *59*, 445–449. [CrossRef] [PubMed]
131. Morgan, R.G. Quality evaluation of clinical records of a group of general dental practitioners entering a quality assurance programme. *Br. Dent. J.* **2001**, *191*, 436–441. [CrossRef] [PubMed]
132. Schou, S.; Holmstrup, P.; Stoltze, K.; Hjørting-Hansen, E.; Fiehn, N.E.; Skovgaard, L.T. Probing around implants and teeth with healthy or inflamed peri-implant mucosa/gingiva: A histologic comparison in cynomolgus monkeys (Macaca fascicularis). *Clin. Oral Implants Res.* **2002**, *13*, 113–126. [CrossRef] [PubMed]
133. Koka, S. The implant-mucosal interface and its role in the long-term success of endosseous oral implants: A review of the literature. *Int. J. Prosthodont.* **1998**, *11*, 421–432. [PubMed]
134. Rakic, M.; Galindo-Moreno, P.; Monje, A.; Radovanovic, S.; Wang, H.-L.; Cochran, D.; Sculean, A.; Canullo, L. How frequent does peri-implantitis occur? A systematic review and meta-analysis. *Clin. Oral Investig.* **2018**, *22*, 1805–1816. [CrossRef] [PubMed]
135. Giraldo, V.M.; Duque, A.; Aristizabal, A.G.; Hernández, R.D.M. Prevalence of Peri-implant Disease According to Periodontal Probing Depth and Bleeding on Probing: A Systematic Review and Meta-Analysis. *Int. J. Oral Maxillofac. Implants* **2018**, *33*, e89–e105. [CrossRef]
136. Lin, C.; Chen, F.; Hariri, A.; Chen, C.; Wilder-Smith, P.; Takesh, T.; Jokerst, J. Photoacoustic Imaging for Noninvasive Periodontal Probing Depth Measurements. *J. Dent. Res.* **2018**, *97*, 23–30. [CrossRef]
137. Moore, C.; Bai, Y.; Hariri, A.; Sanchez, J.B.; Lin, C.-Y.; Koka, S.; Sedghizadeh, P.; Chen, C.; Jokerst, J.V. Photoacoustic imaging for monitoring periodontal health: A first human study. *Photoacoustics* **2018**, *12*, 67–74. [CrossRef]

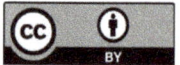

© 2019 by the authors. Licensee MDPI, Basel, Switzerland. This article is an open access article distributed under the terms and conditions of the Creative Commons Attribution (CC BY) license (http://creativecommons.org/licenses/by/4.0/).

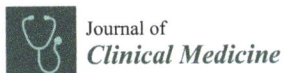

Review

Coupling between Osseointegration and Mechanotransduction to Maintain Foreign Body Equilibrium in the Long-Term: A Comprehensive Overview

Luis Amengual-Peñafiel [1,*], Manuel Brañes-Aroca [2], Francisco Marchesani-Carrasco [3], María Costanza Jara-Sepúlveda [3], Leopoldo Parada-Pozas [4] and Ricardo Cartes-Velásquez [5,6]

1. Dental Implantology Unit, Hospital Leonardo Guzmán, Antofagasta 1240835, Chile
2. Faculty of Sciences, Universidad de Chile, Santiago 7800003, Chile; branesmd.1@vtr.net
3. Clínica Marchesani, Concepción 4070566, Chile; francisco@marchesani.cl (F.M.-C.); mconstanzajara@gmail.com (M.C.J.-S.)
4. Regenerative Medicine Center, Hospital Clínico de Viña del Mar, Viña del Mar 2520626, Chile; dr.polo@ejerciciosalud.cl
5. School of Dentistry, Universidad Andres Bello, Concepción 4300866, Chile; cartesvelasquez@gmail.com
6. Institute of Biomedical Sciences, Universidad Autónoma de Chile, Temuco 4810101, Chile
* Correspondence: luisamengualp@gmail.com; Tel.: +56-9-7569-9469

Received: 10 December 2018; Accepted: 22 January 2019; Published: 25 January 2019

Abstract: The permanent interaction between bone tissue and the immune system shows us the complex biology of the tissue in which we insert oral implants. At the same time, new knowledge in relation to the interaction of materials and the host, reveals to us the true nature of osseointegration. So, to achieve clinical success or perhaps most importantly, to understand why we sometimes fail, the study of oral implantology should consider the following advice equally important: a correct clinical protocol, the study of the immunomodulatory capacity of the device and the osteoimmunobiology of the host. Although osseointegration may seem adequate from the clinical point of view, a deeper vision shows us that a Foreign Body Equilibrium could be susceptible to environmental conditions. This is why maintaining this cellular balance should become our therapeutic target and, more specifically, the understanding of the main cell involved, the macrophage. The advent of new information, the development of new implant surfaces and the introduction of new therapeutic proposals such as therapeutic mechanotransduction, will allow us to maintain a healthy host-implant relationship long-term.

Keywords: oral implants; osseointegration; marginal bone loss; immunomodulation; mechanotransduction

1. Introduction

Titanium dental implants are inserted directly into the bone tissue, a complex and dynamic tissue. This bone tissue not only participates in calcium homeostasis and functions as a hematopoietic organ, but also plays an important role as a regulator of immunity [1].

Recent evidence on foreign body reactions (FBRs) in relation to implantable devices, such as titanium dental implants, reveals that, to achieve a lasting relationship between the implant and the host, titanium implants must have an optimal surface [2], and there must be an adequate healing capacity of the host [3]. Recently, it has been shown that the presence of a titanium implant during bone healing activates the immune system and displays type 2 inflammation, which seems to guide the relationship between the host and the implant [4]. This appears to indicate that osseointegration is a dynamic process, the result of a complex set of reactions in which several mechanisms and pathways of the host interact [1]. If the osseointegration is not altered, a continuous equilibrium occurs in the form of Foreign Body Equilibrium (FBE), which has been documented for 20 years or more in oral implantology [5]. Despite the high rates of survival achieved with titanium dental implants [6], it is necessary to further improve the implant-host relationship to maintain the integrity of the FBE long term; especially when the mechanisms involved in the breakdown of the osseointegration begin to act [7]. Once this occurs the immune system could be activated changing the delicate balance between the osteoblast and the osteoclast, which results in bone resorption [8].

The role of macrophages in osseointegration is greater than expected [1]. Macrophages respond to all implanted materials, which play an essential role in the fate of an implant [9]. Currently, immunomodulation strategies targeting macrophages are being developed around implants, both dental and orthopedic ones; either through new surface treatments [10], the controlled release of specific ions [11] or through specific cytokines [12]. The immunomodulatory effect of the Mesenchymal stem cell (MSC) has also been explored [13], and in this line, the hypothesis of immunomodulation of osseointegration through therapeutic mechanotransduction has recently been proposed, particularly by extracorporeal shock waves therapy (ESWT) [14].

The field of mechanobiology has allowed us to analyze the effects of mechanical forces on cellular processes [15], which has revealed the complex cellular regulation involved in the transduction of mechanical signals [16]. Mechanical stimuli can stimulate the activity not only of bone cells but also MSC [17]. Mechanical stimuli can also change the cellular form and affect the phenotype and function of immune cells, such as macrophage and dendritic cells [18].

This review begins with (i) a discussion of key concepts related to bone tissue and the immune system; (ii) next, we will discuss the FBR, focusing specifically on osseointegration; (iii) to then explore the current strategies of immunomodulation in osseointegrated implants (iv) Finally, we will conclude with a discussion on a topic that may become clinically relevant, the coupling between osseointegration and mechanotransduction to maintain FBE long-term.

2. Bone Tissue and Immune System

The scientific field of osteoimmunology has revealed the vital role of immune cells in the regulation of bone dynamics [19], this has led to the understanding of the existence of different molecular and cellular mechanisms involved in a permanent interaction between bone tissue and the immune system. For this reason, to understand bone healing in general and osseointegration in particular, it is necessary to understand the biology and immunology of bones [20]. Bone is an organ composed of cortical, trabecular, cartilaginous, hematopoietic and connective tissue [21], which is composed by more than 30 different cell populations which reside in the microenvironment of the bone marrow adjacent to an implant. These cell populations, alone or in combination, have the ability to influence the formation and the bone regeneration of the peri-implant environment [2]. In addition, the presence of multiple anatomical and vascular contacts allow for a permanent interaction between the bone tissue and the immune system [22]. In fact, the bone marrow shows structural and functional characteristics that resemble a secondary lymphoid organ. That is why bone marrow is currently considered an immunoregulatory organ, capable of significantly influencing systemic immunity [21].

The cells of the bone tissue and the cells of the immune system share common origins. Osteoclasts (OC) come from stem cells of the monocyte-macrophage cell lineage [22]. However, certain subclasses of circulating monocytes and dendritic cells (DCs) which reside in the bone marrow also have the capacity to transform into OC if they are subjected to certain specific signals [23]. Perhaps this common origin with cells of the immune system could be related to the ability of OCs to recruit CD8 + FoxP3 + T cells and present antigens to them [24,25]. On the other hand, osteoblast (OBs) play a central role in the differentiation of hematopoietic cells [22]. This common origin between osseous and immune cells facilitates understanding of how molecular pathways are involved in bone remodeling (such as in PTH, BMP and Wnt pathway) which also act in regulating the hematopoiesis [26].

Immune cells regulate osteoclastogenesis by three main cytokines: macrophage colony stimulating factor (M-CSF), receptor activator NF kappaB ligand (RANKL) and osteoprotegerin (OPG) [19]. The main element in osteoclastogenesis, the RANKL, can be expressed by activated T lymphocytes, dendritic cells and neutrophils, indicating the participation of these immune cells during osteoclastogenesis [19,21]. The expression of RANKL by activated T cells has been implicated in osteoclastogenesis induced by inflammation, linking adaptive immunity to skeletal biology [27]. This is related to the role of the immune system in several bone diseases, such as osteoporosis, osteoarthritis and rheumatoid arthritis. Several studies have clearly highlighted the role of developing T lymphocytes and the pathophysiology of osteoporosis, which has given birth to a new field of biology called *"immunoporosis"* [28]. Moreover, as the dendritic cells are responsible for the activation of virgin T cells and act as osteoclast precursors, this could be directly involved in osteoclastogenesis induced by inflammation and bone loss [29]. It has been described that persistent inflammation is characterized by the continuous release of proinflammatory cytokines (TNF-a, IL-1a/be IL-6), which is accompanied by a higher RANKL/OPG ratio and an increased osteoclast activity [30]. On the other hand, it has been shown that B cells are an important source of OPG derived from bone marrow, which implies that B cells are one of the main inhibitors of osteoclastogenesis in normal physiology [19].

Macrophages are precursors of osteoclasts, and under the stimulation of M-CSF and RANKL, they can differentiate into osteoclasts during bone remodeling [19]. Bone and bone marrow contain multiple subpopulations of specialized resident macrophages (bone macrophages or osteomacs), which contribute to bone biology and/or hematopoiesis [31]. Macrophages promote osteoblastogenesis in in vitro matrix deposition and they could have an important role in the promotion of bone anabolism, through the provision of trophic support to the osteoblast lineage [32]. In fact, the depletion of macrophages leads to the complete loss of bone formation mediated by osteoblasts in vivo [33]. In addition, they would be important in the reversion phase of a basic multicellular unit (BMU), which separates bone resorption and bone formation [34]. Macrophages are also abundant within the bone callus during the inflammatory phase of bone healing in humans [35], so the presence and diverse functionality of macrophages could allow an important contribution in bone homeostasis and throughout the course of bone healing [32]. Furthermore, the healing of bone fractures is significantly improved in knockout mice lacking T and B cells, which indicates that they may also have a detrimental function during this process. This observation suggests the dual role of immune cells in osteogenesis, through its expression and secretion of a wide range of regulatory molecules [19].

As we have seen, immune cells play an important role in bone homeostasis. Therefore, the insertion of a foreign body into the bone tissue will inevitably be recognized by the immune system, affecting the biological behavior of the bone cells. This event can determine the in vivo destination of an implant or "biomaterial".

3. Foreign Body Reaction and Osseointegration

The interaction between bone tissue and implants involves at least 3 components: immune cells of the host, bone cells of the host and the material [19]. After implantation, the host will experience a response to tissue injury, which will be conditioned by the material present and the degree of the immune response [36].

In general, after a surgical implantation procedure, the damage of the endothelial cells exposes the underlying vascular basement membrane and initiates the coagulation cascade that leads to the formation of a clot of red blood cells-platelets-fibrin. This vascular damage also facilitates the interaction of the implant with blood proteins and interstitial fluids, such as fibrinogen, vitronectin, complement, fibronectin and albumin, which are adsorbed dynamically on the surface of the implant (Vroman effect) in seconds, forming a superficial transient matrix [1,2,7,19,36,37]. This allows physicochemical interactions between the host proteins and the implant's surface, which leads to a change in the molecular conformation of one or more of these host proteins, exposing previously hidden amino acid sequences, which would act as antigenic epitopes [1,7]. Serum factors called "opsonins" will participate in the recognition of the foreign agent, the main ones being immunoglobulin G (IgG) and the complement activated fragment, C3b, allowing for interactions with macrophages through membrane receptors [38]. Hu et al. showed that adsorbed fibrinogen is the main protein responsible for the accumulation of macrophages on the surfaces of implanted biomaterials [39]. It has also been shown that adsorbed fibrinogen exposes two previously hidden amino acids, functioning as epitopes, which allows for interaction with macrophages through the Mac-1 integrin (CD11b/CD18), leading to a proinflammatory environment, modulating the response of the host to the biomaterial in this way [1]. In this same context, it has been suggested that another protein, fibronectin, could participate in the chronic phase of FBR [40].

The complement system seems to play a key role at this early stage [7]. Arvidsson et al. showed that the interaction between titanium and plasma coagulation factors, such as factor XII, could lead to the activation of the complement through the alternative pathway, producing C3b [41]. As is known, immune cells express inactivated C3b/C3b (iC3b) receptors, so that from the early phase of inflammation, the surface of the implant is recognized by the immune system [7]. Recently it has been demonstrated in titanium implants that there is a positive regulation of the C5a-1 receptor (C5aR1) after the inflammatory period, which demonstrates a prolonged activation of innate immunity through the continuous activation of the complement system [4].

After the initial interaction between the blood and the material, acute inflammation begins, which is initiated by the cytokines and chemokines released by the damaged cells, leading to the influx of neutrophils and mononuclear macrophages [19,36]. Neutrophils normally deplete rapidly, undergo apoptosis and disappear from implantation sites within the first two days [19]. The prolonged presence of neutrophils indicates that we are facing active chronic inflammation [36]. This has been observed around titanium implants, probably due to the role of neutrophils in the promotion of vascularization in tissue hypoxia and the ability of the macrophage to suppress the apoptosis of them [4]. It is important to mention that neutrophils, in an effort to degrade the materials, release proteolytic enzymes and reactive oxygen species (ROS), which can corrode the surface of the implanted material [19].

The influx of mononuclear macrophages occurs between 24 and 48 h, which have a phagocytic function that includes the release of proteolytic enzymes that degrade cellular debris and the extracellular matrix (ECM). Currently, these immune cells have aroused great interest among scientists due to their multiple functions in the process of bone healing and high plasticity [19]. Macrophages have been extensively characterized in phenotypes M1 and M2, reflecting the Th1/Th2 nomenclature described for helper T cells [42]. Traditionally, it has been described that M1 proinflammatory macrophages would dominate the early phase of the reparative response and, on the other hand, M2 macrophages (M2a, M2b and M2c), would play a more prominent role during the middle and later stages of the response repair [19]. However, this classification represents only a simplification of the in vivo scenario, since it is very likely that the macrophage phenotype occupies a continuum between the M1 and M2 designations, with transient macrophages with characteristics of both phenotypes present [43]. Therefore, it seems that both phenotypes of macrophages perform essential functions during the process of bone healing, with the macrophage change pattern determining the osteogenesis instead of a specific macrophage phenotype [44].

It has been described that a prolonged M1 polarization phase leads to an increase in fibrosis-enhancing cytokine release pattern by the M2 macrophages, which results in the formation of a fibrocapsule around the biomaterial [19]. This reaction could be related to the "primary failure", which occurs in 1–2% of all dental implants placed, probably due to a series of risk factors that are predisposed to this total failure in osseointegration, like the following: low primary stability, premature loading, traumatic surgery, infection, as well as patient conditions such as smoking or the consumption of some pharmaceutical products [20].

On the contrary, an efficient and timely switch from M1 to M2 macrophage phenotype results in an osteogenic cytokines release and with it the formation of new bone tissue [19]. This second possible reaction is one that would generate the bone encapsulation that allows the commercial use of titanium implants [20]. In commercially pure (c.p.) titanium implants, the presence of the M2 phenotype of the macrophage (most likely M2a) is significantly high, which has been observed as early as 10 days after surgery [4,45]. This indicates that there is an immunomodulated relationship between the titanium implant and the host, which allows the deposit of bone in the implant, and the isolation of this from the space of the bone marrow, through a type of FBR [4]. Albrektsson and colleagues introduce the concept of FBE to describe this phenomenon, osseointegration being considered a mild chronic inflammatory response that allows implant function with a bone-implant interface that remains in a state of equilibrium, susceptible to changes in the environment [5].

Macrophages can swallow particles up to 5 μm, however, if the size of the material or the residue is greater than 50–100 μm, the material is surrounded by macrophages that fuse to form foreign body giant cells (FBGC) [19,46]. This induction of macrophage fusion probably occurs through the secretion of IL-4 and IL-13 by mast cells, basophils, and helper T cells (Th) [40]. It has even been suggested that FBGCs could express phenotypes of M1 and M2 macrophages, depending on the environment, similar to their mononuclear precursors [47]. Although FBGCs are not normally found in healthy tissues, they are abundant around implanted biomaterials, even years after implantation [48]. This is the reason why the presence of FBGC in the interface of the host-implant is an indication of an FBR to the implanted material or device [19,40,46]. Donath et al. described the presence of FGBC on the surface of titanium implants, which were present in multiple cases of FBR through histological studies [49]. It has been seen that the CD11b marker is extremely upregulated at 28 days, demonstrating how macrophages are highly involved in the reaction to titanium implants since this marker has recently been implicated in the fusion of macrophages [4]. For several years, multinucleated giant cells (MNGC) have been described in relation to biomaterials, especially in the case of bone replacement materials, assuming that MNGCs are osteoclasts. However, many studies indicate that these cells actually belong to the cell line of FBGCs, which are of an "inflammatory origin" [47]. It is a fact that osteoclasts can be formed by the fusion of multiple macrophages, and some authors even suggest that macrophages can perform functions of bone resorption [50]. All of the above suggests that FBGS could play a central role in the pathway of bone loss during the FBR [7].

Macrophages and dendritic cells can initiate an adaptive immune response through the presentation of antigens, which can also be particles or ions. When a T cell recognizes an antigen, the T cell is activated (activated TCD4 +) and may have inflammatory secretory profiles (Th1) or anti-inflammatory secretory profiles (Th2) [51]. Recently a constant regulation of CD4 and the negative regulation of CD8, which indicates a reaction of CD4 lymphocytes around the implant, was observed in titanium implants [45]. However, more research is needed to confirm the continued presence of the immune system over time [4].

As we have seen, an implanted device activates the components of the immune system in bone: complement, neutrophils, macrophages and lymphocytes. However, the role of the macrophage in the host-biomaterial relationship is highlighted [4]. Although most implants will be successful, a rejection mechanism may occur. This may be represented by marginal bone loss around the osseointegrated implant, which could be a product of multiple factors such as the implant, the surgical procedure, prosthetic conditions and factors in relation to the patient [20]. The loss of FBE could be the main cause of this peri-implant bone loss. This leaves the door open for the development of different strategies to face the pathology through a deeper understanding of the biology of osseointegration [1].

4. Current Immunomodulation Strategies in Osseointegrated Implants

Titanium is one of the few materials suitable for implantation requirements in the human body, being widely used in oral surgery, maxillofacial surgery, craniofacial surgery and orthopedics. The greater clinical use and popularity of oral implants have led to a growth in demands, with an increasing need for treatments in places where the quality of bone is less than ideal, and in patients with a compromise of scarring products of systemic affections [2]. Although less than 5% of oral implants show failure under optimal clinical conditions. In some cases, through a triad consisting of poor clinical handling, combined with poor implant systems and the treatment of those who are compromised, treating "poor" patients may lead to problems, probably increasing the number of complications [20]. On the other hand, many orthopedic procedures require implants, however, not all implanted devices last forever: up to 15% of the total joint implants require a surgical revision within 15 years of the initial surgery [52]. Therefore, there is a need to improve the biological function and longevity of the implantable devices [20,52].

Recent studies on osseointegrated titanium oral implants demonstrate the presence of the M2 phenotype of the macrophage from the early stage of healing (days) [4,10,45,53]. However, the presence of other chemical elements on the surface of the titanium implant seems to be relevant for the bone balance of osseointegration [2]. Trindade et al. have demonstrated that the bone resorption markers were significantly down-regulated around titanium in turned titanium grade IV implants. Interestingly, the regulation balance of bone resorption RANKL/OPG is suppressed in its entirety, suggesting that bone resorption has been kept to a minimum around Titanium [4]. However, Biguetti et al., using a machined titanium implant of titanium-6 aluminum-4 vanadium alloy, demonstrated the opposite; there was a remarkable remodeling process, evidenced by peaks corresponding to RANKL and OPG, and also an increased area density of osteoclasts. Furthermore, the presence of ten chemical elements in the surface composition of the implants used was determined through an analysis by Energy Dispersive X-ray (EDX): Titanium [Ti], Aluminum [Al], Vanadium [V], Calcium [Ca], Nitrogen [N], Niobium [Nb], Oxygen [O], Phosphorus [P], Sulfur [S] and Zinc [Zn] [53].

In this context, it is noteworthy that c.p. titanium is often alloyed with aluminum and vanadium (Ti6Al4V). However, in some cases, further surface modification procedures such as sand-blasting and acid etching are likely to remove passive layers from the surface of the metal, exposing less stable elements underneath. This could generate an inflammatory response and possible reduction in osteoblast differentiation [2]. Both of these effects can be detrimental to new bone formation and implant integration. However, in relation to the aforementioned, this material has an acceptable clinical success currently [10]. However, the degree of purity of the surfaces is an important issue to consider since there are important studies of oral implants, which reveal the presence of organic and inorganic contaminants onto some surfaces [54,55].

The above could be clinically relevant since, as we know, macrophages respond to all the implanted materials, being fundamental for the fate of an implant [36]. Macrophages are capable of releasing metal ions from solid surfaces in a matter of minutes by dissolucytosis [2]. The fused macrophages in FBGC can remain in the interface biomaterial-tissue, generating a sealed compartment between its surface and the underlying biomaterial, which allows the secretion of different mediators such as ROS, degradative enzymes and acid. Due to this the "frustrated phagocytosis process" being associated with the failure of some implanted devices [48]. Particles, ions, or degradation products from implanted materials or devices may also be recognized as foreign by macrophages and dendritic cells [9,56]. Dendritic cells may also be drawn to the implant site by the recognition of foreign substances, inducing the expansion of CD4 cells [9,21], so that some dental implant could eventually be able to cause a type IV hypersensitivity reaction [57]. Since the bone marrow contains structures in the form of follicles, similar to that observed in lymph nodes or the spleen, although without an organized T and B zone, but these lymphoid follicles can increase in the bone marrow during infections, inflammations and autoimmunity [21].

It has been demonstrated that titanium leakage due to corrosion inevitably results in substantial contact between the foreign material and the tissues. In fact, there was a gradient in titanium intensity from the implant surface and out up to a distance away from it of about 1000 μm [20]. Titanium ions could cause immune responses due to their ability to bind to proteins, such as albumin or transferrin, creating a bioavailable metalloprotein that could serve as an antigen in immunological reactions. Many studies have shown that proinflammatory cytokines such as IL-1β (interleukin 1beta), TNF-α tumor necrosis alpha factor, and GM-CSF (granulocyte-macrophage colony stimulating factor) are jointly regulated after stimulation of a hapten or particles [58]. However, it is likely that this first corrosion is coupled to the acidic environment that inevitably develops after the placement of an implant, a situation that is present until approximately four weeks after surgery when the partial pressure of oxygen has normalized [20]. In all probability at this stage, the released ionic titanium is stabilized by biomolecules such as citrate, an important metal chelator in cellular fluids, forming relatively stable complexes in solutions close to neutral pH [58]. Thereafter it seems likely that titanium corrosion will be quite minimal, provided that there is no more mechanical interruption of the blood flow. The presence of titanium ions in a stage subsequent to osseointegration could generate a synergistic interaction with other negative factors, such as cement particles, leading to marginal bone loss [20].

This scenario where living tissues face the presence of materials in an immunologically active environment allows for a better understanding of the dynamics of osseointegration, and also reveals that the desired FBE in an oral implant can be threatened by clinical conditions [7]. This is why the methods that control the polarization of the macrophage have emerged as an attractive means to reduce inflammatory signaling [19]. It is known that the increase in bone formation correlates with the resolution of the initial inflammatory response. That is, inflammation and osseointegration are inversely proportional [2]. As osseointegration is an immunomodulated inflammatory process, where the immune system is locally up-or down-regulated [57], the precise modulation of postoperative inflammation and the innate immune reaction provide a promising approach for therapeutic purposes [19].

Several immunomodulation strategies have been proposed, mainly through the implanted device, and more recently, the immunomodulation by means of direct stimulation of Human bone marrow-derived mesenchymal stem cell (HBMMSC). This aims to improve integration, avoid fibrosis, prevent bone loss and so increase the useful life of the devices in the human body [14,19,59].

In relation to these immunomodulation strategies through implanted devices, the topographic modification of the titanium dental implant surface has shown a significant positive effect in the speed and degree of osseointegration. In fact, the use of microscale modified implant surfaces has been one of the key factors in increasing the clinical success rate of implants, especially in areas of compromised bone quality [2]. The surface topography of the implant can be optimized at a micro level and nanoscale, influencing properties such as wettability and surface charge, modifying the kinetics of adsorption, the folding of proteins adsorbed onto implant surface and the consequent presentation of bioactive sites to macrophages [51,60]. The geometry of the material may also be relevant for the phenotypic expression of macrophage. It has been demonstrated that micro- and nanopatterned grooves of 400–500 nm wide can influence macrophage elongation, driving macrophages toward an anti-inflammatory, pro-healing phenotype [61]. This interaction of the macrophage with its mechanical environment, that is, the surface of the titanium, is possible through multiple mechanoreceptors on the cell surface, perhaps through integrins [62]. At present, titanium can be alloyed with Zirconium (TiZr). The combination of high-energy and altered surface chemistry (hydrophilic), seems to generate an immunomodulatory effect towards the activation of M2 macrophages, decreasing the presence of FGBC and increasing osseointegration [10].

A growing number of studies report success based on therapies with metal ions such as magnesium, strontium, calcium, among others. These ions can be incorporated into devices, in order to promote osteogenesis coupled with a pro-regenerative immune response. For example, the production of proinflammatory cytokines such as TNF-α, IL-1b, IL-6 and PEG2 has been shown to be reduced in the presence of high concentrations of magnesium, which highlights its role as an immunomodulatory ion [63].

The incorporation of immunomodulatory molecules to the implant constitutes another strategy to modulate the immune response [12,52]. Inflammation could be controlled by the local release of M2 polarizing cytokines such as IL-4, IL-10, IL-13 [64], or the implant could directly inhibit proinflammatory signals, using anti-TNF-α therapy, which are the most potent proinflammatory cytokines that promote the polarization of M1 macrophages [65]. The transcription factor NF-κB has also been pointed out as a possible target to generate implant-mediated immunomodulation. It has been shown that NF-κB decoy can suppress the production of essential chemokines for the recruitment of monocytes, which could avoid the presence of immune cells at the bone-implant interface [66].

In spite of the above-mentioned issues, the biology is more complex. The determination of the appropriate time frame of immunomodulation is critical for optimizing their application. Acute phase inflammation is crucial for proper bone repair after trauma, so the macrophage polarization status also plays a critical role in bone regeneration. As such, the interplay between M1- and M2-dominated microenvironments and the temporal modulation of the transition M1 to M2 provide an interesting line of investigation to pursue new immune-modulatory therapies and improve bone repair and implant integration [52]. One possible method is to utilize a controlled release system to maintain a short period of M1, followed by a transition to M2 polarization via cytokines in a biphasic manner. However, future investigations are necessary [67].

A new therapeutic approach to achieve modulation of the transition from M1 to M2 in the appropriate timeframe could be the MSC of the host, given their innate immunomodulatory capabilities [68]. More than 400 studies have explored the immunomodulatory effect of MSCs for the treatment of various autoimmune conditions, including graft-versus-host disease, diabetes, multiple sclerosis, Crohn's disease, and organ transplantation [69]. In relation to this, a new hypothesis has recently been proposed, that the HBMMSC residing around the peri-implant bone tissue immunomodulate the osseointegration process through the ESWT bio-activation effect. The mechanical stimuli generated by ESWT trigger the release of exosomes by HBMMSCs, generating tolerogenic dendritic cells (Tol-Dcs) and increasing the presence of the M2 phenotype of the macrophage [14].

5. Coupling between Osseointegration and Mechanotransduction to Maintain FBE Long-Term

At present we know that osteogenesis does not depend only on the bone cells of the skeletal system, in fact, there is a multicellular collaboration. Over years, studies have focused on the interaction between bone cells and the material surface, however, now studies in the field of advanced bone materials should involve co-culture systems with the interaction between materials, bone cells, and immune cells. Only then will we know the real osteoimmunomodulatory capacity of the material [19]. However, the complexity becomes even greater when we consider a fourth factor that can become important to maintain the balance of the material-host relationship, the mechanical stimuli. Physical forces also play important roles in embryonic development, tissue homeostasis, and pathogenesis. However, the importance of mechanical signals to control cellular processes has only been recognized more recently. That is why, as interest grows in the field of mechanobiology, new study models are developed to analyze the influence of mechanical forces on cells and tissues [70,71].

The cells are sensitive to shear, tension and compression forces. These mechanical signals have important effects on tissues, such as the production of ECM components [72]. A mechanical alteration can influence gene expression and cellular behavior through the mechanotransduction signal [73]. These mechanical signals would be transmitted by the filaments of the cytoskeleton, such as actin and microtubules, and finally transduced into biochemical signals [74], being the integrins of the cell surface essential for mechanotransduction [75].

The therapeutic mechanotransduction is part of modern Implantology, in fact, good clinical results obtained through progressive loading protocol [76] and immediate loading protocol [77,78], reveal to us that physiological mechanical stimuli can be beneficial to accompany the osseointegration of a dental implant and allow for successful osseointegration [79]. In this sense Duyck et al. demonstrated through a bone chamber model in an animal model that mechanical stimuli are capable of increasing the bone-implant contact (BIC) [80]. However, we also know that mechanical stimuli are key in bone remodeling, so greater trauma can lead to implant failure [20].

At present, ESWT are widely used in the context of therapeutic mechanotransduction. ESWT are supersonic waves, generated by different types of devices, such as electrohydraulic, piezoelectric, electromechanical or pneumatic, which generate transient pressure changes that propagate through the tissues where they are applied [81,82]. ESWT is applied to treat various medical pathologies.

In orthopedics, it is used mainly in the treatment of tendinopathies, the treatment of nonunion in fractures of long bones, avascular necrosis of the femoral head, chronic diabetics, nondiabetic ulcers and ischemic heart disease [83]. In dentistry, ESWT has been used in extracorporeal lithotripsy of salivary stones [84] and painful mielogelosis of the masseter [85]. Recently, Falkensammer et al. used ESWT as a supplement in Orthodontics [86], finding an absence of deleterious effects in the maxillofacial tissues or for pulpal vitality [87].

It has been proposed that the mechanical stimuli generated by ESWT produce an increase in the permeability of the cell membrane, which triggers the release of cytoplasmic ribonucleic acid (RNA) through an active process dependent on exosomes. This event at the cellular level is the one that would produce the effects observed in the accelerated repair of tissues. However, more studies are needed to completely reveal the underlying mechanism [88].

It seems that the bone is programmed to seal immediately any area affecting its integrity, sealing and protecting the marrow content through the restoration of a cortical bone barrier. Therefore, we can assume that the "raw materials" (phosphate, calcium, etc.) could be more available from a source of cortical bone [4]. In this sense, it has been described that oral implants installed in low-density bone tissue (bone type IV) present a higher risk of failure [89]. On the other hand, in patients with osteoporosis, even though there is no difference described to date in the survival rate of oral implants placed in patients with and without osteoporosis, there is an increase in peri-implant bone loss [90]. In orthopedics, it is a proven fact that the fixation of screws and osteosynthesis plates can be hindered in patients with low bone mass and especially with thin cortices. In fact, in osteoporotic fractures, depending on the location, the type of fracture and the surgery performed, the failure rate can reach up to 30% [91]. In this sense, the anabolic effect on the bone described in several studies with the use of ESWT has become particularly attractive [82,92].

Recent research shows that this anabolic bone response through ESWT can also be generated in relation to titanium devices in bone, which could have great therapeutic potential, especially in patients with bone disease. Koolen et al. demonstrated at the histological level that in bone defects reconstructed with a titanium scaffold as a bone substitute show the de novo bone formation after ESWT in rats [93]. In this same line of investigation, Koolen et al. [91] hypothesized that peri-operative shock wave treatment can improve screw fixation and the osteointegration of cortical and cancellous orthopedic screws, especially in osteoporotic patients. They were able to demonstrate in a healthy rodent bones model, that an ESWT immediately after the implantation of titanium screws (Ti6Al4V grade 5) improved screw fixation of the cortical screw, visualized by improved mechanical strength and osseointegration. Another finding was the formation of a neocortex in some animals after treatment. However, the cancellous screw showed no differences in testing after ESWT [91]. In this context, it has been reported that the ESWT not only achieves complete bone healing, but has also been observed to help in the re-attachment of a loose orthopedic screw. This has been observed in a patient with a typical case of non-union treated with ESWT [94].

It has been suggested that these anabolic effects in the bone are due to the fact that shock waves can cause the conversion of progenitor cells into osteogenic precursor cells. Another possibility could be that ESWT induces osteocytic cell death through a mechanism called cavitation. This death of osteocytes could lead to the stimulation of local bone remodeling, activating the osteoblast to produce more osteoid, which could eventually lead to a neocortex [91]. I Osteocytes are important regulators of cellular homeostasis and can act as mechanosensors. In addition, direct contact between dendrites of the osteocytes and the implant surface has been reported after an 8-week osseointegration period in an in vivo model [1]. However, the presence of HBMMSC and immune cells in the peri-implant environment leads us to think that the ESWT could also have a potent immunomodulatory effect in favor of osseointegration [14].

HBMMSC are not only found in the peri-implant environment, but also adhere to the titanium surface [95]. Current evidence indicates that BMMSCs can modulate the immune response by inhibiting polarization induced to M1 macrophages and promote polarization to M2 macrophages through the release of paracrine factors [96]. In addition, HBMMSCs can modulate the immune response through the generation of Tol-DC [97]. This is why the fact that ESWT can act as an effective bioactivator on HBMMSC, increasing its rate of growth, proliferation, migration and reducing apoptosis of these cells, suggests that ESWT could be an adequate tool to express all the potential therapeutic effects of HBMMSC [98]. This evidence suggests that the findings described in relation to ESWT and titanium [91,93,94] are probably a product of the local immunomodulatory effect of HBMMSC [14].

Mechanical signals play an important role in the regulation of immunological and cellular processes in monocytes, macrophages, and dendritic cells [70]. In this sense, recent studies have investigated the anti-inflammatory effect of ESWT in ischemic lesions in the animal model. Scientists have observed that ESWT would regulate the inflammatory reactions reducing the infiltration of inflammatory cells and promoting the differentiation of the M2 macrophage, that is, through the immunomodulation effect [99]. Apparently, the ESWT also exerts direct modulation on the macrophage. It has been demonstrated that the stimulation of macrophages derived from human monocytes with ESWT causes the significant inhibition of some M1 marker genes (CD80, COX2, CCL5) in M1 macrophages and a significant synergistic effect for some M2 marker genes (ALOX15, MRC1, CCL18) in the M2 macrophages. It has also been observed that ESWT affected the production of cytokines and chemokines, inducing, in particular, a significant increase in IL-10 and a reduction in the production of IL-1β [100].

No doubt, infiltrating immune cells play an important role in determining the variable outcome of wound repair in mammals and amphibians. For example, it has been demonstrated that the systemic depletion of macrophages results in a permanent failure in the regenerative capacity of the axolotl, with extensive fibrosis. However, the regenerative capacity of the axolotl is recovered once the macrophage population is restored [101].

While the use of immunomodulatory implants per se (clean implants) generates adequate osseointegration [55], the FBE can be altered under certain clinical conditions, such as overload [1,5,7]. The possibility that we can guide the transition between the M1 inflammatory phase and the M2 anti-inflammatory phase through mechanotransduction makes ESWT a promising therapeutic alternative to improve clinical success in oral implants, maintaining FBE long-term [14]. This could potentially improve the feedback path to the sensory cortex since, as described, the capacity for tactile perception of osseointegrated implants, "osseoperception", increases over time [102]. Furthermore, it has also been proposed that the topical addition of the nerve growth factor (NGF) in oral implants could help to improve this tactile sensitivity in order to minimize occlusal overload [103], and it has been demonstrated that ESWT is effective in increasing the expression of NGF [104].

6. Concluding Remarks

Mechanotransduction can improve the implant-host relationship. However, it is necessary to perform studies at the cellular and molecular level that would allow us to determine both the medical device and the most effective therapeutic range. All of this is in order to improve, maintain and recover the harmony of this triad of elements, i.e., bone cells, immune cells and implants, which finally determines the fate of FBE.

Author Contributions: Writing-Original Draft Preparation, A-P.L.; Writing-Review & Editing, B.-A.M; M.-C.F.; J.-S.M.C.; P.-P.L.; C.-V.R.

Conflicts of Interest: The authors declare no conflict of interest.

References

1. Trindade, R.; Albrektsson, T.; Wennerberg, A. Current concepts for the biological basis of dental implants: Foreign body equilibrium and osseointegration dynamics. *Oral Maxillofac. Surg. Clin. N. Am.* **2015**, *27*, 175–183. [CrossRef] [PubMed]

2. Hamlet, S.; Ivanovski, S. Inflammatory Cytokine Response to Titanium Surface Chemistry and Topography. In *The Immune Response to Implanted Materials and Devices*; Corradetti, B., Ed.; Springer: Cham, Switzerland, 2017; pp. 151–167. ISBN 978-3-319-45433-7.
3. Wennerberg, A.; Albrektsson, T. Current challenges in successful rehabilitation with oral implants. *J. Oral Rehabil.* **2011**, *38*, 286–294. [CrossRef] [PubMed]
4. Trindade, R.; Albrektsson, T.; Galli, S.; Prgomet, Z.; Tengvall, P.; Wennerberg, A. Osseointegration and foreign body reaction: Titanium implants activate the immune system and suppress bone resorption during the first 4 weeks after implantation. *Clin. Implant Dent. Relat. Res.* **2018**, *20*, 82–91. [CrossRef]
5. Albrektsson, T.; Dahlin, C.; Jemt, T.; Sennerby, L.; Turri, A.; Wennerberg, A. Is marginal bone loss around oral implants the result of a provoked foreign body reaction? *Clin. Implant Dent. Relat. Res.* **2014**, *16*, 155–165. [CrossRef] [PubMed]
6. Chrcanovic, B.R.; Kisch, J.; Albrektsson, T.; Wennerberg, A. A retrospective study on clinical and radiological outcomes of oral implants in patients followed up for a minimum of 20 years. *Clin. Implant Dent. Relat. Res.* **2018**, *20*, 199–207. [CrossRef] [PubMed]
7. Trindade, R.; Albrektsson, T.; Tengvall, P.; Wennerberg, A. Foreign Body Reaction to Biomaterials: On Mechanisms for Buildup and Breakdown of Osseointegration. *Clin. Implant Dent. Relat. Res.* **2016**, *18*, 192–203. [CrossRef] [PubMed]
8. Albrektsson, T.; Canullo, L.; Cochran, D.; De Bruyn, H. "Peri-Implantitis": A Complication of a Foreign Body or a Man-Made "Disease". Facts and Fiction. *Clin. Implant Dent Relat. Res.* **2016**, *18*, 840–849. [CrossRef] [PubMed]
9. Scarritt, M.E.; Londono, R.; Badylak, S.F. Host Response to Implanted Materials and Devices: An Overview. In *The Immune Response to Implanted Materials and Devices*; Corradetti, B., Ed.; Springer: Cham, Switzerland, 2017; pp. 1–14. ISBN 978-3-319-45433-7.
10. Hotchkiss, K.M.; Ayad, N.B.; Hyzy, S.L.; Boyan, B.D.; Olivares-Navarrete, R. Dental implant surface chemistry and energy alter macrophage activation in vitro. *Clin. Oral Implants Res.* **2017**, *28*, 414–423. [CrossRef] [PubMed]
11. Chen, Z.; Mao, X.; Tan, L.; Friis, T.; Wu, C.; Crawford, R.; Xiao, Y. Osteoimmunomodulatory properties of magnesium scaffolds coated with β-tricalcium phosphate. *Biomaterials* **2014**, *35*, 8553–8565. [CrossRef]
12. Sato, T.; Pajarinen, J.; Behn, A.; Jiang, X.; Lin, T.H.; Loi, F.; Yao, Z.; Egashira, K.; Yang, F.; Goodman, S.B. The effect of local IL-4 delivery or CCL2 blockade on implant fixation and bone structural properties in a mouse model of wear particle induced osteolysis. *J. Biomed. Mater. Res. A* **2016**, *104*, 2255–2262. [CrossRef]
13. Nojehdehi, S.; Soudi, S.; Hesampour, A.; Rasouli, S.; Soleimani, M.; Hashemi, S.M. Immunomodulatory effects of mesenchymal stem cell-derived exosomes on experimental type-1 autoimmune diabetes. *J. Cell Biochem.* **2018**, *119*, 9433–9443. [CrossRef] [PubMed]
14. Amengual-Peñafiel, L.; Jara-Sepúlveda, M.C.; Parada-Pozas, L.; Marchesani-Carrasco, F.; Cartes-Velásquez, R.; Galdames-Gutiérrez, B. Immunomodulation of Osseointegration Through Extracorporeal Shock Wave Therapy. *Dent. Hypotheses* **2018**, *9*, 45–50. [CrossRef]
15. Van der Meulen, M.C.; Huiskes, R. Why mechanobiology? A survey article. *J. Biomech.* **2002**, *35*, 401–404. [CrossRef]
16. Yusko, E.C.; Asbury, C.L. Force is a signal that cells cannot ignore. *Mol. Biol. Cell* **2014**, *25*, 3717–3725. [CrossRef] [PubMed]
17. Zhao, L.; Wu, Z.; Zhang, Y. Low-magnitude mechanical vibration may be applied clinically to promote dental implant osseointegration. *Med. Hypotheses* **2009**, *72*, 451–452. [CrossRef] [PubMed]
18. Mennens, S.F.B.; van den Dries, K.; Cambi, A. Role for Mechanotransduction in Macrophage and Dendritic Cell Immunobiology. *Results Probl. Cell Differ.* **2017**, *62*, 209–242. [CrossRef] [PubMed]
19. Zetao, C.; Travis, K.; Rachael, M.; Ross, C.; Jiang, C.; Chengtie, W.; Yin, X. Osteoimmunomodulation for the development of advanced bone biomaterials. *Mater. Today* **2016**, *19*, 304–321. [CrossRef]
20. Albrektsson, T.; Chrcanovic, B.; Östman, P.O.; Sennerby, L. Initial and long-term crestal bone responses to modern dental implants. *Periodontol. 2000* **2017**, *73*, 41–50. [CrossRef]
21. Zhao, E.; Xu, H.; Wang, L.; Kryczek, I.; Wu, K.; Hu, Y.; Wang, G.; Zou, W. Bone marrow and the control of immunity. *Cell Mol. Immunol.* **2012**, *9*, 11–19. [CrossRef]

22. Calvi, L.M.; Adams, G.B.; Weibrecht, K.W.; Weber, J.M.; Olson, D.P.; Knight, M.C.; Martin, R.P.; Schipani, E.; Divieti, P.; Bringhurst, F.R.; et al. Osteoblastic cells regulate the haematopoietic stem cell niche. *Nature* **2003**, *425*, 841–846. [CrossRef] [PubMed]
23. Kikuta, J.; Ishii, M. Osteoclast migration, differentiation and function: Novel therapeutic targets for rheumatic diseases. *Rheumatology* **2013**, *52*, 226–234. [CrossRef] [PubMed]
24. Mazo, I.B.; Honczarenko, M.; Leung, H.; Cavanagh, L.L.; Bonasio, R.; Weninger, W. Bone marrow is a major reservoir and site of recruitment for central memory CD8+ T cells. *Immunity* **2005**, *22*, 259–270. [CrossRef] [PubMed]
25. Arboleya, L.; Castañeda, S. Osteoimmunology. *Reumatol. Clin.* **2013**, *9*, 303–315. [CrossRef] [PubMed]
26. Monroe, D.G.; McGee-Lawrence, M.E.; Oursler, M.J.; Westendorf, J.J. Update on Wnt signaling in bone cell biology and bone disease. *Gene* **2012**, *492*, 1–18. [CrossRef] [PubMed]
27. Theill, L.E.; Boyle, W.J.; Penninger, J.M. RANK-L and RANK: T cell, bone loss and mammalian evolution. *Annu. Rev. Immunol.* **2002**, *20*, 795–823. [CrossRef] [PubMed]
28. Srivastava, R.K.; Dar, H.Y.; Mishra, P.K. Immunoporosis: Immunology of Osteoporosis-Role of T Cells. *Front. Immunol.* **2018**, *9*, 657. [CrossRef] [PubMed]
29. Alnaeeli, M.; Park, J.; Mahamed, D.; Penninger, J.M.; Teng, Y.T. Dendritic cells at the osteo-immune interface: Implications for inflammation-induced bone loss. *J. Bone Miner. Res.* **2007**, *22*, 775–780. [CrossRef] [PubMed]
30. Caetano-Lopes, J.; Canhão, H.; Fonseca, J.E. Osteoimmunology-the hidden immune regulation of bone. *Autoimmun. Rev.* **2009**, *8*, 250–255. [CrossRef]
31. Kaur, S.; Raggatt, L.J.; Batoon, L.; Hume, D.A.; Levesque, J.P.; Pettit, A.R. Role of bone marrow macrophages in controlling homeostasis and repair in bone and bone marrow niches. *Semin. Cell Dev. Biol.* **2017**, *61*, 12–21. [CrossRef]
32. Batoon, L.; Millard, S.M.; Raggatt, L.J.; Pettit, A.R. Osteomacs and Bone Regeneration. *Curr. Osteoporos. Rep.* **2017**, *15*, 385–395. [CrossRef]
33. Chang, M.K.; Raggatt, L.J.; Alexander, K.A.; Kuliwaba, J.S.; Fazzalari, N.L.; Schroder, K.; Maylin, E.R.; Ripoll, V.M.; Hume, D.A.; Pettit, A.R. Osteal tissue macrophages are intercalated throughout human and mouse bone lining tissues and regulate osteoblast function in vitro and in vivo. *J. Immunol.* **2008**, *181*, 1232–1244. [CrossRef] [PubMed]
34. Raggatt, L.J.; Wullschleger, M.E.; Alexander, K.A.; Wu, A.C.; Millard, S.M.; Kaur, S.; Maugham, M.L.; Gregory, L.S.; Steck, R.; Pettit, A.R. Fracture healing via periosteal callus formation requires macrophages for both initiation and progression of early endochondral ossification. *Am. J. Pathol.* **2014**, *184*, 3192–3204. [CrossRef] [PubMed]
35. Andrew, J.G.; Andrew, S.M.; Freemont, A.J.; Marsh, D.R. Inflammatory cells in normal human fracture healing. *Acta Orthop. Scand.* **1994**, *65*, 462–466. [CrossRef] [PubMed]
36. Anderson, J.M.; Cramer, S. Perspectives on the inflammatory, healing, and foreign body responses to biomaterials and medical devices. In *Host Response to Biomaterials. The Impact of Host Response on Biomaterial Selection*; Badylak, S., Ed.; Elsevier: New York, NY, USA, 2015; pp. 13–36. ISBN 9780128001967.
37. Hosgood, G. Wound healing. The role of platelet-derived growth factor and transforming growth factor beta. *Vet. Surg.* **1993**, *22*, 490–495. [CrossRef] [PubMed]
38. Anderson, J.M.; Jiang, S. Implications of the Acute and Chronic Inflammatory Response and the Foreign Body Reaction to the Immune Response of Implanted Biomaterials. In *The Immune Response to Implanted Materials and Devices*; Corradetti, B., Ed.; Springer: Cham, Switzerland, 2017; pp. 15–36. ISBN 978-3-319-45433-7.
39. Hu, W.J.; Eaton, J.W.; Ugarova, T.P.; Tang, L. Molecular basis of biomaterial-mediated foreign body reaction. *Blood* **2001**, *98*, 1231–1238. [CrossRef] [PubMed]
40. Christo, S.N.; Diener, K.R.; Bachhuka, A.; Vasilev, K.; Hayball, J.D. Innate Immunity and Biomaterials at the Nexus: Friends or Foes. *BioMed Res. Int.* **2015**. [CrossRef]
41. Arvidsson, S.; Askendal, A.; Tengvall, P. Blood plasma contact activation on silicon, titanium, and aluminum. *Biomaterials* **2007**, *28*, 1346–1354. [CrossRef]
42. Mills, C.D.; Kincaid, K.; Alt, J.M.; Heilman, M.J.; Hill, A.M. M-1/M-2 macrophages and the Th1/Th2 paradigm. *J. Immunol.* **2000**, *164*, 6166–6173. [CrossRef]
43. Mosser, D.M.; Edwards, J.P. Exploring the full spectrum of macrophage activation. *Nat. Rev. Immunol.* **2008**, *8*, 958–969. [CrossRef]

44. Lucas, T.; Waisman, A.; Ranjan, R.; Roes, J.; Krieg, T.; Müller, W.; Roers, A.; Eming, S.A. Differential roles of macrophages in diverse phases of skin repair. *J. Immunol.* **2010**, *184*, 3964–3977. [CrossRef]
45. Trindade, R.; Albrektsson, T.; Tengvall, P.; Wennerberg, A. Bone immune response to Titanium, PEEK and Copper- Osseointegration and the Immune-inflammatory balance. *Clin. Oral Implants Res.* **2018**, *29*, 138. [CrossRef]
46. Anderson, J.M.; Rodriguez, D.T.; Chang, A. Foreign body reaction to biomaterials. *Semin. Immunol.* **2008**, *20*, 86–100. [CrossRef] [PubMed]
47. Barbeck, M.; Booms, P.; Unger, R.; Hoffmann, V.; Sader, R.; Kirkpatrick, C.J.; Ghanaati, S. Multinucleated giant cells in the implant bed of bone substitutes are foreign body giant cells-New insights into the material-mediated healing process. *J. Biomed. Mater. Res. A* **2017**, *105*, 1105–1111. [CrossRef] [PubMed]
48. Scatena, M.; Eaton, K.V.; Jackson, M.F.; Lund, S.A.; Giachelli, C.M. Macrophages: The Bad, the Ugly, and the Good in the Inflammatory Response to Biomaterials. In *The Immune Response to Implanted Materials and Devices*; Corradetti, B., Ed.; Springer: Cham, Switzerland, 2017; pp. 37–62. ISBN 978-3-319-45433-7.
49. Donath, K.; Laass, M.; Günzl, H.J. The histopathology of different foreign body reactions in oral soft tissue and bone tissue. *Virchows Arch. A Pathol. Anat. Histopathol.* **1992**, *420*, 131–137. [CrossRef] [PubMed]
50. Vigneri, A. Macrophage fusion: Molecular mechanisms. *Methods Mol. Biol.* **2008**, *475*, 149–161. [CrossRef]
51. Romagnani, S. T-cell subsets [Th1 versus Th2]. *Ann. Allergy Asthma Immunol.* **2000**, *85*, 9–18. [CrossRef]
52. Lin, T.; Jämsen, E.; Lu, L.; Nathan, K.; Pajarinen, J.; Goodman, S. Modulating Innate Inflammatory Reactions in the Application of Orthopedic Biomaterials. In *Progress in Biology, Manufacturing, and Industry Perspectives*; Li, B., Webster, T., Eds.; Springer: Cham, Switzerland, 2018; pp. 199–218. ISBN 978-3-319-89542-0.
53. Biguetti, C.C.; Cavalla, F.; Silveira, E.M.; Fonseca, A.C.; Vieira, A.E.; Tabanez, A.P.; Rodrigues, D.C.; Trombone, A.P.F.; Garlet, G.P. Oral implant osseointegration model in C57Bl/6 mice: Microtomographic, histological, histomorphometric and molecular characterization. *J. Appl. Oral Sci.* **2018**, *26*, e20170601. [CrossRef]
54. Dohan Ehrenfest, D.M.; Del Corso, M.; Kang, B.; Leclercq, P.; Mazor, Z.; Horowitz, R.A.; Russe, P.; Oh, H.; Zou, D.; Shibli, J.A.; et al. Identification card and codification of the chemical and morphological characteristics of 62 dental implant surfaces. Part 3: Sand-blasted/acid-etched [SLA type] and related surfaces [Group 2A, main subtractive process]. *POSEIDO* **2014**, *2*, 37–55.
55. Clean Implant. Available online: http://www.cleanimplant.com/ (accessed on 25 November 2018).
56. Konttinen, Y.T.; Pajarinen, J.; Takakubo, Y.; Gallo, J.; Nich, C.; Takagi, M.; Goodman, S.B. Macrophage polarization and activation in response to implant debris: Influence by "particle disease" and "ion disease". *J. Long Term Eff. Med. Implants* **2014**, *24*, 267–281. [CrossRef]
57. Albrektsson, T.; Chrcanovic, B.; Mölne, J.; Wennerberg, A. Foreign body reactions, marginal bone loss and allergies to titanium implants. *Eur. J. Oral Implantol.* **2018**, *11*, S37–S46.
58. Høl, P.J.; Kristoffersen, E.K.; Gjerdet, N.R.; Pellowe, A.S. Novel Nanoparticulate and Ionic Titanium Antigens for Hypersensitivity Testing. *Int. J. Mol. Sci.* **2018**, *19*, 1101. [CrossRef]
59. Goodman, S.B.; Gibon, E.; Pajarinen, J.; Lin, T.H.; Keeney, M.; Ren, P.G.; Nich, C.; Yao, Z.; Egashira, K.; Yang, F.; et al. Novel biological strategies for treatment of wear particle-induced periprosthetic osteolysis of orthopaedic implants for joint replacement. *J. R. Soc. Interface* **2014**, *11*, 20130962. [CrossRef]
60. Xu, L.C.; Siedlecki, C.A. Effects of surface wettability and contact time on protein adhesion to biomaterial surfaces. *Biomaterials* **2007**, *28*, 3273–3283. [CrossRef]
61. Luu, T.U.; Gott, S.C.; Woo, B.W.; Rao, M.P.; Liu, W.F. Micro- and Nanopatterned Topographical Cues for Regulating Macrophage Cell Shape and Phenotype. *ACS Appl. Mater. Interfaces* **2015**, *7*, 28665–28672. [CrossRef] [PubMed]
62. Thompson, W.R.; Rubin, C.T.; Rubin, J. Mechanical regulation of signaling pathways in bone. *Gene* **2012**, *503*, 179–193. [CrossRef] [PubMed]
63. Vasconcelos, D.M.; Santos, S.G.; Lamghari, M.; Barbosa, M.A. The two faces of metal ions: From implants rejection to tissue repair/regeneration. *Biomaterials* **2016**, *84*, 262–275. [CrossRef] [PubMed]
64. Martinez, F.O.; Sica, A.; Mantovani, A.; Locati, M. Macrophage activation and polarization. *Front. Biosci.* **2008**, *13*, 453–461. [CrossRef]
65. Gilbert, L.; He, X.; Farmer, P.; Boden, S.; Kozlowski, M.; Rubin, J.; Nanes, M.S. Inhibition of osteoblast differentiation by tumor necrosis factor-alpha. *Endocrinology* **2000**, *141*, 3956–3964. [CrossRef] [PubMed]

66. Lin, T.H.; Pajarinen, J.; Sato, T.; Loi, F.; Fan, C.; Cordova, L.A.; Nabeshima, A.; Gibon, E.; Zhang, R.; Yao, Z.; et al. NF-kappaB decoy oligodeoxynucleotide mitigates wear particle-associated bone loss in the murine continuous infusion model. *Acta Biomater.* **2016**, *41*, 273–281. [CrossRef]
67. Kumar, V.A.; Taylor, N.L.; Shi, S.; Wickremasinghe, N.C.; D'Souza, R.N.; Hartgerink, J.D. Selfassembling multidomain peptides tailor biological responses through biphasic release. *Biomaterials* **2015**, *52*, 71–78. [CrossRef]
68. Viganò, M.; Sansone, V.; d'Agostino, M.C.; Romeo, P.; Perucca Orfei, C.; de Girolamo, L. Mesenchymal stem cells as therapeutic target of biophysical stimulation for the treatment of musculoskeletal disorders. *J. Orthop. Surg. Res.* **2016**, *11*, 163. [CrossRef] [PubMed]
69. Gao, F.; Chiu, S.M.; Motan, D.A.; Zhang, Z.; Chen, L.; Ji, H.L.; Tse, H.F.; Fu, Q.-L.; Lian, Q. Mesenchymal Stem Cell and Immunomodulation: Current Status and Future Prospects. *Cell Death Dis.* **2016**, *7*, e2062. [CrossRef] [PubMed]
70. Guilak, F.; Cohen, D.M.; Estes, B.T.; Gimble, J.M.; Liedtke, W.; Chen, C.S. Control of stem cell fate by physical interactions with the extracellular matrix. *Cell Stem Cell* **2009**, *5*, 17–26. [CrossRef] [PubMed]
71. Carver, W.; Esch, A.M.; Fowlkes, V.; Goldsmith, E.C. The Biomechanical Environment and Impact on Tissue Fibrosis. In *The Immune Response to Implanted Materials and Devices*; Corradetti, B., Ed.; Springer: Cham, Switzerland, 2017; pp. 169–188. ISBN 978-3-319-45433-7.
72. Leung, D.Y.; Glagov, S.; Mathews, M.B. Cyclic stretching stimulates synthesis of matrix components by arterial smooth muscle cells in vitro. *Science* **1976**, *191*, 475–477. [CrossRef] [PubMed]
73. Dunn, S.L.; Olmedo, M.L. Mechanotransduction: Relevance to physical therapist practice—Understanding our ability to affect genetic expression through mechanical forces. *Phys. Ther.* **2016**, *96*, 712–721. [CrossRef] [PubMed]
74. Ingber, D.E. Tensegrity: The architectural basis of cellular mechanotransduction. *Annu. Rev. Physiol.* **1997**, *59*, 575–599. [CrossRef] [PubMed]
75. MacKenna, D.A.; Dolfi, F.; Vuori, K.; Ruoslahti, E. Extracellular signal-regulated kinase and c-Jun NH2-terminal kinase activation by mechanical stretch is integrin-dependent and matrix specific in rat cardiac fibroblasts. *J. Clin. Investig.* **1998**, *101*, 301–310. [CrossRef] [PubMed]
76. Ghoveizi, R.; Alikhasi, M.; Siadat, M.R.; Siadat, H.; Sorouri, M. A radiographic comparison of progressive and conventional loading on crestal bone loss and density in single dental implants: A randomized controlled trial study. *J. Dent.* **2013**, *10*, 155–163.
77. Piattelli, A.; Corigliano, M.; Scarano, A.; Costigliola, G.; Paolantonio, M. Immediate loading of titanium plasma-sprayed implants: An histologic analysis in monkeys. *J. Periodontol.* **1998**, *69*, 321–327. [CrossRef]
78. Huang, H.; Wismeijer, D.; Shao, X.; Wu, G. Mathematical evaluation of the influence of multiple factors on implant stability quotient values in clinical practice: A retrospective study. *Ther. Clin. Risk Manag.* **2016**, *12*, 1525–1532. [CrossRef]
79. Sennerby, L.; Ericson, L.E.; Thomsen, P.; Lekholm, U.; Astrand, P. Structure of the bone-titanium interface in retrieved clinical oral implants. *Clin. Oral Implants Res.* **1991**, *2*, 103–111. [CrossRef] [PubMed]
80. Duyck, J.; Cooman, M.D.; Puers, R.; van Oosterwyck, H.; Sloten, J.V.; Naert, I. A repeated sampling bone chamber methodology for the evaluation of tissue differentiation and bone adaptation around titanium implants under controlled mechanical conditions. *J. Biomech.* **2004**, *37*, 1819–1822. [CrossRef] [PubMed]
81. Ogden, J.A.; Tóth-Kischkat, A.; Schultheiss, R. Principles of shock wave therapy. *Clin. Orthop. Relat. Res.* **2001**, *387*, 8–17. [CrossRef]
82. Van der Jagt, O.P.; Waarsing, J.H.; Kops, N.; Schaden, W.; Jahr, H.; Verhaar, J.A.; Weinans, H. Unfocused extracorporeal shock waves induce anabolic effects in osteoporotic rats. *JBJS* **2011**, *93*, 38–48. [CrossRef] [PubMed]
83. Wang, C.J. Extracorporeal shockwave therapy in musculoskeletal disorders. *J. Orthop. Surg. Res.* **2012**, *7*, 11. [CrossRef] [PubMed]
84. Iro, H.; Schneider, H.T.; Födra, C.; Waitz, G.; Nitsche, N.; Heinritz, H.H.; Benninger, J.; Ell, C. Shockwave lithotripsy of salivary duct stones. *Lancet* **1992**, *339*, 1333–1336. [CrossRef]
85. Kraus, M.; Reinhart, E.; Krause, H.; Reuther, J. Low energy extracorporeal shockwave therapy [ESWT] for treatment of myogelosis of the masseter muscle. *Mund-Kiefer Gesichtschir.* **1999**, *3*, 20–23. [CrossRef]

86. Falkensammer, F.; Rausch-Fan, X.; Schaden, W.; Kivaranovic, D.; Freudenthaler, J. Impact of extracorporeal shockwave therapy on tooth mobility in adult orthodontic patients: A randomized singlecenter placebo-controlled clinical trial. *J. Clin. Periodontol.* **2015**, *42*, 294–301. [CrossRef]
87. Falkensammer, F.; Schaden, W.; Krall, C.; Freudenthaler, J.; Bantleon, H.P. Effect of extracorporeal shockwave therapy [ESWT] on pulpal blood flow after orthodontic treatment: A randomized clinical trial. *Clin. Oral Investig.* **2016**, *20*, 373–379. [CrossRef]
88. Holfeld, J.; Tepeköylü, C.; Reissig, C.; Lobenwein, D.; Scheller, B.; Kirchmair, E.; Kozaryn, R.; Albrecht-Schgoer, K.; Krapf, C.; Zins, K.; et al. Toll-like receptor 3 signalling mediates angiogenic response upon shock wave treatment of ischaemic muscle. *Cardiovasc. Res.* **2016**, *109*, 331–343. [CrossRef]
89. Goiato, M.C.; dos Santos, D.M.; Santiago, J.F.; Moreno, A.; Pellizzer, E.P. Longevity of dental implants in type IV bone: A systematic review. *Int. J. Oral Maxillofac. Surg.* **2014**, *43*, 1108–1116. [CrossRef] [PubMed]
90. De Medeiros, F.C.F.L.; Kudo, G.A.H.; Leme, B.G.; Saraiva, P.P.; Verri, F.R.; Honório, H.M.; Pellizzer, E.P.; Santiago, J.F. Dental implants in patients with osteoporosis: A systematic review with meta-analysis. *Int. J. Oral Maxillofac. Surg.* **2018**, *47*, 480–491. [CrossRef] [PubMed]
91. Koolen, M.K.E.; Kruyt, M.C.; Zadpoor, A.A.; Öner, F.C.; Weinans, H.; van der Jagt, O.P. Optimization of screw fixation in rat bone with extracorporeal shock waves. *J. Orthop. Res.* **2018**, *36*, 76–84. [CrossRef] [PubMed]
92. Van der Jagt, O.P.; Piscaer, T.M.; Schaden, W.; Li, J.; Kops, N.; Jahr, H.; van der Linden, J.C.; Waarsing, J.H.; Verhaar, J.A.; de Jong, M.; Weinans, H. Unfocused extracorporeal shock waves induce anabolic effects in rat bone. *J. Bone Jt. Surg. Am.* **2011**, *93*, 38–48. [CrossRef] [PubMed]
93. Koolen, M.K.E.; Pouran, B.; Öner, F.C.; Zadpoor, A.A.; van der Jagt, O.P.; Weinans, H. Unfocused shockwaves for osteoinduction in bone substitutes in rat cortical bone defects. *PLoS ONE* **2018**, *13*, e0200020. [CrossRef] [PubMed]
94. Loske, A.M. Extracorporeal Shock Wave Therapy, Shock Wave and High Pressure Phenomena. Bone Healing. In *Medical and Biomedical Applications of Shock Waves*; Loske, A.M., Ed.; Springer International Publishing: New York, NY, USA, 2017; p. 222. ISBN 978-3-319-47570-7.
95. Deb, S.; Chana, S. Biomaterials in Relation to Dentistry. *Front. Oral Biol.* **2015**, *17*, 1–12. [CrossRef] [PubMed]
96. Hou, Y.; Zhou, X.; Cai, W.L.; Guo, C.C.; Han, Y. Regulatory effect of bone marrow mesenchymal stem cells on polarization of macrophages. *Zhonghua Gan Zang Bing Za Zhi* **2017**, *25*, 273–278. [CrossRef]
97. English, K.; French, A.; Wood, K.J. Mesenchymal stromal cells: Facilitators of successful transplantation? *Cell Stem Cell* **2010**, *7*, 431–442. [CrossRef]
98. Suhr, F.; Delhasse, Y.; Bungartz, G.; Schmidt, A.; Pfannkuche, K.; Bloch, W. Cell biological effects of mechanical stimulations generated by focused extracorporeal shock wave applications on cultured human bone marrow stromal cells. *Stem Cell Res.* **2013**, *11*, 951–964. [CrossRef]
99. Leu, S.; Huang, T.H.; Chen, Y.L.; Yip, H.K. Effect of Extracorporeal Shockwave on Angiogenesis and Anti-Inflammation: Molecular-Cellular Signaling Pathways. In *Shockwave Medicine*; Wang, C.J., Schaden, W., Ko, J.Y., Eds.; Karger: Basel, Switzerland, 2018; Volume 6, pp. 109–116. [CrossRef]
100. Sukubo, N.G.; Tibalt, E.; Respizzi, S.; Locati, M.; d'Agostino, M.C. Effect of shock waves on macrophages: A possible role in tissue regeneration and remodeling. *Int. J. Surg.* **2015**, *24*, 124–130. [CrossRef]
101. Godwin, J.W.; Pinto, A.R.; Rosenthal, N.A. Macrophages required for regeneration. *Proc. Natl. Acad. Sci. USA* **2013**, *110*, 9415–9420. [CrossRef] [PubMed]
102. Mishra, S.K.; Chowdhary, R.; Chrcanovic, B.R.; Brånemark, P.I. Osseoperception in Dental Implants: A Systematic Review. *J. Prosthodont.* **2016**, *25*, 185–195. [CrossRef] [PubMed]
103. He, H.; Yao, Y.; Wang, Y.; Wu, Y.; Yang, Y.; Gong, P. A novel bionic design of dental implant for promoting its long-term success using nerve growth factor [NGF]: Utilizing nano-springs to construct a stress-cushioning structure inside the implant. *Med. Sci. Monit.* **2012**, *18*, HY42–HY46. [CrossRef] [PubMed]
104. Lee, J.H.; Sung, Y.B.; Jang, S.H. Nerve growth factor expression in stroke induced rats after shock wave. *J. Phys. Ther. Sci.* **2016**, *28*, 3451–3453. [CrossRef] [PubMed]

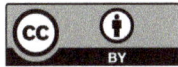

© 2019 by the authors. Licensee MDPI, Basel, Switzerland. This article is an open access article distributed under the terms and conditions of the Creative Commons Attribution (CC BY) license (http://creativecommons.org/licenses/by/4.0/).

www.ingramcontent.com/pod-product-compliance
Lightning Source LLC
LaVergne TN
LVHW070237100526
838202LV00015B/2141

MDPI
St. Alban-Anlage 66
4052 Basel
Switzerland
Tel. +41 61 683 77 34
Fax +41 61 302 89 18
www.mdpi.com

Journal of Clinical Medicine Editorial Office
E-mail: jcm@mdpi.com
www.mdpi.com/journal/jcm